Antimicrobial Resistance: Public Health Challenges

Antimicrobial Resistance: Public Health Challenges

Editor: Sandy Wolford

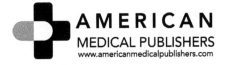

AMERICAN
MEDICAL PUBLISHERS
www.americanmedicalpublishers.com

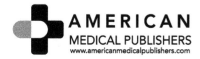

AMERICAN
MEDICAL PUBLISHERS
www.americanmedicalpublishers.com

Cataloging-in-Publication Data

Antimicrobial resistance : public health challenges / edited by Sandy Wolford.
 p. cm.
Includes bibliographical references and index.
ISBN 978-1-63927-887-9
1. Public health. 2. Drug resistance in microorganisms. 3. Medicine, Preventive.
4. Microorganisms—Effect of drugs on. I. Wolford, Sandy.
RA427 .A58 2023
362.1--dc23

American Medical Publishers,
41 Flatbush Avenue,
1st Floor, New York,
NY 11217, USA

ISBN 978-1-63927-887-9 (Hardback)

Contents

Preface

Antimicrobial Resistance (AMR) refers to a phenomenon wherein microorganisms such as bacteria, viruses, fungi, and parasites change or mutate over time in such a manner that they do not respond to medicines. When microorganisms develop such resistance, it makes the treatment of infections difficult which increases the risk of disease spread, severe illness and death. AMR can be caused due to several factors such as inappropriate treatment, prescription errors, self-medication, and the emergence of an increasing number of elderly and immunocompromised population. The overdose of antibiotics causes the resistant bacteria to survive and even multiply. Antimicrobial resistance can be acquired through five mechanisms which are the production of drug-inactivating enzymes, modification of an existing target, acquisition of a target by-pass system, reduced cell permeability, and drug removal from the cell. In order to control AMR, certain actions should be taken into consideration that include running information campaigns for the consumers, broadcasting information, providing training for the healthcare professionals, improving diagnostics for treatment decisions, and issuing treatment guidelines, etc. This book aims to shed light on some of the public health challenges of antimicrobial resistance. It presents researches and studies performed by experts across the globe. The extensive content of this book provides the readers with a thorough understanding of the subject.

This book unites the global concepts and researches in an organized manner for a comprehensive understanding of the subject. It is a ripe text for all researchers, students, scientists or anyone else who is interested in acquiring a better knowledge of this dynamic field.

I extend my sincere thanks to the contributors for such eloquent research chapters. Finally, I thank my family for being a source of support and help.

Editor

1

Confronting Tigecycline-Resistant *Acinetobacter baumannii* via Immunization Against Conserved Resistance Determinants

Ming-Hsien Chiang[1,2†], Ya-Sung Yang[3†], Jun-Ren Sun[4], Yung-Chih Wang[3], Shu-Chen Kuo[5], Yi-Tzu Lee[6,7], Yi-Ping Chuang[8] and Te-Li Chen[2,9]*

[1] Department and Graduate Institute of Biology and Anatomy, National Defense Medical Center, Taipei, Taiwan, [2] Graduate Institute of Life Sciences, National Defense Medical Center, Taipei, Taiwan, [3] Division of Infectious Diseases and Tropical Medicine, Department of Internal Medicine, Tri-Service General Hospital, National Defense Medical Center, Taipei, Taiwan, [4] Institute of Preventive Medicine, National Defense Medical Center, Taipei, Taiwan, [5] National Institute of Infectious Diseases and Vaccinology, National Health Research Institutes, Zhunan, Taiwan, [6] School of Medicine, National Yang-Ming University, Taipei, Taiwan, [7] Department of Emergency Medicine, Taipei Veterans General Hospital, Taipei, Taiwan, [8] Department and Graduate Institute of Microbiology and Immunology, National Defense Medical Center, Taipei, Taiwan, [9] Institute of Clinical Medicine, National Yang-Ming University, Taipei, Taiwan

Correspondence:
Te-Li Chen
tecklayyy@gmail.com
† These authors have contributed equally to this work

Antimicrobial-resistant (AMR) bacterial infections, including those caused by *Acinetobacter baumannii*, have emerged as a clinical crisis worldwide. Immunization with AMR determinants has been suggested as a novel approach to combat AMR bacteria, but has not been validated. The present study targeted tigecycline (TGC) resistance determinants in *A. baumannii* to test the feasibility of this approach. Using bioinformatic tools, four candidates, AdeA, AdeI, AdeK, and TolC, belonging to the resistance-nodulation-division (RND) efflux pump were identified as highly conserved and exposed antigens from 15 *A. baumannii* genomes. Antisera generated from recombinant proteins showed the capability to reserve Hoechst 33342, a substrate of the efflux pump, in bacterial cells. The rTolC antisera had the highest complement-dependent killing and opsonophagocytosis effect compared to the sera from phosphate-buffered saline immunized mice. Among the antisera, anti-rAdeK-specific antisera decreased the minimal inhibitory concentration of TGC in 26.7% of the tested isolates. Immunization with rAdeK significantly potentiated TGC efficacy in treating TGC-resistant *A. baumannii* pneumonia in the murine model. The bacterial load (7.5×10^5 vs. 3.8×10^7, $p < 0.01$) and neutrophil infiltration in the peri-bronchial vasculature region of immunized mice was significantly lower compared to the PBS-immunized mice when TGC was administrated concomitantly. Collectively, these results suggest that active immunization against resistance determinants might be a feasible approach to combat multidrug-resistant pathogens in high risk population.

Keywords: immunization, resistant determinant, *Acinetobacter*, tigecycline, efflux pump

INTRODUCTION

Antimicrobial-resistant (AMR) bacterial infections have emerged as a serious problem in clinical settings worldwide. By 2050, 10 million people may die annually from AMR infections (Jansen et al., 2018). Unfortunately, the launch of new antibiotics is rapidly compromised by the emergence of resistance (Alekshun and Levy, 2007). Therefore, the development of new strategies to combat AMR bacteria is urgently needed.

Recently, vaccine development has been increasingly advocated as a new solution to AMR bacteria (McConnell et al., 2011; Huang et al., 2014; Jansen et al., 2018), especially for those with high risk of acquired infection (Gagneux-Brunon et al., 2018). Vaccine candidates often target capsule polysaccharides and virulent factors that are responsible for disease pathogenesis (Rappuoli et al., 2019). Unfortunately, AMR bacteria-targeting vaccines have not been very successful until now due to the heterogeneity in the expression levels of vaccine antigens in different circulating strains of the target pathogen (Garcia-Quintanilla et al., 2016; Rappuoli et al., 2019). Moreover, the immunity induced by single or multiple antigens, which is usually obtained both *in vitro* or *in vivo*, might be ineffective in protecting the host because the pathobiology in human infection is more complicated and remains obscure (Perez and Bonomo, 2014).

Antibiotic resistance determinants could be considered as potential vaccine candidates (Ni et al., 2017). Although there are variations in these resistance determinants in clinical isolates, this vaccination strategy might still be effective in eradicating resistant strains by means of replacing these strains which have reduced fitness with susceptible strains when vaccination coverage is high (Joice and Lipsitch, 2013; Niewiadomska et al., 2019). This approach has an advantage when the resistance determinants are consistently present *in vitro* and *in vivo* and also possess less selection pressure on bacteria (Niewiadomska et al., 2019). However, this approach has not been validated yet.

The present study tested this idea in *Acinetobacter baumannii*. *A. baumannii* is considered one of the most problematic bacteria by the Infectious Disease Society of America (IDSA) (Boucher et al., 2009) because of the rapid evolution of multidrug and pan-drug resistant strains. Currently, only few strains of this bacteria are still susceptible to last-line antibiotics such as, carbapenem and tigecycline (TGC) (Sun et al., 2013; Ni et al., 2016). In order to maximize the coverage of immunization, the antibiotic resistance determinants used for the vaccine candidate should be the major resistance mechanism of the antibiotic of interest in particular bacterial species. These determinants should be universal in different strains, conserved in sequence homology, and accessible by the immune system. In this aspect, carbapenem resistance determinants are not suitable vaccine candidates, as its major resistance mechanism is production of different classes of carbapenemases (Nordmann and Poirel, 2019), which are very diverse in their protein sequences and structures. On the contrary, the major mechanism for TGC resistance is overexpression of efflux pumps (Sugawara and Nikaido, 2014). These are universal and are conserved in *A. baumannii* strains (Ardehali et al., 2019), and therefore, might

be good vaccine candidates to test this immunization approach. The present study utilized bioinformatics tools to identify conserved and surface-exposed antigens of the chromosomal-encoded resistome of *A. baumannii*. Several protein components of the resistance-nodulation-division (RND) efflux system were identified, which have been associated with TGC resistance in *A. baumannii*. We propose an immunization approach using TGC resistance determinants in a murine pneumonia model to combat multidrug-resistant *A. baumannii*.

MATERIALS AND METHODS

Bioinformatic Tools

Microbial Genome Database (MBGD) was used for comparative analysis of completely sequenced microbial genomes to identify core genes that are universal from 15 *A. baumannii* genomes (**Supplementary Table S1**; Uchiyama et al., 2014). PSORTb 3.0.2 (Yu et al., 2010), CELLO2GO (Yu et al., 2014), or SOSUI-GramN (Imai et al., 2008) were applied to predict the conserved residues and sub-cellular localization of these proteins. Comprehensive Antibiotic Resistance Database (CARD) was used to predict the resistome from raw genome sequence using Resistance Gene Identifier (RGI) software (Jia et al., 2017).

Bacterial Strain Preparation

A. baumannii ATCC17978 reference strain was purchased from the American Type Culture Collection (ATCC). TGC-resistant clinical *A. baumannii* isolates were obtained from Tri-Service General Hospital in Taiwan (Sun et al., 2014). All isolates were identified using conventional biochemical and genomic methods as previously described (Sun et al., 2014).

Construction and Purification of Antigens

Recombinant AdeA (A1S_1751), AdeI (A1S_2735), AdeK (A1S_2737), and TolC (A1S_0255) from ATCC17978 were amplified (the primers are listed in **Supplementary Table S2**) and cloned into a pET-29a expression vector (Vovagen, Darmstadt, Germany) with a 6× polyhistidine tag fused to the C-terminus of the recombinant protein. The resulting plasmids were expressed and purified as described in our previous study (Chiang et al., 2015). Purified proteins were digested with trypsin for subsequent liquid chromatography–mass spectrometry/mass spectrometry (LC-MS/MS) analysis and protein identification was conducted by Mission Biotech Co., Ltd., Taiwan. Sequence similarity comparison of *adeA*, *adeI*, *adeK*, and *tolC* from ATCC17978 and all isolates were analyzed using MEGA7 (Kumar et al., 2016).

Mouse Immunogenicity Assessment and Pneumonia Models

All animal studies were approved by the National Defense Medical Center Institutional Animal Care and Use Committee (NDMC IACUC-17-206). Female C57BL/6 mice (6 weeks old) were bred in a barrier facility under specific pathogen-free conditions. C57BL/6 mice (n = 10/group) were subcutaneously (sc.) immunized with 10 μg of individual recombinant antigens formulated with Complete Freund's Adjuvant/Incomplete Freund's Adjuvant (CFA/IFA) (Invivogen, Hong Kong), on days 0, 14, and 28. Blood samples were collected before the last immunization and tested against each immunogen. Immunoglobulin G (IgG) antibody titers were determined using antigen-specific enzyme-linked immunosorbent assays (ELISAs).

For conducting efficacy studies, immunized mice were challenged intra-tracheally (IT) on day 42 with a lethal dose [3×10^7 colony-forming units (CFUs)] of mid-log phase AB247 strain mixed with 10% porcine mucin (Sigma-Aldrich, MO, United States). The use of porcine mucin is to enhance the infectivity of *A. baumannii* (McConnell et al., 2011). TGC (10 mg/kg/d, q12h., sc.) treatment regimen was adopted from that used in a previous study (Pichardo et al., 2010). After 24 h therapy, the blood, lung, spleen, and kidney were homogenized and plated to evaluate for the CFUs. For histological analysis, the excised lungs were placed in vials containing 4% formaldehyde. The lungs were placed under vacuum overnight, paraffin-embedded, and stained with hematoxylin and eosin (HE). Histological scores were assigned by independent pathologists by evaluating 3–5 fields, according to the following criteria (Noto et al., 2017): 0, no pathology; 1, minimal infiltrates of neutrophils in alveolar spaces; 2, low numbers of neutrophils in alveoli; 3, moderate numbers of neutrophils and hemorrhage in alveoli with occasional lobar involvement and focal necrosis of alveolar-wall neutrophils in bronchioles; 4, marked numbers of neutrophils, consolidation, and widespread alveolar necrosis.

Flow Cytometry

ATCC17978 and clinical isolates from late-log-phase growth ($OD_{600} \approx 1.8$) in Luria-Bertani (LB) cultures were diluted in PBS containing 0.5% (w/v) bovine serum albumin (BSA) as a blocking buffer to an OD_{600} of 0.03. Each specific antiserum was added at a 1:100 dilution with the bacterium. Unbound antibody was removed by washing twice, then fixed by incubating with 4% formaldehyde/PBS for 10 min on ice. A secondary antibody, goat anti-mouse IgG-PE (Invitrogen Corp., Carlsbad, CA, United States) at 0.1 mL per well, was added at a 1:100 dilution and incubated for 30 min. The bacteria were analyzed using a FACSCalibur flow cytometer (BD, Franklin Lakes, NJ, United States). Wash buffer, secondary antibody, or PBS Immunize serum were used as negative controls.

Hoechst 33342 (H33342) Accumulation Assay

H33342 accumulation assays were carried out as described by Richmond et al. (2013). Strains were grown to an OD_{600} of 0.4 and resuspended in PBS at room temperature, and the suspension was adjusted to an OD_{600} of 0.1. Centrifugation steps were carried out at 2500 g. The wells of a black microtiter plate (Corning, Amsterdam, Netherlands) were inoculated with 176 μL of bacterial suspension and 20 μL of 10 μg/mL H33342. After 5 min equilibration, 4 μL of the efflux pump inhibitor, phenylalanine-arginine-β-naphthylamide (PAβN), or specific antisera were added. The fluorescence intensity was recorded every 1 min for 60 min on a SPECTRAmax5 fluorometer (Molecular Devices, Sunnyvale, CA, United States) at excitation and emission wavelengths of 355 and 460 nm, respectively.

Complement and Opsonophagocytosis Bactericidal Assays

ATCC17978 was freshly grown to a final bacterial cell concentration of 10^6 CFU/mL, and aliquoted into 96 well microtiter plates (10 μL, 10^4 cells/well). For complementary studies, 10 μL heat-inactivated or immune sera were mixed with 80 μL of undiluted human complement and added to the wells for 1 h at 37°C. The samples were plated for bacterial enumeration. Bacteriolysis activity was defined as [1 − (CFU immune sera at 60 min/CFU of PBS-immunized antisera at 60 min)] × 100.

For the opsonophagocytic kill assay, RAW 264.7 macrophages were cultured in RPMI 1640 (Irvine Scientific, Santa Ana, CA, United States) with 10% fetal bovine serum (FBS), 1% penicillin/streptomycin, and glutamine (Gemini BioProducts), and 50 μM β-mercaptoethanol (Sigma-Aldrich, St. Louis, MO, United States). RAW 264.7 cells were stimulated with 100 nM PMA (Sigma-Aldrich) for 3 days. RAW 264.7 macrophages (2×10^5/well) and ATCC17978 (1×10^4 CFU/well) were added into the wells along with the heat-inactivated or immune sera (5%). After a 1 h incubation with gentle shaking, the samples were serially diluted and plated. Serum killing rates were counted by comparing the number of reduced CFUs with those observed using PBS-immunized antisera.

RNA Isolation and Quantitative Reverse Transcriptase – PCR

The expression level of *adeA*, *adeI*, *adeK*, and *tolC* were measured by quantitative real-time polymerase chain reaction (PCR) assays as described previously (Rosenfeld et al., 2012). The mRNA expression of *rpoB* from ATCC17978 was used for normalization with specific primers (**Supplementary Table S2**). The relative gene expression was expressed as fold-change calculated by the ΔΔCt method. Gene expression levels ≥ 2-fold compared to that for the reference strain, ATCC17978, were considered significant overexpression. Each experiment was performed in duplicates and at least twice independently.

Minimal Inhibitory Concentration (MIC) Determination by Broth Microdilution Method

The MICs of TGC were determined by broth microdilution methods in Mueller Hilton broth and interpreted according to the Clinical and Laboratory Standards Institute guidelines (CLSI, 2017). Since MIC breakpoints are not established for TGC in *Acinetobacter* spp., we used the Food and Drug Administration breakpoints set for *Enterobacteriaceae* (Pillar et al., 2008). Each experiment was performed in triplicate.

Statistical Analysis

Statistical analyses were performed using GraphPad Prism 7 software. All graphical values were represented as means ± standard error of the mean (SEM). Tests of statistical

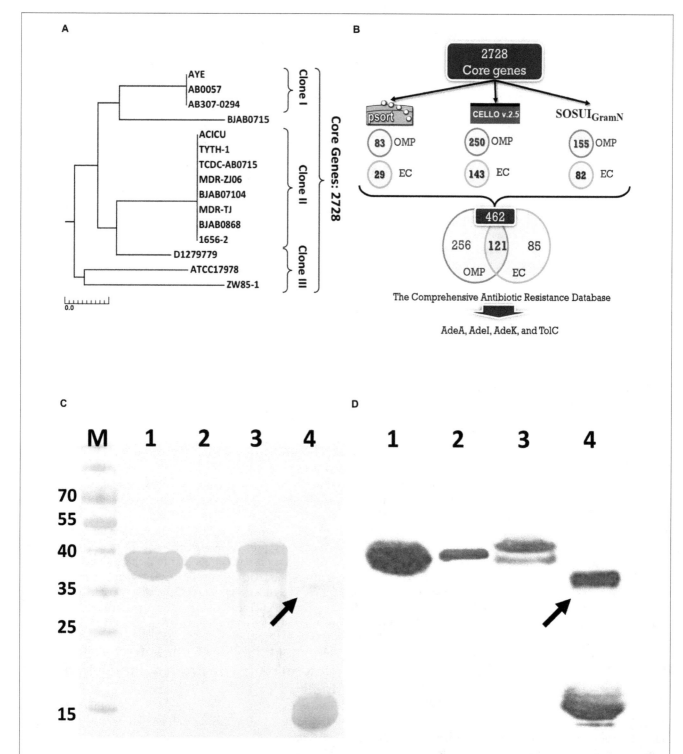

FIGURE 1 | A rational strategy for potential antigen identification and verification from *A. baumannii* genomes. **(A)** The phylogenetic lineage of 15 completely sequenced *A. baumannii* strains analyzed in this study was constructed by the neighbor-joining method performed in MEGA7. Homology core genes were analyzed using the web-based MBGD tool. **(B)** Bioinformatics tools including PSORTb 3.0.2, CELLO2GO, and SOSUI-GramN were utilized to identify 462 non-redundant outer membrane or extracellular proteins from 2728 core genes. Four antimicrobial-resistant genes associated with efflux pumps were identified in the 462-protein datasets based on Comprehensive Antibiotic Resistance Database (CARD) analysis. OMP, outer membrane protein; EC, extracellular protein. **(C)** Purified proteins were analyzed by 12% sodium dodecyl sulfate-polyacrylamide gel electrophoresis. Lane M-standard protein markers, Lane 1-purified rAdeI protein, Lane 2-purified rTolC protein, Lane 3-purified rAdeK, Lane 4-purified rAdeA protein. **(D)** Western blot analysis of purified recombinant proteins using mouse anti-His antibody. The arrow indicates dimerization of rAdeA (confirmed by LC-MS/MS).

significance were performed using one-way analysis of variance and Kruskal–Wallis tests with *post hoc* analysis. Differences were considered significant for $p < 0.05$.

RESULTS

In silico Screening of Conserved Outer Membrane Efflux Pump Proteins and Generation of Recombinant Proteins

Fifteen *A. baumannii* genomes included 12 multidrug resistant strains were used for analysis. The antibiotic susceptibility profiles of these isolates are listed in **Supplementary Table S1**. These strains were grouped by multilocus sequence typing (MLST) (Laure et al., 2010) and three strains belonged to international clone I (IC I), eight to IC II, three to IC III, and the last strain was unclassified, indicating a wide coverage of *A. baumannii* strains (**Figure 1A**). A total of 2728 core genes were identified; among them, 462 non-redundant proteins were predicted to be outer membrane or extracellular proteins. CARD predicted that among the 462 conserved and surface-exposed proteins, four were associated with antibiotic resistance, including AdeA (A1S_1751), AdeI (A1S_2735), AdeK (A1S_2737), and TolC (A1S_0255) and were selected as vaccine candidates (**Figure 1B**). All the proteins belonged to the chromosomally encoded RND efflux pump family and had been associated with resistance to multiple antibiotics, including TGC (Sun et al., 2013). The four recombinant proteins were expressed and purified (**Figure 1C**). The proteins were identified and confirmed by immunoblotting (**Figure 1D**) and LC-MS/MS analysis (**Table 1**).

Polyclonal Antibody Production and Functional Analysis

We then produced antigen-specific polyclonal antibodies from C57BL/6 mice using immunization (**Figure 2A**). All recombinant antigens (rTolC, rAdeK, rAdeI, rAdeA) formulated with CFA/IFA induced strong antigen-specific IgG antibody responses (IgG titers > 10^5, **Figure 2B**) on day 42 after immunization. The results indicated that all four antigens are highly immunogenic. Antigen-specific antisera were used to verify the location of these proteins in the outer surface of bacteria by flow cytometry (**Figure 2C**). Data confirmed that all the antisera could bind on the surface of ATCC17978, with significantly higher intensities than that for the PBS control antisera (**Figure 2D**). *In vitro* complement-dependent and opsonophagocytosis bactericidal

assays were used to assess the potential bacteria-killing activity of each antiserum. The results showed that 2–79% of ATCC17978 were inhibited by these antisera (**Figures 2E,F**). Among them, rTolC-specific antisera had the highest killing efficacy compared to the sera from PBS-immunized mice.

The accumulation of bis-benzamide H33342 dye provides a reliable method to evaluate the effect of agents that can block efflux pumps (Richmond et al., 2013). The fold-change of fluorescence intensity dramatically increased after adding PAβN and specific antisera, except for the PBS antisera control (**Figure 3A**, $p < 0.001$). Notably, fluorescence intensities were slightly decreased after 40 min of antisera treatment.

To examine the synergistic effect of antisera in the MICs range for TGCs in *A. baumannii*, 15 clinical TGC-R *A. baumannii* isolates were tested (**Table 2**). The TGC MICs of all isolates were > 4 mg/L. The sequence similarities of *adeA, adeI, adeK*, and *tolC* were determined (**Table 3**) and the similarities were very high among the isolates (98.2–100%), compared to the ATCC17978 sequence. The quantitative expression levels of *adeA, adeI, adeK,* and *tolC* were also determined. In general, all strains showed more than one pump overexpression phenotype. TGC MICs were significantly reduced after a combination with rAdeK antisera was used (**Figure 3B**), and five of the tested isolates (AB099, AB247, AB294, AB304, AB347) revealed more than fourfold reduction in TGC MICs (**Table 2**), and all five strains had *adeA* overexpression, and similarities in *adeA* sequences was 100% in 4 of the isolates. The similarity in *adeA* sequence of AB099 was 99.8%, with only a single amino-acid substitution (N295T). However, no significant differences were found among the responses of strains to anti-rAdeK antisera regarding their sequence homology (**Table 3**), gene expression level (**Table 2**) and binding ability of antisera to bacterial cells (**Figure 3C**). Furthermore, we examined the synergistic effect of anti-AdeK serum and four antibiotics including amikacin, meropenem, colistin and ampicillin/sulbactam, remained active against different portions of *A. baumannii* isolates. We found that only two isolates demonstrated a twofold reduction in the ampicillin-sulbactam MIC value from 64/32 to 32/16 μg/mL in the presence of anti-AdeK (**Supplementary Table S3**).

TGC Activity Potentiation by rAdeK Immunization in a Mouse Pneumonia Model

According to the *in vitro* data, rAdeK antisera showed the highest capability to potentiate the effect of TGC against TGC-R *A. baumannii,* and also had an addition role to in

---

TABLE 1 | Confirmation of the purified recombinant proteins by liquid chromatography–mass spectrometry/mass spectrometry (LC-MS/MS).

Sample name	Protein name	Accession number	pI	MW (KDa)	Sequence coverage
AdeA	Multidrug RND transporter [*A. baumannii*]	gi| 500174963	5.46	15.714	76%
AdeI	Multidrug RND transporter [*A. baumannii*]	gi| 500185983	9.04	39.778	83%
AdeK	adeC/adeK/oprM family multidrug efflux complex outer membrane factor [*A. baumannii*]	gi| 691007736	9.12	52.770	83%
TolC	RND transporter [*A. baumannii*]	gi| 500183799	9.21	44.273	78%

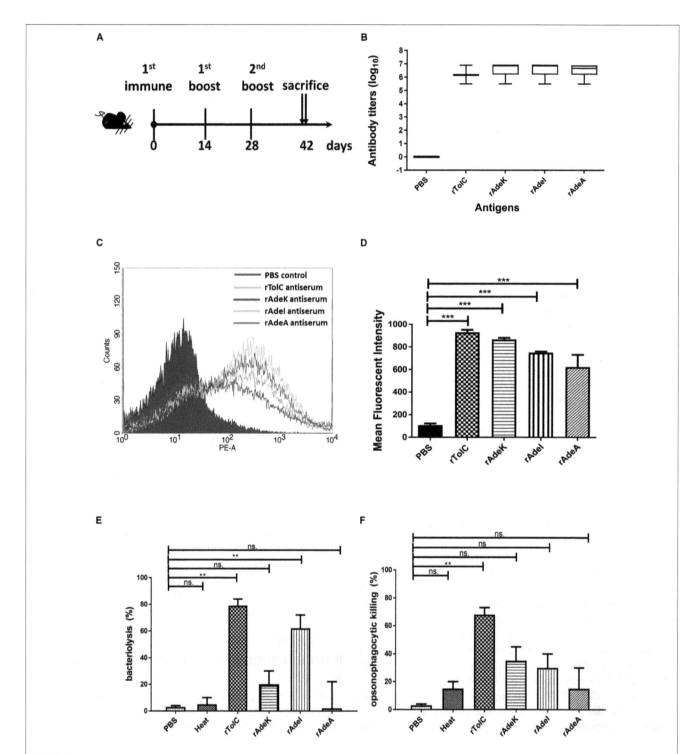

FIGURE 2 | Polyclonal mouse antisera production and characterization. **(A)** Groups of C57BL/6 mice (n = 10) were subcutaneously immunized with either 10 μg of individual antigen (rAdeI, rTolC, rAdeK, and rAdeA) or phosphate-buffered saline (PBS) formulated with Complete Freund's Adjuvant/Incomplete Freund's Adjuvant (CFA/IFA) on days 0, 14, and 28. Blood samples were collected before sacrifice and tested against each antigen. **(B)** Serum IgG antibody titers against each antigen as indicated by enzyme-linked immunosorbent assay. **(C)** Flow cytometry (FACS) analysis demonstrating the surface accessibility of the antigen-specific antisera. Cells from late-log-phase cultures were probed with a control non-specific antibody (shaded histograms) or individual antisera (unshaded histograms). Each histogram shows the fluorescence intensity distribution of >20,000 flow cytometry events. **(D)** Histogram representing quantitative analysis of the binding intensity from FACS studies. Bars indicate the means of at least three independent experiments ± SEM. ***p < 0.001. **(E)** Bacteria inhibition by each antigen-specific mouse antisera at 1:10 dilution, used in the presence of human complement and ATCC17978. **(F)** The complement-dependent opsonophagocytosis assays were performed with mouse antisera (1:10), ATCC17978 and RAW 264.7 macrophages. The results represent the percentage of bacterial survival in the assay after 1 h of incubation at 37°C compared to that in phosphate-buffered saline (PBS)-Immunized antisera. Bars indicate the means of at least three independent experiments ± SEM. ns., non-significance. **p < 0.01, Heat, complement replaced with a heat-inactivated complement.

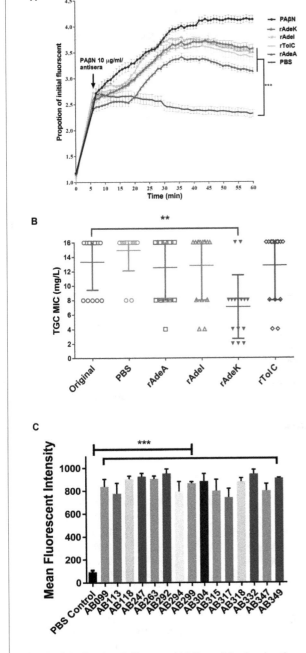

FIGURE 3 | The function of efflux pump inhibition activity of each antiserum. **(A)** Fold changed-H33342 fluorescence values for ATCC17978 following growth in specific antisera and treatment with phenylalanine-arginine beta-naphthylamide (PAβN) (10 μg/mL). Mock-treated cells are also shown (gray line). The assays were performed in triplicates and the error bars show the SEM at 1-min intervals. **(B)** Minimum inhibitory concentration (MIC) of tigecycline-resistant (TGC-R) *A. baumannii* clinical isolates (*n* = 15) compared to original or specific antisera [phosphate-buffered saline (PBS), rAdeA, rAdeI, rAdeK, and rTolC] co-administrated by broth microdilution method. The experiments were performed in triplicates. The *p*-value was determined by Kruskal–Wallis test with Dunn's multiple comparison analysis. **p < 0.01. **(C)** Histogram representing quantitative analysis of the binding intensity between anti-AdeK antisera and isolates from the FACS study. The bars indicate the means of at least three independent experiments ± SEM. ***p < 0.001.

antibody mediated killing, so rAdeK was selected as a vaccine candidate. The protocol for murine pneumonia model is shown in **Figure 4A**. An intratracheal challenge with a clinical isolate of AB247 was performed. AB247 was selected because of its high TGC-resistant phenotype (MIC 16 mg/L) and its significant response in broth microdilution evaluation. The results showed that TGC administration in rAdeK-immunized mice significantly reduced the bacterial load in the lungs compared to that in mice without immunization (**Figure 4B**, *p* < 0.001). The bacterial load was also reduced in the kidney, spleen, and blood, but without statistical significance (**Figures 4C–E**). The histopathology of lung tissues showed that neutrophil infiltration in the peri-bronchial vasculature region was lower in rAdeK-immunization and TGC-treated mice (**Figure 5**) compared to that in other groups. More importantly, there was no evidence of morbidity or mortality among mice during the immunization course, which suggested that rAdeK is safe and suitable for immunization.

DISCUSSION

AMR bacterial infection have been increasing dramatically in recent decades and account for about 80% of all severe bacterial infections (Du et al., 2018). Resistant phenotypes can arise from overexpression of intrinsic efflux activity to effectively respond to antibiotic or toxin related challenges (Du et al., 2018). Inhibition of antimicrobial determinants, such as efflux pump inhibitors (EPIs) is a feasible approach to preserve and improve the clinical performance of antituberculosis agents and overcome crucial drug-resistance challenges (Song and Wu, 2016). The use of EPIs could facilitate the revival of antibiotics and could be suitable for clinical applications. Unfortunately, no EPIs are yet available for clinical use (Abdali et al., 2017). We developed an alternative vaccine strategy targeting an antibiotic efflux pump. We tested this idea in TGC-resistant *A. baumannii*. We found that immunization with the RND efflux pump outer membrane protein, AdeK, interfered with the efflux activity of bacteria and, also induced antibodies with bactericidal effects (**Figure 6**). When co-administrated with TGC therapy, this strategy efficiently attenuated TGC-R *A. baumannii* pneumonia infection. A recent study showed that the combined treatment of anti-outer membrane vesicle serum and antibiotics could increase the intracellular aggregation of antibiotics by affecting porin function (Huang et al., 2019). The strategy significantly improved the antibiotic susceptibility of drug-resistant *A. baumannii* and strengthened the feasibility of combination therapy with vaccine and antibiotics. Accordingly, predominant resistance determinants with high homology, such as MecA, that confer resistance to methicillin in *Staphylococcus aureus* might also be good candidates for this approach.

Efflux-mediated TGC resistance has been extensively investigated in *A. baumannii*, especially in RND efflux pumps such as AdeABC, AdeFGH, AdeIJK, and AcrAB-TolC, in which overexpression leads to a TGC-resistant phenotype (Sugawara and Nikaido, 2014). Moreover, mutations in the *adeR* and *adeS* regulatory genes have been detected in TGC-R clinical isolates with efflux pump overexpression (Sun et al., 2014). Therefore,

TABLE 2 | Minimum inhibitory concentrations (MICs) of clinical isolates and synergistic effects of antigen-specific antisera on tigecycline (TGC) MICs[a].

Strains	Original	rAdeA		rAdeI		rAdeK		rTolC	
	TGC MIC	OE[b]	MIC	OE	MIC	OE	MIC	OE	MIC
AB099	8	+	8	+	4	+	**2**	+	4
AB113	16	+	16	+	16	+	8	+	16
AB118	8	+	8	+	16	−	4	−	8
AB247	16	+	16	+	**4**	+	**2**	−	8
AB263	16	+	16	+	16	+	8	−	16
AB292	8	+	16	+	16	−	16	+	16
AB294	8	+	4	+	4	+	**2**	−	8
AB299	8	+	16	+	8	+	8	−	16
AB304	16	+	8	−	8	+	4	+	16
AB315	16	+	8	+	16	−	8	+	16
AB317	16	+	16	+	16	+	8	+	16
AB318	16	+	16	+	16	+	16	−	16
AB332	16	+	8	+	16	−	8	+	16
AB347	16	+	16	+	16	+	**4**	+	**4**
AB349	16	+	16	+	16	−	8	−	16

[a]*Bold font indicates a fourfold reduction in MIC value. Experiments were performed in triplicate and repeated three times, with similar results.* [b]*OE: overexpression, gene expression level ≥ twofold compared to that of the ATCC17978 reference strain was considered significant overexpression; +, Yes; −, No.*

TABLE 3 | Comparisons of efflux pump protein sequence similarities to *A. baumannii* ATCC 17978.

Strain ID	adeA	adeI	adeK	tolC
AB099	100%	100%	99.80% (N295T)	99.60% (Q85H, K180T)
AB113	99.30% (T138A)	100%	99.80% (G212L)	100%
AB118	99.30% (T138A)	100%	100%	100%
AB247	99.30% (T138A)	100%	100%	100%
AB263	99.30% (T138A)	100%	99.80% (G212C)	100%
AB292	99.30% (T138A)	100%	100%	100%
AB294	99.30% (T138A)	100%	100%	99.60% (E219V, Y220F)
AB299	99.30% (T138A)	100%	100%	100%
AB304	99.30% (T138A)	100%	100%	100%
AB315	99.30% (T138A)	100%	99.80% (L296S)	100%
AB317	99.30% (T138A)	100%	99.80% (Q193H)	99.10% (T293I, R325G, T326S, S327Y)
AB318	99.30% (T138A)	100%	100%	100%
AB332	99.30% (T138A)	100%	100%	100%
AB347	99.30% (T138A)	100%	100%	98.20% (Q163R, N193C, Q195H, Y196D, A201T, A205E, N207D, A213T)
AB349	99.30% (T138A)	100%	100%	100%

inhibition of efflux activity is a promising approach to restore TGC susceptibility. RND efflux systems usually comprise three different components assembling into a functional complex, including outer membrane protein, middle periplasmic protein and inner membrane protein (Du et al., 2018). AdeA and AdeI belonged to the inner membrane protein of the system, whereas AdeK and TolC belonged to the outer membrane protein of the system. The results of kinetic accumulation study in the present study showed that all the antisera could potentially attenuate bisbenzimide H33342 efflux activity in ATCC strains, indicating

H33342 is the substrate of these efflux systems. Decreased accumulation of H33342 after 40 min of antisera treatment (**Figure 3A**) might indicate the activation of the redundant efflux system to extrude H33342. Compared to other antisera, rAdeK antisera efficiently reduced TGC MIC levels in the clinical isolates; this result might indicate the major contribution of AdeIJK in TGC resistance in *A. baumannii* (Rosenfeld et al., 2012). It is interesting that when targeting the same RND system (AdeIJK), different components of the system could have different effects. For example, antisera against AdeK could

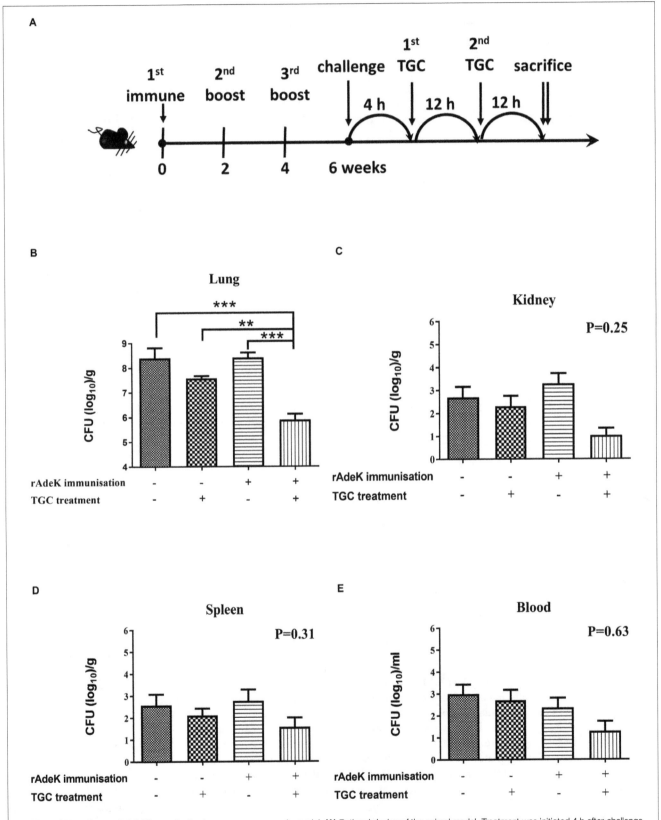

FIGURE 4 | The efficacy of rAdeK immunization in a mouse pneumonia model. **(A)** Rational design of the animal model. Treatment was initiated 4 h after challenge against *A. baumannii* AB247 [tigecycline (TGC) minimum inhibitory concentration of 16 µg/mL], twice a day by subcutaneous injections. Bacterial loads were determined in different organs after the mice were sacrificed and were compared among the four groups. **(B–E)** Bacterial load in the mice lungs **(B)**, kidney **(C)**, spleen **(D)**, and blood **(E)** after 24 h TGC treatment compared among the four groups studied. The bars indicate the means ± the SEM. **$p < 0.01$; ***$p < 0.001$.

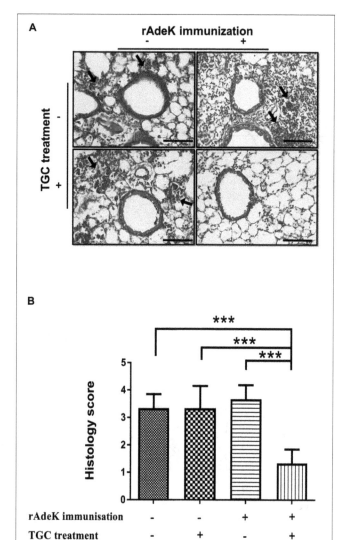

FIGURE 5 | The histology of mouse lung sections in pneumonia model.
(A) Hematoxylin and eosin staining of mouse lung sections obtained from
each group. Images were taken at 40× by light microscopy and represented
sections from three mice per group. The arrows indicate regions of
peri-bronchovascular infiltration. Bars = 100 μm. **(B)** Lung inflammation was
scored, the bars indicate the means of at least three samples ± SEM.
***$p < 0.001$.

(rAdeK vaccinated or TGC-treated group), as *A. baumannii* is a bacterium with low virulence.

In addition to the potentiation of antibiotic treatment, the antisera had other roles as it could enhance the antibody mediated killing of bacteria. In the *in vivo* study, the effect of AdeK immunization might come from two aspects, one is antagonizing the efflux pump against antibiotic extrusion, another is through antibody mediated killing. It is unknown how the antisera of the efflux pump could reverse the antibiotic resistance. It is reported that antibodies may affect the function of specific antigens via conformation changes (Roguin and Retegui, 2003), or that this effect could be a result of blocking the channel of antibiotic extrusion. Some efflux pumps are associated with bacterial virulence and biofilm formation, which are responsible for host cell adhesion and invasion (Du et al., 2018). For example, TolC is a virulence factor associated with toxin translocation in *E. coli* (Lee et al., 2012). In our study, antisera derived from immunization with rTolC conferred significant complement-dependent bactericidal and opsonophagocytic activity. It is worth to determine whether rTolC could be an ideal vaccine candidate in future studies.

The non-responding strains also had similar *adeK* sequence and overexpression level of the gene. Unknown mechanisms for TGC resistance may have been present in the non-responding strains. Li et al. (2016) identified > 50 possible drug efflux pumps that could contribute to multidrug resistance from over 1000 genomes of *A. baumannii* strains. In addition, the antibody might need to be optimized to more effectively block the most critical epitope of the efflux protein. Future research should focus on physical data in three-dimensional structures of efflux pumps and specific antibodies need to be elucidated to understand the structure-function relationships in these pumps (Roguin and Retegui, 2003). Although only 26.7% of strains had reduced TGC MIC after adding antisera, low coverage of the bacteria population (even 1–4%) by immunization with resistant determinants might still be effective in eradicating the resistant population (Niewiadomska et al., 2019).

We examined the effect of the anti-AdeK antisera on amikacin, meropenem, colistin, and ampicillin/sulbactam (**Supplementary Table S3**). These results showed no significant synergistic effect to reverse the resistance against these antibiotics. These was not unexpected, as the major resistant mechanisms of these antibiotics are not through efflux pump. Instead, the major resistance mechanism for amikacin, meropenem and ampicillin/sulbactam is the production of antibiotic modifying or degrading enzymes (Lee et al., 2017), whereas modification or loss of lipopolysaccharide confers colistin resistance in *A. baumannii*.

It is important to note that efflux pumps are conserved not only in *A. baumannii* but also in different bacterial genera. The AdeK protein has sequence homology to efflux proteins in other nosocomial "bad bugs" listed by the Infectious Diseases Society of America (Boucher et al., 2009; **Supplementary Table S4**), thus having the potential of broader coverage and application in the near future. A recent report also supported that AdeK and other 24 resistant determinants are predicted as vaccine candidates to strengthen antibiotic treatments (Ni et al., 2017).

potentiate TGC effects but antisera against *AdeI* could not. This result indicated that the outer membrane component might be a better vaccine candidate than inner membrane protein when combined with antibiotic use. As demonstrated in **Figure 3C**, antisera against rAdeK derived from ATCC17978 could cross-react with all fifteen clinical isolates by flow cytometry assay. The *in vivo* study also demonstrated a good response in AdeK-vaccinated and TGC-treated mice, as they demonstrated less lung inflammation and reduced bacterial load in the lung. The bacteria load in other tissues was also lower in the AdeK-vaccinated and TGC-treated mice, but the difference was not significant. This might be due to the lower bacterial load (about 10^3 CFU/g) in the no treatment or single treatment arms

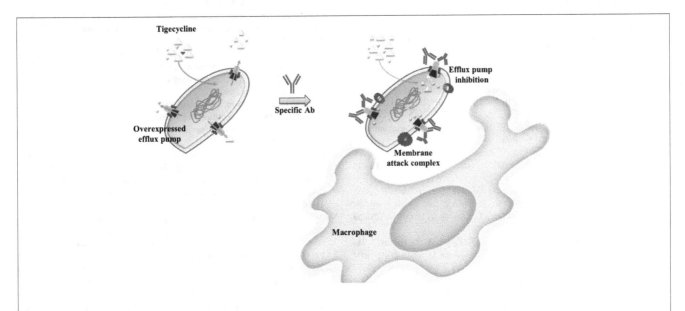

FIGURE 6 | Schematic representation of the proposed mechanism of anti-efflux antibodies-mediated tigecycline efflux inhibition and bactericidal activity. Under overexpressed conditions, activated efflux pumps efficiently remove tigecycline to attenuate antibiotic activity **(left)**. These phenomena might be restored by using an anti-rAdeK antibody as an efflux pump inhibitor. Bactericidal effects might also be induced via complement-mediated lytic membrane attack complex pores and opsonophagocytic activity **(right)**.

CONCLUSION

In conclusion, our results demonstrate that active immunization with antibiotic-resistant determinants may be a promising approach to combat multidrug-resistant pathogens in high-risk population.

ETHICS STATEMENT

The animal study was reviewed and approved by National Defense Medical Center Institutional Animal Care and Use Committee (NDMC IACUC-17-206).

AUTHOR CONTRIBUTIONS

M-HC, T-LC, and Y-PC contributed to the conception and design of the studies. M-HC, Y-SY, S-CK, and Y-PC contributed to the execution of the animal vaccination studies. M-HC, Y-TL, and J-RS carried out the laboratory *in vitro* assays. M-HC, Y-SY, Y-CW, S-CK, Y-TL, Y-PC, and T-LC were involved in the drafting, revision, and approval of the final version of the manuscript.

FUNDING

This work was supported by the Ministry of Science and Technology (Grant Nos. MOST 105-2628-B-016-003-MY2, MOST 105-2314-B-016-039-MY3, MOST 107-2314-B-016-051-MY3, MOST 107-2320-B-016-003, MOST 108-2314-B-016-029, and MOST 109-2320-B-016-002-MY2), Tri-Service General Hospital (Grant Nos. TSGH-C107-098 and TSGH-C108-137). The funders had no role in the study design, data collection and analysis, decision to publish, or preparation of the manuscript.

ACKNOWLEDGMENTS

This study was supported by the ACTION study group. The members of the ACTION study group include Yea-Yuan Chang (National Yang-Ming University Hospital, Yilan, Taiwan), Yuag-Meng Liu (Changhua Christian Hospital, Changhua, Taiwan), S-CK (National Institute of Infectious Diseases and Vaccinology, National Health Research Institute, Miaoli County, Taiwan), Chang-Pan Liu (MacKay Memorial Hospital, Taipei, Taiwan), T-LC (Graduate Institute of Life Sciences, National Defense Medical Center, Taipei, Taiwan), Y-TL (Taipei Veterans General Hospital, Taipei, Taiwan), and Y-SY (National Defense Medical Center, Taipei, Taiwan).

REFERENCES

Abdali, N., Parks, J. M., Haynes, K. M., Chaney, J. L., Green, A. T., Wolloscheck, D., et al. (2017). Reviving antibiotics: efflux pump inhibitors that interact with AcrA, a membrane fusion protein of the AcrAB-TolC multidrug efflux pump. *ACS Infect. Dis.* 3, 89–98. doi: 10.1021/acsinfecdis.6b00167

Alekshun, M. N., and Levy, S. B. (2007). Molecular mechanisms of antibacterial multidrug resistance. *Cell* 128, 1037–1050. doi: 10.1016/j.cell.2007.03.004

Ardehali, S. H., Azimi, T., Fallah, F., Owrang, M., Aghamohammadi, N., and Azimi, L. (2019). Role of efflux pumps in reduced susceptibility to tigecycline in *Acinetobacter baumannii*. *New Microbes. New Infect.* 30:100547. doi: 10.1016/j.nmni.2019.100547

Boucher, H. W., Talbot, G. H., Bradley, J. S., Edwards, J. E., Gilbert, D., Rice, L. B., et al. (2009). Bad bugs, no drugs: no ESKAPE! an update from the infectious diseases society of America. *Clin. Infect. Dis.* 48, 1–12. doi: 10.1086/595011

Chiang, M. H., Sung, W. C., Lien, S. P., Chen, Y. Z., Lo, A. F., Huang, J. H., et al. (2015). Identification of novel vaccine candidates against *Acinetobacter baumannii* using reverse vaccinology. *Hum. Vaccin. Immunother.* 11, 1065–1073. doi: 10.1080/21645515.2015.1010910

CLSI (2017). *M100-S27: Performance Standards for Antimicrobial Susceptibility Testing: 27th Informational Supplement.* Wayne, PA: Clinical and Laboratory Standards Institute.

Du, D., Wang-Kan, X., Neuberger, A., Van Veen, H. W., Pos, K. M., Piddock, L. J. V., et al. (2018). Multidrug efflux pumps: structure, function and regulation. *Nat. Rev. Microbiol.* 16, 523–539.

Gagneux-Brunon, A., Lucht, F., Launay, O., Berthelot, P., and Botelho-Nevers, E. (2018). Vaccines for healthcare-associated infections: present, future, and expectations. *Expert Rev. Vaccin.* 17, 421–433. doi: 10.1080/14760584.2018.1470507

Garcia-Quintanilla, M., Pulido, M. R., Carretero-Ledesma, M., and Mcconnell, M. J. (2016). Vaccines for antibiotic-resistant bacteria: possibility or pipe dream? *Trends Pharmacol. Sci.* 37, 143–152. doi: 10.1016/j.tips.2015.10.003

Huang, W., Yao, Y., Long, Q., Yang, X., Sun, W., Liu, C., et al. (2014). Immunization against multidrug-resistant *Acinetobacter baumannii* effectively protects mice in both pneumonia and sepsis models. *PLoS One* 9:e100727. doi: 10.1371/journal.pone.0100727

Huang, W., Zhang, Q., Li, W., Chen, Y., Shu, C., Li, Q., et al. (2019). Anti-outer membrane vesicle antibodies increase antibiotic sensitivity of pan-drug-resistant *Acinetobacter baumannii*. *Front. Microbiol.* 10:1379. doi: 10.3389/fmicb.2019.01379

Imai, K., Asakawa, N., Tsuji, T., Akazawa, F., Ino, A., Sonoyama, M., et al. (2008). SOSUI-GramN: high performance prediction for sub-cellular localization of proteins in gram-negative bacteria. *Bioinformation* 2, 417–421. doi: 10.6026/97320630002417

Jansen, K. U., Knirsch, C., and Anderson, A. S. (2018). The role of vaccines in preventing bacterial antimicrobial resistance. *Nat. Med.* 24, 10–19. doi: 10.1038/nm.4465

Jia, B., Raphenya, A. R., Alcock, B., Waglechner, N., Guo, P., Tsang, K. K., et al. (2017). CARD 2017: expansion and model-centric curation of the comprehensive antibiotic resistance database. *Nucleic Acids Res.* 45, D566–D573. doi: 10.1093/nar/gkw1004

Joice, R., and Lipsitch, M. (2013). Targeting imperfect vaccines against drug-resistance determinants: a strategy for countering the rise of drug resistance. *PLoS One* 8:e68940. doi: 10.1371/journal.pone.0068940

Kumar, S., Stecher, G., and Tamura, K. (2016). MEGA7: molecular evolutionary genetics analysis version 7.0 *for bigger datasets*. *Mol. Biol. Evol.* 33, 1870–1874. doi: 10.1093/molbev/msw054

Laure, D., Virginie, P., Alexandr, N., Lenie, D., and Sylvain, B. (2010). The population structure of *Acinetobacter baumannii*: expanding multiresistant clones from an ancestral susceptible genetic pool. *PLoS One* 5:e10034. doi: 10.1371/journal.pone.0010034

Lee, C. R., Lee, J. H., Park, M., Park, K. S., Bae, I. K., Kim, Y. B., et al. (2017). Biology of *Acinetobacter baumannii*: pathogenesis, antibiotic resistance mechanisms, and prospective treatment options. *Front. Cell Infect. Microbiol.* 7:55. doi: 10.3389/fcimb.2017.00055

Lee, M., Jun, S. Y., Yoon, B. Y., Song, S., Lee, K., and Ha, N. C. (2012). Membrane fusion proteins of type I secretion system and tripartite efflux pumps share a binding motif for TolC in gram-negative bacteria. *PLoS One* 7:e40460. doi: 10.1371/journal.pone.0040460

Li, L., Hassan, K. A., Brown, M. H., and Paulsen, I. T. (2016). Rapid multiplexed phenotypic screening identifies drug resistance functions for three novel efflux pumps in *Acinetobacter baumannii*. *J. Antimicrob. Chemother.* 71, 1223–1232. doi: 10.1093/jac/dkv460

McConnell, M. J., Domínguez-Herrera, J., Smani, Y., López-Rojas, R., Docobo-Pérez, F., and Pachón, J. (2011). Vaccination with outer membrane complexes elicits rapid protective immunity to multidrug-resistant *Acinetobacter baumannii*. *Infect. Immun.* 79, 518–526. doi: 10.1128/IAI.00741-10

Ni, W., Han, Y., Zhao, J., Wei, C., Cui, J., Wang, R., et al. (2016). Tigecycline treatment experience against multidrug-resistant *Acinetobacter baumannii* infections: a systematic review and meta-analysis. *Int. J. Antimicrob. Agents* 47, 107–116. doi: 10.1016/j.ijantimicag.2015.11.011

Ni, Z., Chen, Y., Ong, E., and He, Y. (2017). Antibiotic resistance determinant-focused *Acinetobacter baumannii* vaccine designed using reverse vaccinology. *Int. J. Mol. Sci.* 18:458. doi: 10.3390/ijms18020458

Niewiadomska, A. M., Jayabalasingham, B., Seidman, J. C., Willem, L., Grenfell, B., Spiro, D., et al. (2019). Population-level mathematical modeling of antimicrobial resistance: a systematic review. *BMC Med.* 17:81. doi: 10.1186/s12916-019-1314-9

Nordmann, P., and Poirel, L. (2019). Epidemiology and diagnostics of carbapenem resistance in gram-negative bacteria. *Clin. Infect. Dis.* 69, S521–S528. doi: 10.1093/cid/ciz824

Noto, M. J., Becker, K. W., Boyd, K. L., Schmidt, A. M., and Skaar, E. P. (2017). RAGE-mediated suppression of interleukin-10 results in enhanced mortality in a murine model of *Acinetobacter baumannii* sepsis. *Infect. Immun.* 85, e954–e916. doi: 10.1128/IAI.00954-16

Perez, F., and Bonomo, R. A. (2014). Vaccines for *Acinetobacter baumannii*: thinking "out of the box". *Vaccine* 32, 2537–2539. doi: 10.1016/j.vaccine.2014.03.031

Pichardo, C., Pachon-Ibanez, M. E., Docobo-Perez, F., Lopez-Rojas, R., Jimenez-Mejias, M. E., Garcia-Curiel, A., et al. (2010). Efficacy of tigecycline vs. *imipenem in the treatment of experimental Acinetobacter baumannii* murine pneumonia. *Eur. J. Clin. Microbiol. Infect. Dis.* 29, 527–531. doi: 10.1007/s10096-010-0890-6

Pillar, C. M., Draghi, D. C., Dowzicky, M. J., and Sahm, D. F. (2008). In vitro activity of tigecycline against gram-positive and gram-negative pathogens as evaluated by broth microdilution and Etest. *J. Clin. Microbiol.* 46, 2862–2867. doi: 10.1128/JCM.00637-08

Rappuoli, R., Black, S., and Bloom, D. E. (2019). Vaccines and global health: in search of a sustainable model for vaccine development and delivery. *Sci. Transl. Med.* 11:eaaw2888. doi: 10.1126/scitranslmed.aaw2888

Richmond, G. E., Chua, K. L., and Piddock, L. J. (2013). Efflux in *Acinetobacter baumannii* can be determined by measuring accumulation of H33342 (bis-benzamide). *J. Antimicrob. Chemother.* 68, 1594–1600. doi: 10.1093/jac/dkt052

Roguin, L. P., and Retegui, L. A. (2003). Monoclonal antibodies inducing conformational changes on the antigen molecule. *Scand. J. Immunol.* 58, 387–394. doi: 10.1046/j.1365-3083.2003.01320.x

Rosenfeld, N., Bouchier, C., Courvalin, P., and Perichon, B. (2012). Expression of the resistance-nodulation-cell division pump AdeIJK in *Acinetobacter baumannii* is regulated by AdeN, a TetR-type regulator. *Antimicrob. Agents Chemother.* 56, 2504–2510. doi: 10.1128/AAC.06422-11

Song, L., and Wu, X. (2016). Development of efflux pump inhibitors in antituberculosis therapy. *Int. J. Antimicrob. Agents* 47, 421–429. doi: 10.1016/j.ijantimicag.2016.04.007

Sugawara, E., and Nikaido, H. (2014). Properties of AdeABC and AdeIJK efflux systems of *Acinetobacter baumannii* compared with those of the AcrAB-TolC system of *Escherichia coli. Antimicrob. Agents Chemother.* 58, 7250–7257. doi: 10.1128/AAC.03728-14

Sun, J. R., Perng, C. L., Lin, J. C., Yang, Y. S., Chan, M. C., Chang, T. Y., et al. (2014). AdeRS combination codes differentiate the response to efflux pump inhibitors in tigecycline-resistant isolates of extensively drug-resistant *Acinetobacter baumannii. Eur. J. Clin. Microbiol. Infect. Dis.* 33, 2141–2147. doi: 10.1007/s10096-014-2179-7

Sun, Y., Cai, Y., Liu, X., Bai, N., Liang, B., and Wang, R. (2013). The emergence of clinical resistance to tigecycline. *Int. J. Antimicrob. Agents* 41, 110–116. doi: 10.1016/j.ijantimicag.2012.09.005

Uchiyama, I., Mihara, M., Nishide, H., and Chiba, H. (2014). MBGD update 2015: microbial genome database for flexible ortholog analysis utilizing a diverse set of genomic data. *Nucleic Acids Res.* 43, D270–D276. doi: 10.1093/nar/gku1152

Yu, C. S., Cheng, C. W., Su, W. C., Chang, K. C., Huang, S. W., Hwang, J. K., et al. (2014). CELLO2GO: a web server for protein subCELlular LOcalization prediction with functional gene ontology annotation. *PLoS One* 9:e99368. doi: 10.1371/journal.pone.0099368

Yu, N. Y., Wagner, J. R., Laird, M. R., Melli, G., Rey, S., Lo, R., et al. (2010). PSORTb 3.0: improved protein subcellular localization prediction with refined localization subcategories and predictive capabilities for all prokaryotes. *Bioinformatics (Oxford, England)* 26, 1608–1615. doi: 10.1093/bioinformatics/btq249

2

Antibiotic Susceptibility, Virulence Pattern and Typing of *Staphylococcus aureus* Strains Isolated from Variety of Infections in India

Shifu Aggarwal[1†], Smrutiti Jena[1†], Sasmita Panda[1†‡], Savitri Sharma[2], Benu Dhawan[3], Gopal Nath[4], N. P. Singh[5], Kinshuk Chandra Nayak[6] and Durg Vijai Singh[1,7]*

[1] Infectious Disease Biology, Institute of Life Sciences, Bhubaneswar, India, [2] Jhaveri Microbiology Centre, LV Prasad Eye Institute, Brien Holden Eye Research Centre, Kallam Anji Reddy Campus, Hyderabad, India, [3] Department of Microbiology, All India Institute of Medical Sciences, New Delhi, India, [4] Department of Microbiology, Institute of Medical Sciences, Banaras Hindu University, Varanasi, India, [5] Department of Microbiology, Faculty of Medical Sciences, University of Delhi, New Delhi, India, [6] Institute of Life Sciences, Bhubaneswar, India, [7] Department of Biotechnology, Central University of South Bihar, Gaya, India

*Correspondence:
Durg Vijai Singh
durg_singh@yahoo.co.in;
singhdv@ils.res.in;
dvsingh@cusb.ac.in

Staphylococcus aureus is one of the major causes of nosocomial infections. This organism produces powerful toxins and cause superficial lesions, systemic infections, and several toxemic syndromes. A total of 109 *S. aureus* strains isolated from a variety of infections like ocular diseases, wound infection, and sputum were included in the study. Minimum inhibitory concentration (MIC) was determined against 8 antimicrobials. PCR determined the presence of 16S rRNA, *nuc*, *mecA*, czrC, *qacA/B*, *pvl*, and toxin genes in *S. aureus* isolates. Pulse-field gel electrophoresis (PFGE), multi-locus sequence typing (MLST), SCC*mec*, *spa*-, and *agr*-typing and serotyping determined the diversity among them. All isolates of *S. aureus* were resistant to two or more than two antibiotics and generated 32 resistance patterns. These isolates were positive for 16S rRNA and *S. aureus*-specific *nuc* gene, but showed variable results for *mecA*, czrC, and qacA/B and *pvl* genes. Of the 32 methicillin-resistant *S. aureus* (MRSA), 13 strains carried SCC*mec* type V, seven type IV, two type III, and nine carried unreported type UT6. Of the 109 strains, 98.2% were positive for *hlg*, 94.5% for *hla*, 86.2% for *sei*, 73.3% for *efb*, 70.6% for *cna*, 30.2% for *sea*, and 12.8% for *sec* genes. Serotypes VII and VI were prevalent among *S. aureus* strains. PFGE analysis grouped the 109 strains into 77 clusters. MLST classified the strains into 33 sequence types (ST) and eight clonal complexes (CCs) of which 12 were singletons, and two belong to new allelic profiles. Isolates showed 46 *spa*-types that included two new spa-types designated as t14911 and t14912. MRSA and methicillin-susceptible *S. aureus* (MSSA) isolates were diverse in terms of antibiotic resistance pattern, toxin genotypes, SCC*mec* types, serotypes and PFGE, MLST, and spa-types. However, few isolates from eye infection and wound infection belong to CC239, ST239, and *spa*-type t037/t657. The study thus suggests that *S. aureus* strains are multidrug resistant, virulent, and diverse irrespective of sources and place of isolation. These findings necessitate the continuous surveillance of multidrug-resistant and virulent *S. aureus* and monitoring of the transmission of infection.

Keywords: antibiotic susceptibility, virulence, MLST, *spa*-typing, PFGE, biofilm, *Staphylococcus aureus*

INTRODUCTION

Staphylococcus aureus commensal to human skin and mucous membranes could cause nosocomial (Lindsay and Holden, 2004) and systemic infections (Jarraud et al., 2002). The isolation of methicillin-resistant *S. aureus* (MRSA) from ocular infections varies from 3 to 30% in a hospital in India and other countries (Shanmuganathan et al., 2005; Freidlin et al., 2007). MRSA strains belonging to ST5, ST72, and ST88 and isolated from severe eye infections in India were resistant to all antibiotics except tetracycline, chloramphenicol, and cefazolin (Nadig et al., 2012). Godebo et al. (2013) showed that 94.5% of *S. aureus* isolated from wound infection were resistant to penicillin, 91.8% to ampicillin, and 76.7% to oxacillin.

Several studies have shown the presence of toxin genes among MRSA. The presence of the *sea* gene in MRSA varies from country to country (Mehrotra et al., 2000; Kim et al., 2006; Wang et al., 2013). However, *hla* gene was present in all isolates (Shukla et al., 2010). MRSA isolated from conjunctivitis in Nigeria belonging to ST88 and SCC*mec* type IV were positive for *pvl* gene (Ghebremedhin et al., 2009). However, *pvl* gene positive methicillin-susceptible *S. aureus* (MSSA) strains belonged to ST30 (D'Souza et al., 2010). *S. aureus* carrying the *pvl* gene and belonging to ST239, ST5, and ST88 was reported from a teaching hospital in China (Liu et al., 2009). MSSA belonging to ST121 and *spa*-type 287 isolated from community-acquired pneumonia in young patients carried the virulence genes (*cna* and *bbp*) and *pvl* (Baranovich et al., 2010). The role of virulence genes in *S. aureus* pathogenesis may vary from one infection type to another type of infections. Dhawan et al. (2015) reported the isolation of SCC*mec* type IV and V clones of MRSA in an Indian hospital. Several other workers also showed a decrease in SCC*mec* III MRSA isolation but increased SCC*mec* IV and V MRSA isolation (Hsu et al., 2005; D'Souza et al., 2010). Multidrug-resistant isolates belonging to ST239 and SCC*mec* type III were slowly replaced by multidrug-susceptible ST22 (SCC*mec* type IV) and ST772 (SCC*mec* type V) in hospitals (D'Souza et al., 2010).

Several molecular biology techniques like multi-locus sequence typing (MLST), pulse-field gel electrophoresis (PFGE), SCC*mec* typing, and *spa*-typing have been used to study epidemiology and clonal diversity of *S. aureus* (Maslow et al., 1993; Norazah et al., 2001; Ghaznavi-Rad et al., 2011). However, not a single technique alone could discriminate the bacteria because of differences in the degree of typeability, reproducibility, and discriminatory power (Tenover et al., 1994). Overall analysis of different typing techniques can provide information on diversity of the isolates that can be useful for outbreak investigations. In India, *S. aureus* is rated as one of the major pathogen causing a variety of infections and showing

resistance to several antibiotics; however, not much information is available on their antibiotic susceptibility, virulence profile, and genomic diversity. In this study, our aim was to determine the antibiotic susceptibility pattern, virulence profiles, and genomic diversity among MRSA and MSSA isolated from patients with a variety of infections, including ocular diseases and collected from different parts of India from 2007 to 2015. Genetic, serotype, and phenotypic data were used to determine whether isolates from a variety of infections had similar characteristics.

MATERIALS AND METHODS

Bacterial Strains

A total of 109 *S. aureus* strains isolated from patients visited/admitted to hospitals with infections in different part of India between July 2007 and November 2015 were included in the study. These isolates were from LV Prasad Eye Institute, Bhubaneswar (*n* = 54), comprised of microbial keratitis (*n* = 18), eyelid abscess (*n* = 8), endophthalmitis (*n* = 5), Steven Johnson syndrome with bacterial keratitis (*n* = 9), suture-related infections (*n* = 3), and other ocular infection (*n* = 5); LV Prasad Eye Institute, Hyderabad (*n* = 10) comprised of cornea scrapping (*n* = 5), pus from eye (*n* = 4), and suture-related infections (*n* = 1); Institute of Medical Sciences, Banaras Hindu University, Varanasi (*n* = 21) comprised of wound infection (*n* = 16) and unknown sources (*n* = 5); All India Institute of Medical Sciences, New Delhi (wound infection *n* = 10); and University College of Medical Sciences, Delhi (wound infection *n* = 9). Also, five isolates were from the conjunctiva of the asymptomatic healthy volunteers LV Prasad Eye Institute, Bhubaneswar. We conducted the study following the guidelines mentioned in the Declaration of Helsinki. We identified all the 109 isolates by using biochemical tests including Gram staining, catalase production, fermentation of glucose and mannitol, and ID32 STAPH strips using ATB™ NEW v.1.0.0 software on an ATB™ reader (bioMerieux, France) (Panda et al., 2014). The amplification of the *S. aureus nuc* gene confirmed the identity of isolates (Hirotaki et al., 2011). We used *S. aureus* ATCC 25293 and *S. aureus* ATCC 29213 as quality control strains for antibiotic susceptibility testing, and *S. aureus* ATCC 25923 and ATCC 43300 as a reference for serotyping, PFGE, MLST, and *spa*-typing.

Coagulase Gene Typing

Coagulation-inhibition test with coagulase type I–VIII-specific antisera (staphylococcal coagulase antiserum kit; Denka Seiken, Inc., Tokyo, Japan) was conducted to determine the coagulase type of *S. aureus* following the manufacturer's instructions (Goh et al., 1992). Briefly, a single colony for each test strain was suspended in BHI broth (Becton Dickinson Co.) and incubated at 37°C for overnight. Then centrifuged the culture and 0.1 ml of the supernatant used as test antigen. Distributed an aliquot (0.1 ml) of the test antigen into ten tubes followed by addition of 0.1-ml aliquots of anticoagulase types I–VIII sera to first eight tubes, except 9th and 10th tubes which were used as positive and negative controls and incubated at 37°C for 1 h. After that, 0.2 ml of diluted rabbit plasma was added to each tube and incubated at 37°C for 1 h. Visual inspection judged the coagulation of plasma after 2, 4, 24, and 48 h and accordingly, strains were typed based on results obtained with staphylocoagulase reaction showing coagulation inhibition.

Minimum Inhibitory Concentration (MIC) Determination

Minimum inhibitory concentrations (MICs) of oxacillin, chloramphenicol, vancomycin, tetracycline, gentamicin, erythromycin, clindamycin, and trimethoprim were determined by broth microdilution methodology as recommended by the CLSI breakpoints. The 96-well plates were incubated at 37°C and were read for turbidity after 24 h.

Polymerase Chain Reaction (PCR) Assays

The presence of genes encoding for methicillin resistance (*mecA*), the nuclease (*nuc*), Panton-Valentine leukocidin (*pvl*), cadmium resistance (*czrC*), and quaternary ammonium resistance (*qacA/B*) was determined by hexaplex PCR (Panda et al., 2014). PCR identified the presence of *msrA, ermA, ermC* (erythromycin resistance), *tetK* (tetracycline resistance) genes (Duran et al., 2012). Also, PCR determined the presence of gene encoding for resistance to aminoglycosides [*aac (6')/aph (2), aph (3'-III)*] by the method described earlier (Schmitz et al., 1999). The presence of *catpC221, catpC223*, and *catpC194* (chloramphenicol resistance) was determined by PCR as described by Argudín et al. (2011). The *mphC* (clindamycin resistance) gene was detected by PCR method described earlier (Panda et al., 2016).

SCC*mec* Typing

Two PCRs, MPCR1 and MPCR2 were used to detect the presence of *mec* complex, *ccr* complex, and SCC*mec* type among *S. aureus* (Kondo et al., 2007).

Virulence Gene Profile and Accessory Gene Regulator (*Agr*) Typing

PCR determined the presence of Staphylococcal enterotoxin (SE) genes encoding for *seA, seC*, and *seI* (Monday and Bohach, 1999; Jarraud et al., 2002). Also, the presence of hemolysin genes, *hlA* and *hlG*, was determined by PCR (Mitchell et al., 2010; Paniagua-Contreras et al., 2012). PCR was used to detect the presence of collagen adhesion (*cna*) and extracellular fibrinogen binding protein (*efb*) among *S. aureus* strains (Zecconi et al., 2006). The presence of intracellular adhesion genes (*icaA, icaD*) was

determined by PCR as described by Arciola et al. (2001). PCR amplification was carried out to determine the presence of *agr* alleles using group-specific primers as described by Gilot et al. (2002).

Pulsed-Field Gel Electrophoresis (PFGE)

Pulsed-field gel electrophoresis of *S. aureus* genomic DNA digested with *Sma*I (NEB) was carried out by the protocol described for *S. aureus* by Centre for Disease Control and Prevention. The dendrogram of similarity showing the clustering of the isolates according to banding patterns was generated with Bionumerics software, version 7.1 (Applied Maths, Belgium) using the Dice index and the un-weighted pair group method with arithmetic average (UPGMA) with 0.5% optimization and 1% position tolerance. Isolates showing similarity coefficient of up to 80% were considered belonging to similar pulsotype (Van Belkum et al., 2007).

Multi-Locus Sequence Typing (MLST)

The internal fragments of seven housekeeping genes, viz., *arcC, gmk, aroE, glpF, pta, tpi,* and *yqil* were amplified by PCR method described earlier (Enright and Spratt, 1999). The amplified products were purified (ExoSAP; Affymetrix, Cleveland, OH, United States) and both strands sequenced using an ABI sequencer model 3500 (Life Technologies, Marsiling, Singapore) at the sequencing facility of the Institute of Life Sciences (Bhubaneswar, India). The nucleotide sequences were aligned using Mega 5.2 software. After manually comparing with reported alleles, STs were assigned accordingly. Sequencing was performed in biological duplicates to confirm the presence of novel alleles.

The advanced cluster analysis was performed to define the clonal complexes (CCs) by using Bionumerics software, version 7.1 (Applied Maths, Belgium). A minimum spanning tree (MST) was constructed using the MLST data and partitions were created to form clusters. The similarity in at least six alleles grouped isolates of *S. aureus* in one CC. The central ST of each separation was used to designate a CC.

Spa-Typing

PCR amplified the polymorphic X region of *Staphylococcus* protein A (*spa*) gene following the conditions mentioned earlier (Nelson et al., 2007). Amplified products were purified, and both strands were sequenced using an ABI sequencer model 3500 (Life Technologies, Marsiling, Singapore) at the sequencing facility of the Institute of Life Sciences (Bhubaneswar, India). The nucleotide sequences were aligned using Mega 5.2 software. Repeat succession in the polymorphic X-region assigned the *spa*-types, and accordingly the MST was generated using Bionumerics 7 software (Applied Maths, Belgium) using gap creation cost 250%, gap extension cost 50%, duplicate production cost 25%, duplicate expansion cost 25%, and maximum duplication three repeats.

Statistical Analysis

We performed principal coordinates analysis (PCoA) and discriminant analysis (DA) using PAST program v2.17 for the antibiotic resistance genes and virulence genes in MRSA and MSSA isolates with regard to sources of isolation (Hammer et al., 2001). We carried out the DA using default values to confirm the hypothesis of whether MRSA and MSSA isolates are different.

RESULTS

Hexaplex PCR

All the isolates of *S. aureus* were positive for 16S rRNA and *S. aureus*-specific *nuc* genes. Hexaplex PCR discriminates between MSSA and MRSA isolates. Thirty-one of 109 (29.4%) methicillin-resistant strains were positive for the *mecA* gene, and 77 (70.6%) methicillin sensitive isolates were negative for the *mecA* gene. One of the methicillin-resistant strains of *S. aureus* was negative for the *mecA* gene. Among 109 isolates, 43 (39.4%) isolates comprising 23 of the 77 (29.9%) MSSA and 20 of the 31 (64.5%) MRSA isolates were positive for *pvl* gene. Of the 31 MRSA isolates, two (6.5%) strains were positive for the *czrC* gene and four (12.9%) isolates were positive for *qacA/B* gene, and remaining isolates were negative for both *czrC* and *qacA/B* genes (data not shown).

Coagulase Serotyping

Serotyping classified *S. aureus* isolates into I–VIII serotypes by using coagulase typing scheme. Twelve of the 109 (11%) strains belong to serotype I, 11 (10%) to serotype II, nine (8%) to serotype III, 14 (12.8%) to serotype IV, 12 (11%) to serotype V, 19 (17.4%) to serotype VI, 20 (18.3%) to serotype VII, and 12 (11%) to serotype VIII, respectively. Nine of 31 (29%) MRSA belong to serotype VI and 17 of 78 (21.8%) and MSSA isolates belong to serotype VII (**Table 1**). Nine of the 24 (37.5%) isolates from wound infection belong to serotype VI and 16 of 64 (25%) isolates from eye infection belonged to serotype VII.

Antibiotic Resistance Genes

One hundred two of the 109 *S. aureus* isolates were multidrug resistant showing resistance to two or more antibiotics. All the strains were susceptible to vancomycin when tested by broth microdilution assay. Thirty-one isolates of *S. aureus* were resistant to oxacillin and carried the *mecA* gene; however, one isolate of *S. aureus* resistant to oxacillin was negative by PCR for the *mecA* gene. The remaining 77 isolates were sensitive to oxacillin and negative by PCR for the *mecA* gene (**Table 1**).

Ninety-five isolates of *S. aureus* resistant to chloramphenicol carried *cat: pC221* gene; however, 86 isolates carried *cat: pC223* and 37 isolates carried *cat: pC194* gene, respectively. Twenty isolates carried all the three genes tested; however, 83 isolates were positive for *cat: pC221* and *cat: pC223* and 37 isolates for *cat: pC221* and *cat: pC194* genes, respectively (**Table 1**). One of the isolates sensitive to chloramphenicol was negative by PCR for all three genes. In contrast, 15 strains of *S. aureus* susceptible to chloramphenicol were positive for *cat: pC221* and 14 for *cat: pC223* genes, respectively.

Twenty-nine isolates were phenotypically resistant to tetracycline of which 29 isolates were positive for *tetK*, 25 for *tetL*, and 28 for *tetM* genes. Twenty-five strains carried all the three genes tested; however, three strains carried *tetK* and *tetM* genes and one isolate *tetL* and *tetM* genes. In contrast, 76 isolates sensitive to tetracycline were positive for the *tetM* gene, 66 for *tetL*, and 29 for *tetK* genes. Among them, 27 isolates carried all the three genes, six had *tetK* and *tetM*, and 39 strains had *tetL* and *tetM* genes, respectively. One isolate sensitive to tetracycline was negative by PCR for all three genes tested (**Table 1**).

A total of 54 isolates were resistant to gentamicin of which 45 isolates were positive for *aac(6')/aph(2')* and *aph (3'-III)* genes and nine isolates for *aph (3'-III)* gene only. In contrast, 43 gentamycin sensitive isolates showed positive results for *aac(6')/aph(2')* and *aph (3'-III)*, seven isolates for *aac(6')/aph(2')*, and two isolates for *aph (3'-III)* genes. However, 56 isolates sensitive to gentamicin were negative by PCR for *aac(6')/aph(2')* and *aph (3'-III)* genes (**Table 1**).

Of the 91 isolates of *S. aureus* showing resistance to macrolides carried erythromycin resistance genes. Twenty-eight isolates carried all the erythromycin resistance genes, namely, *msrA*, *ermA*, and *ermC*. Fifty-one isolates were positive for two genes, of which 30 isolates carried *msrA* and *ermC* genes, and 21 strains had *ermA* and *ermC* genes. Besides, 12 isolates were positive for a single gene of which five isolates carried the *ermC* gene, and seven isolates had *msrA* gene. In contrast, two of the 10 erythromycin sensitive isolates carried *msrA* and *ermC* genes, four strains possess *msrA* and *ermC* genes, and three isolates had the *ermC* gene. Of the 64 isolates carrying the *mphC* gene, 22 isolates were phenotypically resistant to clindamycin (**Table 1**). None of the 17 strains showing sensitivity to erythromycin carried any of the erythromycin resistance genes. One of the resistant isolate not carrying any of the erythromycin resistant genes is likely to be mediated by an as-yet-unknown mechanism.

Similarly, 74 isolates were resistant to trimethoprim of which 45 isolates were positive for *dfrA*, *dfrB*, and *dfrG* genes, 27 strains for *dfrB* and *dfrG* genes, and one isolate each for *dfrB* and *dfrG* genes, respectively. In contrast, 34 isolates sensitive to trimethoprim were also positive for *dfrA*, *dfrB*, and *dfrG* genes; however, one strain was positive for the *dfrG* gene (**Table 1**).

D-Test and Macrolide Resistance

Ninety of 109 (89.9%) *S. aureus* isolates that exhibited erythromycin resistance were evaluated for MLSB resistance phenotype, namely, iMLSB, cMLSB and MSB. Seventy eight of 90 (79.5%) isolates were erythromycin-resistant but clindamycin susceptible were tested for D-test. We found 14 isolates (10 MRSA and four MSSA) showed iMLSB phenotype, and 12 (two MRSA and 10 MSSA) had MSB phenotype. Seven erythromycin-resistant isolates comprising six MRSA and one MSSA had cMLSB phenotype. The remaining 45 isolates (14 MRSA and 31 MSSA) did not show any MLSB phenotypes.

Among MRSA and MSSA showing cMLSB resistance phenotype, three of six MRSA isolates possessed the *ermA* and *ermC* genes and one each possessed *ermC* gene, *msrA*, *ermC*, *mphC* genes, and *ermC* and *mphC* genes. One MSSA isolate was positive for *msrA*, *ermA*, and *ermC* genes. On the hand, one

TABLE 1 | Antibiotic resistance patterns and presence of antibiotic resistance genes in *Staphylococcus aureus* isolates from different parts of India.

Phenotypic antibiotic resistance pattern	Number of isolates showing presence of gene(s) encoding for																	
	MRSA	MSSA	mecA	aac(6')/aph(2)	aph(3'III)	msrA	ermA	ermC	mphC	tetK	tetL	tetM	cat::pC221	cat::pC223	cat::pC194	dfrA	dfrB	dfrG
OX, CHL, TET, GEN, ERY, CL, TMP	10	0	10	10	10	–	10	10	10	10	10	10	10 (3)	–	10	10	10	10
OX, CHL, ERY, TMP	0	1	–	1	–	1	–	1 (1)	1	–	–	1	1 (1)	–	1	–	–	1
CHL, ERY, TMP	0	11	–	11	11	–	11 (3)	11	11	–	11	11	11 (3)	11	–	11	11	11
CHL, TMP	0	6	–	6	–	–	–	+	–	–	6	6	6 (2)	–	6	–	6	6
OX, CHL, TET, ERY, TMP	3	0	3	3	3	3	3 (1)	3	3	3	3	3	3 (1)	–	–	–	3	3
OX, CHL, GEN, ERY, TMP	11	0	11	11	11	11	11 (5)	11	11	–	11	11	11 (2)	11	11	–	11	11
OX, CHL, TET, GEN, ERY, TMP	5	0	5	5 (1)	5	5	–	5	5	5	5	5	5 (1)	5	–	5	5	5
ERY, CL, TMP	0	1	–	–	1	1	1	1	2 (1)	–	–	–	–	–	–	–	1	–
CHL, ERY, CL, TMP	0	2	–	2	2	–	–	2 (1)	2 (1)	–	–	2	2 (1)	2	–	2	2	2
CHL, ERY, **CL**	0	13	–	13	13	13	13 (9)	13	13 (1)	13	13	13	13 (3)	13	–	13	13	13
CHL	0	3	–	–	–	3	–	3	3	3	3	3	3	3	–	3	3	3
CHL, TET, GEN, ERY, **CL**, TMP	0	3	–	–	3	3	–	3	3	3	–	33	3	3	–	3	3	3
CHL, TET, GEN, ERY, TMP	0	1	–	1	1	–	–	1	1	1	–	–	1 (1)	–	–	–	–	–
CHL, GEN, ERY, CL, TMP	0	2	–	2 (1)	2	–	–	2 (2)	2 (2)	2	2	2	2	2	–	–	2	2
CHL, GEN, ERY, **CL**, TMP	0	7	–	7 (2)	7	7 (3)	–	–	–(3)	7	7	7	7	7	7	7	7	7
CHL, TET, GEN, ERY, CL, TMP	0	1	–	1 (1)	1	–	–	–	1 (1)	1	–	–	1	1 (1)	–	1	1	1
CHL, GEN, ERY	0	3	–	3	3	3 (1)	–	3 (1)	–	1	3	3	3	–	–	3	3	3
CHL, TET, GEN, ERY	0	3	–	3 (2)	3	3	–	3 (1)	–	3	3	3	3	–	–	3	3	3
GEN, ERY, CL, TMP	0	1	–	1 (1)	1	–	–	1	1	1	–	1	1	1	–	1	1	1
GEN, ERY	0	2	–	–	2 (1)	2	–	2 (1)	–	–	2	2	2	2	–	2	2	2
ERY	0	4	–	4	4	4	–	4 (2)	–	4	–	4	4	4	–	4	4	4
ERY, TMP	0	3	–	3	3	3	–	3 (3)	–	–	3	3	3	3	–	3	3	3
OX, CHL, GEN, **ERY**	1	0	1	–	1	–	–	–(1)	–	–	1	1	1	1	–	1	1	1
CHL, TET, **ERY**, TMP	0	2	–	2	2	–	–	2 (1)	–	2	2	2	2 (1)	2	–	2	2	2
CHL, ERY, CL	0	1	–	–	1	1	–	1 (1)	1	–	1	1	1	1	–	1	1	1
GEN, ERY, TMP, **CHL**	0	1	–	1	1	1	–	1	–	–	1	1	1 (1)	–	–	–	1	1
CHL, CL, TMP	0	2	–	2	2	2	–	2	2	–	2	2	2	2	–	–	2	2
TET, TMP	0	1	–	1	1	1	–	1	–	1	1	1	1	1	–	–	11	1
ERY, CL, **CHL**	0	1	–	1	1	1	–	1	1 (1)	1	1	1	1 (1)	–	–	1	1	1
TET, GEN, **CL**, ERY	0	2	–	–	2	2	–	2	–(1)	–	–	2	2	2	–	2	2	2
OX, CHL, ERY, **CL**, **CL**, TMP	1	0	1	1	1	1	–	1	–(1)	1	1	1	1	1	–	1	1	1
CHL, TET, GEN	0	1	–	1	1	–	–	–	–	–	1 (1)	1	1	–	–	–	1	1

MRSA: methicillin-resistant Staphylococcus aureus; MSSA: methicillin-susceptible Staphylococcus aureus; OX: oxacillin; GEN: gentamicin; ERY: erythromycin; TET: tetracycline; CL: clindamycin; CHL: chloramphenicol; TMP: trimethoprim. Isolates showing phenotypic resistance to given antibiotic(s) are shown in bold. Number in brackets indicate phenotypic sensitive isolates.

TABLE 2 | Result of D-test obtained with MRSA and MSSA isolates showing presence of erythromycin resistance genes and its correlation with MLSB phenotypes among *Staphylococcus aureus*.

Erythromycin resistance and MSB phenotypes	Phenotype (%)	Gene combinations									
		msrA	ermA	ermC	mphC	msrA, ermC	ermA, ermC	ermC, mphC	msrA, ermA, ermC	msrA, ermC, mphC	msrA, ermA, ermC, mphC
MRSA (n=32)											
ER-S, CL-S	10 (31.25%)	0	0	0	0	3 (30%)	0	1 (10%)	1 (10%)	3 (30%)	1 (10%)
ER-R, CL-S (MSB phenotype)	2 (6.25%)	0	0	0	0	1 (50%)	0	0	0	1 (50%)	0
ER-R, CL-R (cMLSB phenotype)	6 (18.75%)	0	0	1 (16.6 %)	0	0	3 (50%)	1 (16.6%)	0	1 (16.6%)	0
ER-R, CL-D (iMLSB phenotype)	10 (31.25%)	0	0	6 (60%)	0	0	1 (10%)	0	1 (10%)	1 (10%)	0
MSSA (n=77)											
ER-S, CL-S	52 (67.5%)	3 (5.7%)	1 (1.9%)	16 (30.7 %)	1 (1.9%)	20 (38.4%)	0	4 (7.6%)	0	4 (7.6%)	0
ER-R, CL-S (MSB phenotype)	12 (15.5%)	0	1 (8.3%)	1 (8.3%)	2 (16.6 %)	6 (50%)	0	0	0	0	0
ER-R, CL-R (cMLSB phenotype)	1 (1.29%)	0	0	0	0	0	0	0	1 (100%)	0	0
ER-R, CL-D (iMLSB phenotype)	4 (5.19%)	0	0	1 (25%)	0	3 (75%)	0	0	0	0	0

S: sensitive; R: resistance; ER: erythromycin; CL: clindamycin.

TABLE 3 | Distribution of SCCmec types among *S. aureus* strains isolated from wound and ocular infection.

			Distribution of SCCmec types among *S. aureus* strains isolated from wound and ocular infection			
SCCmec type	Recombinase complex	*mecA* complex	Source of infection			Total no. of isolates (*n* = 109)
			Wound (*n* = 34)	Ocular (*n* = 69)	Unknown (*n* = 6)	
III	ccrC1, ccrAB3	Class A	2	0	0	2 (1.8%)
IV	ccrAB2	Class B	7	0	0	7 (6.4%)
V	ccrC1	Class C2	5	4	4	13 (11.9%)
UT6	ccrC1	Class A	5	3	1	9 (8.2%)
Untypable-1	ccrC1	–	1	0	0	1 (0.91%)
Untypable-2	ccrAB4	–	0	1	0	1 (0.91%)
Untypable-3	ccrAB1	–	0	14	0	14 (12.8%)
Untypable-4	ccrAB2	–	0	1	0	1 (0.91%)
Untypable-5	ccrAB3	–	0	1	0	1 (0.91%)

of the two MRSA isolates showing MSB phenotype had *msrA*, *ermC* genes and other strain had *msrA*, *ermC*, and *mphC* genes (**Table 2**). Of the 12 MSSA, six isolates contained *msrA* and *ermC* genes, one isolate each contained *ermC* and *ermA* genes, respectively, two strains had *mphC* gene. The remaining isolates did not carry any of the genes tested. Of the 10 MRSA, six isolates with iMLSB phenotype had *ermC* gene. One isolate each carried *msrA*, *ermA*, and *ermC* genes, *ermA*, *ermC* genes, *msrA*, *ermC*, and *mphC* genes, respectively. The remaining one isolate did not possess any of the resistance genes. Of the four MSSA isolates that showed iMLSB phenotype, three strains were positive for *msrA*, *ermC* genes, and one isolate was positive for *ermC* gene (**Table 2**).

Of the 109 *S. aureus* isolates tested for the presence of MLSB resistance genes, 102 isolates carried one or more *erm* genes. Three strains carried all the erythromycin resistance genes, namely, *msrA*, *ermA*, and *ermC*. Fifty-one isolates were positive for two genes, of which 46 isolates carried *msrA* and *ermC* genes, and five had *ermA* and *ermC* genes. Besides, 37 isolates were positive for a single gene of which 34 isolates carried the *ermC* gene, two isolates had *ermA* gene, and three isolates had the *msrA* gene (**Table 2**). In contrast, four of the 13 erythromycin-sensitive isolates carried *msrA* and *ermC* genes. One strain each had the *ermC* gene and *msrA* gene. The remaining isolates did not carry any resistance genes. Twelve of the 21 *mphC* gene-positive isolates showed phenotypic resistant to clindamycin. The remaining nine isolates were sensitive to clindamycin (**Table 2**). Eight erythromycin-resistant strains did not carry any of the erythromycin-resistant genes is likely to be mediated by an as-yet-unknown mechanism.

SCCmec Typing

The presence of the *mec* complex and *ccr* complex classified *S. aureus* strains into different SCCmec types. Thirty-one MRSA isolates showed four known SCCmec types of which 13 (40.6%) belong to type V, nine (28.1) belong to type UT6, seven (21.9%) belong to type IV, and two (6.3%) belong to type III (**Table 3**). One isolate showing phenotypic resistance to methicillin but negative for *mecA* gene carried C1 type of *ccr* complex but lack *mec* complex. Of the 32 methicillin-sensitive isolates lacking the *mec* complex, 14 isolates carried *ccrA1B1*, one strain possesses

ccrA4B4, and 17 isolates had *ccrA3B3* and *ccrA4B4* type of *ccr* complex, respectively (**Table 3**).

Toxin Gene Profiles

Of the 109 isolates, 34 (31.2%) isolates harbored *sea* gene, 14 (12.8%) isolates *sec* gene, 93 (85.3%) isolates *sei* gene, 76 (69.7%) *cna* gene, 101 (92.6%) isolates *hla* gene, 107 (98%) isolates *hlg* gene, and 84 (77%) isolates carried *efb* gene, respectively. All the isolates, except one isolate, was positive for the *hlg*, and carried multiple virulence genes (**Table 4**).

Ninety-one isolates comprising 26 MRSA and 65 MSSA were positive for both *icaA* and *icaD* genes, but five strains containing three MRSA and two MSSA were negative for both *icaA* and *icaD* genes. Two of the three MRSA isolates were positive for *icaA* gene, and another strain was positive for *icaD* gene. Similarly, nine of the 10 MSSA isolates were positive for *icaD* gene and one isolate for *icaA* gene, respectively (**Table 4**).

Also, a total of 25 toxin genes combinations was obtained with 109 strains belonging to 77 PFGE patterns, 32 sequence types (STs), 46 *spa*-types, and five *agr*-types. Twenty-three isolates belonging to five MRSA and 18 MSSA showed a toxin pattern comprising *sei-cna-hla-hlg-efb* genes. On the other hand, five MRSA and two MSSA showed another virulence pattern composed of *sea-sec-sei-cna-hla-hlg-efb* genes. The remaining isolates showed 23 different virulence gene patterns (**Table 4**).

Agr-Typing

Of 109 *S. aureus* strains, 40 (36.7%) isolates belong to *agr*-I, 31 (28.4%) isolates to *agr*-III, 18 (16.5%) to *agr*-II, and seven (6.4%) belong to *agr*-IV; however, 13 (11.9%) isolates were not typeable by the method employed (**Table 4**). Of the 32 MRSA isolates, 20 (62.5%) belong to *agr*-I, five (15.6%) to *agr*-II, three (9.4%) to *agr*-III, and remaining isolates were untypeable. On the other hand, 28 of 77 (36.4%) MSSA isolates belong to *agr*-III, 20 (25.9%) to *agr*-I, 13 (16.9%) to *agr*-II, seven (9%) to *agr*-IV, and nine (11.7%) isolates were untypeable. There was a good correlation between virulence patterns and specific molecular types (**Table 4**). The *sea-sei-cna-hla-hlg-efb* was the dominant virulence pattern shown by MRSA belonged to SCCmec type UT6, and *agr* type I, followed by *sei-hla-hlg-efb* and *sei-cna-hla-hlg-efb* pattern showed

TABLE 4 | Source, clonal complex, sequence-, *spa*-, SSC*mec*-, and *agr*-types and virulence profiles of *S. aureus* isolated from different parts of India.

Source (isolate number)	CC/ST, *spa*-type	SCC*mec* type	*agr* type	*pvl* gene	*icaA/icaD*	Serotypes	Virulence pattern
MRSA (*n* = 32)							
Wound infection (2095)	239/239, t037	III	1	–	+/+	II	*sei-cna-hla-hlg-efb*
Wound infection (2103)					+/+	IV	*sea-sei-cna-hla-hlg-efb*
Wound infection (2656)	239/239,t037	UT6	1	–	+/+	IV	*sea-sei-cna-hla-hlg-efb*
Wound infection (22/248)					+/+	III	*sea-cna-hla*
Wound infection (UC650)					+/+	IV	*sea-cna-hla-hlg-efb*
Wound infection (UC858)					–/–	V	*sea-hla-hlg-efb*
Wound infection (UC1079)	239/239,t2952	UT6	1	–	+/+	I	*sea-sei-cna-hla-hlg-efb*
Wound infection (2658)	239/241,t037	UT6	1	–	+/+	IV	*sei-cna-hlg-efb*
Eye infection (P844628, N307002)	239/239, t037	UT6	1	–	+/+ ±	IV	*sei-cna-hla-hlg*
Eye infection (P853836)	239/239, t037	UT6	1	–	±	V	*sea-cna-hla-hlg-efb*
Wound infection (2380,2452)	772/772, t657	V	None	+	+/+ +/+	VI	*sea-sec-sei-cna-hla-hlg-efb*
Wound infection (UC609)	772/772, t657	V	2	+	+/+	VI	*sea-sec-sei-cna-hla-hlg-efb*
Wound infection (22/252)	772/Unk, t657	V	None	+	–/–	VI	*sea-sec-sei-cna-hla-hlg-efb*
Eye infection (845)	772/772, t345	V	3	+	–/+	I	*sea-sec-sei-cna-hla-hlg-efb*
Eye infection (1295)	2884/88, t2526	V	2	+	+/+	III	*sei-hla-hlg-efb*
Eye infection (1690)	5/5, t442	V	1	–	+/+	IV	*sei-hla-hlg-efb*
Eye infection (1820)	772/772, t657	V	1	+	+/+	VII	*sea-sec-sei-cna-hla-hlg-efb*
Unknown (1189)	772/772, t657	V	2	+	+/+	VI	*sec-sei-cna-hla-hlg-efb*
Unknown (1192,1249)	772/772, t345	V	2	+	+/+ +/+	VII VI	*sea-sei-cna-hla-hlg-efb* / *sec-sei-cna-hla-hlg-efb*
Unknown (2654)	772/772, t345	V	1	+	+/+	VI	*sea-sei-cna-hla-hlg-efb*
Wound infection (284)	Singleton 4/2642, t064	V	1	–	+/+	IV	*hla-hlg-efb*
Wound infection (221)	30/30, t012	IV	3	+	+/+	VI	*sei-cna-hla-hlg-efb*
Wound infection (27/231)	30/503, t012	IV	3	+	+/+	VII	*sei-cna-hla-hlg*
Wound infection (296)	22/22, t005	IV	1	+	+/+	I	*sec-sei-cna-hla-hlg*
Wound infection (293)	22/1414, t1328	IV	1	+	+/+	I	*sei-cna-hla-hlg*
Wound infection (UC104)	22/22, Unk	IV	1	+	+/+	II	*sei-cna-hla-hlg-efb*
Wound infection (UC101)	22/22, t091				+/+		
Wound infection (UC463)	22/22, t309	IV	1	+	–/–	III	*sec-sei-cna-hla-hlg-efb*
Wound infection (2518)*	121/120, t272		NT	+	+/+	VI	*sea-sei-cna-hla-hlg-efb*
MSSA (*n* = 77)							
Wound infection (2130)	772/772, t345		2	+	+/+	VI	*sec-cna-hla-hlg-efb*
Wound infection (2164)	772/772, t1839	UT*	None	+	+/+	VI	*sea-sec-sei-cna-hla-hlg-efb*
Wound infection (2493)	772/1, t386		4	+	+/+	VI	*sei-cna-hla-hlg-efb*
Eye infection (N309852)	772/1, t098		3	–	+/+	VII	*sea-cna-hla-hlg*
Eye infection (518)	772/1, t693	UT*	3	–	+/+	VII	*sea-sei-cna-hla-hlg-efb*
Eye infection (535,1636)	772/1, t127	UT*	3	–	+/+ +/+	VII V	*sea-sei-cna-hlg-efb*
Eye infection (831)	772/1, t127	UT*	3	–	+/+	II	*sea-sei-cna-hla-hlg-efb*
Eye infection (1361)	772/1, t128	UT*	3	–	+/+	VII	*sea-sec-sei-hla-hlg-efb*
Eye infection (1321)	772/1, t177	UT*	3	–	+/+	VII	*sea-sei-cna-hla-hlg-efb*
Eye infection (1476)	772/1, t127		3	–	+/+	VIII	*sea-sei-cna-hla-hlg-efb*
Eye infection (1881)					+/+	I	
Eye infection (1503)	772/1, t127		3	–	+/+	VI	*sei-cna-hla-hlg-efb*
Eye infection (975)	772/1, t8078		3	–	+/+	VI	*sei-hla-hlg-efb*
Eye infection (1214)	772/772, t657		3	+	+/+	VI	*sea-sec-sei-cna-hla-hlg*
Healthy conjunctiva (N11OD)	772/1, t948	UT*	None	–	+/+	I	*sea-sei-cna-hla-hlg-efb*
Healthy conjunctiva (N12OD)	772/1, t948		3	–	+/+	IV	*sea-cna-hla-hlg-efb*
Wound infection (2151)	30/714, t021		3	+	+/+	VI	*sei-cna-hla-hlg-efb*
Wound infection (2413)	30/1482, t386		3	+	+/+	IV	*sei-cna-hla-hlg-efb*

(Continued)

TABLE 4 | Continued

Source (isolate number)	CC/ST, *spa*-type	*SCCmec* type	*agr* type	*pvl* gene	*icaA/icaD*	Serotypes	Virulence pattern
Eye infection (1196)	30/938, t021		3	+	+/+	IV	*sei-cna-hla-hlg-efb*
Eye infection (1850)					+/+	V	
Wound infection (2488)	121/121, t159		4	−	+/+	II	*sei-cna-hla-hlg-efb*
Eye infection (P832812)	121/121, t3204		4	+	+/+	V	*cna-hla-hlg*
Eye infection (P706434)	121/1964, t272		4	−	+/+	V	*sei-cna-hla-hlg*
Eye infection (917)	121/2160, t159		4	+	+/+	V	*cna-hla-hlg-efb*
Unknown (2657)	2884/2884, t4104		3	+	+/+	III	*hla-hlg-efb*
Eye infection (149)	2884/88, t5562		3	+	−/+	VI	*sei-hla-hlg-efb*
Eye infection (1764Y)	2884/88, t448		3	+	+/+	VIII	*sea-sei-hla-hlg-efb*
Eye infection (504, 1035, 1271)	5/5, t442		2	−	+/+	II	*sei-cna-hla-hlg-efb*
					+/+		*sei-hla-hlg-efb*
					+/+		*sei-hlg*
Eye infection (N303284)			None	−	+/+	I	*sei-cna-hla-hlg*
Eye infection (843)			2	−	+/+	VIII	*sei-hlg-efb*
Eye infection (1042)			2	−	+/+	VII	*sei-hla-hlg-efb*
Eye infection (1766, 1862)			1	−	+/+	VIII	*sei-hla-hlg*
					+/+		*sei-hla-hlg-efb*
Eye infection (1867)			1	−	+/+	VII	*sei-hla-hlg-efb*
Eye infection (1103)	5/5, t14912		2	−	+/+	V	*sei-hla-hlg-efb*
Eye infection (1306)	5/83, t442		2	−	+/+	II	*sei-hla-hlg-efb*
Eye infection (1424)	5/5, 8179		2	−	−/+	VI	*sei-hla-hlg-efb*
Healthy conjunctiva (N9OD)	5/5, t010		2	−	+/+	VII	*sei-hla-hlg-efb*
Wound infection (17/201)	813/813, t10579		1	−	+/+	VII	*sei-cna-hla-hlg*
Wound infection (262)	813/291, t1149		1	−	+/+	VII	*hlg*
Eye infection (186)	22/22, t310		1	+	+/+	II	*sei-cna-hla-hlg-efb*
Healthy conjunctiva (N61OD)	22/22, t948	UT*	1	+	+/+	VII	*sea-sei-hla-hlg-efb*
Eye infection (481)	Singleton 1/580, t14911		None	−	−/+	V	*sei-cna-hla-hlg-efb*
Eye infection (N297214)	Singleton 2/45, t302		1	−	+/+	VII	*cna-hla-hlg*
Wound infection (2417)	Singleton 3/Unk, t021		None	−	−/−	VI	*sei-hla-hlg-efb*
Eye infection (1525,1545)	Singleton 5/72, t148		1	−	−/+	VI	*sei-hla-hlg*
			None	−	−/+	V	*sei-cna-hla-hlg-efb*
Wound infection (1/229, 861)	Singleton 6/789, t091		1	−	−/−	III	*sei-cna-hla-hlg*
			None	−	+/+	III	*sei-cna-hla-hlg-efb*
Wound infection (379)	Singleton 6/789, t2505		None	−	+/+	III	*sei-cna-hla-hlg-efb*
Eye infection (1603)	Singleton 6/789, t091		1	−	+/+	V	*sei-hla-hlg-efb*
Eye infection (1320)	Singleton 7/6, t657		1	−	+/+	III	*sei-cna-hla-hlg-efb*
Eye infection (1428)	Singleton 7/6, t4285		1	−	−/+	VIII	*sea-sei-cna-hla-hlg-efb*
Eye infection (1698)	Singleton 7/6, t12406		1	−	+/+	VIII	*sea-sei-cna-hla-hlg-efb*
Healthy conjunctiva (N21OS)	Singleton 8/15, t084		2	−	+/+	IV	*sei-hla-efb*
Wound infection (2508)	Singleton 9/2885, t15579		4	+	+/+	III	*sei-cna-hla-hlg-efb*
Wound infection (2653)	Singleton 10/672, t3841		2	−	±	I	*sei-hla-hlg-efb*
Eye infection (N259615, N289378, 1049, 1506)	Singleton 10/672, t3841		1	−	+/+	I	*sei-cna-hla-hlg*
			None	−	+/+	I	*cna-hla-hlg*
			1	−	+/+	VII	*sei-hla-hlg-efb*
			1	−	+/+	VIII	*sei-hla-hlg-efb*
Eye infection (188, 1164, 1355, 1670)	Singleton 10/672, t1309		I	−	+/+	I	*sei-hla-hlg-efb*
			I	−	−/+	II	*sei-hla-hlg-efb*
			I	−	+/+	I	*sei-cna-hla-hlg-efb*
			1	−	+/+	VIII	*sei-cna-hla-hlg*
Eye infection (884,1333)	Singleton 11/2233, t2663		3	+	+/+	VII	*sei-cna-hlg-efb*
					+/+		
Eye infection (1716OD, 1758)			3	+	+/+	IV	*sei-cna-hla-hlg*
					+/+		

(Continued)

TABLE 4 | Continued

Source (isolate number)	CC/ST, spa-type	SCCmec type	agr type	pvl gene	icaA/icaD	Serotypes	Virulence pattern
Eye infection (1716OS, 1769)			3	+	−/+	VIII	sei-cna-hla-hlg
			4		+/+		
Eye infection (915, 1366, 1729)			3	+	+/+	VII	sei-cna-hla-hlg-efb
		UT*	3	+	−/+	VII	sei-hla-hlg
			3	−	+/+	VIII	sea-sei-cna-hla-hlg-efb

MRSA: methicillin-resistant Staphylococcus aureus; MSSA: methicillin-sensitive Staphylococcus aureus; CC: clonal complex; ST: sequence type; SSC: Staphylococcal cassette chromosome; agr: accessory gene regulator; Unk: unknown; UT: untypeable; NT: non-typeable; *Isolates with ccrAIB1 complex but lack mec complex; pvl: Panton-valentine leucocidin; icaA: intracellular adhesion gene A; icaD: intracellular adhesion gene D; sea: staphylococcal enterotoxin A; sec: staphylococcal enterotoxin C; sei: staphylococcal enterotoxin I; cna: collagen adhesion; hlyA: hemolysin A; hlyG: hemolysin G; efb: extracellular fibronectin binding protein.

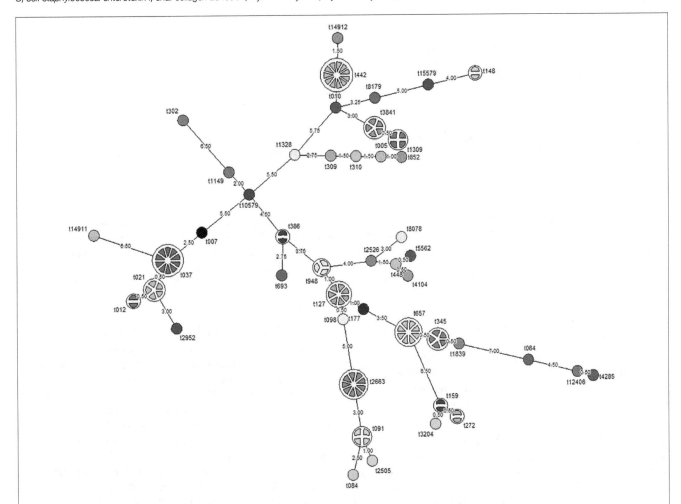

FIGURE 1 | Minimum spanning tree (MST) showing 109 S. aureus isolates typed by spa-typing. Each node represents one spa-type, and the corresponding spa-type is given beside the node. The number of disks in a node indicates the number of isolates having a particular spa-type. The number provided on the string depicts the phylogenetic distance between two nodes. Length ≤ 1 is represented by dotted lines and more than one by solid lines.

by MSSA isolates belonged to agr type I and III, respectively (**Supplementary Table S1**).

Spa-Typing

Analysis of the aligned sequence of the polymorphic X region of spa gene using the spa-typing plug-in tool of Bionumerics 7 software showed 46 spa-types (**Figure 1**). MST analysis classified the strains into six major clusters, seven minor clusters, and

30 singletons. We designated cluster as a minor cluster that contained less than five but more than two strains. Of the 109 S. aureus isolates, 11 (10%) isolates belong to spa-type t442, 10 (9%) to t037, nine (8.2%) to t2663, eight (7.3%) to t657, six (5.5%) to t127, five (4.5%) isolates each to t345 and t3841, and four isolates each belong to t021, t091, and t1309. In addition, four (3.6%) isolates belong to t1309, three (2.7%) isolates belong to t948, and two (1.8%) each belong to t148, t386, t012, t159, and

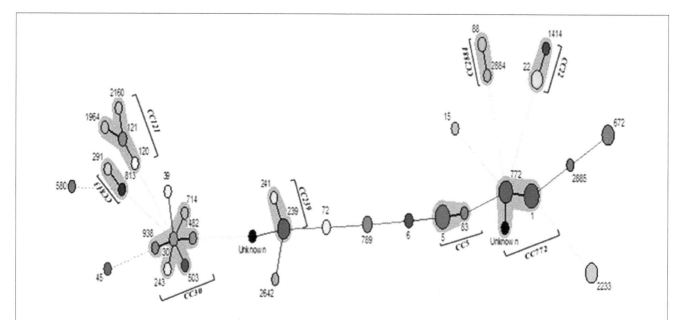

FIGURE 2 | Minimum spanning tree (MST) showing the relationship between different STs assigned by the analysis of MLST data. Each node represents one sequence type, and the corresponding ST is given beside the node. The size of each node is directly proportional to the number of isolates included in that ST. Bold lines connect types that are identical for six loci, solid lines connecting types identical for ≥four but ≤six locus, and dotted lines connecting STs differing from each other by ≥four genes out of seven gene locus.

t272, respectively. Moreover, one isolate each of 30 strains belong to single *spa*-types, namely, t15579, t8179, t14912, t010, t852, t005, t310, t309, t1328, t302, t1149, t10579, t007, t14911, t2952, t693, t2526, t8078, t5562, t448, t4104, t177, t098, t084, t2505, t3204, t1839, t064, t12406, and t4285 (**Figure 1**). Whereas 10 of 32 (31.2%) MRSA isolates belong to t037, 11 of 77 (14.3%) MSSA isolates belong to t442. *S. aureus* strain ATCC 25923 showed *spa*-type t948 along with three test isolates. We found two novel *spa*-types, namely, t14911 and t14912 among *S. aureus* strains after submission of nucleotide sequences to the Ridom *spa* server. *Spa*-type t14912 showed a close association with major *spa*-type t442, but 14911 *spa*-type was diverse and unrelated. One of the isolates was not assigned any *spa*-type (**Figure 1**).

Multi-Locus Sequence Typing (MLST)

Multi-locus sequence typing of 109 *S. aureus* isolates showed 32 STs, eight CCs, and 12 singletons (**Figure 2**). The major ST comprised of ST1 (12.8%), ST5 (11.9%), ST772 (11%) followed by ST239 (9.2%), ST672 (8.3%), and ST2233 (8.3%). Also, we found two new allelic profiles designated as unknown not reported earlier among *S. aureus* strains (**Supplementary Table S2**). Of the eight CCs, CC5 contained 14 isolates, CC22 had eight isolates, CC30 had six isolates, CC121 contained five isolates, CC239 had 11 isolates, CC772 had 26 isolates, CC813 had two isolates, and CC2884 contained four isolates, respectively. Of the major CCs, CC30 contained five STs, namely, ST30, ST503, ST714, ST938, and ST1482, CC121 contained four STs, namely, ST120, ST121, ST1964, ST2160, and CC772 had three STs, namely, ST772, ST1, and new unknown ST (**Figure 2**). Seven of the 32 (21.8%) of MRSA strains belong to ST239, *spa*-type t037, and SCC*mec* type UT6. However, 14 (18.2%) of MSSA strains possessing ST1

belong to different *spa*-types, namely, t127, t948, t177, t693, t098, and t386, of which few strains carry *ccr* complex but devoid of *mec* complex (**Table 4**). However, few isolates from eye infection and wound infection belong to CC239, ST239, and *spa*-type t037/t657. Reference strain of *S. aureus* ATCC25923 belonged to ST30 and CC30.

Pulsed-Field Gel Electrophoresis

*Sma*I-digested genomic DNA of *S. aureus* yielded bands classifying the 109 strains into 77 pulsotypes that includes two identical pairs (12 and 19A), three major clusters (1, 3, and 19), 17 minor clusters (14, 15, 17, 19, 20, 22, 24, 25, 28, 32, 57, 58, 63, 67, 69, 71, and 73), and 56 singletons. Four isolates were untypeable by the method employed. We found a total of 24 PFGE patterns among 32 MRSA isolates, of which one isolate was untypeable. Similarly, 77 MSSA isolates showed 53 PFGE patterns, of which three MSSA isolates were untypeable (**Figure 3**). MSSA isolates belonging to the major pulsotype 19 contained seven subtypes 19A, 19B, 19C, 19D, 19E, 19F, and 19G. These isolates were mostly from ocular infection and belong to ST1, *agr* type III, except one subtype 19G which belongs to ST6 and *agr* type I. *S. aureus* strain ATCC 25923 showed pulsotype 14. A dendrogram was generated using Bionumerics 7 software and percentage similarity with a cut-off of 80% and dice coefficients.

Statistical Analysis

Principal coordinates analysis segregates MRSA and MSSA isolates, except for few isolates with 25.75% of explained variance for antibiotic resistance genes (**Figure 4A**) and 26% for virulence genes (**Figure 5A**). We used axis one for the highest percentage of representation. DA graph showed that MRSA isolates grouped within more positive values, whereas MSSA isolates grouped within negative values for both antibiotic resistance genes and virulence genes (**Figures 4B, 5B**). Predominant biomarkers were determined by calculating the coefficient of discriminant function and considered when the value was equal to 0.5 or >0.5. For antibiotic resistance genes, MRSA isolates are discriminating in the biomarker of resistance to *ermA* (0.8407), *mphC* (2.0167), *tetK* (2.3495), *tetL* (2.0604), and *dfrA* (1.3116), whereas the MSSA isolates were discriminating in resistance to *aac(6')/aph(2)* (−0.351), *aph3* (−2.7179), *ermC* (−0.8473), *tetM* (−0.522), *cat:pC221* (−2.421), *cat:pC223* (−6.601), *dfrB* (−0.443), and *dfrG* (−0.603). For virulence genes, MRSA isolates are discriminating in the biomarker of resistance to *icaA* (0.67169), *seA* (0.68593), *seC* (2.3245), *cnA* (0.90744), and *hlA* (0.54797). On the other hand, MSSA isolates were discriminating in resistance to *icaD* (−2.1945), *seI* (−0.58795), and *hlG* (−1.4999). PCoA and discriminant function of antibiotic resistance and virulence genes of *S. aureus* isolates with source and place of isolation was heterologous and complex (data not shown).

DISCUSSION

We used hexaplex PCR for detection of MRSA and MSSA isolates along with the presence of *mecA*, *pvl*, *czrC*, and *qacA/B* genes. We found a good correlation between oxacillin resistance and the presence of the *mecA* gene. However, one isolate showing resistance to oxacillin and lack *mecA* gene indicate the occurrence of different mechanism of methicillin resistance. Twenty of 31 MRSA and 23 of 77 MSSA isolates were positive for *pvl* gene indicating the prevalence of *pvl* gene among MRSA strains from the wound and eye infections. This finding is in contrast to those who did not find such correlation among clinical isolates (Shittu et al., 2011); therefore, it cannot be used as a reliable marker for MRSA. The presence of *czrC* and *qacA/B* genes among the number of MRSA isolates indicates their possible association with the *mecA* gene; however, further investigation is required to authenticate these findings.

Coagulase gene typing has been used to characterize *S. aureus* strains. Hwang and Kim (2007) showed the presence of coagulase

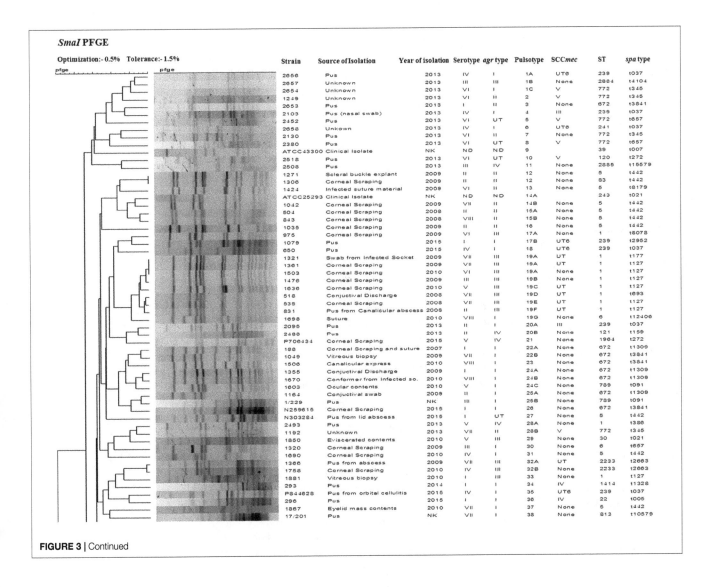

FIGURE 3 | Continued

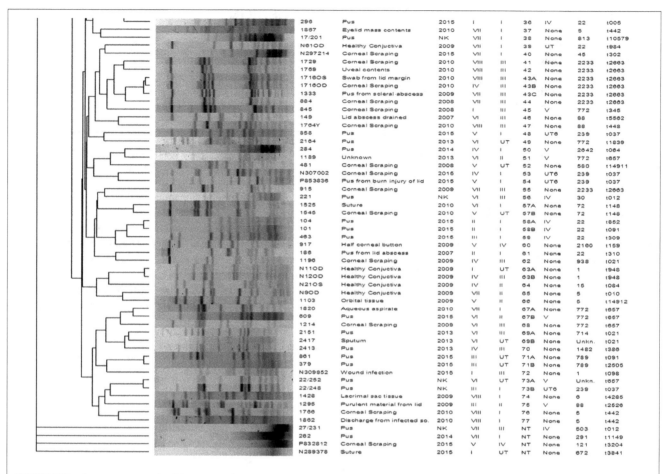

FIGURE 3 | Dendrogram representation (Dice coefficient) for macro-restriction banding patterns of *S. aureus* strains isolated from different sources with ATCC reference strains, generated by pulsed-field gel electrophoresis of total chromosomal DNA digested with *Sma*I restriction enzyme and correlation between their pulsotype, ST, *spa*-type, SCC*mec* type, and *agr* type with information regarding their source and year of isolation.

serotype II among 54.4% MRSA and serotype VII among 30.9% MSSA. In contrast, we found serotype VII was present among 22% of MSSA isolates and serotype VI in 28.1% of MRSA isolates. These observations thus suggest that there is a difference in the presence of serotypes with regard to MRSA and MSSA.

Genetic determinants study among *S. aureus* showed a good correlation between resistance to aminoglycosides, chloramphenicol, clindamycin, erythromycin, trimethoprim, and tetracycline, and the presence of corresponding resistance genes. In this study, we found 85.3% strains showing resistance to chloramphenicol carried the *pC221* gene; however, some of these strains also carried either *pC223* or *pC194* or both genes. Although one of 109 strains sensitive to chloramphenicol did not carry any of these genes, 13.8% strains showing sensitivity to chloramphenicol carried either *pC221* or *pC223* genes. These observations thus suggest that chloramphenicol sensitive strains carrying antibiotic resistance genes can develop resistance against this drug on exposure.

The aminoglycoside-modifying enzyme, encoded by *aac (6')-aph(2")* gene, is responsible for resistance against aminoglycosides (Vanhoof et al., 1994). Besides, two other genes encoding for *aph(3.III)* and *ant(4, IV)* are accountable for

aminoglycoside resistance, but their frequency is less compared to *aac(6')-aph(2")* among staphylococci (Busch-SØRensen et al., 1996). In this study, we found 41.3% *S. aureus* possesses both *aac(6')-aph(2")* and *aph (3, III)* genes and 8.3% contained *aph (3, III)* gene and showed phenotypic resistance to gentamycin. These findings thus suggest that there are strains which harbor aminoglycoside resistance genes other than *aac(6')-aph(2")* and few strains had *aph (3, III)* only. At least 47.7% strains of *S. aureus* that were sensitive to aminoglycosides contain either *aph (3, III)* or aac(6')-aph(2") or both; however, three strains susceptible to gentamycin lack resistance genes. These findings are in contrast to those workers who reported that all aminoglycoside-resistant strains carried *aac(6')-aph(2")* (Price et al., 1981; Lovering et al., 1988; Dornbusch et al., 1990; Vanhoof et al., 1994; Martineau et al., 2000). The presence of aminoglycoside resistance gene among gentamycin sensitive isolates of *S. aureus* indicates that there is likely hood development of aminoglycoside resistance among *S. aureus* upon exposure to these drugs.

Similarly, 83.4% strains of *S. aureus* resistant to erythromycin harbored any of the four genes, namely, *ermA*, *ermB*, *ermC*, and *msrA*; however, an strain sensitive to erythromycin did not

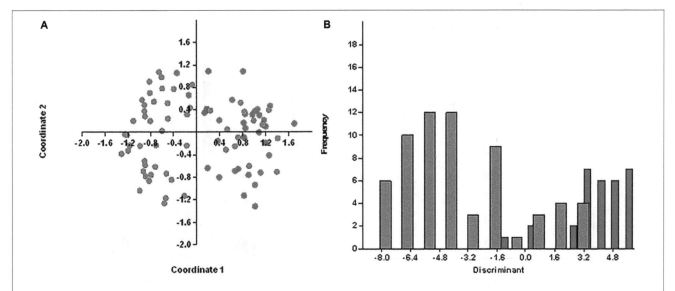

FIGURE 4 | Results obtained by statistical analysis using antibiotic resistance genes. **(A)** Principle component analysis (PCoA) of methicillin-resistant *S. aureus* (MRSA, red) and methicillin-susceptible *S. aureus* (MSSA, green). **(B)** Discriminant analysis of MRSA (red) and MSSA (green). Negative values belong to MSSA isolates and positive values to MRSA isolates.

carry any of the genes. Previously, it was reported that the *ermA* gene is dominant among erythromycin resistance genes in *S. aureus* (Kaur and Chate, 2015). In contrast, we found the presence of the *ermC* gene in 83.4% strains compared to 49% of *ermA* gene. Kaur and Chate (2015) reported that majority of MRSA strains showed constitutive MLSB (cMLSB) resistance; however, two isolates had inducible MLSB (iMLSB) phenotype. In this study, 64.5% MRSA and 37.1% MSSA strains belong to iMLSB phenotype; however, 35.4% of MRSA and 43.5% of MSSA strains belong to cMLSB phenotype. This difference could be due to less number of MRSA isolates used in the study, and MSSA isolates were multidrug resistant. Seventeen strains showing sensitivity to erythromycin harbored one of the resistance genes, and one of the strains resistant to erythromycin did not possess any of the resistance genes to indicate that these strains are likely to develop resistance and mediated by an unknown mechanism.

About trimethoprim resistance, 67.8% strains harbored any of the three genes, namely, *dfrA*, *dfrB*, and *dfrG*. The remaining strains showing sensitivity to trimethoprim also carried all or one of the three genes. In this study, 73 of 74 trimethoprim resistance strains possess *dfrG* and *dfrB* genes; 45 strains carried the *dfrA* gene. These findings are in contrast to those who reported the presence of the *dfrG* gene in 92% strains, *dfrA* in 7% strains, and one strain carried a *dfrB* among trimethoprim resistance strains in a travel-associated skin and soft tissue infection study in Europe (Nurjadi et al., 2015).

Like other antibiotic resistance, 26.6% phenotypic resistance strains carried one or all the three tetracycline resistance genes, namely, *tetK*, *tetL*, and *tetM*. One of the strains sensitive to tetracycline was devoid of carrying any genes. However, the majority (69.7%) strain showing sensitivity to tetracycline carried one or all three resistance genes indicating that these isolates could develop resistance after exposure to an antibiotic. From

this study, it is clear that erythromycin and gentamicin were least active; however, vancomycin and clindamycin were the most effective drugs. These results corroborate the finding of Pai et al. (2010), who also reported that vancomycin and clindamycin are the most effective drugs.

SCC*mec* type V was predominant type among MRSA strains followed by SCC*mec* type UT6, IV, and III, respectively. This finding is similar to Nadig et al. (2012), who also reported the prevalence of SCC*mec* type V among isolates from eye infections. To our knowledge, we are the first to inform of the presence of SCC*mec* type UT6 among *S. aureus* from India. The combination of SCC*mec* IV, V, and *pvl* gene was reported as the genetic markers for a community-associated MRSA (Bhutia et al., 2015). Similarly, our study showed the presence of SCC*mec* V (40.6%), IV (21.9%), and *pvl* (64.5%); therefore it can be used as a marker for hospital-associated infections. However, new UT6 SCC*mec* type is emerging in India. Many untypeable strains carried *ccr* complex but no *mec* complex. This observation thus suggests the ability of such strains to acquire *mec* complex and became a known or unknown SCC*mec* type.

A total of 25 unique toxin combination was found among *S. aureus* strains, of which at least one toxin gene was present in a given strain. Sotto et al. (2008) reported the presence of *sei* and *sea* genes in *S. aureus* isolated from diabetic foot ulcer. Similarly, we found the presence of *sei* and *sea* genes in both MRSA and MSSA strains. Although we noted the high percentage of *hlg* (98%) and *hla* (92.6%) among in *S. aureus* comprising both MSSA and MRSA, other workers reported the presence of these genes in mupirocin resistant in MRSA isolates in China (Liu et al., 2012). Moreover, the distribution of virulence genes with regards to source and place of isolation was complex. Gowrishankar et al. (2016) reported the isolation of 84% MRSA strains carrying *icaADBC* genes from patients with pharyngitis. Also, in this

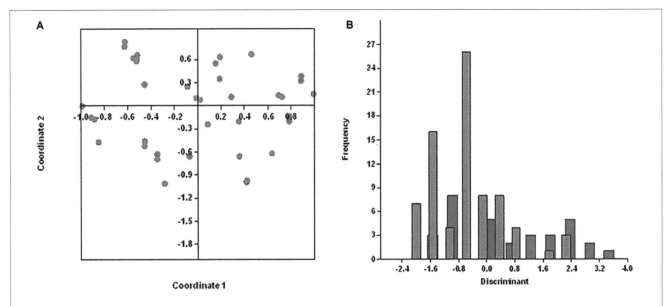

FIGURE 5 | Results obtained by statistical analysis using virulence genes. **(A)** Principle component analysis (PCoA) of methicillin-resistant *S. aureus* (MRSA, red) and methicillin-susceptible *S. aureus* (MSSA, green). **(B)** Discriminant analysis of MRSA (red) and MSSA (green). Negative values belong to MSSA isolates and positive values to MRSA isolates.

study, 81.3% MRSA and 84.4% MSSA carrying *icaA/icaD* genes were isolated from the eye and wound infections (**Supplementary Table S3**). Absence of *icaA/icaD* genes in *S. aureus* strains was similar to those of the previous report (Agarwal and Jain, 2013).

Several molecular genotyping tools are used to trace the origin of the strain, and distribution of CC with regard to methicillin-resistant, methicillin-sensitive, sources and place of isolation. We determined the population structure of *S. aureus* isolated from ocular and wound infections from different parts of India using MLST, *agr*-typing, *spa*-typing, and PFGE.

Multi-locus sequence typing analysis showed the presence of six major ST(s) comprising ST1, ST5, ST772, ST239, ST672, and ST2233, respectively. While ST239-MRSA-UT6 was the typical type among MRSA isolates from wound infection, ST772-MRSA-V were from eye infections (Nadig et al., 2012). Similarly, ST772-SCCmec-V were reported slowly replacing multidrug resistant ST239-SCCmec-III in Asian studies (D'Souza et al., 2010). This finding is in contrast to Suzuki et al. (2012), who reported the presence of ST5 and ST764 among MRSA strains from the infected eye and healthy conjunctiva sacs. Also, Mohammadi et al. (2014) showed emergence of SCCmec-III with variable antimicrobial resistance profiles in Iran. We found ST772-MRSA-V with *spa*-type t345 and t657 belonging to dominant CC772 among wound infection isolates. Besides, we reported two new *spa*-types among *S. aureus* strains from India.

There were eight CCs, namely, CC30, CC121, CC772, CC813, CC239, CC28841, CC22, and CC5 present among *S. aureus* represents different PFGE clusters. CC30 and CC121 comprising different STs were almost equally distributed among MRSA and MSSA isolates. Whereas CC772-ST772 was dominant among MRSA, CC772-ST1 was prevalent among MSSA isolates. Similarly, CC239-ST239 and CC22-ST22 were prevalent among

MRSA isolates and CC5-ST5, CC813-ST813, and CC28841-ST28841 were more commonly found in MSSA isolates. The prevalent CC among Varanasi isolates (mostly wound infection) were CC772 followed by CC239 besides the presence of CC30, and CC121. However, isolates from wound infection from Delhi showed varied results. Whereas AIIMS isolates showed CC CC30, CC22, and CC813, UCMS isolates showed the presence of CC239 and CC22 CCs. Interestingly isolates from Hyderabad (eye infection) had CC239 but isolates from Bhubaneswar (eye infection) showed the presence of CC772, CC5, CC2884, and CC30.

Mobasherizadeh et al. (2019) reported the prevalence of CC5 and CC30 and other CCs among MRSA isolates isolated from nasal carriage in Iranian hospitals. Similarly, CC8, CC121, CC1, CC45, and CC5 were reported in MRSA isolates from Malaysia (Ghasemzadeh-Moghaddam et al., 2011). These observations indicate the existence of different CCs in India and Asian countries. MLST and *spa*-typing was better than PFGE and toxin genotyping a finding unusual from those who reported a good correlation between various typing schemes. Overall, there was diversity in genotypes, antimicrobial resistance, and virulence determinants among MRSA and MSSA strains.

From this study, it is clear that *S. aureus* strains sensitive to antibiotics but carried antibiotic resistance genes could develop resistance upon exposure to antibiotic(s), and vancomycin and clindamycin were the most effective drugs. ST239-SCCmec UT6/t035 were dominant clones among *S. aureus*. There was diversity in genotypes, antimicrobial resistance, and virulence determinants among MRSA and MSSA strains, therefore suggests continuous surveillance of multidrug-resistant strains circulating in the community/hospitals in India, to take adequate measures to control the infection.

ETHICS STATEMENT

The studies involving human participants were reviewed and approved by the Institutional Review Board (IRB) of LV Prasad Eye Institute (LEC/08/110/2009) and by the Institute Ethics Sub-Committee (IESC) of All India Institute of Medical Sciences, New Delhi (IESC/T-34/2013), and the data were analyzed anonymously and reported. The patients/participants provided their written informed consent to participate in this study.

AUTHOR CONTRIBUTIONS

SA, SJ, SS, and DS conceived the experiments. SA, SJ, and SP conducted the experiments. SA, SJ, SP, SS, BD, GN, NS, and DS analyzed the results. KN performed statistical analysis. SA, SJ, and DS wrote the manuscript. All authors reviewed and approved the manuscript.

FUNDING

This study was supported by the Department of Science and Technology (Grant No. SR/SO/HS-117 to DS). This study, in part, was also supported by the fund contributed by the Department of Biotechnology, New Delhi, to the Institute of Life Sciences, Bhubaneswar. The funder had no role in study design, data collection and analysis, decision to publish, or preparation of the manuscript.

ACKNOWLEDGMENTS

SA and SJ are grateful to the Institute of Life Sciences, Bhubaneswar and Department of Science and Technology, New Delhi, respectively for providing Senior Research Fellowship.

REFERENCES

Agarwal, A., and Jain, A. (2013). Glucose & sodium chloride induced biofilm production & ica operon in clinical isolates of staphylococci. Indian J. Med. Res. 138:262.

Arciola, C. R., Baldassarri, L., and Montanaro, L. (2001). Presence of icaA and icaD genes and slime production in a collection of Staphylococcal strains from catheter-associated infections. J. Clin. Microbiol. 39, 2151–2156. doi: 10.1128/JCM.39.6.2151-2156.2001

Argudín, M., Tenhagen, B.-A., Fetsch, A., Sachsenröder, J., Käsbohrer, A., Schroeter, A., et al. (2011). Virulence and resistance determinants of German Staphylococcus aureus ST398 isolates from nonhuman sources. Appl. Environ. Microbiol. 77, 3052–3060. doi: 10.1128/AEM.02260-10

Baranovich, T., Zaraket, H., Shabana, I., Nevzorova, V., Turcutyuicov, V., and Suzuki, H. (2010). Molecular characterization and susceptibility of methicillin-resistant and methicillin-susceptible Staphylococcus aureus isolates from hospitals and the community in Vladivostok, Russia. Clin. Microbiol. Infect. 16, 575–582. doi: 10.1111/j.1469-0691.2009.02891.x

Bhutia, K. O., Singh, T., Adhikari, L., and Biswas, S. (2015). Molecular characterization of community-& hospital-acquired methicillin-resistant & methicillin-sensitive Staphylococcus aureus isolates in Sikkim. Indian J. Med. Res. 142:330. doi: 10.4103/0971-5916.166600

Busch-SØRensen, C., SØNmezoglu, M., Frimodt-Moller, N., Hojbjerg, T., Miller, G. H., and Espersen, F. (1996). Aminoglycoside resistance mechanisms in Enterobacteriaceae and Pseudomonas spp. from two Danish hospitals: correlation with type of aminoglycoside used. Apmis 104, 763–768. doi: 10.1111/j.1699-0463.1996.tb04940.x

Dhawan, B., Rao, C., Udo, E., Gadepalli, R., Vishnubhatla, S., and Kapil, A. (2015). Dissemination of methicillin-resistant Staphylococcus aureus SCCmec type IV and SCCmec type V epidemic clones in a tertiary hospital: challenge to infection control. Epidemiol. Infect. 143, 343–353. doi: 10.1017/S095026881400065X

Dornbusch, K., Miller, G., Hare, R., Shaw, K., and Group, E. S. (1990). Resistance to aminoglycoside antibiotics in gram-negative bacilli and staphylococci isolated from blood. Report from a European collaborative study. J. Antimicrob. Chemother. 26, 131–144. doi: 10.1093/jac/26.1.131

D'Souza, N., Rodrigues, C., and Mehta, A. (2010). Molecular characterization of methicillin-resistant Staphylococcus aureus with emergence of epidemic clones of sequence type (ST) 22 and ST 772 in Mumbai, India. J. Clin. Microbiol. 48, 1806–1811. doi: 10.1128/JCM.01867-09

Duran, N., Ozer, B., Duran, G. G., Onlen, Y., and Demir, C. (2012). Antibiotic resistance genes & susceptibility patterns in staphylococci. Indian J. Med. Res. 135:389.

Enright, M. C., and Spratt, B. G. (1999). Multilocus sequence typing. Trends Microbiol. 7, 482–487. doi: 10.1016/S0966-842X(99)01609-1

Freidlin, J., Acharya, N., Lietman, T. M., Cevallos, V., Whitcher, J. P., and Margolis, T. P. (2007). Spectrum of eye disease caused by methicillin-resistant Staphylococcus aureus. Am. J. Ophthalmol. 144, 313–315. doi: 10.1016/j.ajo.2007.03.032

Ghasemzadeh-Moghaddam, H., Ghaznavi-Rad, E., Sekawi, Z., Yun-Khoon, L., Aziz, M. N., Hamat, R. A., et al. (2011). Methicillin-susceptible Staphylococcus aureus from clinical and community sources are genetically diverse. Int. J. Med. Microbiol. 301, 347–353. doi: 10.1016/j.ijmm.2010.10.004

Ghaznavi-Rad, E., Goering, R., Shamsudin, M. N., Weng, P., Sekawi, Z., Tavakol, M., et al. (2011). mec-associated dru typing in the epidemiological analysis of ST239 MRSA in Malaysia. Eu. J. Clin Microbiol. Infect Dis. 30, 1365–1369. doi: 10.1007/s10096-011-1230-1

Ghebremedhin, B., Olugbosi, M., Raji, A., Layer, F., Bakare, R., König, B., et al. (2009). Emergence of a community-associated methicillin-resistant Staphylococcus aureus strain with a unique resistance profile in Southwest Nigeria. J. Clin. Microbiol. 47, 2975–2980. doi: 10.1128/JCM.00648-09

Gilot, P., Lina, G., Cochard, T., and Poutrel, B. (2002). Analysis of the genetic variability of genes encoding the RNA III-activating components Agr and TRAP in a population of Staphylococcus aureus strains isolated from cows with mastitis. J. Clin. Microbiol. 40, 4060–4067. doi: 10.1128/JCM.40.11.4060-4067.2002

Godebo, G., Kibru, G., and Tassew, H. (2013). Multidrug-resistant bacterial isolates in infected wounds at Jimma University Specialized Hospital, Ethiopia. Annals Clin. Microbiol. Antimicrob. 12:17. doi: 10.1186/1476-0711-12-17

Goh, S.-H., Byrne, S., Zhang, J., and Chow, A. (1992). Molecular typing of Staphylococcus aureus on the basis of coagulase gene polymorphisms. J. Clin. Microbiol. 30, 1642–1645.

Gowrishankar, S., Kamaladevi, A., Balamurugan, K., and Pandian, S. K. (2016). In vitro and in vivo biofilm characterization of methicillin-resistant *Staphylococcus aureus* from patients associated with pharyngitis infection. *Biomed. Res. Int.* 2016, 1–14. doi: 10.1155/2016/1289157

Hammer, Ø, Harper, D., and Ryan, P. (2001). Paleontological statistics software: package for education and data analysis. *Palaeontol. Electron.* 4:9.

Hirotaki, S., Sasaki, T., Kuwahara-Arai, K., and Hiramatsu, K. (2011). Rapid and accurate identification of human-associated staphylococci by use of multiplex PCR. *J. Clin. Microbiol.* 49, 3627–3631. doi: 10.1128/JCM.00488-11

Hsu, L.-Y., Koh, T.-H., Singh, K., Kang, M.-L., Kurup, A., and Tan, B.-H. (2005). Dissemination of multisusceptible methicillin-resistant *Staphylococcus aureus* in Singapore. *J. Clin. Microbiol.* 43, 2923–2925. doi: 10.1128/JCM.43.6.2923-2925.2005

Hwang, S.-M., and Kim, T.-U. (2007). Changes in coagulase serotype of *Staphylococcus aureus* isolates in Busan, 1994-2005. *Korean J. Microbiol.* 43, 346–350.

Jarraud, S., Mougel, C., Thioulouse, J., Lina, G., Meugnier, H., Forey, F., et al. (2002). Relationships between *Staphylococcus aureus* genetic background, virulence factors, *agr* groups (alleles), and human disease. *Infect. immun.* 70, 631–641. doi: 10.1128/IAI.70.2.631-641.2002

Kaur, D. C., and Chate, S. S. (2015). Study of antibiotic resistance pattern in methicillin resistant *Staphylococcus aureus* with special reference to newer antibiotic. *J. Glob. Infect. Dis.* 7, 78–84. doi: 10.4103/0974-777X.157245

Kim, J.-S., Song, W., Kim, H.-S., Cho, H. C., Lee, K. M., Choi, M.-S., et al. (2006). Association between the methicillin resistance of clinical isolates of *Staphylococcus aureus*, their staphylococcal cassette chromosome *mec* (SCC*mec*) subtype classification, and their toxin gene profiles. *Diagn. Microbiol. Infect. Dis.* 56, 289–295. doi: 10.1016/j.diagmicrobio.2006.05.003

Kondo, Y., Ito, T., Ma, X. X., Watanabe, S., Kreiswirth, B. N., Etienne, J., et al. (2007). Combination of multiplex PCRs for staphylococcal cassette chromosome *mec* type assignment: rapid identification system for *mec*, *ccr*, and major differences in junkyard regions. *Antimicrob. Agents Chemother.* 51, 264–274. doi: 10.1128/AAC.00165-06

Lindsay, J. A., and Holden, M. T. (2004). *Staphylococcus aureus*: superbug, super genome? *Trends Microbiol.* 12, 378–385. doi: 10.1016/j.tim.2004.06.004

Liu, Q., Han, L., Li, B., Sun, J., and Ni, Y. (2012). Virulence characteristic and MLST-*agr* genetic background of high-level mupirocin-resistant, MRSA isolates from Shanghai and Wenzhou, China. *PLoS One* 7:e37005. doi: 10.1371/journal.pone.0037005

Liu, Y., Wang, H., Du, N., Shen, E., Chen, H., Niu, J., et al. (2009). Molecular evidence for spread of two major methicillin-resistant *Staphylococcus aureus* clones with a unique geographic distribution in Chinese hospitals. *Antimicrob. Agents Chemother.* 53, 512–518. doi: 10.1128/AAC.00804-08

Lovering, A., Bywater, M., Holt, H., Champion, H., and Reeves, D. (1988). Resistance of bacterial pathogens to four aminoglycosides and six other antibacterials and prevalence of aminoglycoside modifying enzymes, in 20 UK centres. *J. Antimicrob. Chemother.* 22, 823–839. doi: 10.1093/jac/22.6.823

Martineau, F., Picard, F. J., Lansac, N., Ménard, C., Roy, P. H., Ouellette, M., et al. (2000). Correlation between the resistance genotype determined by multiplex PCR assays and the antibiotic susceptibility patterns of *Staphylococcus aureus* and *Staphylococcus epidermidis*. *Antimicrob. Agents Chemother.* 44, 231–238. doi: 10.1128/aac.44.2.231-238.2000

Maslow, J. N., Mulligan, M. E., and Arbeit, R. D. (1993). Molecular epidemiology: application of contemporary techniques to the typing of microorganisms. *Clin. Infect. Dis.* 17, 153–162. doi: 10.1093/clinids/17.2.153

Mehrotra, M., Wang, G., and Johnson, W. M. (2000). Multiplex PCR for detection of genes for *Staphylococcus aureus* enterotoxins, exfoliative toxins, toxic shock syndrome toxin 1, and methicillin resistance. *J. Clin. Microbiol.* 38, 1032–1035.

Mitchell, G., Séguin, D. L., Asselin, A.-E., Déziel, E., Cantin, A. M., Frost, E. H., et al. (2010). *Staphylococcus aureus* sigma B-dependent emergence of small-colony variants and biofilm production following exposure to *Pseudomonas aeruginosa* 4-hydroxy-2-heptylquinoline-N-oxide. *BMC Microbiol.* 10:33. doi: 10.1186/1471-2180-10-33

Mobasherizadeh, S., Shojaei, H., Azadi, D., Havaei, A. A., and Rostami, S. (2019). Molecular characterization and genotyping of methicillin-resistant *Staphylococcus aureus* in nasal carriage of healthy Iranian children. *J. Med. Microbiol.* 68, 374–378. doi: 10.1099/jmm.0.000924

Mohammadi, S., Sekawi, Z., Monjezi, A., Maleki, M.-H., Soroush, S., Sadeghifard, N., et al. (2014). Emergence of SCC*mec* type III with variable antimicrobial resistance profiles and *spa* types among methicillin-resistant *Staphylococcus aureus* isolated from healthcare- and community-acquired infections in the west of Iran. *Int. J. Infect. Dis.* 25, 152–158. doi: 10.1016/j.ijid.2014.02.018

Monday, S. R., and Bohach, G. A. (1999). Use of multiplex PCR to detect classical and newly described pyrogenic toxin genes in staphylococcal isolates. *J. Clin. Microbiol.* 37, 3411–3414.

Nadig, S., Velusamy, N., Lalitha, P., Kar, S., Sharma, S., and Arakere, G. (2012). *Staphylococcus aureus* eye infections in two Indian hospitals: emergence of ST772 as a major clone. *Clin. Ophthalmol.* 6, 165–173. doi: 10.2147/OPTH.S23878

Nelson, J. L., Rice, K. C., Slater, S. R., Fox, P. M., Archer, G. L., Bayles, K. W., et al. (2007). Vancomycin-intermediate *Staphylococcus aureus* strains have impaired acetate catabolism: implications for polysaccharide intercellular adhesin synthesis and autolysis. *Antimicrob. Agents Chemother.* 51, 616–622. doi: 10.1128/AAC.01057-06

Norazah, A., Liew, S., Kamel, A., Koh, Y., and Lim, V. (2001). DNA fingerprinting of methicillin-resistant *Staphylococcus aureus* by pulsed-field gel electrophoresis (PFGE): comparison of strains from 2 Malaysian hospitals. *Singapore Med. J.* 42, 015–019.

Nurjadi, D., Schäfer, J., Friedrich-Jänicke, B., Mueller, A., Neumayr, A., Calvo-Cano, A., et al. (2015). Predominance of *dfrG* as determinant of trimethoprim resistance in imported *Staphylococcus aureus*. *Clin. Microbiol. Infect.* 21, 1095.e5–1095.e9. doi: 10.1016/j.cmi.2015.08.021

Pai, V., Rao, V. I., and Rao, S. P. (2010). Prevalence and antimicrobial susceptibility pattern of methicillin-resistant *Staphylococcus aureus* [MRSA] isolates at a tertiary care hospital in Mangalore South India. *J. Lab. Physicians* 2:82. doi: 10.4103/0974-2727.72155

Panda, S., Kar, S., Choudhury, R., Sharma, S., and Singh, D. V. (2014). Development and evaluation of hexaplex PCR for rapid detection of methicillin, cadmium/zinc and antiseptic-resistant staphylococci, with simultaneous identification of PVL-positive and-negative *Staphylococcus aureus* and coagulase negative staphylococci. *FEMS Microbiol. Lett.* 352, 114–122. doi: 10.1111/1574-6968.12383

Panda, S., Kar, S., Sharma, S., and Singh, D. V. (2016). Multidrug-resistant *Staphylococcus haemolyticus* isolates from infected eyes and healthy conjunctivae in India. *J. Glob. Antimicrob. Res.* 6, 154–159. doi: 10.1016/j.jgar.2016.05.006

Paniagua-Contreras, G., Sáinz-Espuñes, T., Monroy-Pérez, E., Rodríguez-Moctezuma, J. R., Arenas-Aranda, D., Negrete-Abascal, E., et al. (2012). Virulence markers in *Staphylococcus aureus* strains isolated from hemodialysis catheters of Mexican patients. *Adv. Microbiol.* 2:476. doi: 10.4236/aim.2012.24061

Price, K., Kresel, P., Farchione, L., Siskin, S., and Karpow, S. (1981). Epidemiological studies of aminoglycoside resistance in the USA. *J. Antimicrob. Chemother.* 8(Suppl. A), 89–105. doi: 10.1093/jac/8.suppl-A.89

Schmitz, F.-J., Fluit, A. C., Gondolf, M., Beyrau, R., Lindenlauf, E., Verhoef, J., et al. (1999). The prevalence of aminoglycoside resistance and corresponding resistance genes in clinical isolates of staphylococci from 19 European hospitals. *J. Antimicrob. Chemother.* 43, 253–259. doi: 10.1093/jac/43.2.253

Shanmuganathan, V., Armstrong, M., Buller, A., and Tullo, A. (2005). External ocular infections due to methicillin-resistant *Staphylococcus aureus* (MRSA). *Eye* 19, 284–291. doi: 10.1038/sj.eye.6701465

Shittu, A. O., Okon, K., Adesida, S., Oyedara, O., Witte, W., Strommenger, B., et al. (2011). Antibiotic resistance and molecular epidemiology of *Staphylococcus aureus* in Nigeria. *BMC Microbiol.* 11:92. doi: 10.1186/1471-2180-11-92

Shukla, S. K., Karow, M. E., Brady, J. M., Stemper, M. E., Kislow, J., Moore, N., et al. (2010). Virulence genes and genotypic associations in nasal carriage, community-associated methicillin-susceptible and methicillin-resistant USA400 *Staphylococcus aureus* isolates. *J. Clin. Microbiol.* 48, 3582–3592. doi: 10.1128/JCM.00657-10

Sotto, A., Lina, G., Richard, J.-L., Combescure, C., Bourg, G., Vidal, L., et al. (2008). Virulence potential of *Staphylococcus aureus* strains isolated from diabetic foot ulcers: a new paradigm. *Diabetes Care* 31, 2318–2324. doi: 10.2337/dc08-1010

Suzuki, T., Hayashi, S., and Ohashi, Y. (2012). Genotypic characterization of *staphylococcus aureus* isolates from eyes with keratitis. *Invest. Ophthalmol. Vis. Sci.* 53, 6139–6139.

Tenover, F. C., Arbeit, R., Archer, G., Biddle, J., Byrne, S., Goering, R., et al. (1994). Comparison of traditional and molecular methods of typing isolates of *Staphylococcus aureus*. *J. Clin. Microbiol.* 32, 407–415.

Van Belkum, A., Tassios, P., Dijkshoorn, L., Haeggman, S., Cookson, B., Fry, N., et al. (2007). Guidelines for the validation and application of typing methods for use in bacterial epidemiology. *Clin. Microbiol. Infect.* 13, 1–46. doi: 10.1111/j.1469-0691.2007.01786.x

Vanhoof, R., Godard, C., Content, J., and Nyssen, H. (1994). Detection by polymerase chain reaction of genes encoding aminoglycoside-modifying enzymes in methicillin-resistant *Staphylococcus aureus* isolates of epidemic phage types. *J. Med. Microbiol.* 41, 282–290. doi: 10.1099/00222615-41-4-282

Wang, L., Hu, Z., Hu, Y., Tian, B., Li, J., Wang, F., et al. (2013). Molecular analysis and frequency of *Staphylococcus aureus* virulence genes isolated from bloodstream infections in a teaching hospital in Tianjin. *China Genet. Mol. Res.* 12, 646–654. doi: 10.4238/2013.March.11.12

Zecconi, A., Cesaris, L., Liandris, E., Dapra, V., and Piccinini, R. (2006). Role of several *Staphylococcus aureus* virulence factors on the inflammatory response in bovine mammary gland. *Microb. Pathogen.* 40, 177–183. doi: 10.1016/j.micpath.2006.01.001

3

Characterization of KPC-Producing *Serratia marcescens* in an Intensive Care Unit of a Brazilian Tertiary Hospital

*Roumayne L. Ferreira[1†], Graziela S. Rezende[1†], Marcelo Silva Folhas Damas[1†],
Mariana Oliveira-Silva[2], André Pitondo-Silva[2], Márcia C. A. Brito[3],
Eduardo Leonardecz[1], Fabiana R. de Góes[4], Emeline Boni Campanini[1], Iran Malavazi[1],
Anderson F. da Cunha[1] and Maria-Cristina da Silva Pranchevicius[1]**

[1] *Departamento de Genética e Evolução, Universidade Federal de São Carlos, São Carlos, Brazil,* [2] *Programas de Pós-graduação em Odontologia e Tecnologia Ambiental, Universidade de Ribeirão Preto, Ribeirão Preto, Brazil,* [3] *Laboratório Central de Saúde Pública do Tocantins, Palmas, Brazil,* [4] *Instituto de Ciências Matemáticas e de Computação, Universidade de São Paulo, São Carlos, Brazil*

*Correspondence:
Maria-Cristina da Silva Pranchevicius
mcspranc@gmail.com

[†] *These authors have contributed equally to this work*

Serratia marcescens has emerged as an important opportunistic pathogen responsible for nosocomial and severe infections. Here, we determined phenotypic and molecular characteristics of 54 *S. marcescens* isolates obtained from patient samples from intensive-care-unit (ICU) and neonatal intensive-care-unit (NIUC) of a Brazilian tertiary hospital. All isolates were resistant to beta-lactam group antibiotics, and 92.6% (50/54) were not susceptible to tigecycline. Furthermore, 96.3% showed intrinsic resistance to polymyxin E (colistin), a last-resort antibiotic for the treatment of infections caused by MDR (multidrug-resistant) Gram-negative bacteria. In contrast, high susceptibility to other antibiotics such as fluoroquinolones (81.5%), and to aminoglycosides (as gentamicin 81.5%, and amikacin 85.2%) was found. Of all isolates, 24.1% were classified as MDR. The presence of resistance and virulence genes were examined by PCR and sequencing. All isolates carried KPC-carbapenemase (bla_{KPC}) and extended spectrum beta-lactamase bla_{TEM} genes, 14.8% carried bla_{OXA-1}, and 16.7% carried $bla_{CTX-M-1group}$ genes, suggesting that bacterial resistance to β-lactam antibiotics found may be associated with these genes. The genes SdeB/HasF and SdeY/HasF that are associated with efflux pump mediated drug extrusion to fluoroquinolones and tigecycline, respectively, were found in 88.9%. The aac(6′)-Ib-cr variant gene that can simultaneously induce resistance to aminoglycoside and fluoroquinolone was present in 24.1% of the isolates. Notably, the virulence genes to (i) pore-forming toxin (*ShlA*); (ii) phospholipase with hemolytic and cytolytic activities (*PhlA*); (iii) flagellar transcriptional regulator (*FlhD*); and (iv) positive regulator of prodigiosin and serratamolide production (*PigP*) were present in 98.2%. The genetic relationship among the isolates determined by ERIC-PCR demonstrated that the vast majority of isolates were grouped in a single cluster with 86.4% genetic similarity. In addition, many isolates showed 100% genetic similarity to each other, suggesting that the *S. marcescens* that circulate in this ICU are closely related. Our results suggest that the antimicrobial resistance to many drugs currently used to treat ICU and NIUC patients, associated with the high frequency of resistance and virulence genes is a worrisome phenomenon. Our findings emphasize the importance of active surveillance plans for infection control and to prevent dissemination of these strains.

Keywords: *Serratia marcescens*, intensive care units, KPC, virulence and resistance genes, ERIC-PCR

INTRODUCTION

Serratia marcescens is a Gram-negative bacillus that naturally resides in the soil and water and produces a red pigment at room temperature. Although previously considered non-pathogenic, this species has emerged as a prominent opportunistic pathogen found in nosocomial outbreaks in neonatal intensive care Units (NICUs), intensive care units (ICUs) and other hospital units over the last few decades (Enciso-Moreno et al., 2004; Moradigaravand et al., 2016; Ghaith et al., 2018).

The true occurrence of *S. marcescens* is still underestimated (Zingg et al., 2017). In NICUs, studies have showen that infected newborns are a potential source of *S. marcescens* (Cristina et al., 2019), although there is a constant increase of *S. marcescens* bacteremia across all age groups (Vetter et al., 2016; Phan et al., 2018). *S. marcescens* increasingly adapts to hospital environments (Yoon et al., 2005; Gastmeier, 2014). It accounts for 15% of all isolates from nosocomial infections (Raymond and Aujard, 2000). Although it is difficult to identify the source of *S. marcescens* during outbreaks, it is the third most frequent pathogen identified (Gastmeier et al., 2007), and more than one clone can be usually identified (David et al., 2006; Montagnani et al., 2015; Dawczynski et al., 2016).

Serratia marcescens associated with hospital outbreaks or epidemic events are commonly resistant to several antibiotics (Moradigaravand et al., 2016; Cristina et al., 2019). In fact, one important feature of *S. marcescens* is its resistance to narrow-spectrum penicillins and cephalosporins; nitrofurantoin; tetracycline; macrolides; cefuroxime; cephamycins; fluoroquinolone, and colistin (Stock et al., 2003; Liou et al., 2014; Moradigaravand et al., 2016; Sandner-Miranda et al., 2018). The resistance to some of these molecules may be intrinsic to this specie and is explained by either the presence of resistance genes on the chromosome or by the acquisition of such genes via horizontal transfer. It is noteworthy that the latter mechanism is considered the most important event that leads to multiple antibiotic resistance (von Wintersdorff et al., 2016; Sandner-Miranda et al., 2018).

Extended-spectrum β-lactamases (ESBLs) are a group of bacterial enzymes that can be rapidly transferred via plasmid exchange (Rawat and Nair, 2010) causing resistance to a broad range of β-lactams (Naas et al., 2008). Carbapenemases are the most versatile family of β-lactamases able to hydrolyze carbapenems and many other β-lactams (Jeon et al., 2015) including penicillins, cephalosporins, and monobactams (Anderson et al., 2007; Marschall et al., 2009). In general, bacteria carrying the bla_{KPC} and/or ESBLs genes usually harbor other resistance genes associated with several classes of antimicrobials (Tzouvelekis et al., 2012; Cao et al., 2014; Ribeiro et al., 2016).

Since *S. marcescens* has been acquiring a range of ESBLs and commonly exhibit co-resistance to many other classes of antibiotics, the infections caused by these multidrug-resistant (MDR) isolates impair therapy and limit treatment options (Yu et al., 1998; Mostatabi et al., 2013; Herra and Falkiner, 2018).

In this study, we investigated the phenotypic characteristics regarding antimicrobial resistance and the genotypic traits of *S. marcescens* isolated from a tertiary care hospital's ICUs including the search for resistance and virulence genes as well as the genetic relationship among the isolates. Our report describes MDR profile and KPC-producing *S. marcescens* isolates and highlight the importance of monitoring *S. marcescens* infection and the need of constant surveillance to support continuous and effective measures to prevent the spread of these strains.

MATERIALS AND METHODS

Study Design and Bacterial Isolates

From February 2014 to June 2015, a total of 54 *S. marcescens* were isolated of clinical specimens collected from 45 patients admitted to intensive-care-unit (ICU) and neonatal intensive care unit (NICU) of a tertiary care government hospital in Palmas, Tocantins, Brazil. Since 2013, there has been an increase in detection of *S. marcescens* isolates from hospital inpatients, and in 2015, the hospital reported an apparent *S. marcescens* outbreak that occurred from July to August 2015. Appropriate intervention measures were established, such as reviewing the infection control policies, hand antisepsis practices and determination of trends of isolation of *S. marcescens* over time. To trace the source of the infection, bacteria were isolated from various samples obtained from clinical indications of infections during the patients' ICU stay.

As part of the control measures, surveillance cultures were obtained from tracheal aspirate and rectal swabs from all ICU patients, on admission (within the first 24 h) and during the stay (once a week). Blood, wound, catheter tip, drain, sputum, urine, rectal swab, and tracheal aspirate samples were primarily sent to the hospital's laboratory, processed and cultured by standard microbiological techniques. The blood samples were inoculated first in blood culture bottles (Hemoprov-NewProv, Brazil). All clinical samples, including blood culture bottles giving positive signals were cultured onto MacConkey agar (Probac, Brazil), blood agar (Probac, Brazil), and chocolate blood agar (Probac, Brazil). Plates were incubated at 37°C for up to 48 h. *S. marcescens* were identified by Gram staining, cultural characteristics in MacConkey agar (Probac, Brazil), blood agar (Probac, Brazil), and biochemical tests (Bactray I, II,III; Laborclin, Brazil). The antimicrobial susceptibility profile was determined by Kirby-Bauer disk diffusion method. All *S. marcescens* isolates and the microbiological reports prepared at the hospital were sent to the Central Laboratory of Public Health of Tocantins (LACEN-TO) for further phenotypic validations.

Bacterial Identification and Antimicrobial Susceptibility Test

Once samples were received at LACEN, bacterial identification and antimicrobial susceptibility tests were performed by the Vitek 2 system (Biomerieux, France), according to Clinical and Laboratory Standards Institute guidelines (CLSI, 2019). All 54 *S. marcescens* isolates were screened for susceptibility against 16 antimicrobial agents: ampicillin (AMP), ampicillin/sulbactam (SAM), piperacillin/tazobactam (TZP), cefuroxime (CXM), cefoxitin (FOX), ceftazidime (CAZ), ceftriaxone (CRO), cefepime (FEP), ertapenem (ETP), imipenem (IPM), meropenem (MEM), amikacin (AMK), gentamicin (GEN), ciprofloxacin (CIP), tigecycline (TGC), and colistin (CST). Broth microdilution method was performed to determine tigecycline and colistin minimum inhibitory concentration (MICs) and results were interpreted based on the European Committee on Antimicrobial Susceptibility Testing (EUCAST, 2018) criteria, available at https://www.eucast.org/fileadmin/src/media/PDFs/EUCAST_files/Breakpoint_tables/v_8.1_Breakpoint_Tables.pdf. All isolates were tested for carbapenemase production by Modified Hodge test, synergy test and ethylenediaminetetraacetic acid (EDTA) test under the CLSI guidelines (CLSI, 2019) as described elsewhere (Miriagou et al., 2010; Nordmann et al., 2011; Okoche et al., 2015; Ferreira et al., 2019). Multidrug-resistance *S. marcescens* isolates were classified by non-susceptibility to at least one agent of three or more antimicrobial categories (Magiorakos et al., 2012). *S. marcescens* is intrinsically resistant to AMP, SAM, CXM, FOX, and CST; therefore, these antibiotics were not included in the MDR classification (Magiorakos et al., 2012).

Genomic DNA Extraction

Isolates of *S. marcescens* were subcultured on Brain Heart Infusion (BHI) agar (Oxoid, United Kingdom) and incubated for 24 h at 37°C. All samples were submitted to genomic DNA extraction using the Wizard Genomic DNA Purification Kit (Promega, Madison, WI, United States), according to manufacture's instructions.

Detection of Antibiotic-Resistance

Polymerase chain reaction (PCR) was performed for detection of β-lactamase genes (bla_{TEM}, $bla_{SHV variants}$, $bla_{OXA-1, 4 and 30}$, $bla_{CTX-M-1 group}$), carbapenemase genes (bla_{KPC}, bla_{IMP}, bla_{VIM}, bla_{NDM}, bla_{OXA-48}) (Ferreira et al., 2019), plasmid mediated quinolone resistance (PMQR) gene ($aac(6')$-Ib-cr) (Wong et al., 2014; Mitra et al., 2019), resistance-nodulation-division (RND) efflux pumps (*SdeB*, *SdeY*), and outer membrane gene (*HasF*, a *TolC* homolog) involved in energy-dependent efflux of antimicrobial agents (Kumar and Worobec, 2005b). The genes were amplified using specific primers designed to follow the conditions described in the references from **Table 1**. All primers were synthesized by Exxtend (Brazil). Amplicons were

analyzed by gel electrophoresis in 1.0% agarose and visualized under ultraviolet (UV) light.

Virulence Gene Detection

The presence of four virulence genes were assessed by PCR: genes *PigP*, a positive regulator of prodigiosin and serratamolide production; *FlhD*, a flagellar transcriptional regulator; *ShlA*, a pore-forming toxin with hemolytic activity; *PhlA*, a phospholipase A with hemolytic activity. The primers sequences amplicon sizes and annealing temperatures are listed in **Table 1**. Amplicons were analyzed by gel electrophoresis in 1.0% agarose and visualized under ultraviolet (UV) light.

Sequence Analysis of Antibiotic-Resistance Markers and Virulence Genes

One amplicon of each studied gene was randomly selected for confirmation of identity by DNA sequencing using an automated sequencer (ABI 3500xL Genetic Analyzer; Applied Biosystems, Foster City, CA, United States). After amplification, we extracted the PCR products from agarose gels using the Illustra GFX PCR DNA (GE Healthcare), which were purified using the Gel Band Purification Kit (GE Healthcare), both according to manufacturer's instructions. Obtained sequences were edited with Bioedit v7.0.5 (Hall, 1999), compared with the nr database using the Blastn tool[1] and submitted to the GenBank database. Genes and their respective accession numbers: bla_{CTX} – MK576103; bla_{KPC} – MK576104; bla_{OXA} – MK576105; bla_{TEM} – MK576106; *SdeB* – MN583232; *SdeY* – MN583233; *HasF* – MN583234; $aac(6')$-Ib-cr – MN583235; *FlhD* – MN583236; *PigP* – MN583237; *ShlA* – MN583238; *PhlA* – MN583239). Access to genetic heritage was approved by the National System for the Management of Genetic Heritage (SisGen n° AFF27ED).

Enterobacterial Repetitive Intergenic Consensus Polymerase Chain Reaction

Enterobacterial repetitive intergenic consensus PCR (ERIC-PCR) analysis was performed to evaluate the genetic similarity among the 54 *S. marcescens* isolates using the primers and conditions previously described by Versalovic et al. (1994). PCR reactions were performed using the enzyme TaKaRa Ex Taq DNA Polymerase (Takara Bio, Kusatsu, Japan). The BioNumerics program version 5.1 (AppliedMaths, Keistraat, Belgium) was used to construct the unweighted pair group mean method (UPGMA) similarity dendrogram with Dice's similarity coefficient, following Ferreira et al. (2019).

Statistical Analyses

In the analysis of contingency tables, we used Fisher's exact test and/or Barnard's exact test. Maximum likelihood did not present superior efficiency in relation to the previous methods (data not show). It was used logistic regression model with two predictor variables x_1 and x_2. Statistical software R was used in all data analysis.

---

[1] https://blast.ncbi.nlm.nih.gov/

TABLE 1 | Sequences of primes used for detection of resistance markers.

Gene	Sequence (5'-3'), F/R	TM (°C)	Amplicon size (bp)	References
blaKPC	CGTCTAGTTCTGCTGTCTTG CTTGTCATCCTTGTTAGGCG	61.3	797	Poirel et al., 2011
blaTEM	TGCGGTATTATCCCGTGTTG TCGTCGTTTGGTATGGCTTC	63	296	Xiong et al., 2007
blaCTX−M−1group,	ACAGCGATAACGTGGCGATG TCGCCCAATGCTTTACCCAG	64	216	Li and Li, 2005
blaSHVvariants	AGCCGCTTGAGCAAATTAAAC ATCCCGCAGATAAATCACCAC	55.6	712	Dallenne et al., 2010
blaOXA−1	GGCACCAGATTCAACTTTCAAG GACCCCAAGTTTCCTGTAAGTG	63	563	Dallenne et al., 2010
blaOXA−48	GCGTGGTTAAGGATGAACAC CATCAAGTTCAACCCAACCG	55	438	Poirel et al., 2011
blaIMP	CTACCGCAGCAGAGTCTTTGC ACAACCAGTTTTGCCTTACC	55	587	Martins et al., 2007
blaVIM	AAAGTTATGCCGCACTCACC TGCAACTTCATGTTATGCCG	55	865	Yan et al., 2001
blaNDM	GCAGCTTGTCGGCCATGCGGGC GGTCGCGAAGCTGAGCACCGCAT	60	782	Doyle et al., 2012
mcr-1	CGGTCAGTCCGTTTGTTC CTTGGTCGGTCTGTAGGG	51.6	309	Liu et al., 2015
aac(6')-Ib-cr	ATGACTGAGCATGACCTTGC TTAGGCATCACTGCGTGTTC	55.4	519	Platell et al., 2011
SdeB	AGATGGCCGATAAGCTGTTG CAGCGTCCAGCTTTCATACA	55.4	200	Hornsey et al., 2010
SdeY	TCCATCAACGAAGTGGTGAA GTTTATCGAGAAGCCGAACG	55.5	200	Hornsey et al., 2010
HasF	CATGTCGAAATGGCGCCAAC TTGTAGGCGTTGATGCTGCT	57.5	785	Hornsey et al., 2010
PigP	GAACATGTTGGCAATGAAAA ATGTAACCCAGGAATTGCAC	53.4	207	Srinivasan et al., 2017
FlhD	TGTCGGGATGGGGAATATGG CGATAGCTCTTGCAGTAAATGG	57	307	Salini and Pandian, 2015
ShlA	AGCGTGATCCTCAACGAAGT TGCGATTATCCAGAGTGCTG	55.4	217	Aggarwal et al., 2017
PhlA	GGGGACAACAATCTCAGGA ACGCCAACAACATACTGCTTG	55.4	207	Aggarwal et al., 2017

Ethical Considerations

In our study, we did not use/collect human genetic material and biological samples. Strains were part of the collection of the Central Laboratory of Public Health, (LACEN-TO), a health-care facility that is a reference in diagnosis in the state of Tocantins, Brazil. It was a retrospective study, and epidemiological data were obtained from a database or similar, which will be kept confidential in accordance with the with the terms of Resolution 466/12 of the National Health Council. These epidemiological data were also provided by LACEN-TO. Informed consent was not required according to resolution 466/12 concerning research involving humans of the National Health Council (Conselho Nacional de Saúde/Ministério da Saúde, Brasília, Brazil, 2012). The study was approved by the Committee of Ethics in Human Research of the Federal University of São Carlos (no. 1.088.936). Permission to conduct the study was also obtained from the Health Department of the State of Tocantins (Secretaria de Saúde do Estado do Tocantins – SESAU) and LACEN/TO.

RESULTS

Serratia marcescens Isolates

A total of 54 *S. marcescens* strains were isolated from 39 ICU and 6 NICU patients' samples at a tertiary hospital located in city of Palmas, Tocantins state. In six patients, 5 from ICU and 1 from NCIU, *S. marcescens* was isolated in more than one infection site. The prevalence of *S. marcescens* strains by age group was the following: 0–1 day (12.96%; $n = 7$), 18–59 years (38.89%, $n = 21$), 60 years or more (48.15%, $n = 26$). The median age of patients was 57.0 years (range, 0–93 years). *S. marcescens* strains were more frequently found in male (68.5%, $n = 37$)

than in female (31.5%, $n = 17$) patients (**Figure 1A**). Forty-three samples (79%) were from tracheal aspirate (33%, $n = 18$), rectal swab, (22%, $n = 12$), and blood (24%, $n = 13$) cultures, while 11 (21%) came from wound (9%, $n = 5$), catheter tip (4%, $n = 2$), surgical drain (4%, $n = 2$), sputum (2%, $n = 1$), and urine (2%, $n = 1$) cultures (**Figure 1B**). Antibiotic resistance profiles of *S. marcescens* isolated from the abovementioned different sites showed that all strains were resistant to β-lactams antibiotics. In addition, colistin (CST) and tigecycline (TGC) non-susceptibility pattern of *S. marcescens* per site of isolation was statistically significant ($p < 0.01$) in several organs (tracheal aspirate, blood, rectal swab, and wound) when compared with amikacin (AMK), gentamicin (GEN), and ciprofloxacin (CIP) antibiotics (**Figure 1C**).

Antimicrobial Resistance Profile and Genetic Markers for Antibiotic-Resistance and Virulence Patterns

Serratia marcescens strains showed high-levels of resistance to all β-lactams (100%, $n = 54$) (TZP, CAZ, CRO, FEP, ETP, IPM, MEM), including high-levels of intrinsic resistance to β-lactams (AMP, SAM, CXM, FOX) (100%, $n = 54$) and colistin (CST) (96.3%, $n = 52$). Resistance to tigecycline (TGC) *S. marcescens* was found in nearly all isolates (92.6%; $n = 50$). However, for the antibiotics classes fluoroquinolones (CIP) (81.5%, $n = 44$) and aminoglycosides such as gentamicin (GEN) (81.5%, $n = 44$), amikacin (AMK) (85.2%, $n = 46$) (**Figure 2A**), high susceptibility profile was detected. In contrast, MDR was observed in 24.1% ($n = 13$) of the isolates, and the most common MDR profile was related to β-lactams-glycylcycline-aminoglycosides-quinolone (14.8%, $n = 8$), followed by β-lactams-glicylcycline-quinolone (5.6%, $n = 3$), and (β-lactams-glicylcycline-aminoglycosides 3.7%, $n = 2$).

All 54 tested isolates harbored KPC-carbapenemase (bla_{KPC}) and ESBL (bla_{TEM}) genes. The ESBL-encoding genes bla_{OXA-1} was detected in 14.8% (8/54), and the $bla_{CTX-M-1group}$ in 16.7% (9/54). However, the bla_{SHV} variants, bla_{IMP}, bla_{OXA-48}, bla_{NDM}, bla_{VIM}, and mcr-1 genes were not detected. The aac(6')-Ib-cr variant gene that can induce simultaneous resistance against aminoglycoside and fluoroquinolone was found in 13 (24.1%) strains. The RND pump efflux encoding genes SdeY and SdeB were identified in all strains while the outer membrane component gene (HasF) was present in 48 (88.9%). Thus, the coexistence of SdeY/HasF genes and SdeB/HasF was observed in 49 (88.9%) strains (**Figure 2B**). Finally, with the exception of one strain (Sm40), the virulence-associated genes PigP, FlhD, ShlA, and PhlA were regularly distributed among *S. marcescens* strains, which were detected in 98.2% of all strains (**Figure 2B**).

Resistance Phenotype-Genotype Correlation and Genetic Markers for Virulence Factors

The correlation between the results of phenotypic and genotypic detection and the presence of virulence genes is shown in **Figure 3**.

All isolates carried bla_{KPC} and conferred resistance to all beta-lactam, including carbapenem antibiotics. Furthermore, all detectable bla genes in $bla_{CTX-M-1}$ bla_{OXA-1}, and bla_{TEM} group presented ESBL phenotype. Of the 13 isolates with aac(6')-Ib-cr gene, 9 (69.2%) were non-susceptible to gentamicin, 7 (53.9%) to amikacin, and 8 (61.5%) to ciprofloxacin. Among the 49 (88.9%) HasF-positive isolates, 44 (81.5%) were non-susceptible to tigecycline.

ERIC-PCR

The ERIC-PCR results indicated that the majority of the isolates presented a rate of genetic similarity above 85% (**Figure 4**). Almost all strains (96.3%) were grouped into a large cluster named B cluster, sharing 86.4% of genetic similarity. In addition, the B cluster was separated into two sub-clusters named B1, with 21 isolates, and B2, with 31 isolates, sharing a genetic similarity of 96.1% and 100%, respectively. Although the cluster B1 presented two subgroups with 4 and 17 isolates, they showed 100% genetic similarity in each one. Interestingly, two strains (Sm38 and Sm40) were grouped separately within the A cluster and presented 71.4% of genetic similarity (**Figure 4**).

DISCUSSION

Serratia marcescens is a prominent opportunistic pathogen that frequently causes infections in intensive care, surgical and dialysis units (Krishnan et al., 1991; Martineau et al., 2018). In Brazil, there are only few studies on *S. marcescens* (Ribeiro et al., 2013; Silva et al., 2015). Therefore, we here describe the presence of MDR *S. marcescens* isolates producing KPC-carbapenemase (bla_{KPC}) and extended spectrum beta-lactamase (bla_{TEM}, $bla_{CTX-M-1group}$ e bla_{OXA-1}, 4and 30) in the state of Tocantins, Brazil. Tocantins, located southeast of the Northern Region, is the newest state of Brazil and shares borders with six states presenting intensive migration flow.

Serratia marcescens were isolated mainly from male patients with 60 or more years of age, similarly to previous studies that demonstrated advanced age male patients as presenting a higher risk of contracting *S. marcescens* infections (Ulu-Kilic et al., 2013; Kim et al., 2015; O'Horo et al., 2017). Samples with higher amounts of *S. marcescens* were those from tracheal aspirate, followed by blood, rectal swab, and wounds. Our findings corroborate studies by Kim et al. (2015) and Liou et al. (2014) that reported the respiratory tract as the main route of infection for *S. marcescens*. Other studies have also reported *S. marcescens* in other sites as bloodstream (Seeyave et al., 2006) and wounds (Us et al., 2017), demonstrating the versatility of these strains in colonizing the host and affecting a wide variety of physiological system.

In addition to the intrinsic resistance to the antibiotics AMP, SAM, CXM, FOX, and CST, we found multidrug-resistant (MDR) *S. marcescens* isolates to beta-lactam, glycylcycline, and/or aminoglycoside and quinolone group antibiotics. This is in line with other studies that have also reported MDR *S. marcescens* mainly to beta-lactam, aminoglycoside, and quinolone antibiotics groups (Stock et al., 2003), in hospital

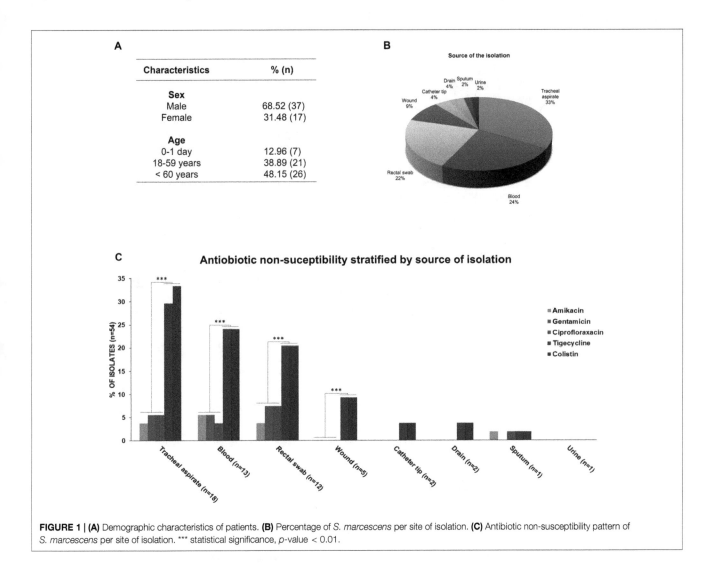

FIGURE 1 | (A) Demographic characteristics of patients. **(B)** Percentage of *S. marcescens* per site of isolation. **(C)** Antibiotic non-susceptibility pattern of *S. marcescens* per site of isolation. *** statistical significance, *p*-value < 0.01.

environment (Merkier et al., 2013), and particularly in critically ill patients and neonatal intensive care units (Maragakis et al., 2008). We also observed a significant resistance to colistin and tigecycline in several colonization sites, as shown by a previous study (Silva et al., 2017).

All the *S. marcescens* strains tested here were resistant to β-lactams, including carbapenems antibiotics. Resistance to carbapenems used to be uncommon among *Serratia* species (Stock et al., 2003), but many resistant strains have now emerged throughout the world (Lin et al., 2016). Although few studies have related resistance to carbapenems in *S. marcescens* in Brazil (Milisavljevic et al., 2004; da Costa Guimarães et al., 2013; Ribeiro et al., 2013), Silva et al. (2015) obtained similar results. They have isolated *S. marcescens* resistant to imipenem, meropenem and ertapenem in samples from different infection sites of ICU patients in another Brazilian locality. Both results are troubling. Infections caused by carbapenem-resistant bacteria often do not respond to conventional treatment (Okoche et al., 2015), as produced carbapenemases hydrolyze not only carbapenems but also penicillins, cephalosporins and monobactams

(Queenan and Bush, 2007). The most common carbapenem resistance of *S. marcescens* in Brazil is due to the production of carbapenamases, especially the KPC-2 type (da Costa Guimarães et al., 2013; Ribeiro et al., 2013), that is encoded by the gene bla_{KPC-2}.

Enterobacteriaceae, such as *S. marcescens*, have the genes bla_{TEM-1} and bla_{SHV-1}; these genes express classical class A beta-lactamases, encoded by plasmid that hydrolyze first generation penicillins and cephaloporins (Bush, 2010). We found gene bla_{TEM} in all isolates while gene $bla_{SHVvariants}$ was not detected. It is noteworthy that even though *S. marcescens* also carries the gene bla_{CTX-M} (Yu et al., 2003; Kim et al., 2005; Tenover et al., 2013), few of our strains had the gene. Some strains also carried the genes bla_{OXA-1}, 4 and 30, that have been reported in few studies in Brazil or in other countries, either alone or associated with extended spectrum beta-lactamases genes (ESBL) (bla_{TEM}, bla_{SHV} e bla_{CTX-M}) in *S. marcescens* strains. Although there are discrepancies in frequency rate and in genotyping of ESBL-producing *S. marcescens* (Cheng et al., 2006), the observed beta-lactam antibiotic resistance may have also been caused by the genes bla_{TEM}, bla_{CTX-M}, and

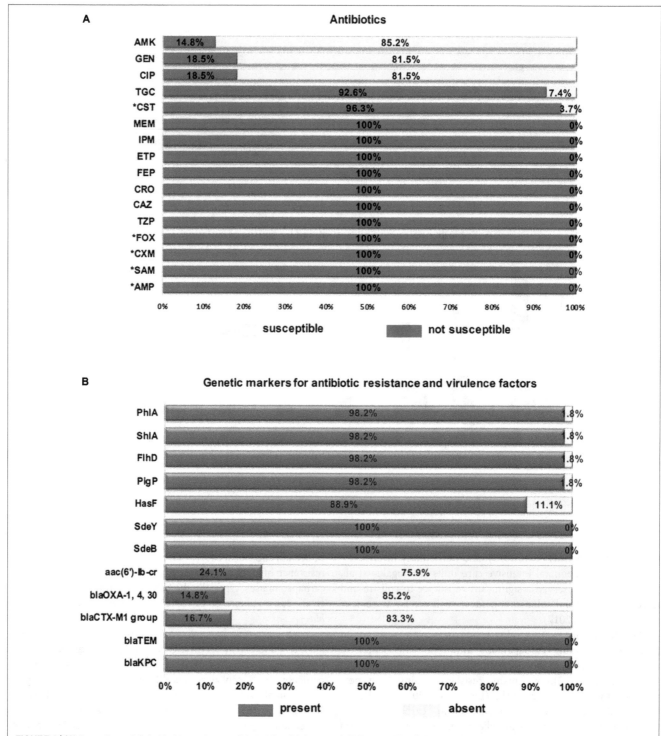

FIGURE 2 | (A) Percentage of clinical isolates not susceptible to 16 antibiotics tested. AMP (ampicillin), SAM (ampicillin-sulbactam), TZP (piperacillin-tazobactam), CXM (cefuroximeaxetil), FOX (cefoxitin), CAZ (ceftazidime), CRO (ceftriaxone), FEP (cefepime), ETP (ertapenem), IPM (imipenem), MEM (meropenem), AMK (amikacin), GEN (gentamicin), CIP (ciprofloxacin), TGC (tigecycline), CST (colistin); * intrinsic resistance to antibiotics. **(B)** Percentage of genetic markers for resistance and virulence genes. *bla*$_{KPC}$, *bla*$_{TEM}$, *bla*$_{CTX-M1}$, aac(6')-lb-cr: resistance genes; *SdeB*, *SdeY*, *HasF*: efflux pump and outer membrane component genes; *PigP*, *FlhD*, *ShlA*, *PhlA*: virulence genes.

bla$_{OXA}$, since the production of broad-spectrum beta-lactamases enzymes (TEM-1, TEM-2, SHV-1, OXA-1) generate resistant to ampicillin, ticarcillin, piperacillin, piperacillin/tazobactam and cephalosporin antibiotics, and the enzymes CTX-M have hydrolytic activity against cefotaxime (Levy and Marshall, 2004; Sugumar et al., 2014).

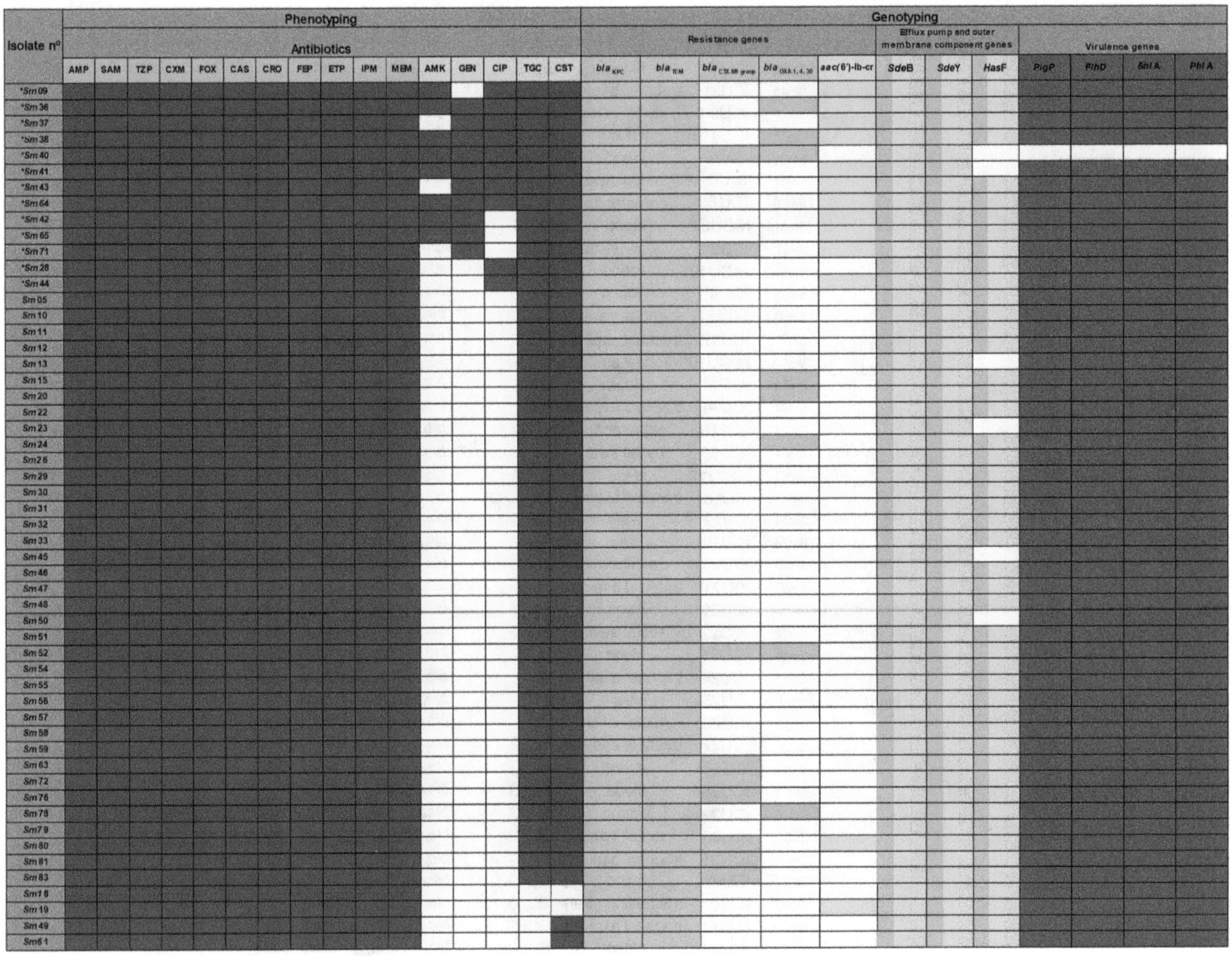

FIGURE 3 | Phenotyping and genotyping of *Serratia marcescens* isolates. Sm represents *Serratia marcescens* and numbers represent identifications of strains. *Sm is classified as multidrug resistant (MDR) strains. AMP (ampicillin), SAM (ampicillin-sulbactam), TZP (piperacillin-tazobactam), CXM (cefuroximeaxetil), FOX (cefoxitin), CAZ (ceftazidime), CRO (ceftriaxone), FEP (cefepime), ETP (ertapenem), IPM (imipenem), MEM (meropenem), AMK (amikacin), GEN (gentamicin), CIP (ciprofloxacin). *Serratia marcescens* are intrinsically resistant to TGC (tigecycline) and CST (colistin). AMP, SAM, CXM, FOX, and CST antibiotics were not included in the MDR classification. The bla_{IMP}, bla_{OXA-48}, bla_{NDM}, bla_{VIM}, bla_{SHV} variants and mcr-1 genes were not detected. Blue box correlates with AMP, SAM, TZP, CXM, FOX, CAZ, CRO, FEP, ETP, IPM, MEM. Green box correlate with AMK, GEN, CIP. Multicolored box (*HasF*) correlates with CIP and TGC. Brown box shows number of *S. marcescens* caring virulence genes.

In our study, most strains of *S. marcescens* were only sensitive to aminoglycosides (gentamicin and amikacin) and fluoroquinolone (ciprofloxacin). Aminoglycosides are the oldest antibiotics that have been used less frequently in the last years, thus possibly preserving activity against some resistant bacteria that cause difficult to cure infections (Falagas et al., 2008; Gad et al., 2011). The observed low resistance to ciprofloxacin (18.18%) is in agreement with the results obtained by Sheng et al. (2002) who observed 20–30% resistance to quinolone in *S. marcescens* isolates. However, it is important to consider that *S. marcescens* is highly adaptable, so rates of resistance to fluoroquinolones diverge considerably among institutions (Young et al., 1980; Mahlen, 2011; Sader et al., 2014), including within Brazilian ones.

Resistance to fluoroquinolones may be caused by alterations in the target enzymes DNA gyrase and topoisomerase IV, and by acquisition of the transferable plasmid-mediated quinolone resistance (PMQR) determinants qnr, qepA, aac(6')-Ib-cr, and oqxAB (Veldman et al., 2011; Poirel et al., 2012; Moradigaravand et al., 2016). The gene aac(6')-Ib-cr, a variant gene of the aminoglycoside acetyltransferase, was also present in most of strains that presented fluoroquinolone and/or aminoglycoside resistance. This finding is consistent with others studies that have shown that aac(6')-Ib-cr may be associated with antibacterial resistance against fluoroquinolone and aminoglycoside (Kim et al., 2009, 2011) antibiotics.

Three RND-type efflux have been reported in *S. marcescens*, namely SdeAB (Kumar and Worobec, 2005a), SdeCDE (Kumar and Worobec, 2005a; Begic and Worobec, 2008), and SdeXY (Chen et al., 2003). SdeAB and SdeXY interact with HasF (an outer membrane component, TolC homolog gene) contributing to resistance against a wide variety of antimicrobial agents

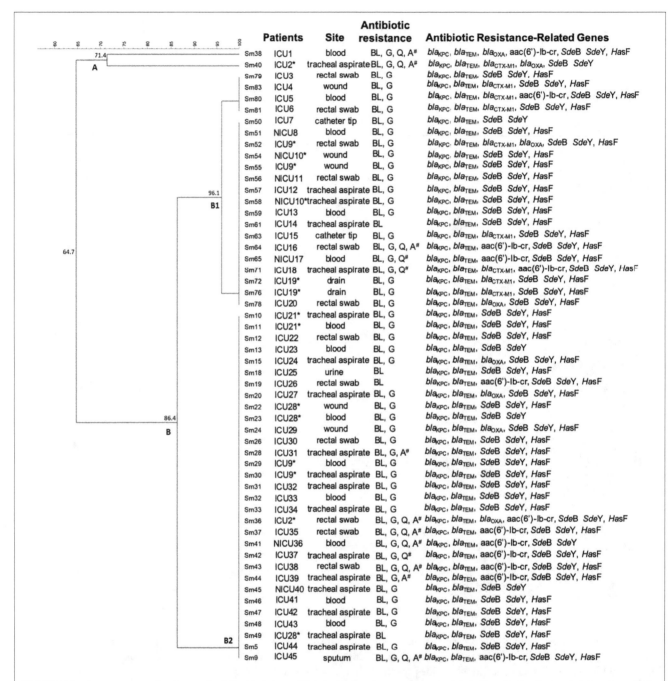

FIGURE 4 | Dendrogram representing the genetic relationship between 54 strains of *Serratia marcescens* associated with patient localization, isolation site, antibiotic resistance, and virulence genes. ICU: Intensive Care Unit. NICU: Neonatal Intensive Care Unit. *Patients presenting *S. marcescens* in more than one infection site. # multidrug resistance (MDR) pattern.

(Begic and Worobec, 2008; Hornsey et al., 2010). Although we did not analyze the genes *SdeA* e *SdeX*, the genes *SdeB* and *SdeX* were present in all strains and the gene *HasF* was also found in most strains. Drug extrusion by efflux pumps as *SdeAB-HasF* comprises one of the main mechanisms for fluoroquinolones antibiotic resistance (Dalvi and Worobec, 2012). Additionally, Hornsey et al. (2010) has shown the intrinsic activity of the *SdeXY-HasF* efflux pump is responsible for the lower

susceptibility to ciprofloxacin. Thus, in addition to the presence of the genes *aac(6′)*-Ib-cr [associated with plasmid-mediated quinolone resistance (PMQR)], the genes *SdeB*, *SdeY*, and *HasF* that encode RND-type efflux pump may have contributed to the observed ciprofloxacin resistance.

Our data shows high prevalence of tigecycline-resistant *S. marcescens* strains and *SdeY* and *HasF* genes. The reduced sensitivity of *S. marcescens* to tigecycline may be related to the up-regulation of the *SdeXY-HasF* efflux pump (Hornsey et al., 2010). Although the gene *SdeX* was not analyzed, our findings strongly suggest that these genes may be responsible for the high tigecycline resistance.

Many bacteria produce virulence factors as hydrolytic enzymes and toxins that enable host invasion, bacterial proliferation and inhibit host defense mechanisms, sometimes resulting in host death (Aggarwal et al., 2017). *S. marcescens* strains were also evaluated for the presence of toxin genes *ShlA* and *phlA*, and all but the *Sm*40 strain carried these genes. Our findings are in agreement with other studies that reported the presence these genes in *S. marcescens* (strain SEN) (Aggarwal et al., 2017). *FlhDC* has been proposed as a regulator controlling flagellum biogenesis, biofilm formation, cell septation and expression of virulence factors during swarming (Givskov et al., 1995; Fraser and Hughes, 1999; Chilcott and Hughes, 2000; Lin et al., 2010). In our study, the presence of *FlhC* was not analyzed but the gene *FlhD* was present in almost all isolates. *S. marcescens* produces biosurfactant serrawettin and red pigment prodigiosin used in surfaces colonization (Hejazi and Falkiner, 1997). *PigP* is a positive regulator of prodigiosin production that regulates swarming and hemolysis through serratamolide production (Fineran et al., 2005; Shanks et al., 2013). In our study, *PigP* gene was found in almost all isolates (98.15%). Overall, our results suggest that the combination of these virulence genes could have contributed to the pathogenicity of *S. marcescens* strains.

The dendrogram based on ERIC-PCR fingerprint analysis demonstrated that the vast majority of isolates are closely related, sharing a genetic similarity of 86.4% (except for two strains). In addition, many isolates showed 100% similarity to each other. A study conducted by Ferreira-Firmo et al. (2019) evaluated nine *S. marcescens* from different clinical sources and three hospitals in Northeast Brazil showed a greater genetic diversity among the studied strains. Lin et al. (2016) studied 83 carbapenem-resistant *S. marcescens* isolates recovered from Zhejiang Provincial 501 People's Hospital, China, from which they found 63 blaKPC-2 positive strains sharing nine different profiles. Our results demonstrate the predominance of few genetic profiles grouped together, with similarity above 85%, indicating that, although bacteria have been isolated from different patients and devices, the circulating *S. marcescens* in this hospital is highly genetically related.

Our study has some limitations worth noting. There was a high number of *S. marcescens* isolated from rectal swabs and tracheal aspirate, and both cultures are recommended for surveillance in ICU and NICU patients. However, microbiological reports sent to LACEN were not clear regarding how many of these samples were analyzed for both clinical and surveillance purposes. This study was further limited by the duration of the research, which was relatively short (2014–2015), and by conventional phenotypic and genotypic techniques, that have their own particular strengths and limitations in detecting MDR strains. Nonetheless, we intend to extend the analysis period of *S. marcescens* isolates, and

whole genome sequencing to type relevant MDR strains must be performed. We expect that this study broadens our understanding on epidemiology, antibiotic resistance, and putative virulence factors of these strains, and provides relevant information for the prevention and management of *S. marcescens* infections.

In conclusion, *S. marcescens* represents a problem for public health (Kurz et al., 2003) and the resistance pattern exhibited by clinical isolates along with the transmission to other clones show the importance of researching factors associated with the increase in frequency and/or emergence of infections caused by *S. marcescens* in Brazilian hospitals. The occurrence of antibiotic-resistant bacteria considerably varies according to country, region and susceptible population, and the mitigation of this problem in ICUs is especially associated with actions to control the spreading of such drug-resistant bacteria (Ko et al., 2002; Hou et al., 2015). Thus, it is crucial to eliminate sources of resistance development and associated reservoirs as well as to overtake standardized sanitation and enforce mandatory notification to gather important data for continuous risk assessment evaluation and effective decision making to control these species in hospital environments.

ETHICS STATEMENT

The studies involving human participants were reviewed and approved by the Committee of Ethics in Human Research of the Federal University of São Carlos (no. 1.088.936). In this work, all *Serratia marcescens* and the anonymous archival data related patient age, gender, and sample type were obtained from the Central Laboratory of Public Health of Tocantins (LACEN/TO, data's owner). Permission to conduct the present study was obtained from the Health Department of the State of Tocantins (Secretaria da Saúde do Estado do Tocantins – SESAU) and LACEN/TO. Patient consent was not required, since the data presented in this study do not relate to any specific person or persons. Written informed consent from the participants' legal guardian/next of kin was not required to participate in this study in accordance with the national legislation and the institutional requirements.

AUTHOR CONTRIBUTIONS

RF, GR, MD, MO-S, MB, and M-CP performed the experiments. FG and EL aided with statistical analysis. EC aided with the sequencing analysis and the sequence submission to the NCBI platform. M-CP conceived and supervised the study. M-CP, AC, IM, and AP-S wrote the manuscript and analyzed the data. MO-S performed ERIC-PCR.

FUNDING

This work was supported by the Fundação de Amparo a Pesquisa do Estado de São Paulo (FAPESP grants 2020/05699-6 to M-CP and FAPESP grant 2013/22581-5 to AP-S) and Conselho Nacional de Desenvolvimento Científico e Tecnológico (CNPq, grant 2013/485873 to M-CP). This study was partially financed by the Fundação de Amparo á Pesquisa do Estado de São Paulo-Brazil (FAPESP) as a fellowship to MD (FAPESP fellowship 2018/24213-7), and by the Coordenação de Aperfeiçoamento de Pessoal de Nível Superior – Brazil (CAPES) – Finance Code 001 as a fellowship to GR, FG, and EC.

ACKNOWLEDGMENTS

The authors thank the Laboratório Central de Saúde Pública do Tocantins, Palmas, TO, Brazil (LACEN-TO) who kindly provided the *S. marcescens* strains, and to Secretaria de Saúde do Estado do Tocantins (SESAU-TO) for facilitating the development of project.

REFERENCES

Aggarwal, C., Paul, S., Tripathi, V., Paul, B., and Khan, M. A. (2017). Characterization of putative virulence factors of *Serratia marcescens* strain SEN for pathogenesis in *Spodoptera litura*. *J. Invertebr. Pathol.* 143, 115–123. doi: 10.1016/j.jip.2016.12.004

Anderson, K. F., Lonsway, D. R., Rasheed, J. K., Biddle, J., Jensen, B., McDougal, L. K., et al. (2007). Evaluation of methods to identify the *Klebsiella pneumoniae* Carbapenemase in *Enterobacteriaceae*. *J. Clin. Microbiol.* 45, 2723–2725. doi: 10.1128/JCM.00015-07

Begic, S., and Worobec, E. A. (2008). Characterization of the *Serratia marcescens* SdeCDE multidrug efflux pump studied via gene knockout mutagenesis. *Can. J. Microbiol.* 54, 411–416. doi: 10.1139/w08-019

Bush, K. (2010). The coming of age of antibiotics: discovery and therapeutic value. *Ann. N. Y. Acad. Sci.* 1213, 1–4. doi: 10.1111/j.1749-6632.2010.05872.x

Cao, X., Xu, X., Zhang, Z., Shen, H., Chen, J., and Zhang, K. (2014). Molecular characterization of clinical multidrug-resistant *Klebsiella pneumoniae* isolates. *Ann. Clin. Microbiol. Antimicrob.* 13:16. doi: 10.1186/1476-0711-13-16

Chen, J., Kuroda, T., Huda, M. N., Mizushima, T., and Tsuchiya, T. (2003). An RND-type multidrug efflux pump SdeXY from *Serratia marcescens*. *J. Antimicrob. Chemother.* 52, 176–179. doi: 10.1093/jac/dkg308

Cheng, K., Chuang, Y., Wu, L., Huang, G., and Yu, W. (2006). Clinical experiences of the infections caused by extended-spectrum beta-lactamase-producing *Serratia marcescens* at a medical center in Taiwan. *Jpn. J. Infect. Dis.* 59, 147–152.

Chilcott, G. S., and Hughes, K. T. (2000). Coupling of flagellar gene expression to flagellar assembly in *Salmonella enterica* serovar typhimurium and *Escherichia coli*. *Microbiol. Mol. Biol. Rev.* 64, 694–708. doi: 10.1128/mmbr.64.4.694-708. 2000

CLSI (2019). *Performance Standards for Antimicrobial Susceptibility Testing. CLSI Supplement M100*, 29th Edn. Wayne, PA: Clinical and Laboratory Standards Institute.

Cristina, M. L., Sartini, M., and Spagnolo, A. M. (2019). *Serratia marcescens* Infections in Neonatal Intensive Care Units (NICUs). *Int. J. Environ. Res. Public Health* 16:E610. doi: 10.3390/ijerph16040610

da Costa Guimarães, A. C., Almeida, A. C. S., Nicoletti, A. G., Vilela, M. A., Gales, A. C., and Morais, M. M. C. (2013). Clonal spread of carbapenem-resistant *Serratia marcescens* isolates sharing an IncK plasmid containing blaKPC-2. *Int. J. Antimicrob. Agents* 42, 369–370. doi: 10.1016/j.ijantimicag.2013. 05.017

Dallenne, C., Da Costa, A., Decre, D., Favier, C., and Arlet, G. (2010). Development of a set of multiplex PCR assays for the detection of genes encoding important

ß-lactamases in *Enterobacteriaceae*. *J. Antimicrob. Chemother.* 65, 490–495. doi: 10.1093/jac/dkp498

Dalvi, S. D., and Worobec, E. A. (2012). Gene expression analysis of the SdeAB multidrug efflux pump in antibiotic-resistant clinical isolates of *Serratia marcescens*. *Indian J. Med. Microbiol.* 30, 302–307. doi: 10.4103/0255-0857. 99491

David, M. D., Weller, T. M., Lambert, P., and Fraise, A. P. (2006). An outbreak of *Serratia marcescens* on the neonatal unit: a tale of two clones. *J. Hosp. Infect.* 63, 27–33. doi: 10.1016/j.jhin.2005.11.006

Dawczynski, K., Proquitté, H., Roedel, J., Edel, B., Pfeifer, Y., Hoyer, H., et al. (2016). Intensified colonisation screening according to the recommendations of the German Commission for Hospital Hygiene and Infectious Diseases Prevention (KRINKO): identification and containment of a *Serratia marcescens* outbreak in the neonatal intensive care unit, Jena, Germany, 2013–2014. *Infection* 44, 739–746. doi: 10.1007/s15010-016-0922-y

Doyle, D., Peirano, G., Lascols, C., Lloyd, T., Church, D. L., and Pitout, J. D. (2012). Laboratory detection of *Enterobacteriaceae* that produce carbapenemases. *J. Clin. Microbiol.* 50, 3877–3880. doi: 10.1128/JCM.02117-12

Enciso-Moreno, J. A., Pernas-Buitrón, N., Ortiz-Herrera, M., and Coria-Jiménez, R. (2004). Identification of *Serratia marcescens* populations of nosocomial origin by RAPD-PCR. *Arch. Med. Res.* 35, 12–17. doi: 10.1016/j.arcmed.2003. 07.005

EUCAST (2018). The European Committee on Antimicrobial Susceptibility Testing . 2018. Breakpoint tables for Interpretation of MICs and Zone Diameters. Available online at: https://www.eucast.org/fileadmin/src/media/PDFs/EUCAST_files/Breakpoint_tables/v_8.1_Breakpoint_Tables.pdf

Falagas, M. E., Grammatikos, A. P., and Michalopoulos, A. (2008). Potential of old-generation antibiotics to address current need for new antibiotics. *Expert Rev. Anti Infect. Ther.* 6, 593–600. doi: 10.1586/14787210.6.5.593

Ferreira, R. L., Silva, B. C. M., Rezende, G. S., Nakamura-Silva, R., Pitondo-Silva, A., Campanini, E. B., et al. (2019). High prevalence of multidrug-resistant *Klebsiella pneumoniae* harboring several virulence and β-Lactamase encoding genes in a Brazilian intensive care unit. *Front. Microbiol.* 9:3198. doi: 10.3389/fmicb.2018. 03198

Ferreira-Firmo, E., Beltrão, E. M. B., da Silva, F. R. F., Alves, L. C., Brayner, F. A., Veras, D. L., et al. (2019). Association of blaNDM-1 with blaKPC-2 and aminoglycoside-modifying enzymes genes among *Klebsiella pneumoniae*, *Proteus mirabilis* and *Serratia marcescens* clinical isolates in Brazil. *J. Glob. Antimicrob. Resist.* doi: 10.1016/j.jgar.2019.08.026 [Epub ahead of print].

Fineran, P. C., Slater, H., Everson, L., Hughes, K., and Salmond, G. P. (2005). Biosynthesis of tripyrrole and beta-lactam secondary metabolites in *Serratia*: integration of quorum sensing with multiple new regulatory components in the control of prodigiosin and carbapenem antibiotic production. *Mol. Microbiol.* 56, 1495–1517. doi: 10.1111/j.1365-2958.2005.04660.x

Fraser, G. M., and Hughes, C. (1999). Swarming motility. *Curr. Opin. Microbiol.* 2, 630–635.

Gad, G. F., Heba, A., Mohamed, and Hossam, M. A. (2011). aminoglycoside resistance rates, phenotypes, and mechanisms of Gram-negative bacteria from infected patients in upper Egypt. *PLoS One* 6:e17224. doi: 10.1371/journal.pone.0017224

Gastmeier, P. (2014). *Serratia marcescens*: an outbreak experience. *Front. Microbiol.* 5:81. doi: 10.3389/fmicb.2014.00081

Gastmeier, P., Loui, A., Stamm-Balderjahn, S., Hansen, S., Zuschneid, I., Sohr, D., et al. (2007). Outbreaks in neonatal intensive care units-they are not like others. *Am. J. Infect. Control* 35, 172–176. doi: 10.1016/j.ajic.2006.07.007

Ghaith, D. M., Zafer, M. M., Ismail, D. K., Al-Agamy, M. H., Bohol, M. F. F., Al-Qahtani, A., et al. (2018). First reported nosocomial outbreak of *Serratia marcescens* harboring bla IMP-4 and bla VIM-2 in a neonatal intensive care unit in Cairo, Egypt. *Infect. Drug Resist.* 11, 2211–2217. doi: 10.2147/IDR.S174869

Givskov, M., Eberl, L., Christiansen, G., Benedik, M. J., and Molin, S. (1995). Induction of phospholipase- and flagellar synthesis in *Serratia liquefaciens* is controlled by expression of the flagellar master operon flhD. *Mol. Microbiol.* 15, 445–454. doi: 10.1111/j.1365-2958.1995.tb02258.x

Hall, T. A. (1999). BioEdit: a user-friendly biological sequence alignment editor and analysis program for Windows 95/98/NT. *Nucleic Acids Symp. Ser.* 41, 95–98.

Hejazi, A., and Falkiner, F. R. (1997). Serratia marcescens. *J. Med. Microbiol.* 46, 903–912.

Herra, C., and Falkiner, F. R. (2018). *Serratia marcescens. In: Antimicrobe Microbes.* Available online at: http://www.antimicrobe.org/b26.asp (accessed June 8, 2019).

Hornsey, M., Ellington, M. J., Doumith, M., Hudson, S., Livermore, D. M., and Woodford, N. (2010). Tigecycline resistance in *Serratia marcescens* associated with up-regulation of the SdeXY-HasF efflux system also active against ciprofloxacin and cefpirome. *J. Antimicrob. Chemother.* 65, 479–482. doi: 10.1093/jac/dkp475

Hou, X. H., Song, X. Y., Ma, X. B., Zhang, S. Y., and Zhang, J. Q. (2015). Molecular characterization of multidrug-resistant *Klebsiella pneumoniae* isolates. *Braz. J. Microbiol.* 46, 759–768. doi: 10.1590/S1517-838246320140138

Jeon, J., Lee, J., Lee, J., Park, K., Karim, A., Lee, C., et al. (2015). Structural basis for carbapenem-hydrolyzing mechanisms of carbapenemases conferring antibiotic resistance. *Int. J. Mol. Sci.* 16, 9654–9692. doi: 10.3390/ijms16059654

Kim, E. S., Jeong, J. Y., Jun, J. B., Choi, S. H., Lee, S. O., Kim, M. N., et al. (2009). Prevalence of aac(6')-Ib-cr encoding a ciprofloxacin-modifying enzyme among *Enterobacteriaceae* blood isolates in Korea. *Antimicrob. Agents Chemother.* 53, 2643–2645. doi: 10.1128/AAC.01534-08

Kim, J., Lim, Y.-M., Jeong, Y.-S., and Seol, S.-Y. (2005). Occurrence of CTX-M-3, CTX-M-15, CTX-M-14, and CTX-M-9 Extended-Spectrum -Lactamases in *Enterobacteriaceae* Clinical Isolates in Korea. *Antimicrob. Agents Chemother.* 49, 1572–1575. doi: 10.1128/AAC.49.4.1572-1575.2005

Kim, S. B., Jeon, Y. D., Kim, J. H., Kim, J. K., Ann, H. W., Choi, H., et al. (2015). Risk factors for mortality in patients with *Serratia marcescens* bacteremia. *Yonsei Med. J.* 56:348. doi: 10.3349/ymj.2015.56.2.348

Kim, Y. T., Jang, J. H., Kim, H. C., Kim, H., Lee, K. R., Park, K. S., et al. (2011). Identification of strain harboring both aac(6')-Ib and aac(6')-Ib-cr variant simultaneously in *Escherichia coli* and *Klebsiella pneumoniae*. *BMB Rep.* 4, 262–266. doi: 10.5483/BMBRep.2011.44.4.262

Ko, W. C., Paterson, D. L., Sagnimeni, A. J., Hansen, D. S., Von Gottberg, A., Mohapatra, S., et al. (2002). Community-acquired *Klebsiella pneumoniae* bacteremia: global differences in clinical patterns. *Emerg. Infect Dis.* 8, 160–166. doi: 10.3201/eid0802.010025

Krishnan, P. U., Pereira, B., and Macaden, R. (1991). Epidemiological study of an outbreak of *Serratia marcescens* in a haemodialysis unit. *J. Hosp. Infect.* 18, 57–61. doi: 10.1016/0195-6701(91)90093-n

Kumar, A., and Worobec, E. A. (2005a). Cloning, sequencing, and characterization of the SdeAB multidrug efflux pump of *Serratia marcescens*. *Antimicrob Agents Chemother.* 49, 1495–1501. doi: 10.1128/AAC.49.4.1495-1501.2005

Kumar, A., and Worobec, E. A. (2005b). HasF, a TolC-homolog of *Serratia marcescens*, is involved in energy-dependent efflux. *Can. J. Microbiol.* 51, 497–500. doi: 10.1139/w05-029

Kurz, C. L., Chauvet, S., Andrès, E., Aurouze, M., Vallet, I., Michel, G. P., et al. (2003). Virulence factors of the human opportunistic pathogen *Serratia marcescens* identified by in vivo screening. *EMBO J.* 22, 1451–1460. doi: 10.1093/emboj/cdg159

Levy, S. B., and Marshall, B. (2004). Antibacterial resistance worldwide: causes, challenges and responses. *Nat. Med.* 10, S122–S129. doi: 10.1038/nm1145

Li, H., and Li, J. B. (2005). Detection of five novel CTX-M-type extended spectrum beta-lactamases with one to three CTX-M-14 point mutations in isolates from Hefei, Anhui province, China. *J. Clin. Microbiol.* 43, 4301–4302. doi: 10.1128/JCM.43.8.4301-4302.2005

Lin, C. S., Horng, J. T., Yang, C. H., Tsai, Y. H., Su, L. H., Wei, C. F., et al. (2010). RssAB-FlhDC-ShlBA as a major pathogenesis pathway in *Serratia marcescens*. *Infect. Immun.* 78, 4870–4881. doi: 10.1128/IAI.00661-10

Lin, X., Hu, Q., Zhang, R., Hu, Y., Xu, X., and Lv, H. (2016). Emergence of *Serratia marcescens* isolates possessing carbapenem-hydrolysing ß-lactamase KPC-2 from China. *J. Hosp. Infect.* 94, 65–67. doi: 10.1016/j.jhin.2016.04.006

Liou, B. H., Duh, R. W., Lin, Y. T., Lauderdale, T. L., and Fung, C. P. (2014). Taiwan surveillance of antimicrobial resistance (TSAR) hospitals. *J. Microbiol. Immunol. Infect.* 47, 387–393. doi: 10.1016/j.jmii.2013.04.003

Liu, Y. Y., Wang, Y., Walsh, T. R., Yi, L. X., Zhang, R., Spencer, J., et al. (2015). Emergence of plasmid mediated colistin resistance mechanism MCR-1 in animals and human beings in China: a microbiological and molecular biological study. *Lancet Infect.* 16, 161–168. doi: 10.1016/S1473-3099(15)00424-7

Magiorakos, A.-P., Srinivasan, A., Carey, R. B., Carmeli, Y., Falagas, M. E., Giske, C. G., et al. (2012). Multidrug-resistant, extensively drug-resistant and pandrug-resistant bacteria: an international expert proposal for interim standard definitions for acquired resistance. *Clin. Microbiol. Infect.* 18, 268–281. doi: 10.1111/j.1469-0691.2011.03570.x

Mahlen, S. D. (2011). *Serratia* infections: from military experiments to current practice. *Clin. Microbiol. Rev.* 24, 755–791. doi: 10.1128/CMR.00017-11

Maragakis, L. L., Winkler, A., Tucker, M. G., Cosgrove, S. E., Ross, T., Lawson, E., et al. (2008). Outbreak of multidrug-resistant *Serratia marcescens* infection in a neonatal intensive care unit. *Infect. Control Hosp. Epidemiol.* 29, 418–423. doi: 10.1086/587969

Marschall, J., Tibbetts, R. J., Dunne, W. M., Frye, J. G., Fraser, V. J., and Warren, D. K. (2009). Presence of the KPC carbapenemase gene in *Enterobacteriaceae* causing bacteremia and its correlation with in vitro carbapenem susceptibility. *J. Clin. Microbiol.* 47, 239–241. doi: 10.1128/JCM.02123-08

Martineau, C., Li, X., Lalancette, C., Perreault, T., Fournier, E., Tremblay, J., et al. (2018). *Serratia marcescens* outbreak in a neonatal intensive care unit: new insights from next-generation sequencing applications. J. Clin. Microbiol. 56:e00235-18. doi: 10.1128/JCM.00235-18

Martins, A. F., Zavascki, A. P., Gaspareto, P. B., and Barth, A. L. (2007). Dissemination of *Pseudomonas aeruginosa* producing SPM-1-like and IMP-1-like metallo-beta-lactamases in hospitals from southern Brazil. *Infection* 35, 457–460. doi: 10.1007/s15010-007-6289-3

Merkier, A. K., Rodríguez, C., Togneri, A., Brengi, S., Osuna, C., and Pichel, M. (2013). Outbreak of a cluster with epidemic behavior due to *Serratia marcescens* after colistin administration in a hospital setting. *J. Clin. Microbiol.* 51, 2295–2302. doi: 10.1128/JCM.03280-12

Milisavljevic, V., Wu, F., Larson, E., Rubenstein, D., Ross, B., Drusin, L. M., et al. (2004). Molecular epidemiology of *Serratia marcescens* outbreaks in two neonatal intensive care units. *Infect. Control Hosp. Epidemiol.* 25, 719–721. doi: 10.1086/502466

Miriagou, V., Cornaglia, G., Edelstein, M., Galani, I., Giske, C. G., Gniadkowski, M., et al. (2010). Acquired carbapenemases in Gram-negative bacterial pathogens: detection and surveillance issue. *Clin. Microbiol. Infect.* 16, 112–122. doi: 10.1111/j.1469-0691.2009.03116.x

Mitra, S., Mukherjee, S., Naha, S., Chattopadhyay, P., Dutta, S., and Basu, S. (2019). Evaluation of co-transfer of plasmid-mediated fluoroquinolone resistance genes and bla NDM gene in *Enterobacteriaceae* causing neonatal septicaemia. *Antimicrob. Resist. Infect. Control* 8:46. doi: 10.1186/s13756-019-0477-7

Montagnani, C., Cocchi, P., and Lega, L. (2015). *Serratia marcescens* outbreak in a neonatal intensive care unit: crucial role of implementing hand hygiene among external consultants. *BMC Infect. Dis.* 15:11. doi: 10.1186/s12879-014-0734-6

Moradigaravand, D., Boinett, C. J., Martin, V., Peacock, S. J., and Parkhill, J. (2016). Recent independent emergence of multiple multidrug-resistant *Serratia marcescens* clones within the United Kingdom and Ireland. *Genome Res.* 26, 1101–1109. doi: 10.1101/gr.205245.116.Freely

Mostatabi, N., Farshad, S., and Ranjbar, R. (2013). Molecular evaluations of extended spectrum β-lactamase producing strains of *Serratia* isolated from blood samples of the patients in Namazi Hospital, Shiraz, Southern Iran. *Iran. J. Microbiol.* 5, 328–333.

Naas, T., Cuzon, G., Villegas, M.-V., Lartigue, M.-F., Quinn, J. P., and Nordmann, P. (2008). Genetic structures at the origin of acquisition of the beta-lactamase bla KPC gene. *Antimicrob. Agents Chemother.* 52, 1257–1263. doi: 10.1128/AAC.01451-07

Nordmann, P., Naas, T., and Poirel, L. (2011). Global Spread of Carbapenemase-producing *Enterobacteriaceae*. *Emerg. Infect. Dis.* 17, 1791–1798. doi: 10.3201/eid1710.110655

O'Horo, J., Mahler, S. B., Gardner, B., and Berbari, E. F. (2017). *Serratia* and Surgical Site Infections: risk factors and Epidemiology. *Open Forum Infect. Dis.* 4, S650–S650. doi: 10.1093/ofid/ofx163.1730

Okoche, D., Asiimwe, B. B., Katabazi, F. A., Kato, L., and Najjuka, C. F. (2015). Prevalence and characterization of carbapenem-resistant *Enterobacteriaceae* Isolated from Mulago National Referral Hospital, Uganda. *PLoS One* 10:e0135745. doi: 10.1371/journal.pone.0135745

Phan, H. T. T., Stoesser, N., Maciuca, I. E., Toma, F., Szekely, E., Flonta, M., et al. (2018). Illumina short-read and MinION long-read WGS to characterize the molecular epidemiology of an NDM-1 *Serratia marcescens* outbreak in Romania. *J. Antimicrob. Chemother.* 73, 672–679. doi: 10.1093/jac/dkx456

Platell, J. L., Cobbold, R. N., Johnson, J. R., Heisig, A., Heisig, P., Clabots, C., et al. (2011). Commonality among fluoroquinolone-resistant sequence type ST131 extraintestinal *Escherichia coli* isolates from humans and companion animals in Australia. *Antimicrob Agents Chemother.* 55, 3782–3787. doi: 10.1128/AAC.00306-11

Poirel, L., Cattoir, V., and Nordmann, P. (2012). Plasmid-mediated quinolone resistance; interactions between Human, Animal, and Environmental Ecologies. *Front. Microbiol.* 3:24.

Poirel, L., Dortet, L., Bernabeu, S., and Nordmann, P. (2011). Genetic features of blaNDM-1-Positive *Enterobacteriaceae*. *Antimicrob. Agents Chemother.* 55, 5403–5407. doi: 10.1128/AAC.00585-11

Queenan, A. M., and Bush, K. (2007). Carbapenemases: the Versatile betalactamases. *Clin. Microbiol. Rev.* 20, 440–458. doi: 10.1128/CMR.00001-07

Rawat, D., and Nair, D. (2010). Extended-spectrum ß-lactamases in gram negative bacteria. *J. Glob. Infect. Dis.* 2, 263–274. doi: 10.4103/0974-777X.68531

Raymond, J., and Aujard, Y. (2000). Nosocomial infections in pediatric patients: a European, multicenter prospective study. European study group. *Infect. Control Hosp. Epidemiol.* 21, 260–263. doi: 10.1086/501755

Ribeiro, P. C. S., Monteiro, A. S., Marques, S. G., Monteiro, S. G., Monteiro-Neto, V., Coqueiro, M. M. M., et al. (2016). Phenotypic and molecular detection of the blaKPC gene in clinical isolates from inpatients at hospitals in São Luis, MA, Brazil. *BMC Infect. Dis.* 16:737. doi: 10.1186/s12879-016-2072-3

Ribeiro, V. B., Andrade, L. N., Linhares, A. R., Barin, J., Darini, A. L. D. C., Zavascki, A. P., et al. (2013). Molecular characterization of *Klebsiella pneumoniae* carbapenemase-producing isolates in southern Brazil. *J. Med. Microbiol.* 62, 1721–1727. doi: 10.1099/jmm.0.062141-0

Sader, H. S., Farrell, D. J., Flamm, R. K., and Jones, R. N. (2014). Antimicrobial susceptibility of Gram-negative organisms isolated from patients hospitalized in intensive care units in United States and European hospitals (2009–2011). *Diagn. Microbiol. Infect. Dis.* 78, 443–448. doi: 10.1016/j.diagmicrobio.2013.11.025

Salini, R., and Pandian, S. K. (2015). Interference of quorum sensing in urinary pathogen *Serratia marcescens* by *Anethum graveolens*. *Pathog. Dis.* 73:ftv038. doi: 10.1093/femspd/ftv038

Sandner-Miranda, L., Vinuesa, P., Cravioto, A., and Morales-Espinosa, R. (2018). The genomic basis of intrinsic and acquired antibiotic resistance in the genus *Serratia*. *Front. Microbiol.* 9:828. doi: 10.3389/fmicb.2018.00828

Seeyave, D., Desai, N., Miller, S., Rao, S. P., and Piecuch, S. (2006). Fatal delayed transfusion reaction in a sickle cell anemia patient with *Serratia marcescens* sepsis. *J. Natl. Med. Assoc.* 98, 1697–1699.

Shanks, R. M. Q., Lahr, R. M., Stella, N. A., Arena, K. E., Brothers, K. M., Kwak, D. H., et al. (2013). A *Serratia marcescens* PigP homolog controls prodigiosin biosynthesis, swarming motility and hemolysis and is regulated by cAMP-CRP and HexS. *PLoS One* 8:e57634. doi: 10.1371/journal.pone.0057634

Sheng, W. H., Chen, Y. C., Wang, J. T., Chang, S. C., Luh, K. T., and Hsieh, W. C. (2002). Emerging fluoroquinolone-resistance for common clinically important gram-negative bacteria in Taiwan. *Diagn. Microbiol. Infect. Dis.* 43, 141–147. doi: 10.1016/S0732-8893(02)00381-4

Silva, D. D. C., Rampelotto, R. F., Lorenzoni, V. V., Santos, S. O. D., Damer, J., Hörner, M., et al. (2017). Phenotypic methods for screening carbapenem-resistant *Enterobacteriaceae* and assessment of their antimicrobial susceptibility profile. *Rev. Soc. Bras. Med. Trop.* 50, 173–178. doi: 10.1590/0037-8682-0471-2016

Silva, K. E., Cayô, R., Carvalhaes, C. G., Sacchi, F. P. C., Rodrigues-Costa, F., Da Silva, A. C. R., et al. (2015). Coproduction of KPC-2 and IMP-10 in Carbapenem-Resistant *Serratia marcescens* isolates from an outbreak in a Brazilian teaching hospital. *J. Clin. Microbiol.* 53, 2324–2328. doi: 10.1128/JCM.00727-15

Srinivasan, R., Mohankumar, R., Kannappan, A., Karthick Raja, V., Archunan, G., Karutha Pandian, S., et al. (2017). Exploring the anti-quorum sensing and antibiofilm efficacy of phytol against *Serratia marcescens* associated acute pyelonephritis infection in Wistar rats. *Front. Cell. Infect. Microbiol.* 7:498. doi: 10.3389/fcimb.2017.00498

Stock, I., Grueger, T., and Wiedemann, B. (2003). Natural antibiotic susceptibility of strains of *Serratia marcescens* and the *S. liquefaciens* complex: *S. liquefaciens* sensu stricto, *S. proteamaculans* and *S. grimesii*. *Int. J. Antimicrob. Agents* 22, 35–47. doi: 10.1016/s0924-8579(02)00163-2

Sugumar, M., Kumar, K. M., Manoharan, A., Anbarasu, A., and Ramaiah, S. (2014). Detection of OXA-1 β-lactamase gene of *Klebsiella pneumoniae* from blood stream infections (BSI) by conventional PCR and in-silico analysis to understand the mechanism of OXA mediated resistance. *PLoS One* 9:e91800. doi: 10.1371/journal.pone.0091800

Tenover, F. C., Canton, R., Kop, J., Chan, R., Ryan, J., Weir, F., et al. (2013). Detection of Colonization by Carbapenemase-Producing Gram-Negative Bacilli in Patients by Use of the Xpert MDRO Assay. *J. Clin. Microbiol.* 51, 3780–3787. doi: 10.1128/JCM.01092-13

Tzouvelekis, L. S., Markogiannakis, A., Psichogiou, M., Tassios, P. T., and Daikos, G. L. (2012). Carbapenemases in *Klebsiella pneumoniae* and Other *Enterobacteriaceae*: an Evolving Crisis of Global Dimensions. *Clin. Microbiol. Rev.* 25, 682–707. doi: 10.1128/CMR.05035-11

Ulu-Kilic, A., Parkan, O., Ersoy, S., Koc, D., Percin, D., Onal, O., et al. (2013). Outbreak of postoperative empyema caused by *Serratia marcescens* in a thoracic surgery unit. *J. Hosp. Infect.* 85, 226–229. doi: 10.1016/j.jhin.2013.07.008

Us, E., Kutlu, H. H., Tekeli, A., Ocal, D., Cirpan, S., and Memikoglu, K. O. (2017). Wound and soft tissue infections of *Serratia marcescens* in patients receiving wound care: a health care–associated outbreak. *Am. J. Infect. Control* 45, 443–447. doi: 10.1016/j.ajic.2016.11.015

Veldman, K., Cavaco, L. M., Mevius, D., Battisti, A., Franco, A., Botteldoorn, N., et al. (2011). International collaborative study on the occurrence of plasmid-mediated quinolone resistance in *Salmonella enterica* and *Escherichia coli* isolated from animals, humans, food and the environment in 13 European countries. *J. Antimicrob. Chemother.* 66, 1278–1286. doi: 10.1093/jac/dkr084

Versalovic, J., Schneider, M., De Bruijn, F. J., and Lupski, J. R. (1994). Genomic fingerprinting of bacteria using repetitive sequence-based polymerase chain reaction Meth. *Mol. Cell. Biol.* 5, 25–40. doi: 10.1128/JCM.43.1.199-207.2005

Vetter, L., Schuepfer, G., Kuster, S. P., and Rossi, M. (2016). A Hospital-wide Outbreak of *Serratia marcescens*, and Ishikawa's "Fishbone" Analysis to Support Outbreak Control. *Qual. Manag. Health Care* 25, 1–7. doi: 10.1097/QMH.0000000000000078

von Wintersdorff, C. J., Penders, J., van Niekerk, J. M., Mills, N. D., Majumder, S., van Alphen, L. B., et al. (2016). Dissemination of antimicrobial resistance in microbial ecosystems through horizontal gene transfer. *Front. Microbiol.* 19:173. doi: 10.3389/fmicb.2016.00173

Wong, M. H., Chan, E. W., Liu, L. Z., and Chen, S. (2014). PMQR genes oqxAB and aac(6')Ib-cr accelerate the development of fluoroquinolone resistance in *Salmonella typhimurium*. *Front. Microbiol.* 5:521. doi: 10.3389/fmicb.2014.00521

Xiong, Z., Li, T., Xu, Y., and Li, J. (2007). Detection of CTX-M-14 extended-spectrum β-lactamase in *Shigella sonnei* isolates from China. *J. Infect.* 55, e125–e128. doi: 10.1016/j.jinf.2007.07.017

Yan, B. C., Westfall, B. A., and Orlean, P. (2001). Ynl038wp (Gpi15p) is the *Saccharomyces cerevisiae* homologue of human Pig-Hp and participates in the first step in glycosylphosphatidylinositol assembly. *Yeast* 18, 1383–1389. doi: 10.1002/yea.783

Yoon, H. J., Choi, J. Y., Park, Y. S., Kim, C. O., Kim, J. M., Yong, D. E., et al. (2005). Outbreaks of Serratia marcescens bacteriuria in a neurosurgical intensive care unit of a tertiary care teaching hospital: a clinical, epidemiologic, and laboratory perspective. *Am. J. Infect. Control* 33, 595–601. doi: 10.1016/j.ajic.2005.01.010

Young, V. M., Moody, M. R., and Morris, M. J. (1980). Distribution of *Serratia marcescens* serotypes in cancer patients. *J. Med. Microbiol.* 13, 333–339. doi: 10.1099/00222615-13-2-333

Yu, W. L., Lin, C. W., and Wang, D. Y. (1998). *Serratia marcescens* bacteremia: clinical features and antimicrobial susceptibilities of the isolates. *J. Microbiol. Immunol. Infect.* 31, 171–179.

Yu, W. L., Wu, L. T., Pfaller, M. A., Winokur, P. L., and Jones, R. N. (2003). Confirmation of extended-spectrum beta-lactamase-producing *Serratia marcescens*: preliminary report from Taiwan. *Diagn. Microbiol. Infect. Dis.* 45, 221–224. doi: 10.1016/s0732-8893(02)00539-4

Zingg, W., Soulake, I., Baud, D., Huttner, B., Pfister, R., Renzi, G., et al. (2017). Management and investigation of a *Serratia marcescens* outbreak in a neonatal unit in Switzerland - the role of hand hygiene and whole genome sequencing. *Antimicrob. Resist. Infect. Control* 6:125. doi: 10.1186/s13756-017-0285-x

4

Clinical Impact of Antibiotics for the Treatment of *Pseudomonas aeruginosa* Biofilm Infections

Elodie Olivares[1,2]*, Stéphanie Badel-Berchoux[3], Christian Provot[2,3], Gilles Prévost[1], Thierry Bernardi[2,3] and François Jehl[1]

[1] University of Strasbourg, CHRU Strasbourg, Fédération de Médecine Translationnelle de Strasbourg, EA7290, Institut de Bactériologie, Strasbourg, France, [2] BioFilm Pharma SAS, Saint-Beauzire, France, [3] BioFilm Control SAS, Saint-Beauzire, France

*Correspondence:
Elodie Olivares
elodie.olivares@biofilmpharma.com

Bacterial biofilms are highly recalcitrant to antibiotic therapies due to multiple tolerance mechanisms. The involvement of *Pseudomonas aeruginosa* in a wide range of biofilm-related infections often leads to treatment failures. Indeed, few current antimicrobial molecules are still effective on tolerant sessile cells. In contrast, studies increasingly showed that conventional antibiotics can, at low concentrations, induce a phenotype change in bacteria and consequently, the biofilm formation. Understanding the clinical effects of antimicrobials on biofilm establishment is essential to avoid the use of inappropriate treatments in the case of biofilm infections. This article reviews the current knowledge about bacterial growth within a biofilm and the preventive or inducer impact of standard antimicrobials on its formation by *P. aeruginosa*. The effect of antibiotics used to treat biofilms of other bacterial species, as *Staphylococcus aureus* or *Escherichia coli*, was also briefly mentioned. Finally, it describes two *in vitro* devices which could potentially be used as antibiotic susceptibility testing for adherent bacteria.

Keywords: biofilms, antibiotic tolerance, biofilm-related infections, *Pseudomonas aeruginosa*, clinical laboratory technique, MBEC assay, antibiofilmogram

INTRODUCTION

Bacterial biofilm was defined for the first time in 1978 as a structured community of microorganisms adhering to a surface and producing an extracellular matrix of polysaccharides (Costerton et al., 1978). It represents a particular behavior of bacteria triggered by the proximity of a surface and involving complex signaling networks, including quorum sensing (QS). Its discovery was attributed to the microscope inventor, Antoni Van Leeuwenhoek who observed bacteria clusters on dental plaque in 1684. He wrote in a report for the Royal Society of London: "The number of these animalcules in the scurf of a man's teeth are so many that I believe they exceed the number of men in a kingdom" (Biofilms: The Hypertextbook, 2011).

Nowadays, it is well-recognized that biofilms play an ecological role and have a significant impact in medicine by the development of healthcare-associated infections. The National Institutes of Health (NIH) estimated that bacterial biofilms are involved in 65% of microbial diseases and in more than 80% of chronic infections (Jamal et al., 2018). Sessile cells can colonize indwelling medical devices as any type of catheters, contact lenses, heart valves, and protheses. Their presence on retrieved infected implants is easily detectable by laboratory methods. Indeed, bacterial colony outgrowths can be revealed by culturing techniques but can also be directly visualized by microscopy methodologies (Dibartola et al., 2017). Biofilm formation is equally involved in non-device-associated infections as periodontitis, osteomyelitis, and chronic infections (Srivastava and Bhargava, 2016). *Pseudomonas aeruginosa* biofilms are particularly deadly in cystic fibrosis (CF) patients. They also have a relevant impact on clinical outcomes of patients with chronic wounds (Mulcahy et al., 2014). Relevant animal models are now available to study the involvement of *P. aeruginosa* sessile cells *in vivo* infections. Diabetic wounds were mimicked in mice by Watters et al. (2013) and a porcine model allowed replicating the development of bacterial infections in CF lungs (Pezzulo et al., 2012).

A specific feature of sessile cells is their inherent tolerance to antimicrobials. Despite this basic knowledge, classical antibiotic susceptibility testing, providing the minimal inhibitory concentration (MIC) of molecules, is performed on non-adherent bacteria. Results collected according to antibiogram methods cannot predict the therapeutic success of the corresponding antibiotic therapies against biofilms. Furthermore, it is now well-recognized that low doses of antibiotics, encountered during continuous and fluctuating treatments, can stimulate biofilm establishment and are partly responsible for biofilm-specific antimicrobial tolerance.

Currently, no guidelines exist to help clinicians treat this kind of infections, although they are involved in the majority of untreatable clinical cases. Therefore, it appears urgent to develop a susceptibility test specific to biofilm or to validate a new-existing method for a routine use in diagnostic labs.

This review summarizes the basic knowledge about the growth of bacteria within a biofilm and the main steps of its formation. The tolerance features of sessile microorganisms to antimicrobial molecules were also detailed as well as the beneficial or deleterious effects of antibiotics for biofilm treatment. Available diagnostic tools for the selection of appropriate therapies against adherent bacteria are discussed herein.

THE BACTERIAL BIOFILM

A Community Way of Life

The growth of bacteria within biofilms is a natural process. The entirety of microorganisms could be sessile and live attached to a surface. This community mode is different from the planktonic growth, in which bacteria are isolated and mobile in the environment. The sessile cells differ from the planktonic ones by their morphology, physiology, and gene expression. The ability to adhere and grow on a surface as a biofilm is a survival strategy allowing the colonization of the environment by microorganisms. Bacteria continuously switch from a planktonic phenotype to a sessile one. This state variation is strategic for the cell as it allows a rapid adaptation to environmental conditions (Lebeaux and Ghigo, 2012).

The use of microscope can highlight a specific mushroom-like structure, especially for *P. aeruginosa* biofilms. They are mainly composed of microorganism clusters, delimited by aqueous channels. These latter separate bacterial microcolonies and allow the flow of oxygen and nutriments in the deepest areas of the biofilm as well as the elimination of degradation products. Nevertheless, it appears hard to generalize the composition, structure and features of biofilms owing to the wide range of environments and bacterial species. External factors, as medium composition and/or genetic properties of bacteria, contribute to the perpetual structure variation of the sessile population.

The key step of biofilm development is the synthesis of the extracellular matrix. It incorporates all the elements apart the bacterial cells. By forming up to 90% of its total organic matter, the matrix is the main structural component of the bacterial biofilm. It is highly hydrated and mainly composed of exopolysaccharides, proteins, nucleic acids, and minerals (Limoli et al., 2015). Its composition depends on the bacterial species and growth conditions. It allows strengthening of the biofilm structure while keeping a high flexibility. It also plays a protective role as it enhances the tolerance of bacteria to antimicrobials by creating a physical barrier that limits their diffusion to other environmental factors (UV, pH, and osmotic pressure variations, desiccation, etc.).

During the early development of the bacterial structure, it has been highlighted that extracellular DNA (eDNA) is essential for the adhesion of microorganisms and for their intercellular cohesion (Whitchurch et al., 2002). Quantitatively, in the biofilm matrix of *P. aeruginosa*, eDNA is six times more abundant than proteins and eighteen times more abundant than carbohydrates. Its origin was confirmed as being genomic. Nucleic acids can arise either from the lysis of a part of sessile cells or from an active secretion by living bacteria through merging membrane vesicles (Okshevsky and Meyer, 2015).

Development of a Mixed Environment

Bacterial biofilm can be formed in a few hours. Its general development consists of five main steps (Dufour et al., 2010). Mobile free-floating bacteria detect an available conditioned surface through environmental signals as pH variation, oxygen and nutriment concentrations, temperature, and osmolarity, etc. They are transported by physical forces or bacterial appendages (i.e., flagella). The flagellum is as much required in the surface arrival as in the biofilm formation initiation since mutants defective in its synthesis are not able to adhere (O'Toole and Kolter, 1998). In the same way, a complete but inactive flagellum does not allow the establishment of the biofilm (Vallet et al., 2001).

The increasing proximity of the support, which is conditioned by the fluids and flows to where it is exposed, allows the initial adhesion of bacterial cells by physicochemical and electrostatic interactions. At this stage, the adhesion is reversible (**Figure 1**). Besides the environmental influence, this attachment is strongly influenced by the nature of the surface itself. A rough and/or hydrophobic surface boosts the adhesion of microorganisms, contrary to a smooth and/or hydrophilic support. Furthermore, the organic molecules, which are present at the surface, also condition the cell attachment.

Following this first step, which can occur few seconds after the initial contact with the surface, a second stage of adhesion happens, allowing the strengthening of the bacteria-surface bonds by the implication of bacterial compounds, such as type IV pili or more generally, surface adhesins. The surface binding, becoming irreversible, enables subsequently the multiplication of adherent bacteria, and the formation of microcolonies.

As for the flagella, *P. aeruginosa* mutants defective in the production of type IV pili adhere to a surface by the formation of a cell monolayer but are not able to gather in microcolonies. This data confirms that the microcolony formation is a process

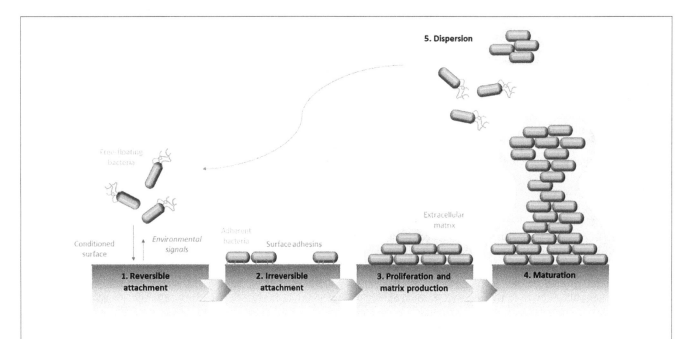

FIGURE 1 | Schematic representation of the five main steps defining the *Pseudomonas aeruginosa* biofilm development. The biofilm formation begins by the initial attachment of mobile bacterial cells to the surface and is followed by the irreversible adhesion of bacteria, which form a monolayer along the surface. Therefore, biofilm maturation is characterized by the matrix production and the formation of three-dimensional structures. Finally, the biofilm dispersion reflects its life end.

requiring bacterial mobility and not only a clonal growth from a bacterial cell (O'Toole and Kolter, 1998). In general, bacterial structures involved in the mobility of microorganisms are needed for the initial step of biofilm formation. They allow the approach and the colonization of the surface. The use of DNA microarrays on biofilms formed by the PAO1 strain, on sterilized granite pebbles in a continuous-culture model, showed that genes required for the synthesis of bacterial surface structures are repressed as soon as biofilm formation is initiated (Whiteley et al., 2001). They are no longer necessary for biofilm development and move on to compounds allowing its structuring and differentiation. It was shown that QS is involved in the structural steps of the biofilm. Analysis of *P. aeruginosa* wild type and *lasI* mutant highlighted an architectural difference in both biofilms (thinner and less heterogeneous for the mutant one) (Davies et al., 1998).

The first maturation step of biofilm development is defined by the production of the extracellular matrix. It allows a mechanical cohesion between bacterial cells and favors the switch from a "free life" to a "static life." Its composition fluctuates in space and time and determines the spatial configuration of the biofilm.

As for the gene inactivation of extracellular structures, studies on *P. aeruginosa* showed that bacteria have a "sense of touch," namely the ability to detect the presence of a surface and to combine a specific gene expression. During the first stages of adhesion, the transcription of genes involved in the alginate synthesis is activated to organize the matrix production after the formation of microcolonies (Davies and Geesey, 1995). More recent works showed that this gene regulation is directly dependent on the cyclic di-GMP (c-di-GMP), a central messenger present in the cytoplasm of bacterial cells, which controls the transition between the planktonic life and biofilm

establishment and whose intracellular concentration is affected by environmental stimuli (Donné and Dewilde, 2015).

If growth conditions are optimal, a second phase of biofilm maturation occurs, defined by a growth in thickness. Therefore, the mature biofilm shows a complex 3D-structure. It can acquire a typical "mushroom-like" shape formed by bacterial columns on the basement of cells and in which bacteria are mobile. The whole biofilm is surrounded by an extracellular matrix. Through this structure, channels remain and allow the transfer of oxygen and nutriments required for the growth of sessile bacteria. Gradients of oxygen and pH also set up from the top to the bottom of the biofilm. These variations of concentrations within the biofilm lead to metabolic activity and growth differences of bacteria even in a monomicrobial community, their activity being increased at the surface and reduced at its center. These physicochemical differences lead to a physiological heterogeneity of microorganisms and generate the formation of environmental microniches constituted by bacterial subpopulations that are genetically identical but physiologically distinct (concerning the tolerance against antimicrobials for instance).

The final step of the biofilm formation cycle is its destructuring. Biofilm dispersion can be initiated by various factors as mechanical disruptions (abrasion), enzymatic degradations (enzyme secretion determined by QS) or even a lack in nutriments or an overpopulation (McDougald et al., 2011). Fractions of bacteria are removed from the community and are spread in the environment. Newly mobile and adherent individual cells will be able to explore and colonize new surfaces by the establishment of a new biofilm. A new cycle of adhesion/maturation can get back.

Biofilms must be considered as an elaborate and dynamic organization which constantly evolve to get used to its environment. The passing through the sessile state to the planktonic one plays a considerable role in the transmission of bacteria from environmental reserves to the host and also in the transmission between hosts and in the infection propagation in the individual (biofilm metastasis).

BACTERIA UNDER SHELTER

The main advantage of the sessile way of life is the modification of the adherent bacteria in regard to their susceptibility to mechanisms of immune defenses and antimicrobials. Indeed, a single planktonic cell is vulnerable to the action of antibodies or phagocytes and is fairly sensitive to antibiotics. Conversely, bacteria that are embedded in a biofilm structure can be tolerant to the host immune system, antimicrobials, and biocide molecules (Høiby et al., 2011). Indeed, we usually talk about biofilm tolerance to antibiotics rather than resistance.

The resistance can be defined as the ability of a microorganism to grow when an antimicrobial compound is present in the environment. Resistance mechanisms are heritable and avoid the antibiotic interaction with its target. On the contrary, the term tolerance must be used for bacteria, which are able to survive in high concentrations of antimicrobials, but with a suspended growth. This feature, specific to the sessile bacterial life, is reversible, phenotypical, and non-inherited. A bacterial cell from a biofilm, which is resuspended in liquid medium, will get back an *in vitro* susceptibility to antimicrobials.

Inefficiency of Immune System

The size of the bacterial biofilm is the first brake to the phagocytosis process. Even in immunocompetent individuals, components of the immune system are seldom effective against biofilm infections. During the innate immune response, macrophages and neutrophils are rapidly activated following the direct contact with bacteria (i.e., through the O-antigen of the bacterial lipopolysaccharide (LPS) or the alginate for *P. aeruginosa*). Then, the immediate immune response triggers an important accumulation of neutrophils around the biofilm structure associated with an oxygen exhaustion, which is due to an active stimulation of the oxidative metabolism, as the molecular oxygen is reduced in superoxide (Watters et al., 2016).

The phagocytic cells penetrate with difficulty the extracellular matrix. They are slowed down and become more vulnerable to the inactivation by bacterial enzymes. Besides, the extended lysis of neutrophils leads to the overflow of harmful compounds in the medium, which are responsible for consecutive tissue damages. The host immune response is the main cause of the healthy tissue degradation surrounding the bacterial infection.

Concerning the memory of the immune system response, it has been reported that specific antibodies against bacterial compounds as the elastase, the LPS or the flagellum are secreted in CF patients. These data show that antigenic determinants were neutralized during chronic lung infection. Unfortunately, it has been demonstrated that these antibodies contribute to the formation of immune complexes, which are precipitated into the parenchyma and lead to complement activation and opsonization

of neutrophils, namely in an indirect way, to the nearby tissue degradation (Jensen et al., 2010).

General Tolerance to Antimicrobials

Biofilm tolerance to external aggressions, notably to antibiotic treatments, is one of its exceptional features. It is well-known that the MIC of an antimicrobial, which is effective on sessile bacteria, is 10 to 1,000 times more concentrated that the one which would be active on their planktonic version (Schurek et al., 2012). This decreased antimicrobial susceptibility can have several causes. It can be inherent to the own organization of the biofilm (structure and functioning) but can also be acquired by transmission of resistance factors.

Given its complex architecture, the biofilm itself creates a protective environment for bacterial cells. It can be seen as an "innate" tolerance. As for compounds of the host immune system, the extracellular matrix forms a mechanical barrier limiting antibiotic diffusion within the biofilm and their access to microorganisms. The electrostatic charges or some matrix components bind antimicrobial molecules and trap them. The general high viscosity of the polymeric matrix can also prevent the antibiotics from reaching their effective concentrations in the deeper layers of the bacterial community. Consequently, bacteria in the outer layers of the biofilm die following an antimicrobial treatment, while those in the deeper layers have time to react (Paraje, 2011). This invasion delay should be enough to allow a progressive physiological adaptation of bacteria exposed to antimicrobials (expression of resistance genes, secretion of inactivating enzymes...). For instance, it has been demonstrated that alginate and eDNA in the biofilm matrix of *P. aeruginosa* could link aminoglycosides and play a role in the sessile bacterial tolerance to tobramycin (Hentzer et al., 2001). Similarly, an extracytoplasmic process of antibiotic sequestration by periplasmic glucans was highlighted. The locus *ndvB* was identified as being required for the production of cyclic glucans (Mah et al., 2003). The authors showed that polymers physically bound antimicrobial compounds in the periplasm, leading to the diffusion slowdown of antibiotics into the cells and preventing them from reaching their action sites. Nevertheless, this global diffusion barrier, specific of the biofilm matrix and the sessile cells, appears to be strain- and antibiotic-dependent. By itself, it cannot explain the radical tolerance of biofilms against antimicrobial agents.

In view of their own biofilm organization, bacterial metabolism plays an important part in antibiotic tolerance. The concentration gradients of metabolites, oxygen, and nutriments within the mature biofilm create bacterial niches that are less metabolically active. For example, in *P. aeruginosa* microcolonies, the oxygen is consumed faster at the surface than it diffuses into the deeper layers of the biofilm. Its graduated diffusion leads to the formation of hypoxic areas in the bacterial community (Serra and Hengge, 2014). Some of microorganisms could get back to a stationary phase in lowering their growth and multiplication rates as an induced stress response. This reduced metabolism of sessile cells is partly responsible for the tolerance associated with the biofilm, as the action mode of the majority of antimicrobials targets metabolic processes in growing bacteria (replication, transcription, translation, or cell wall synthesis). Lots of works have validated the advantageous efficacy of antimicrobials on active bacteria, which are located in external areas of the biofilm. However, parallel studies showed that other types of molecules, such as SDS, EDTA, or chlorhexidine could conversely act on bacterial cells in stationary phase of growth, located in the internal niches (Ciofu et al., 2015).

The activation of efflux pumps by bacteria embedded in the extracellular matrix can also contribute to the inefficiency of antimicrobials in actively discharging them outside the biofilm structure before they can reach their target. These membrane transporters can be specific of a class of antibiotics or responsible for multidrug resistance. In Gram-negative bacteria as *P. aeruginosa*, efflux pumps are usually composed of a pump located in the inner membrane, an outer membrane factor, and a periplasmic fusion protein. The association of cell impermeability with the expression of the efflux system MexAB-OprM leads partly to the inherent resistance of the bacillus to antibiotics. The expression of some of them was demonstrated as being specific to the biofilm mode (Zhang and Mah, 2008).

The bacterial density and the spatial proximity of microorganisms within a mature biofilm promote the gene exchange and the resistance plasmid transmission. The horizontal gene transfer could be 1,000-fold more important in a bacterial community than between planktonic cells. Due to the starved local environment within the biofilm, bacteria are also subjected to random mutations and genetic rearrangements. This generation of bacterial variants, favored by natural selection, leads to a chromosomal resistance (Poole, 2012). The mutation frequency can be stimulated by environmental factors, as the presence of reactive oxygen species from the lung inflammatory response. These reagents, in damaging DNA, cause mutations in bacteria and lead to the diversity of bacterial phenotypes in the biofilm (Rodríguez-Rojas et al., 2012). Finally, by combination of several of these mechanisms, sessile bacteria rapidly became multiresistant.

It also demonstrated the existence of a "persister" bacterial population which could constitute a reserve allowing the infection relaunch after elimination of peripheral planktonic and sessile cells (Stewart, 2002).

The "Persister Cells" Enigma

Persisters are regular cells exhibiting a specific non-growing phenotype, combined with an excessive tolerance to antibiotic concentrations. Their existence was firstly described in the 1940s (Bigger, 1944). The transcription downregulation of genes involved in motility and energy production was highlighted for these isolated bacteria. Consequently, as they are in a dormant state, antimicrobials are able to bind to their target molecules but not to impair their initial function (Lewis, 2005).

The presence of persisters can be easily detected in bacterial cultures by a process of biphasic death, further to an exposition to bactericidal antibiotic concentrations. Firstly, a lethal dose of antimicrobials will rapidly eradicate the sensitive bacterial population. A much slower second phase of death follows, reflecting the poor killing of persister cells. Finally, the end of antimicrobial treatment will allow the renewal of the

bacterial community by regeneration of persister survivors (Conlon et al., 2015).

Each bacterium shows the capacity to be differentiated in a persister cell, but few of them are really observed during the early exponential phase of growth. Indeed, the genuine persister population is formed during the mid-exponential phase and finally, they reach up to 1% of the overall population at the stationary phase. This phenotypic conversion can be induced by environmental stimuli or stresses, as antibiotic exposure, which are predictive of immediate threats for cells, or they may be preexisting in the bacterial population (Harms et al., 2016; Fisher et al., 2017). It is assumed that stochastic modifications in genes can lead to the phenotypic switch along with the over-expression of specific toxin-antitoxin (TA) module proteins. Typically, the toxin portions are neutralized by their antitoxins, but under cellular stresses, proteases must be over-expressed and degrade the antitoxin proteins. In that case, the toxin modules are free to exert their toxic action on bacteria. The expression of many other compounds implicated in the persister phenotype can be induced by environmental stimuli. The signaling pathway of the SOS response and the alarmone ppGpp, two stringent responses to stress, also appears to be associated with the persistence of bacteria (Del Pozo, 2018).

EFFECTIVENESS OF CONVENTIONAL ANTIBIOTICS

Despite the intensive tolerance of the biofilm to antimicrobials, certain conventional antibiotics still demonstrate activity against bacterial cells growing in the biofilm state.

In a recent study, Otani et al. (2018) showed that sub-MICs of ceftazidime reduce biofilm volume, inhibit twitching motility, and repress gene expression involved in bacterial adhesion and matrix production of *P. aeruginosa* PAO1. Roudashti et al. (2017) had previously noticed this effect of cephalosporin on motility and biofilm formation for the same strain.

Similarly, other common antimicrobials were described as being effective on biofilm behavior of *P. aeruginosa*. Subinhibitory doses of piperacillin/tazobactam altered the pathogenic potential of various clinical and laboratory strains of *P. aeruginosa* in reducing bacterial adhesion, in decreasing biofilm formation, swimming, and twitching motility and conversely in increasing the susceptibility of cells to oxidative stress (Fonseca, 2004). Indeed, one early step of biofilm formation which can be targeted for the prevention of chronic infection is bacterial adhesion to a surface. The process of twitching motility contributes to this part of virulence of sessile microorganisms. Wozniak and Keyser (2004) noticed that clarithromycin substantially inhibited cell translocation of *P. aeruginosa* through its type IV pilus as well as altered its biofilm architecture at sub-MIC levels. Another control strategy against bacterial biofilm is QS disruption. Azithromycin, ceftazidime, and ciprofloxacin showed, at subinhibitory concentrations, QS-inhibitory activities in bacteria (Skindersoe et al., 2008). This beneficial effect of the macrolide was also emphasized in an experimental urinary tract infection model. Antibiotic concentrations below the MIC could inhibit the production of QS molecules, leading to the complete clearance of *P. aeruginosa* from the mouse kidneys (Bala et al., 2011). Azithromycin was also described as being able to prevent PAO1 biofilm formation in a flow cell biofilm model (Gillis and Iglewski, 2004).

Continuous treatment of colistin (25 µg/ml) turned out to be effective against the non-dividing central part of a *P. aeruginosa* biofilm growing in a flow chamber for 4 days. Associated with ciprofloxacin (60 µg/ml), which can kill metabolically active cells in the surface layers, this combination therapy showed a clinical efficacy for the early eradication treatment of bacteria in CF patients (Høiby et al., 2010). In a more recent study, the association of minimal biofilm inhibitory concentrations (MBICs) of fosfomycin with tobramycin ($\geq$1024 µg/ml and from 8 to 32 µg/ml, respectively) has been demonstrated to be synergistic against CF isolates in *in vitro* models (Díez-Aguilar et al., 2018). Overall, the aminoglycosides usually prescribed in CF (amikacin and tobramycin) showed a preventive action on the early adhesion of clinical *P. aeruginosa* strains at various concentrations (sub-MICs, MICs, and so-called PK/PD doses) (Olivares et al., 2017).

The efficacy of antibiotic lock solution (meropenem, levofloxacin, and colistin) on *P. aeruginosa* clinical and reference strains was also confirmed. The antibiotic lock technique (ALT), using antimicrobial molecules, prevented bacterial regrowth in an *in vitro* antibiotic lock model. The efficacy of ALT to eliminate *P. aeruginosa* biofilms should be improved when the three antibiotics were used in combination with clarithromycin (Ozbek and Mataraci-Kara, 2016).

Finally, all the cited publications attest that some conventional molecules can still be active on *P. aeruginosa* in the context of chronic infections, in preventing its growth within the biofilm. Nevertheless, a lot of these studies were carried out on the reference PAO1 strain. To confirm the clinical effectiveness of antimicrobial treatments, antibiotic susceptibility testing must be performed on clinical isolates, and clinical trials must be planned.

Concerning the positive effect of classic antimicrobial therapies on other sessile pathogens, MICs and minimal bactericidal concentrations (MBCs) of rifampicin have demonstrated an activity against biofilms of *Staphylococcus epidermidis* and *Staphylococcus aureus* isolates associated with device infections, especially when it is used in association with other molecules as fusidic acid, vancomycin or ciprofloxacin in an *in vitro* biofilm model (Saginur et al., 2006). More recently, adherent staphylococci involved in skin and soft tissue infections were described as being more or less susceptible to multiples of tedizolid MICs and other comparator agents (vancomycin, linezolid, and daptomycin) (Delpech et al., 2018). The use of daptomycin-lock therapy (50 mg/ml) also showed a therapeutic advantage for the 24 h-treatment of a long-term catheter-related bloodstream infections by coagulase-negative *S. epidermidis* in a rabbit model (Basas et al., 2018). Similarly, subinhibitory concentrations of fluoroquinolones were able to reduce the number of sessile cells to prevent the adhesion of the corresponding *S. epidermidis* strains and to alter biofilm morphology (Szczuka et al., 2017).

This overall review of publications, dealing with the anti-biofilm property of conventional antimicrobials, can be completed with studies using *Escherichia coli*, another bacterial specie well-characterized for its capacity to form biofilm structures. In a recent article, Klinger-Strobel et al. (2017) noticed that colistin concentrations from 4 to 16 mg/l could reduce the amount of adherent *E. coli* bacteria and exert a matrix-reducing effect on biofilms in formation. Similarly, Butini et al. (2018) investigated the anti-biofilm property of gentamicin-eluting bone graft substitute against bacterial species involved in bone and implant-associated infections. Calcium sulfate bone graft substitutes served as local antibiotic delivery carrier, and gentamicin is one of the most used molecules for the treatment of bone-related infections. Therefore, they demonstrated that 12 µg/ml of released gentamicin were able to prevent *E. coli* adhesion and 23 µg/ml of the molecule could eliminate a 24 h-old biofilm. These data are promising as the applied concentrations are achievable for local treatment in bone and soft tissues. In another recent publication, a mupirocin spray was formulated and tested against *E. coli* strains, in a context of wound and surgical site infections. Inhibition and disruption of formed biofilms were achieved with a single and a sub-actual dose of the antibiotic spray (1 mg per spray or 1 mg per 50 mg of ointment), compared to the commercialized mupirocin ointment (Bakkiyaraj et al., 2017). Results showed that both formulations had an anti-biofilm action on *E. coli* sessile cultures in tissue culture plates but microscope studies provided complementary evidences that it remained more individual adherent cells with ointment formulation than for treatment with the antibiotic spray. Authors concluded that this efficacy on biofilm prevention and disruption was comparable with that of the ointment. Nevertheless, the spray use seemed beneficial as it included an easy application: while the ointment was removed from the application site upon washing, the spray formulation significantly resisted removal after a single wash.

Finally, for the treatment of recurrent urinary tract infections (UTIs) associated with the presence of biofilm, the use of amikacin, ciprofloxacin, and third-generation cephalosporins could be recommended. Indeed, various concentrations of these molecules, selected according the bioavailability of antibiotics in human urine, showed the ability to significantly reduce biofilm biomass in a study of 116 *E. coli* strains of UTIs (González et al., 2017).

Even if it seems that antimicrobials can be effective on prematurely adherent bacteria, a small percentage of persister cells develop a high tolerance to antibiotics and are typically involved in infection relapses. Moreover, the biofilm must be considered as a single compartment with its own pharmacokinetic parameters. This will influence local antibiotic concentration and its metabolization in the biofilm (Cao et al., 2015). All these combined factors lead to the recommended use of high doses of antimicrobials for long periods, which cannot always be practicable in patients because of severe systemic side effects.

Biofilm tolerance to antimicrobials is complex and above all multifactorial. A now long list of studies demonstrate that low doses of antimicrobials at the infection site might increase the selection of mutagenesis and the risk of biofilm formation initiation induction (Ciofu et al., 2017).

INDUCTION OF BIOFILM FORMATION BY ANTIMICROBIALS

At high concentrations, antibiotics appear to be perfect bacterial killers. Their original function in the environment is fighting and inhibiting the growth of competitors (Linares et al., 2006). The production of antimicrobials by bacteria themselves allows the killing of predators. This application of the classical Darwinian principle supports the idea that they allow the competing colonization of soil by microorganisms. However, antibiotic molecules constitute only a small part of organic compounds produced by bacteria. Consequently, it can be assumed that they can affect the general modulation metabolic function in bacteria, as other signaling analogous (rhamnolipids, peptides, and QS signals, etc.). Supporting this assumption, phylogenetic analyses revealed that antimicrobial resistant genes were present in bacterial genomes millions of years before the modern use of antibiotics. A similar example concerns the metagenomic study of Alaskan soils, which demonstrated the existence of an ancient and varied collection of β-lactamase genes, whereas this antimicrobial family is not detected in the environment (Aminov, 2009).

In activating specific gene transcription, antimicrobial compounds seem to act as signaling molecules, regulating the homeostasis of bacterial communities. As sessile cells are significantly less sensitive to antimicrobials, biofilm formation would be a strategic evolution of bacterial populations to counteract non-lethal doses of antibiotics produced by soil microorganisms. This implies that antimicrobials can also be beneficial for the survival of susceptible planktonic cells in nature. Therefore, they can permit a more efficient colonization of heterogeneous environments. Especially at subinhibitory levels, antibiotics modulate bacterial virulence, stress response, motility, and biofilm formation (Song et al., 2016).

The first report describing the ability of low doses of antibiotics to interfere with bacterial functions was made by Gardner (1940). In the presence of subinhibitory concentrations of penicillin, numerous gram-negative, and positive pathogens formed elongated filaments.

Since then, similar studies introducing the structure modification of bacterial cells by antibiotics were published. *P. aeruginosa* showed the most morphological changes as bacteria reacted to meropenem and biapenem in forming a "bulge" midway along them (Horii et al., 1998). The authors also described a relationship between the induction of a new morphology and the amount of endotoxin released by bacteria. The modification of the bacterial size and shape was explained by the fact that antibiotic molecules inhibit the Penicillin-Binding-Proteins 2 and 3 (PBP-2 and PBP-3). They are involved in the assembly of the bacteria cell wall by the catalysis of the terminal stages of the peptidoglycan network. These proteins are the primary target of β-lactam antibiotics in Gram-negative bacteria. The inactivation of PBP-1 leads to bacteria lysis, whereas the inhibition of PBP-2 and PBP-3 is associated with either spherical cells or filamentous bacteria. These effects of antimicrobials onto the bacterial morphology were also observed in experimental infections in mice (Yokochi et al., 2000).

More precisely, the authors highlighted a relationship between the shape of bacteria and their susceptibility to phagocytosis. Induced round bacteria were phagocytosed by peritoneal cells, whereas long filaments were not. Finally, it appeared that the morphological reorganization of bacteria is a reversible process as when antibiotics were no longer present, the induced spherical or filamentous population converts back to the normal bacillary form (Monahan et al., 2014). This transition is a strategy to survive antibiotic exposure as the biofilm formation.

Furthermore, exposure of *P. aeruginosa* strains to sub-MICs of ciprofloxacin leads to the selection of pre-existing mutants with high level resistance (Jørgensen et al., 2013). The analysis of the strains selected by subinhibitory doses of the fluoroquinolone showed phenotypic changes in bacteria, as decreased protease activity and swimming motility, down-regulation of the type III secretion system and higher levels of quorum-sensing signals (Wassermann et al., 2016). In some cases, this implies that antibiotic therapies may expose patients to detrimental side-effects by accelerating pathogen adaptation and raising the risk of antimicrobial tolerance and spread in the commensal bacterial flora if bacteria are exposed to low antibiotic concentrations.

The first study demonstrating the real "inducer" property of antimicrobials on biofilm formation at subinhibitory concentrations dates back to 1988 (Schadow et al., 1988). The adherence of coagulase-negative staphylococci was increased to 65% after rifampicin treatment. Since then, numerous works focusing on the effect of low antibiotic doses on biofilm formation were published.

Although several studies have shown that aminoglycoside antibiotics act as antagonists of biofilm formation *in vitro* (see previous section of this paper), opposite data were collected and highlighted the ability of the same molecules to significantly induce the sessile growth of a variety of bacterial species. Hoffman et al. (2005) described the effect of subinhibitory doses of aminoglycosides in *P. aeruginosa* and *E. coli* biofilms. They showed that these antibiotics stimulated the expression of the *arr* gene, which encodes a phosphodiesterase whose substrate is the c-di-GMP. Reinforcing this idea, induction of biofilm formation after an exposure to sub-MICs of aminoglycosides was detected among half of a *P. aeruginosa* clinical isolate collection (Elliott et al., 2010).

Imipenem, a carbapenem molecule, was also able to substantially influence the expression of 34 genes in the common reference PAO1 strain. When subinhibitory concentrations of this antibiotic were applied to bacterial cultures, the alginate gene cluster, the main component of the biofilm matrix of *P. aeruginosa* was more than 10-fold induced (Bagge et al., 2004). The corresponding polysaccharide amount in biofilms was quantified by the authors and they found that the alginate level in the matrix of stimulated-biofilms was 20-fold higher than the one of the non-exposed controls.

Induction phenomenon of biofilm formation by antimicrobials was also described for other bacterial species. The use of β-lactam antibiotics at sub-MIC concentrations leads to the induction of the bacterial adhesion by a community-associated Methicillin-Resistant *S. aureus* (MRSA) strain and clinical isolates (Ng et al., 2014). All of the antimicrobial molecules tested in this study exhibited a biphasic dose-response curve. Authors also described an inversely proportional relationship between the biofilm amount and the susceptibility of bacteria to methicillin: the more sensitive the strain to antibiotic, the lower is the concentration required to induced biofilm. Biofilm formation of a clinical isolate of *Enterococcus faecalis*, which commonly underlies prosthetic valve endocarditis and multiple device infections, was also significantly increased by low concentrations of ampicillin, ceftriaxone, oxacillin, and fosfomycin. This enhancement of biofilm establishment appeared to be specific of molecules inhibiting cell wall synthesis (Yu et al., 2017). Additionally, a collection of ninety-six clinical isolates of *S. epidermidis*, which originate from various samples as wounds, catheters, sputum, etc., was recovered by He et al. (2016). The authors described that 27% of erythromycin-resistant strains exhibited biofilm induction by 0.25 MIC of the molecule. The induction intensity ranged from 1.11-fold to more than twofold (He et al., 2016).

A more complete review article written by Kaplan (2011) gathers studies showing that subinhibitory concentrations of antimicrobial molecules can act as agonists of bacterial biofilms *in vitro*.

Biological responses of bacterial species are strain- and dose-dependent. Some molecules can promote the biofilm formation at high levels and conversely be antagonists and repress its establishment at lower doses. Nonetheless, this dose-response relationship cannot be generalized as it can be inverted, depending on the considered antibiotic, which is used in the treatment for a specific laboratory or clinical strain. The discovery of this ecological function of antibiotics is essential as, in a clinical context, the induction of biofilm formation by low concentrations of antibiotics would contribute to the failure of antimicrobial therapies in case of biofilm-related infections. It can be speculated that this is a common phenomenon as microorganisms are usually under fluctuating doses of antibiotics during a chemotherapy.

Clinical Tools Available for the Diagnosis and Treatment of Biofilm Infections

Traditionally, clinical microbiology laboratories have focused on the culture of isolated bacterial strains and provide their susceptibility to antibiotics in defining the breakpoints and the PK/PD parameters under planktonic growth conditions. The corresponding antibiotic therapies, based on non-adherent microorganisms, are often associated with treatment failures and/or recurrence of the infection. No guidelines are offered to clinicians to successfully treat biofilm infections, which can result to false-negative data if the samples do not significantly represent the main infection.

Besides, there is still no available standardized tool to detect easily the presence of sessile cells in a clinical sample and allow determination of their specific antibiotic susceptibility. As biofilm bacteria are inherently more tolerant to antimicrobials, the establishment of the corresponding breakpoints to predict therapeutic success is needed. New methods monitoring the effect/response of biofilm cells to antibiotic therapy must

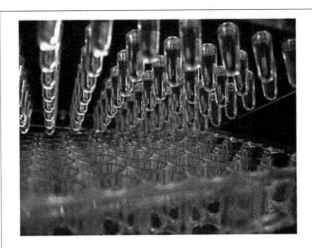

FIGURE 2 | Regular MBEC with 96-well plate. Photography adapted from Parker et al. (2014).

be designed. Currently, two technologies were developed but not yet standardized for a rapid routine use in hospital laboratories: the Calgary device (also called MBEC assay) and the Antibiofilmogram®.

The Calgary biofilm device consists of a two-part reaction vessel (Ceri et al., 1999). A lid, composed of 96 pegs, forms the first and top component. The bottom component of the device is a standard 96-well plate, in which the pegs are designed to sit into each well. The microplate contains the medium allowing the growth of bacteria, which is set up in 96 equivalent biofilms at each peg site (**Figure 2**). Biofilm susceptibility testing is performed in transferring the lid with bacterial biofilms to a standard 96-well plate containing serial dilutions of antibiotics. The minimal biofilm eradication concentration (MBEC) is defined as the minimal concentration of antibiotic that prevents visible growth in the recovery medium used to collect sessile cells.

Moskowitz et al. (2004) evaluated the *in vitro* activity of twelve antimicrobials on a large number of CF sessile clinical isolates of *P. aeruginosa* using a modified Calgary device protocol. The MBICs of the antimicrobial agents were much higher than the corresponding conventional MICs. In a context of biofilm infections, this suggests that the use of broth microdilution susceptibility testing or other standard methods to guide therapy may not contribute to improve clinical outcomes. Quite the reverse, devices simulating biofilm growth conditions might guide therapy more effectively. To verify this hypothesis, clinical trials were already conducted. Unfortunately, no evidence that biofilm susceptibility testing performed with the Calgary device was more efficient than conventional techniques in terms of clinical outcomes was provided (Waters and Ratjen, 2017). Yau et al. (2015) introduced the first randomized controlled trial evaluating the utility of biofilm antimicrobial susceptibility testing in the treatment of CF pulmonary exacerbations. They concluded that the choice of antibiotic therapies based on biofilm behavior of bacteria did not improve clinical outcomes and did not decrease pulmonary bacterial loads. They explained the lack of Calgary method efficacy by an oversimplification

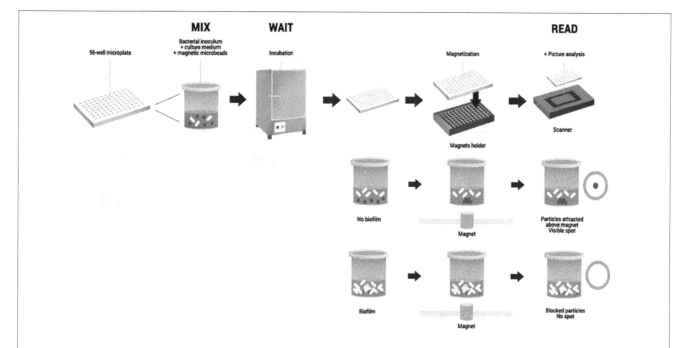

FIGURE 3 | Schematic representation of the Antibiofilmogram® principle. The initial bacterial suspension is loaded in a 96-well microplate with the microbead solution. After incubation, the plate is magnetized during 1 min. If bacterial cells preserve a free-floating form, the beads are attracted by the magnetic field and form a spot. Conversely, if bacteria adhere to the well bottom, beads are embedded in the biofilm in formation and consequently, no spot is visible. Schematic adapted from Azeredo et al. (2017).

of the sessile growth conditions. Biofilm formation on a lid composed of 96 plastic pegs could not recreate the environment *in vivo*, in which sessile cells grow and express specific properties. Moreover, the determination of antimicrobial susceptibility of a selected isolate could underestimate the microbial diversity response to antibiotics.

The Antibiofilmogram® (ATBFG) method was specifically designed to investigate early steps of biofilm development, by rapidly screening antibiotic effective against sessile bacteria. Its functioning principle is based on the potential immobilization of magnetic microbeads by bacteria forming a biofilm in the well bottom of a microplate (Chavant et al., 2007).

Briefly, a given bacterial culture is mixed with the microbead suspension and loaded in the plate (**Figure 3**). Afterward, it is incubated and submitted to a magnetic field at a desired time point, without staining and/or washing stages. The formation of a brown spot in the bottom of wells reveals the free migration of beads during plate magnetization and so, the remaining-free state of bacteria. Conversely, the absence of visible spots reflects the bead blockage by a pre-forming biofilm (Olivares et al., 2016). The main advantage of this methodology is its capacity to collect data within a couple of hours, allowing comparison of antibiotic susceptibility of sessile bacteria to the results of classical antibiograms. But as for the Calgary method, the ATBFG is an *in vitro* assay, which does not provide information about structure or thickness of the mature biofilms.

Results of ATBFG performed on 29 clinical strains of *S. aureus* isolated from bone and joint infections (BIJs) were also published (Tasse et al., 2016). On the basis of antibiotic breakpoint values, the authors defined effective antimicrobial

molecules against adhesion of the majority of *S. aureus* strains (rifampicin, linezolid, clindamycin, and fusidic acid), others inefficient against bacterial adherence (fosfomycin, ofloxacin, daptomycin, and gentamicin) and some of them whose efficacy was strain-dependent (cloxacillin, vancomycin, and teicoplanin). Data validity was confirmed by *in vivo* assays (catheter-related infections in the mouse). Results showed that serum concentrations of cloxacillin, corresponding to the MBICs determined by ATBFG (either 2 or 4 µg/ml), allowed reduction to 3 log the bacterial biomasses colonizing the catheters for three clinical strains, whereas the simple MICs of the antibiotic were inefficient on biofilm formation.

In a CF context, the use of ATBFG on clinical *P. aeruginosa* strains also showed the capacity of two aminoglycosides (amikacin and tobramycin) to prevent bacterial adhesion at concentrations close to the MICs (Olivares et al., 2017). Only *in vitro* assays were performed in this study but an inter-method reproducibility was conducted through Crystal Violet staining and a tissue culture system, which validated the inhibitory effect of the antimicrobials on the early adhesion of *P. aeruginosa* isolates.

CONCLUDING REMARKS

As demonstrated in previous sections, the treatment of bacterial infections with chemically distinct antibiotics can lead to a variety of responses from sessile bacteria. Despite the increased tolerance of microorganisms toward antimicrobials, some molecules are always effective against newly adherent bacteria. In clinical practice, it is recommended that when possible, as for the diabetic foot for instance, to resort to topical administration to provide high local concentrations to the infection site without systemic side-effects.

Disappointingly, numerous studies have also described that low doses of antibiotics can significantly induce biofilm formation *in vitro* for a variety of bacterial species. The plausibility of this phenomenon *in vivo* must be considered as bacterial pathogens are exposed to sub-MIC concentrations of antimicrobials during a clinical therapy with fluctuating dosing regimens. More researches on antibiotic-induced biofilm formation are required to elucidate the involved mechanisms. Clinical trials that verify the relevance of this process in patients and the potential relationship with therapy failure will also be highly helpful. The prospect of complementary assays evaluating the susceptibility of free and sessile cells to antibiotics would also allow the optimization of the general use of antimicrobials in the treatment of biofilm-related infections.

AUTHOR CONTRIBUTIONS

EO wrote the manuscript. All authors read and approved the submitted version.

FUNDING

This study was received funding from the BioFilm Pharma SAS. The funder was not involved in the study design, collection, analysis, interpretation of data, and the writing of this article or the decision to submit it for publication. This study was supported by the 15th Fonds Unique Interministériel (FUI).

ACKNOWLEDGMENTS

We thank BioFilm Pharma SAS for the financial support.

REFERENCES

Aminov, R. I. (2009). The role of antibiotics and antibiotic resistance in nature. *Environ. Microbiol.* 11, 2970–2988. doi: 10.1111/j.1462-2920.2009.01972.x

Azeredo, J., Azevedo, N. F., Briandet, R., Cerca, N., Coenye, T., Costa, A. R., et al. (2017). Critical review on biofilm methods. *Crit. Rev. Microbiol.* 43, 331–351. doi: 10.1080/1040841X.2016.1208146

Bagge, N., Schuster, M., Hentzer, M., Ciofu, O., Givskov, M., Greenberg, E. P., et al. (2004). *Pseudomonas aeruginosa* biofilms exposed to imipenem exhibit changes in global gene expression and β-Lactamase and alginate production. *Antimicrob. Agents Chemother.* 48, 1175–1187. doi: 10.1128/AAC.48.4.1175-1187.2004

Bakkiyaraj, D., Sritharadol, R., Padmavathi, A. R., Nakpheng, T., and Srichana, T. (2017). Anti-biofilm properties of a mupirocin spray formulation against *Escherichia coli* wound infections. *Biofouling* 33, 591–600. doi: 10.1080/08927014.2017.1337100

Bala, A., Kumar, R., and Harjai, K. (2011). Inhibition of quorum sensing in *Pseudomonas aeruginosa* by azithromycin and its effectiveness in urinary tract infections. *J. Med. Microbiol.* 60, 300–306. doi: 10.1099/jmm.0.025387-0

Basas, J., Palau, M., Ratia, C., Del Pozo, J. L., Martín-Gómez, M. T., Gomis, X., et al. (2018). High-dose daptomycin is effective as an antibiotic lock therapy in a rabbit model of *Staphylococcus epidermidis* catheter-related infection. *Antimicrob. Agents Chemother.* 62:e01777-17. doi: 10.1128/AAC.01777-17

Bigger, J. W. (1944). Treatment of staphylococcal infections with penicillin by intermittent sterilisation. *The Lancet* 244, 497–500. doi: 10.1016/S0140-6736(00)74210-3

Biofilms: The Hypertextbook (2011). Available at: http://www.hypertextbookshop.com/biofilmbook/v004/r003Test/index.html (accessed December 15, 2016).

Butini, M. E., Cabric, S., Trampuz, A., and Di Luca, M. (2018). *In vitro* anti-biofilm activity of a biphasic gentamicin-loaded calcium sulfate/hydroxyapatite bone graft substitute. *Colloids Surf. B Biointerfaces* 161, 252–260. doi: 10.1016/j.colsurfb.2017.10.050

Cao, B., Christophersen, L., Thomsen, K., Sønderholm, M., Bjarnsholt, T., Jensen, P. Ø., et al. (2015). Antibiotic penetration and bacterial killing in a *Pseudomonas aeruginosa* biofilm model. *J. Antimicrob. Chemother.* 70, 2057–2063. doi: 10.1093/jac/dkv058

Ceri, H., Olson, M. E., Stremick, C., Read, R. R., Morck, D., and Buret, A. (1999). The calgary biofilm device: new technology for rapid determination of antibiotic susceptibilities of bacterial biofilms. *J. Clin. Microbiol.* 37, 1771–1776.

Chavant, P., Gaillard-Martinie, B., Talon, R., Hébraud, M., and Bernardi, T. (2007). A new device for rapid evaluation of biofilm formation potential by bacteria. *J. Microbiol. Methods* 68, 605–612. doi: 10.1016/j.mimet.2006.11.010

Ciofu, O., Rojo-Molinero, E., Macià, M. D., and Oliver, A. (2017). Antibiotic treatment of biofilm infections. *APMIS* 125, 304–319. doi: 10.1111/apm.12673

Ciofu, O., Tolker-Nielsen, T., Jensen, P. Ø, Wang, H., and Høiby, N. (2015). Antimicrobial resistance, respiratory tract infections and role of biofilms in lung infections in cystic fibrosis patients. *Adv. Drug Deliv. Rev.* 85, 7–23. doi: 10.1016/j.addr.2014.11.017

Conlon, B. P., Rowe, S. E., and Lewis, K. (2015). Persister cells in biofilm associated infections. *Adv. Exp. Med. Biol.* 831, 1–9. doi: 10.1007/978-3-319-09782-4_1

Costerton, J. W., Geesey, G. G., and Cheng, K. J. (1978). How bacteria stick. *Sci. Am.* 238, 86–95. doi: 10.1038/scientificamerican0178-86

Davies, D. G., and Geesey, G. G. (1995). Regulation of the alginate biosynthesis gene *algC* in *Pseudomonas aeruginosa* during biofilm development in continuous culture. *Appl. Environ. Microbiol.* 61, 860–867.

Davies, D. G., Parsek, M. R., Pearson, J. P., Iglewski, B. H., Costerton, J. W., and Greenberg, E. P. (1998). The involvement of cell-to-cell signals in the development of a bacterial biofilm. *Science* 280, 295–298. doi: 10.1126/science.280.5361.295

Del Pozo, J. L. (2018). Biofilm-related disease. *Expert Rev. Anti Infect. Ther.* 16, 51–65. doi: 10.1080/14787210.2018.1417036

Delpech, P., ALeryan, M., Jones, B., Gemmell, C., and Lang, S. (2018). An *in vitro* evaluation of the efficacy of tedizolid: implications for the treatment of skin and soft tissue infections. *Diagn. Microbiol. Infect. Dis.* 91, 93–97. doi: 10.1016/j.diagmicrobio.2018.01.006

Dibartola, A. C., Swearingen, M. C., Granger, J. F., Stoodley, P., and Dusane, D. H. (2017). Biofilms in orthopedic infections: a review of laboratory methods. *APMIS* 125, 418–428. doi: 10.1111/apm.12671

Díez-Aguilar, M., Morosini, M. I., Köksal, E., Oliver, A., Ekkelenkamp, M., and Cantón, R. (2018). Use of calgary and microfluidic BioFlux systems to test the activity of fosfomycin and tobramycin alone and in combination against cystic fibrosis *Pseudomonas aeruginosa* biofilms. *Antimicrob. Agents Chemother.* 62:e01650-17. doi: 10.1128/AAC.01650-17

Donné, J., and Dewilde, S. (2015). The challenging world of biofilm physiology. *Adv. Microb. Physiol.* 67, 235–292. doi: 10.1016/bs.ampbs.2015.09.003

Dufour, D., Leung, V., and Lévesque, C. M. (2010). Bacterial biofilm: structure, function, and antimicrobial resistance. *Endod. Topics* 22, 2–16. doi: 10.1111/j.1601-1546.2012.00277.x

Elliott, D., Burns, J. L., and Hoffman, L. R. (2010). Exploratory study of the prevalence and clinical significance of tobramycin-mediated biofilm induction in *Pseudomonas aeruginosa* isolates from cystic fibrosis patients. *Antimicrob. Agents Chemother.* 54, 3024–3026. doi: 10.1128/AAC.00102-10

Fisher, R. A., Gollan, B., and Helaine, S. (2017). Persistent bacterial infections and persister cells. *Nat. Rev. Microbiol.* 15, 453–464. doi: 10.1038/nrmicro.2017.42

Fonseca, A. P. (2004). Effect of subinhibitory concentration of piperacillin/tazobactam on *Pseudomonas aeruginosa*. *J. Med. Microbiol.* 53, 903–910. doi: 10.1099/jmm.0.45637-0

Gardner, A. D. (1940). Morphological effects of penicillin on bacteria. *Nature* 146, 837–838. doi: 10.1038/146837b0

Gillis, R. J., and Iglewski, B. H. (2004). Azithromycin retards *Pseudomonas aeruginosa* biofilm formation. *J. Clin. Microbiol.* 42, 5842–5845. doi: 10.1128/JCM.42.12.5842-5845.2004

González, M. J., Robino, L., Iribarnegaray, V., Zunino, P., and Scavone, P. (2017). Effect of different antibiotics on biofilm produced by uropathogenic *Escherichia coli* isolated from children with urinary tract infection. *Pathog. Dis.* 75:ftx053. doi: 10.1093/femspd/ftx053

Harms, A., Maisonneuve, E., and Gerdes, K. (2016). Mechanisms of bacterial persistence during stress and antibiotic exposure. *Science* 354:aaf4268. doi: 10.1126/science.aaf4268

He, H.-J., Sun, F.-J., Wang, Q., Liu, Y., Xiong, L.-R., and Xia, P.-Y. (2016). Erythromycin resistance features and biofilm formation affected by subinhibitory erythromycin in clinical isolates of *Staphylococcus epidermidis*. *J. Microbiol. Immunol. Infect.* 49, 33–40. doi: 10.1016/j.jmii.2014.03.001

Hentzer, M., Teitzel, G. M., Balzer, G. J., Heydorn, A., Molin, S., Givskov, M., et al. (2001). Alginate overproduction affects *Pseudomonas aeruginosa* biofilm structure and function. *J. Bacteriol.* 183, 5395–5401. doi: 10.1128/JB.183.18.5395-5401.2001

Hoffman, L. R., D'Argenio, D. A., MacCoss, M. J., Zhang, Z., Jones, R. A., and Miller, S. I. (2005). Aminoglycoside antibiotics induce bacterial biofilm formation. *Nature* 436, 1171–1175. doi: 10.1038/nature03912

Høiby, N., Bjarnsholt, T., Givskov, M., Molin, S., and Ciofu, O. (2010). Antibiotic resistance of bacterial biofilms. *Int. J. Antimicrob. Agents* 35, 322–332. doi: 10.1016/j.ijantimicag.2009.12.011

Høiby, N., Ciofu, O., Johansen, H. K., Song, Z., Moser, C., Jensen, P. Ø, et al. (2011). The clinical impact of bacterial biofilms. *Int. J. Oral Sci.* 3, 55–65. doi: 10.4248/IJOS11026

Horii, T., Kobayashi, M., Sato, K., Ichiyama, S., and Ohta, M. (1998). An *in vitro* study of carbapenem-induced morphological changes and endotoxin release in clinical isolates of gram-negative bacilli. *J. Antimicrob. Chemother.* 41, 435–442. doi: 10.1093/jac/41.4.435

Jamal, M., Ahmad, W., Andleeb, S., Jalil, F., Imran, M., Nawaz, M. A., et al. (2018). Bacterial biofilm and associated infections. *J. Chin. Med. Assoc.* 81, 7–11. doi: 10.1016/j.jcma.2017.07.012

Jensen, P. Ø, Givskov, M., Bjarnsholt, T., and Moser, C. (2010). The immune system vs. *Pseudomonas aeruginosa* biofilms. *FEMS Immunol. Med. Microbiol.* 59, 292–305. doi: 10.1111/j.1574-695X.2010.00706.x

Jørgensen, K. M., Wassermann, T., Jensen, P. Ø, Hengzuang, W., Molin, S., Høiby, N., et al. (2013). Sublethal ciprofloxacin treatment leads to rapid development of high-level ciprofloxacin resistance during long-term experimental evolution of *Pseudomonas aeruginosa*. *Antimicrob. Agents Chemother.* 57, 4215–4221. doi: 10.1128/AAC.00493-13

Kaplan, J. B. (2011). Antibiotic-induced biofilm formation. *Int. J. Artif. Organs* 34, 737–751. doi: 10.5301/ijao.5000027

Klinger-Strobel, M., Stein, C., Forstner, C., Makarewicz, O., and Pletz, M. W. (2017). Effects of colistin on biofilm matrices of *Escherichia coli* and *Staphylococcus aureus*. *Int. J. Antimicrob. Agents* 49, 472–479. doi: 10.1016/j.ijantimicag.2017.01.005

Lebeaux, D., and Ghigo, J.-M. (2012). Infections associées aux biofilms - Quelles perspectives thérapeutiques issues de la recherche fondamentale?? *Med. Sci.* 28, 727–739. doi: 10.1051/medsci/2012288015

Lewis, K. (2005). Persister cells and the riddle of biofilm survival. *Biochemistry* 70, 267–274. doi: 10.1007/s10541-005-0111-6

Limoli, D. H., Jones, C. J., and Wozniak, D. J. (2015). Bacterial extracellular polysaccharides in biofilm formation and function. *Microbiol. Spectr.* 3, doi: 10.1128/microbiolspec.MB-0011-2014

Linares, J. F., Gustafsson, I., Baquero, F., and Martinez, J. L. (2006). Antibiotics as intermicrobial signaling agents instead of weapons. *Proc. Natl. Acad. Sci. U.S.A.* 103, 19484–19489. doi: 10.1073/pnas.0608949103

Mah, T.-F., Pitts, B., Pellock, B., Walker, G. C., Stewart, P. S., and O'Toole, G. A. (2003). A genetic basis for *Pseudomonas aeruginosa* biofilm antibiotic resistance. *Nature* 426, 306–310. doi: 10.1038/nature02122

McDougald, D., Rice, S. A., Barraud, N., Steinberg, P. D., and Kjelleberg, S. (2011). Should we stay or should we go: mechanisms and ecological consequences for biofilm dispersal. *Nat. Rev. Microbiol.* 10, 39–50. doi: 10.1038/nrmicro2695

Monahan, L. G., Turnbull, L., Osvath, S. R., Birch, D., Charles, I. G., and Whitchurch, C. B. (2014). Rapid conversion of *Pseudomonas aeruginosa* to a spherical cell morphotype facilitates tolerance to carbapenems and penicillins but increases susceptibility to antimicrobial peptides. *Antimicrob. Agents Chemother.* 58, 1956–1962. doi: 10.1128/AAC.01901-13

Moskowitz, S. M., Foster, J. M., Emerson, J., and Burns, J. L. (2004). Clinically feasible biofilm susceptibility assay for isolates of *Pseudomonas aeruginosa* from patients with cystic fibrosis. *J. Clin. Microbiol.* 42, 1915–1922. doi: 10.1128/JCM.42.5.1915-1922.2004

Mulcahy, L. R., Isabella, V. M., and Lewis, K. (2014). *Pseudomonas aeruginosa* biofilms in disease. *Microb. Ecol.* 68, 1–12. doi: 10.1007/s00248-013-0297-x

Ng, M., Epstein, S. B., Callahan, M. T., Piotrowski, B. O., Simon, G. L., Roberts, A. D., et al. (2014). Induction of MRSA biofilm by low-dose β-Lactam antibiotics: specificity, prevalence and dose-response effects. *Dose Response* 12, 152–161. doi: 10.2203/dose-response.13-021.Kaplan

Okshevsky, M., and Meyer, R. L. (2015). The role of extracellular DNA in the establishment, maintenance and perpetuation of bacterial biofilms. *Crit. Rev. Microbiol.* 41, 341–352. doi: 10.3109/1040841X.2013.841639

Olivares, E., Badel-Berchoux, S., Provot, C., Jaulhac, B., Prévost, G., Bernardi, T., et al. (2016). The BioFilm ring test: a rapid method for routine analysis of *Pseudomonas aeruginosa* biofilm formation kinetics. *J. Clin. Microbiol.* 54, 657–661. doi: 10.1128/JCM.02938-15

Olivares, E., Badel-Berchoux, S., Provot, C., Jaulhac, B., Prévost, G., Bernardi, T., et al. (2017). Tobramycin and amikacin delay adhesion and microcolony formation in *Pseudomonas aeruginosa* cystic fibrosis isolates. *Front. Microbiol.* 8:1289. doi: 10.3389/fmicb.2017.01289

Otani, S., Hiramatsu, K., Hashinaga, K., Komiya, K., Umeki, K., Kishi, K., et al. (2018). Sub-minimum inhibitory concentrations of ceftazidime inhibit *Pseudomonas aeruginosa* biofilm formation. *J. Infect. Chemother.* 24, 428–433. doi: 10.1016/j.jiac.2018.01.007

O'Toole, G. A., and Kolter, R. (1998). Flagellar and twitching motility are necessary for *Pseudomonas aeruginosa* biofilm development. *Mol. Microbiol.* 30, 295–304. doi: 10.1046/j.1365-2958.1998.01062.x

Ozbek, B., and Mataraci-Kara, E. (2016). Comparative *in vitro* efficacies of various antipseudomonal antibiotics based catheter lock solutions on eradication of *Pseudomonas aeruginosa* biofilms. *J. Chemother.* 28, 20–24. doi: 10.1179/1973947814Y.0000000212

Paraje, M. G. (2011). "Antimicrobial resistance in biofilms," in *Science Against Microbial Pathogens: Communicating Current Research and Technological Advances*, ed. A. Méndez-Vilas, (Badajoz: Formatex Research Center), 736–744.

Parker, A. E., Walker, D. K., Goeres, D. M., Allan, N., Olson, M. E., and Omar, A. (2014). Ruggedness and reproducibility of the MBEC biofilm disinfectant efficacy test. *J. Microbiol. Methods* 102, 55–64. doi: 10.1016/j.mimet.2014.04.013

Pezzulo, A. A., Tang, X. X., Hoegger, M. J., Abou Alaiwa, M. H., Ramachandran, S., Moninger, T. O., et al. (2012). Reduced airway surface pH impairs bacterial killing in the porcine cystic fibrosis lung. *Nature* 487, 109–113. doi: 10.1038/nature11130

Poole, K. (2012). Stress responses as determinants of antimicrobial resistance in Gram-negative bacteria. *Trends Microbiol.* 20, 227–234. doi: 10.1016/j.tim.2012.02.004

Rodríguez-Rojas, A., Oliver, A., and Blázquez, J. (2012). Intrinsic and environmental mutagenesis drive diversification and persistence of *Pseudomonas aeruginosa* in chronic lung infections. *J. Infect. Dis.* 205, 121–127. doi: 10.1093/infdis/jir690

Roudashti, S., Zeighami, H., Mirshahabi, H., Bahari, S., Soltani, A., and Haghi, F. (2017). Synergistic activity of sub-inhibitory concentrations of curcumin with ceftazidime and ciprofloxacin against *Pseudomonas aeruginosa* quorum sensing related genes and virulence traits. *World J. Microbiol. Biotechnol.* 33:50. doi: 10.1007/s11274-016-2195-0

Saginur, R., Stdenis, M., Ferris, W., Aaron, S. D., Chan, F., Lee, C., et al. (2006). Multiple combination bactericidal testing of staphylococcal biofilms from implant-associated infections. *Antimicrob. Agents Chemother.* 50, 55–61. doi: 10.1128/AAC.50.1.55-61.2006

Schadow, K. H., Simpson, W. A., and Christensen, G. D. (1988). Characteristics of adherence to plastic tissue culture plates of coagulase-negative staphylococci exposed to subinhibitory concentrations of antimicrobial agents. *J. Infect. Dis.* 157, 71–77. doi: 10.1093/infdis/157.1.71

Schurek, K. N., Breidenstein, E. B. M., and Hancock, R. E. W. (2012). "*Pseudomonas aeruginosa*: a persistent pathogen in cystic fibrosis and hospital-associated infections," in *Antibiotic Discovery and Development*, eds T. J. Dougherty, and M. J. Pucci, (New York, NY: Springer), 679–715. doi: 10.1007/978-1-4614-1400-1_21

Serra, D. O., and Hengge, R. (2014). Stress responses go three dimensional - the spatial order of physiological differentiation in bacterial macrocolony biofilms. *Environ. Microbiol.* 16, 1455–1471. doi: 10.1111/1462-2920.12483

Skindersoe, M. E., Alhede, M., Phipps, R., Yang, L., Jensen, P. O., Rasmussen, T. B., et al. (2008). Effects of antibiotics on quorum sensing in *Pseudomonas aeruginosa. Antimicrob. Agents Chemother.* 52, 3648–3663. doi: 10.1128/AAC.01230-07

Song, T., Duperthuy, M., and Wai, S. N. (2016). Sub-optimal treatment of bacterial biofilms. *Antibiotics* 5:E23. doi: 10.3390/antibiotics5020023

Srivastava, S., and Bhargava, A. (2016). Biofilms and human health. *Biotechnol. Lett.* 38, 1–22. doi: 10.1007/s10529-015-1960-8

Stewart, P. S. (2002). Mechanisms of antibiotic resistance in bacterial biofilms. *Int. J. Med. Microbiol.* 292, 107–113. doi: 10.1078/1438-4221-00196

Szczuka, E., Jabłońska, L., and Kaznowski, A. (2017). Effect of subinhibitory concentrations of tigecycline and ciprofloxacin on the expression of biofilm-associated genes and biofilm structure of *Staphylococcus epidermidis. Microbiology* 163, 712–718. doi: 10.1099/mic.0.000453

Tasse, J., Croisier, D., Badel-Berchoux, S., Chavanet, P., Bernardi, T., Provot, C., et al. (2016). Preliminary results of a new antibiotic susceptibility test against biofilm installation in device-associated infections: the antibiofilmogram§. *Pathog. Dis.* 74: ftw057. doi: 10.1093/femspd/ftw057

Vallet, I., Olson, J. W., Lory, S., Lazdunski, A., and Filloux, A. (2001). The chaperone/usher pathways of *Pseudomonas aeruginosa*: identification of fimbrial gene clusters (cup) and their involvement in biofilm formation. *Proc. Natl. Acad. Sci. U.S.A.* 98, 6911–6916. doi: 10.1073/pnas.111551898

Wassermann, T., Meinike Jørgensen, K., Ivanyshyn, K., Bjarnsholt, T., Khademi, S. M. H., Jelsbak, L., et al. (2016). The phenotypic evolution of *Pseudomonas aeruginosa* populations changes in the presence of subinhibitory concentrations of ciprofloxacin. *Microbiology* 162, 865–875. doi: 10.1099/mic.0.000273

Waters, V., and Ratjen, F. (2017). Standard versus biofilm antimicrobial susceptibility testing to guide antibiotic therapy in cystic fibrosis. *Cochrane Database Syst. Rev.* 10:CD009528. doi: 10.1002/14651858.CD009528.pub4

Watters, C., DeLeon, K., Trivedi, U., Griswold, J. A., Lyte, M., Hampel, K. J., et al. (2013). *Pseudomonas aeruginosa* biofilms perturb wound resolution and antibiotic tolerance in diabetic mice. *Med. Microbiol. Immunol.* 202, 131–141. doi: 10.1007/s00430-012-0277-7

Watters, C., Fleming, D., Bishop, D., and Rumbaugh, K. P. (2016). Host responses to biofilm. *Prog. Mol. Biol. Transl. Sci.* 142, 193–239. doi: 10.1016/bs.pmbts.2016.05.007

Whitchurch, C. B., Tolker-Nielsen, T., Ragas, P. C., and Mattick, J. S. (2002). Extracellular DNA required for bacterial biofilm formation. *Science* 295:1487. doi: 10.1126/science.295.5559.1487

Whiteley, M., Bangera, M. G., Bumgarner, R. E., Parsek, M. R., Teitzel, G. M., Lory, S., et al. (2001). Gene expression in *Pseudomonas aeruginosa* biofilms. *Nature* 413, 860–864. doi: 10.1038/35101627

Wozniak, D. J., and Keyser, R. (2004). Effects of subinhibitory concentrations of macrolide antibiotics on *Pseudomonas aeruginosa. CHEST J.* 125, 62S–69S. doi: 10.1378/chest.125.2_suppl.62s

Yau, Y. C. W., Ratjen, F., Tullis, E., Wilcox, P., Freitag, A., Chilvers, M., et al. (2015). Randomized controlled trial of biofilm antimicrobial susceptibility testing in cystic fibrosis patients. *J. Cyst. Fibros.* 14, 262–266. doi: 10.1016/j.jcf.2014.09.013

Yokochi, T., Narita, K., Morikawa, A., Takahashi, K., Kato, Y., Sugiyama, T., et al. (2000). Morphological change in *Pseudomonas aeruginosa* following antibiotic treatment of experimental infection in mice and its relation to susceptibility to phagocytosis and to release of endotoxin. *Antimicrob. Agents Chemother.* 44, 205–206. doi: 10.1128/aac.44.1.205-206.2000

Yu, W., Hallinen, K. M., and Wood, K. B. (2017). Interplay between antibiotic efficacy and drug-induced lysis underlies enhanced biofilm formation at subinhibitory drug concentrations. *Antimicrob. Agents Chemother.* 62:e01603-17. doi: 10.1128/AAC.01603-17

Zhang, L., and Mah, T.-F. (2008). Involvement of a novel efflux system in biofilm-specific resistance to antibiotics. *J. Bacteriol.* 190, 4447–4452. doi: 10.1128/JB.01655-07

5

In vitro Activity and Heteroresistance of Omadacycline against Clinical *Staphylococcus aureus* Isolates from China Reveal the Impact of Omadacycline Susceptibility by Branched-Chain Amino Acid Transport System II Carrier Protein, Na/Pi Cotransporter Family Protein, and Fibronectin-Binding Protein

Bing Bai[1,2†], Zhiwei Lin[1,2†], Zhangya Pu[3†], Guangjian Xu[1,2†], Fan Zhang[1,2], Zhong Chen[1,2], Xiang Sun[1], Jinxin Zheng[1], Peiyu Li[1,2], Qiwen Deng[1,2]* and Zhijian Yu[1,2]*

[1] Department of Infectious Diseases and Shenzhen Key Lab of Endogenous Infections, Shenzhen Nanshan People's Hospital and the 6th Affiliated Hospital of Shenzhen University Health Science Center, Shenzhen, China, [2] Quality Control Center of Hospital Infection Management of Shenzhen, Shenzhen Nanshan People's Hospital, Guangdong Medical University, Shenzhen, China, [3] Key Laboratory of Viral Hepatitis of Hunan Province, Department of Infectious Diseases, Xiangya Hospital, Central South University, Changsha, China

Correspondence:
Qiwen Deng
qiwendeng@hotmail.com
Zhijian Yu
yuzhijiansmu@163.com

[†] These authors have contributed equally to this work

Omadacycline (Omad), a new tetracycline (Tet)-class broad-spectrum aminomethylcycline, has been reported to exhibit excellent potency against Gram-positive bacteria, including *Staphylococcus aureus* and Enterococci. The aim of this study was to evaluate the *in vitro* activity and heteroresistance characteristics of Omad in clinical *S. aureus* isolates from China and investigate Omad resistance mechanisms. A sample of 263 non-duplicate clinical *S. aureus* isolates [127 methicillin-resistant (MRSA) and 136 methicillin-sensitive (MSSA)] were collected retrospectively. Our data indicated that Omad exhibited excellent *in vitro* activity against both MRSA and MSSA. Omad heteroresistance frequencies were 3.17% (4/126) in MRSA and 12.78% (17/133) in MSSA. No mutations in Tet target sites, (five 16SrRNA copies and 30S ribosomal protein S10) were present in heteroresistance-derived clones, whereas Tet target site mutations contribute to induced Omad resistance in *S. aureus in vitro*. RNA sequencing (RNA-Seq) revealed that overexpression of branched-chain amino acid transport system II carrier protein and Na/Pi cotransporter family protein contributes to Omad heteroresistance emergence. Whole-genome sequencing demonstrated that the genetic mutation of fibronectin-binding protein (FnBP) could increase the Omad MIC. In conclusion, Omad heteroresistance risk should be considered in clinical isolates with

MICs $\geq$ 0.5 mg/L and Omad susceptibility in *S. aureus* may be affected by efflux pump proteins (i.e., a branched-chain amino acid transport system II carrier protein and an Na/Pi cotransporter family protein), and FnBP.

Keywords: omadacycline, *Staphylococcus aureus*, antimicrobial activity, multilocus sequence typing, tetracycline specific resistance genes

INTRODUCTION

Staphylococcus aureus is a pervasive human pathogen that causes infectious diseases ranging in severity from superficial skin abscesses to bacteremia and septic shock (Calfee, 2017). Although the incidence of methicillin-resistant *S. aureus* (MRSA) infection appears to be declining worldwide, the incidence of bacteremia and severe community-acquired infection caused by methicillin-susceptible *S. aureus* (MSSA) continues to be an important human health threat (Bal et al., 2017). Both MRSA and MSSA infections remain a major clinical problem exacerbated by the ongoing evolution and transmission of traits engendering resistance or reduced susceptibility to current last-line antimicrobial agents, including linezolid, daptomycin, tigecycline (Tig), and vancomycin. Thus, there remains an urgent need for the development of new antimicrobial agents (Bal et al., 2017; Calfee, 2017).

Omadacycline [7-dimethylamino, 9-(2,2-dimethyl-propyl)-aminomethylcycline; Omad] is a recently developed semisynthetic aminomethylcycline belonging to the tetracycline (Tet) family (Pfaller et al., 2017a). It has extraordinarily broad-spectrum antimicrobial activity against Gram-positive and -negative bacteria, including difficult-to-treat multidrug resistant bacteria, such as MRSA and vancomycin-resistant *enterococci* (Pfaller et al., 2017a). Like other Tet drugs, Omad is a potent inhibitor of the bacterial ribosome that inhibits bacterial protein synthesis by binding 30S ribosomal subunits during translation (Draper et al., 2014; Honeyman et al., 2015; Heidrich et al., 2016; Villano et al., 2016). Omad has the advantage of being minimally affected by classical Tet resistance mechanisms, including efflux pumps and ribosomal protection mechanisms. Omad also exhibits lower minimum inhibitory concentration (MIC) values against multidrug resistant bacteria than minocycline and Tig (Draper et al., 2014; Honeyman et al., 2015; Heidrich et al., 2016; Villano et al., 2016), making it a novel potential last-resort antibiotic for difficult-to-treat bacteria infections (Noel et al., 2012; Macone et al., 2014; Pfaller et al., 2017b; Zhang et al., 2018).

Heteroresistance means that there are population-wide variable responses to antibiotics. Several reports, including the earliest studies describing the phenomenon, applied this definition without specifying a particular antibiotic concentration range (El-Halfawy and Valvano, 2013, 2015). Previously, we obtained MICs and heteroresistance occurrence data for the new generation Tet-class drug erevacycline in clinical *S. aureus* isolates from China, underscoring the importance and necessity of investigating the characteristics of new-generation Tet derivatives (Zhang et al., 2018; Zheng et al., 2018). There are

limited data regarding Omad activity against clinical *S. aureus* isolates from China. Heteroresistance development in last-resort antibiotics can hinder efficacy and, ultimately, lead to treatment failure (Claeys et al., 2016; Zhang et al., 2018; Zheng et al., 2018). Thus, it is important to establish potential factors associated with Omad heteroresistance development.

Reduced susceptibility to Tig, an archetype new-generation Tet-class drug, in several species of bacteria has been associated with genetic mutations affecting 30S ribosomal subunits, including altered copy numbers of genes encoding 16S rRNA and 30S ribosomal proteins S3 and S10 (Nguyen et al., 2014; Lupien et al., 2015; Grossman, 2016; Argudin et al., 2018). Tig resistance has been related to regulators of cell envelop proteins, including efflux pumps (e.g., SoxS, MarA, RamA, and Rob) in Gram-negative enterobacteria and MepR/MepA in *S. aureus* (Nguyen et al., 2014; Grossman, 2016; Linkevicius et al., 2016; Dabul et al., 2018). The possible influences of 30S ribosomal subunit mutations and the overexpression of efflux proteins on Omad heteroresistance and resistance in *S. aureus* has not been resolved and needs to be further studied.

The main purpose of this study was to investigate the *in vitro* antimicrobial activity of Omad and to use population analysis profile (PAP) analysis to evaluate the occurrence of Omad heteroresistance in *S. aureus* isolates from China. We examined Omad heteroresistance mechanisms in *S. aureus* by conducting polymerase chain reaction (PCR) experiments to detect genetic mutations in 30S ribosome units, administering efflux protein inhibitors (Zhang et al., 2018; Zheng et al., 2018), and conducting RNA sequencing (RNA-Seq) studies. Furthermore, we used *in vitro* induction of resistance under Omad pressure and next generation sequencing (NGS) to compare Omad-sensitive and -resistant isolates and uncover molecular factors involved in Omad resistance.

MATERIALS AND METHODS

Bacterial Isolates

A total of 263 non-duplicate clinical *S. aureus* isolates (127 MRSA and 136 MSSA) were collected from Shenzhen Nanshan People's Hospital, a tertiary hospital with 1,200 beds in China, between 2008 and 2016. The specimen sources are summarized in **Supplementary Figure S1**. *S. aureus* ATCC29213 was used as a quality control organism. All procedures involving human participants were performed in accordance with the ethical standards of Shenzhen University and the 1964 Helsinki declaration and its later amendments, or comparable ethical standards. For this type of study, formal consent is not required.

Antimicrobial Susceptibility

Staphylococcus aureus antimicrobial susceptibilities to a panel of antibiotics (i.e., amikacin, erythromycin, ciprofloxacin, rifampicin, Tet, tobramycin, vancomycin, linezolid, nitrofurantoin, amoxicillin/clavulanate, and quinupristin) with the VITEK 2 system (BioMérieux, Marcy l'Etoile, France) and susceptibility breakpoints based on CLSI guidelines (2016). Omad was obtained from The Medicines Company (Med Chem Express, Monmouth Junction, NJ, United States). Omad MICs were determined with the agar dilution method according to CLSI guidelines (Klionsky et al., 2016). We employed three Omad MIC levels ($\leq$0.25 mg/L, 0.5 mg/L, and $\geq$1 mg/L) in our antimicrobial susceptibility analysis. The following Acute Bacterial Skin and Skin Structure Infections Omad susceptibility breakpoints recommended by FDA criteria were adopted: $\leq$0.5 mg/L for susceptibility, 1 mg/L for intermediate status, and $\geq$2 mg/L for resistance.

PAP Development

Omad heteroresistance in *S. aureus* was determined by PAP development as described previously (Zhang et al., 2018; Zheng et al., 2018) with a MIC cut-off criterion of $\leq$0.5 mg/L. Briefly, 50-μL aliquots (108 bacterial colony forming units) were spread onto Müller-Hinton broth plates containing serial dilutions of Omad (in mg/L): 0.5, 1, 2, and 3. Colonies were counted on Omad-containing plates after 24 h of incubation at 37°C. According to the criteria described above, we defined 2 mg/L as the susceptibility breakpoint for PAP determination of *S aureus*. For Omad-resistant subpopulations detected among Omad-susceptible *S. aureus* isolate colonies grown on agar plates with 2 mg/L Omad with a detection limit of $\geq$5 colony forming units/ml, the parental isolates were considered to have Omad heteroresistance. Two heteroresistance-derived colonies were selected randomly from plates and their Omad and Tig MICs were measured by agar dilution according to CLSI guidelines and then subjected to PCRs, efflux inhibition, and transcriptional analysis (Zhang et al., 2018).

Polymerase Chain Reaction

Genomic DNA was extracted from isolates with Lysis Buffer for Microorganisms to Direct PCR (Takara Bio Inc., Japan). Tet resistance genes encoding Tet(K), Tet(L), Tet(M), and Tet(O) were detected by PCR analysis as described previously (Bai et al., 2018). The presence of 30S ribosomal subunit mutations, including five separate copies of the 16S rRNA gene, the genes encoding the 30S ribosomal proteins S3 and S10, and the genes encoding recombinase (RecB) and fibronectin-binding protein (FnBP) were analyzed by PCR and sequence alignment (primer sequences listed in **Supplementary Table S1**). Multi-locus sequence typing (MLST) was conducted to identify the distributions of sequence types (STs) among MRSA

and MSSA isolates. PCR conditions recommended for locus amplification[1] were employed.

Efflux Inhibition

The role of efflux pumps in Omad heteroresistance was evaluated with the efflux pump inhibitors phenylalanine-arginine-β-naphthylamide (PaβN) and carbonyl cyanidem-chlorophenylhydrazine (CCCP; both from Sigma). Omad MICs were determined by the agar dilution method in the presence and absence of 50 mg/L PaβN or 16 mg/L CCCP. Inhibition was confirmed based on a $\geq$4-fold MIC reduction (Osei Sekyere and Amoako, 2017; Zhang et al., 2018).

In vitro Induction of Omad-Resistance Under Omad Pressure

Seven parental *S. aureus* isolates, including six clinical isolates (MSSAs: CHS221, CHS165, and 149. MRSAs: CHS759, CHS810, and CHS820) and a well-characterized antibiotic-susceptible MS4 strain, were used to select Omad-resistant isolates. These isolates were subcultured serially in Mueller-Hinton broth containing gradual increasing Omad concentrations with the initial concentration being MIC equivalents followed by successive increases to 2$\times$, 4$\times$, 8$\times$, and 16$\times$ MICs (Yao et al., 2018), with four passages at each concentration. Isolates from the passages of each concentration were stored at $-$80°C in Mueller-Hinton broth containing 40% glycerol for subsequent Tet-target site genetic mutation detection, subsequent MIC assays, next generation sequencing, and PCR analysis. Killing curves were performed on the CHS221 (wild-type MSSA strain), CHS221-O (Omad heteroresistance MSSA strain), CHS221-1Δ: (Omad resistance MSSA strain), CHS759 (wild-type MRSA strain), CHS759-O (Omad heteroresistance MRSA strain), and CHS759-1Δ: (Omad resistance MRSA strain). Tubes containing Omad at concentrations corresponding to 0 and 4 mg/L were inoculated with a suspension of each test strain, yielding to a final bacterial density of 8 $\times$ 106 cfu/ml. The killing curves shown Omad-resistant strain could grow well at concentrations corresponding to 4 mg/L (**Supplementary Figure S2**).

RNA-Seq

Wild-type strain CHS221 (S221) and its heteroresistance-derived *S. aureus* isolate CHS221-O (S221-O1) were grown and prepared for total RNA extraction with TRIzol reagent (Invitrogen, Carlsbad, CA, United States) as described previously (Zheng et al., 2018). RNA-Seq of the aforementioned parental and heteroresistance-derived isolates was performed as reported previously (Lin et al., 2017). Raw data (raw reads) of fastq format were firstly processed through in-house perl scripts. In this step, clean data (clean reads) were obtained by removing reads containing adapter, reads containing ploy-N and low quality reads from raw data. All the downstream analyses were based on the clean data with high quality. The raw data from the samples were analyzed in Subread software; raw counts for each group

---

[1]http://www.mlst.com/server

were normalized and processed in the EdgeR Bioconductor software package. 1.3-fold differences in expression level by RNA-Sequencing were considered to be differentially expressed genes (DEGs). The RNA sequencing outcomes for two strains were deposited in the NCBI database (BioProject accession number PRJNA505108).

Quantitative Real Time (qRT)-PCR Analysis

We selected 30 DEGs based on our RNA-Seq results and employed qRT-PCR to compare transcriptional expression levels between the parental and heteroresistance-derived strains as described in detail previously (Zheng et al., 2018). The transcriptional expression levels of the eight candidates genes (USA300HOU_RS00705, USA300 HOU_RS03535, USA300 HOU_RS01625, USA300 HOU_RS00550, USA300HOU_RS13205, USA300HOU_RS13945, USA300HOU_RS10505, and USA300HOU_RS00660) were further analyzed and compared among the CHS165 (MSSA), 149 (MSSA), CHS759 (MRSA), CHS810 (MRSA), and CHS820 (MRSA) parental strains and their derivative heteroresistant and resistant strains. Total RNA of bacteria was extracted using the RNeasyH Mini Kit (QIAGEN, Hilden, Germany) following the manufacturer's instructions. The extracted RNA was reverse transcribed into cDNA using iScript reverse transcriptase (Bio-Rad, Hercules, CA, United States) with incubation for 5 min at 25°C, followed by 30 min at 42°C and 5 min at 85°C. Subsequently, qRT-PCRs were performed using SYBR green PCR reagents (Premix EX TaqTM, Takara Biotechnology, Dalian, China) in the Mastercycler realplex system (Eppendorf AG, Hamburg, Germany) with amplification conditions of 95°C for 30 s, 40 cycles of 95°C for 5 s and 60°C for 34 s, followed by melting curve analysis. The control gene *gyrB* was used to normalize gene expression. Threshold cycle (Ct) numbers were determined by detection system software and analyzed with the $2^{-\Delta\Delta Ct}$ method and three replicates have been made. The qRT-PCR primers used are listed in **Supplementary Table S2**.

Next Generation Sequencing

An Omad resistant *S. aureus* strain, MS4O8, was derived from an Omad-susceptible isolate, MS4. Chromosomal DNA was extracted from MS4O8 cells for NGS. Nextera shotgun libraries and whole genome sequencing were performed by Novogene Company (Beijing, China). Illumina PE150 sequencing data were mapped against the CP009828 *S. aureus* MS4 strain reference genome in bwa mem software (v0.7.5a)[2] with standard parameters. Small nucleotide polymorphisms and small insertions/deletions were detected in MS408 cells, relative to MS4, in MUMmer (version 3.23). A custom script was used to detect substitutions, insertions, and deletions that might be impacting protein coding regions. Binary alignment/map files of the sequenced strains were deposited in the NCBI database (BioProject accession number PRJNA511962).

_____

[2]http://biobwa.sourceforge.net/

Gene Overexpression

Full-length candidate genes, including USA300HOU_RS00550 (encodes a Na/Pi cotransporter family protein), USA300HOU_RS01625 (encodes a branched-chain amino acid transport system II carrier protein), USA300HOU_RS03535, USA300HOU_Tet(K), NI36_12460 (FnBP), and NI36_00170 (RecB), were amplified with extra double enzyme sites from total DNA extracted from USA300HOU and MS4 isolates. RecB-M is RecB with a mutation (R10R, I23V, I23N, H24N, H24Q, V29L, and V35M) and FnBP-M is FnBP with a mutation (T672S and I665V). RecB-M and FnBP-M DNA fragments were amplified from MS4O8 by PCR. The candidate gene fragments were each integrated into separate pIB166 vectors, and their encoded target protein were induced with 2 mM chromium chloride (Wu et al., 2012). The primers used for vector constructs in this study are listed in **Supplementary Table S3**. Positively vector transformed *S. aureus* clones were selected with chloramphenicol and verified by PCR and Sanger sequencing. The overexpression plasmids were transformed separately into three to five Omad-sensitive isolates and their integrations was confirmed by PCR and Sanger sequencing. Candidate gene transcriptional levels were measured by qRT-PCR, as described above. Omad and Tig MICs for these derivatives were determined and heteroresistance occurrence in these derivatives was tested by PAP analysis under Omad pressure as described above.

Statistical Analysis

Continuous data were analyzed with Student's *t*-tests and one-way factorial analyses of variance (ANOVAs) in SPSS software package (version 17.0, Chicago, IL, United States). *P*-values < 0.05 were regarded as statistically significant.

RESULTS

In vitro Activity of Omad Against Clinical *S. aureus* Isolates

Of the 127 MRSA isolates examined, 46 (36.22%), 80 (62.99%), and 1 (0.78%) were found to have Omad MIC levels of ≤0.25 mg/L (sensitive), 0.5 mg/L (sensitive), and 1 mg/L (intermediate), respectively. Of the 136 MSSA isolates examined, 23 (16.91%), 110 (80.88%), and 3 (2.20%) were categorized into these levels, respectively. Thus, there were higher frequencies of MSSA isolates than MRSA isolates with Omad MICs in the 0.5 and ≥1 mg/L levels. We analyzed the distribution of the above three Omad MIC levels among strains with sensitive and intermediate status relative to other common antibiotics (amikacin, erythromycin, ciprofloxacin, rifampicin, Tet, tobramycin, nitrofurantoin, quinupristin, and amoxicillin/clavulanate, vancomycin, and linezolid). The frequencies of isolates at each Omad MIC level found to be resistant to these antibiotics are reported in **Table 1**, together with the resistance breakpoints used. All *S. aureus* isolates in this study were susceptible to vancomycin and linezolid, and all of the MSSA isolates were susceptible to

TABLE 1 | *Staphylococcus aureus* antibiotic resistance and correspondence to Omad MIC level.

Class	Drug	Resistance rate (%)	Total N	MIC breakpoint (mg/L)	N	Omad MIC level (mg/L), N		
						≤0.25	0.5	1
MRSA	Total		127	–	127	46	80	1
	Amikacin	51.61	124	≤16	60	24	36	0
				32	3	0	3	0
				≥64	61	20	42	1
	Erythromycin	99.21	127	≤0.5	1	1	0	0
				1–4	1	1	0	0
				≥8	125	44	80	1
	Ciprofloxacin	52.84	123	≤1	58	24	34	0
				2	1	0	1	0
				≥4	64	19	44	1
	Rifampicin	15.87	126	≤1	106	39	66	1
				≥4	20	6	14	0
	Tet	69.29	127	≤4	39	20	19	0
				8	15	6	9	0
				≥16	73	20	52	1
	Tobramycin	52.84	123	≤4	58	23	35	0
				≥16	65	21	43	1
	Nitrofurantoin	3.17	126	≤32	122	43	78	1
				64	2	1	1	0
				≥128	2	1	1	0
	Quinupristin	2.50	120	≤1	117	42	74	1
				2	1	0	1	0
				≥4	2	1	1	0
MSSA	Total		136	–	136	23	110	3
	Amikacin	5.30	132	≤16	124	21	100	3
				32	5	0	5	0
				≥64	2	0	2	0
	Erythromycin	83.58	134	≤0.5	22	1	21	0
				1–4	3	0	3	0
				≥8	109	21	85	3
	Ciprofloxacin	10.76	130	≤1	116	21	93	2
				≥4	14	0	13	1
	Rifampicin	4.51	133	≤1	127	21	104	2
				≥4	6	1	4	1
	Tet	50	136	≤4	68	21	47	0
				8	9	0	8	1
				≥16	59	2	55	2
	Tobramycin	45.60	125	≤4	68	14	52	2
				8	1	0	1	0
				≥16	56	5	51	0
	Nitrofurantoin	0.74	134	≤32	133	22	108	3
				64	1	0	1	0
	Quinupristin	2.5	120	≤1	116	20	94	2
				2	1	0	1	0
				≥4	2	0	2	0

amoxicillin/clavulanate. Interestingly, as reported in **Table 1**, Tet-resistant MRSA were more frequent than Tet-resistant MSSA, and Omad MICs $\geq$ 0.5 mg/L were more frequent among MSSA isolates than among MRSA isolates, suggesting a non-conformity in the antimicrobial susceptibility dynamics of Tet and Omad. The characteristics of *S. aureus* with

Omad MICs of 1 mg/L are summarized in **Supplementary Table S4**. Briefly, no genetic mutations in 30S ribosome units were detected and efflux pump inhibition reversed Omad resistance, as evidenced by significant reductions in MICs to $\leq$0.03 mg/L with CCCP and to 0.25–1 mg/L with PAβN.

Omad MICs of *S. aureus* Isolates Harboring Tet-Resistance Genes

The frequencies of genes encoding the Tet-resistance factors Tet(M), Tet(L), Tet(K), and Tet(O), alone and in combination, in MRSA and MSSA isolates are reported in **Supplementary Table S5**. There were 109 *S. aureus* isolates harboring at least one Tet-resistance factor gene; their MIC$_{90}$ values were consistently 0.5 mg/L. Omad exhibited excellent *in vitro* activity against both Tet-resistance gene carrying and non-carrying *S. aureus* isolates. Omad MICs for both MRSA and MSSA harboring Tet-resistance factors were ≤0.5 mg/L for all isolates, with the exception of three Tet(K) gene-carrying isolates (1 MRSA and 2 MSSA), indicating that overexpression of Tet(K) might impact Omad susceptibility. It is noteworthy that the Omad MIC values obtained for all 46 MSSA isolates carrying the Tet(K) gene, Tet(L) gene, or both were ≥0.5 mg/L. Meanwhile, of the 63 MRSA isolates with the Tet(M) gene, Tet(K) gene, Tet(L) gene, or some combination of these genes, just 47 (74.60%) had Omad MIC values ≥0.5 mg/L.

Clonality of Omad MIC Distribution in Clinical *S. aureus* Isolates

MLST results for the 263 isolates are summarized in **Supplementary Figure S3**. To evaluate the relationship of ST clonality with Omad MIC distribution, we examined ST distributions relative to Tet and Omad MICs (**Supplementary Table S6**). Omad MICs ≥ 0.5 mg/L were found for 72.58% (45/62) of ST239-MRSA, 57.5% (23/40) of ST59-MRSA, and 57.14% (4/7) of ST1-MRSA isolates. Meanwhile, Omad MICs ≥ 0.5 mg/L were found for 89.66% (26/29) of ST7-MSSA, 89.47% (17/19) ST59-MSSA, 76.92% (10/13) of ST398-MSSA, 85.71% (6/7) of ST88-MSSA, and 71.43% (5/7) of ST120-MSSA isolates. Hence, Omad sensitivity differed between MRSA and MSSA of the same ST (e.g., ST59-MRSA vs. ST59-MSSA). MLST indicated that 72/81 (88.89%) MRSA isolates with Omad MICs ≥ 0.5 mg/L belonged to the top three MRSA STs (ST239, ST59, and ST1), whereas only 52/113 (46.12%) of MSSA isolates with Omad MICs ≥ 0.5 mg/L belonged to the top three MSSA STs (**Supplementary Table S6** and **Table 1**), revealing a more pronounced clustering of Omad MIC creep in the top three MRSA STs than in the top three MSSA STs (nearly 90% vs. less than half).

Omad Heteroresistance Frequency and Mechanism in *S. aureus*

Omad heteroresistance was identified in 0.0% (0/46) of MRSA with an Omad MIC ≤ 0.25 mg/L and 3.75% (3/80) of MRSA with an Omad MIC of 0.5 mg/L. Omad heteroresistance was identified in 0.0% (0/30) of MSSA with an Omad MIC ≤ 0.25 mg/L and 17.48% (18/103) of MSSA with an Omad MIC of 0.5 mg/L. We determined the Omad and Tig MICs of two clones from each heteroresistant subpopulation and found that their Omad MICs were in the range of 1–8 mg/L and their Tig MICs were in the range of 2–8 mg/L (shown in **Supplementary Table S7** and data for six isolates subjected to *in vitro* resistance induction are shown in **Table 2**). Moreover, no genetic mutations were found in 30S ribosomal subunit genes (five 16SrRNA gene copies, 30S

ribosomal protein S3 and S10 genes) in heteroresistance-derived clones (**Table 2** and **Supplementary Table S7**). In efflux pump inhibition experiments, Omad MICs in heteroresistance-derived *S. aureus* clones were reduced to ≤0.03 mg/L by CCCP and reduced to 0.25–1 mg/L by PAβN (**Supplementary Table S7**).

Association of Selected Candidate Genes With Omad Heteroresistance

Efflux pump inhibition experiments indicated that efflux pumps or membrane proteins might participate in the development of heteroresistance. Therefore, RNA-Seq was performed and unigene transcription levels were compared between the parental strain CHS221 (S221) and its heteroresistant derivative CHS221-O1 (S221-O). Ninety six DEGs were found by this approach between S221 and S221-O, including 58 upregulated and 38 down-regulated genes in the derivative strain (**Supplementary Figure S4**). KEGG pathway analysis showed that the pathways most frequently linked to DEGs were related to phosphate ion transport (3 DEGs), inorganic anion transport (3 DEGs), dihydrofolate reductase activity (2 DEGs), and glycine biosynthesis process (2 DEGs).

Subsequent qRT-PCRs for 30 candidate genes were carried out to test the accuracy of our transcriptomic analyses implicated eight efflux-pump encoding DEGs in heteroresistance. The expression levels of these eight candidate genes determined by RNA-Seq and qRT-PCR are shown in **Table 3**. The results of qRT-PCRs performed to quantitate transcription in six *S. aureus* strain groups—inclusive of parental strains, their heteroresistance derivatives, and resistant isolates (**Table 2**)—enabled us to probe the relationship of their expression levels with Omad susceptibility (**Figure 1**). The data suggest that transcription levels of the three candidate genes USA300HOU_RS03535, USA300HOU_RS01625 (encodes a Na/Pi cotransporter family protein), and USA300HOU_RS00550 (encodes a branched-chain amino acid transport system II carrier protein) may impact heteroresistance occurrence.

Mechanism of Omad-Induced Resistance in *S. aureus* Under Omad Pressure

To evaluate Omad resistance mechanisms and Omad-Tig cross-resistance, *in vitro* induction experiments were carried out under Omad pressure with the following Omad-resistant *S. aureus*: CHS221 (MSSA), CHS165 (MSSA), 149 (MSSA), CHS759 (MRSA), CHS810 (MRSA), CHS820 (MRSA), and MS4. The Omad-resistant isolates were characterized with respect to MICs and resistance mechanisms (**Table 2**). Importantly, increasing Omad MICs were accompanied by increasing Tig MICs in Omad-resistant *S. aureus* isolates, indicating that Omad-Tig cross-resistance can be induced under Omad pressure. Moreover, upregulation of Omad MICs was related to increasing numbers of 16SrRNA copies with a genetic mutation. The mutation sites varied among the five 16SrRNA copies, with high frequencies of the T170G polymorphism in RR1, A1124G in RR2, C810T in RR3, and G1036A in RR4. Leu47His and Tyr87His amino acid

TABLE 2 | Antimicrobial susceptibility and resistance mechanism of seven groups of parental, heteroresistant, and Omad-induced resistant strains.

Strain	MIC (mg/L)		Mutation(s)								
	Tig	Omad	RR1	RR2	RR3	RR4	RR5	S3	S10	RecB	FnBP
CHS221 (S221)	0.5	0.5	W	W	W	W	W	W	W	W	W
CHS221-O (S221-O*)	4	8	W	W	W	W	W	W	W	W	W
CHS221-1Δ	32	32	W	A1124G	C810T	G1036A	G1248C	W	MeT48Ile	W	W
CHS221-2	32	32	G848T	A1124G	C810T A1281G	G1036A	A854C	W	MeT48Ile	W	W
CHS165	0.5	0.5	W	W	W	W	W	W	W	W	W
CHS165-O*	4	8	W	W	W	W	W	W	W	W	T672S,
CHS165-1Δ	32	32	T170G	G848A A1124G	C810T	G1036A	G1248C	W	LeT47His	W	T672S, I665V
CHS165-2	32	32	T170G	G77A A1124G	C810T G848C	G1036A	G742A C1247T	W	LeT47His	W	T672S, I665V
149	0.25	0.5	W	W	W	W	W	W	W	W	W
149-O*	8	4	W	W	W	W	W	W	W	W	W
149-1 Δ	64	64	W	A1124G	C810T	G1036A	W	W	LeT47His	W	W
149-2	>64	128	W	A1124G	C810T G848C	G1036A	C1247T	W	LeT47His	W	W
CHS759	0.25	0.5	W	W	W	W	W	W	W	W	W
CHS759-O*	4	4	W	W	W	W	W	W	W	W	W
CHS759-1Δ	32	32	G1036A	A1124G G1036A	C810T G848C	G185A G1036A	G1248C G1036A	W	Met48Thr	W	I665V
CHS759-2	32	32	W	A1124G G1036A	C810T A1281G	G185A G1036A	C1036T	W	Let47Let Tyr87His	W	I665V
CHS810	0.25	0.5	W	W	W	W	W	W	W	W	W
CHS810-O*	4	4	W	W	W	W	W	W	W	W	W
CHS810-1Δ	32	32	T170G	A1124G	C810T	G185A	T1257C G1248C	W	Tyr87His	W	W
CHS810-2	32	32	T170G	A1124G	C810T	G185A G1036A	A79G T1257C	W	Tyr87His	W	T672S,
CHS820	0.25	0.5	W	W	W	W	W	W	W	W	W
CHS820-O*	4	2	W	W	W	W	W	W	W	W	W
CHS820-1Δ	64	128	T170G	A1124G	C810T	G185A G1036A	A79G	W	Tyr87His	W	W
CHS820-2	64	128	T170G G848C	A1124G	C810T A1281G	G185A G1036A	A79G G848C	W	Tyr87His	W	W
MS4	0.125	0.125	W	W	W	W	W	W	W	W	W
MS4-O2	4	4	T170G G783A	W	C810T A1281G	W	T1257C	W	W	W	T672S,
MS4-O8	4	4	T170G C1041T	G848A T1124C	C810T T1281C	W	W	W	Asp60Tyr	RecB-M	T672S, I665V

Parental isolates are isolated with shading; * and Δ represent heteroresistant and Omad-induced resistant strain, respectively (see qRT-PCR in **Figure 1**); RR1-7 are 16s rRNA gene copies; S3 and S10 are 30S ribosome proteins; W, wild-type (no mutation).

substitutions in the 30S ribosomal protein S10 were relatively frequent in Omad-resistant bacteria.

Candidate Genes Related to Omad Resistance in NGS

To identify the genetic mutations that correlate with Omad resistance, whole genome sequencing of MS4O8 was performed and variants relative to MS4 were detected by NGS in MUMmer, version 3.23 (**Supplementary Table S8** and **Table 4**). Non-synonymous mutations were found in NI36_11090 (encodes 30S ribosomal protein S10), NI36_12460 (*fnbp* encoding FnBP protein), and NI36_ 00170 (*recB* encoding recombinase). Mutations affecting these three genes also emerged in our induced Omad-resistance experiment above (**Table 2**). Notably, 30S ribosomal protein S10 has been widely reported to be associated with Tet-class resistance and the impact of FnBP and RecB protein on Omad susceptibility need to be further verified.

Relationship Between Candidate Genes Overexpression and Omad Susceptibility

The impacts of following candidate genes on Omad susceptibility in Omad-sensitive *S. aureus* isolates was conducted: USA300HOU_RS03535, USA300HOU_RS01625 (encodes a branched-chain amino acid transport system II carrier protein), USA300HOU_RS00550 (encodes a Na/Pi cotransporter family protein), *tet*(K), NI36_12460/NI36_12465 (*fnbp*), and NI36_00170 (*recB*). The former three were candidately implicated in Omad heteroresistance in our qRT-PCR experiments. Meanwhile, *tet*(K) was found frequently among *S. aureus* isolates with an Omad MIC of 1 mg/L, and the proteins

encoded by *fnbp* and *recB* have been hypothesized to participate in antimicrobial resistance evolution.

The overexpression plasmids pRS00550, pRS01625, pRS03535, pTet(K), pRecB, pRecB-M, pFnBP, and pFnBP-M, where -M suffix indicates a mutated variant, were transformed into clinical isolates with low expression of the target gene (**Supplementary Tables S9, S10**). Stable overexpression of the candidate genes was confirmed by qRT-PCR (**Supplementary Figure S5**). The influence of the overexpression of these six genes on Omad susceptibility was reported in **Table 5**. Briefly, although RS00550, RS01625, and RS03535 did not elevate Omad or Tig MICs in the absence of antibiotic pressure, PAP experiments showed that RS00550 or RS01625 overexpression could lead to Omad heteroresistance compared with negative findings in controls (**Table 5**). RS00550 and RS01625 homology analysis results are reported in **Supplementary Tables S11, S12**.

Overexpression of *tet*(K) did not elevate Omad or Tig MICs and had no apparent contribution to heteroresistance development in *S. aureus*. The overexpression of *fnbp* (NI36_12 460) and its mutated type led to MIC creep (**Table 5**), supporting the possibility that FnBPs may participate in Omad resistance development. Homology analysis results for *fnbp* are shown in **Supplementary Table S13**. Overexpression of *recB* and its mutants did not impact Omad susceptibility in *S. aureus*.

DISCUSSION

The presently observed low Omad MICs in this study support the supposition that Omad should be considered a prospective preferential choice for *S. aureus* infection treatment. Omad MICs $\geq$ 0.5 mg/L were more frequent among MSSA than MRSA in this study, and moreover, Tet-specific resistance genes, particularly *tet*(K) and *tet*(L), were found to be more common among MSSA than MRSA isolates, indicating that Omad may have greater efficacy against MRSA than MSSA. Our Omad MICs were higher than previously reported, perhaps due to regional variation and environmental factors (Villano et al., 2016; Pfaller et al., 2017a). We also obtained higher MICs for the new-generation Tet-class drug eravacycline in isolates from China than had been reported for isolates from the United States and Europe, suggesting that Tet-class drug MIC dynamics should monitored across global regions with particular attention to MIC creep in China (Zhang et al., 2018; Zheng et al., 2018).

Major mechanisms of Tet resistance in both Gram-positive and -negative microorganisms have been linked to ribosomal protection proteins and efflux pumps, most of which can be overcome with new generation tetracyclines, including Tig and Omad (Jones et al., 2006; Noel et al., 2012; Draper et al., 2014; Macone et al., 2014; Honeyman et al., 2015; Grossman, 2016; Heidrich et al., 2016; Villano et al., 2016; Pfaller et al., 2017b; Argudin et al., 2018; Zhang et al., 2018). In this study, we obtained low Omad MICs for *S. aureus*, even among isolates harboring a ribosomal protection protein, namely Tet(M), or an efflux pump factor, namely Tet(K) and Tet(L), uncovering an apparent advantage of using Omad to overcome Tet-specific resistance mechanisms, particularly those mediated by Tet(M), Tet(K), and

TABLE 3 | Transcriptional expression levels of eight DEGs between S221-O and S221 analyzed by RNA-Seq and qRT-PCR.

Gene_ID	Gene description	Relative increase in transcription in S221-O compared to S221	
		qRT-PCR	Fold change in RNA-Seq
USA300HOU_RS00705	Cell wall-anchored protein SasD	1.42 ± 0.12	2.73
USA300HOU_RS03535	Membrane protein	1.73 ± 0.14	2.83
USA300HOU_RS01625	Branched-chain amino acid transport system II carrier protein	2.77 ± 0.21	2.84
USA300HOU_RS00550	Na/Pi cotransporter family protein	1.18 ± 0.06	2.90
USA300HOU_RS13205	Amino acid permease	1.32 ± 0.11	2.97
USA300HOU_RS13945	PTS transporter subunit IIC	1.42 ± 0.07	3.29
USA300HOU_RS10505	hypothetical protein	5.73 ± 0.65	3.42
USA300HOU_RS00660	MFS transporter	3.27 ± 0.22	3.43

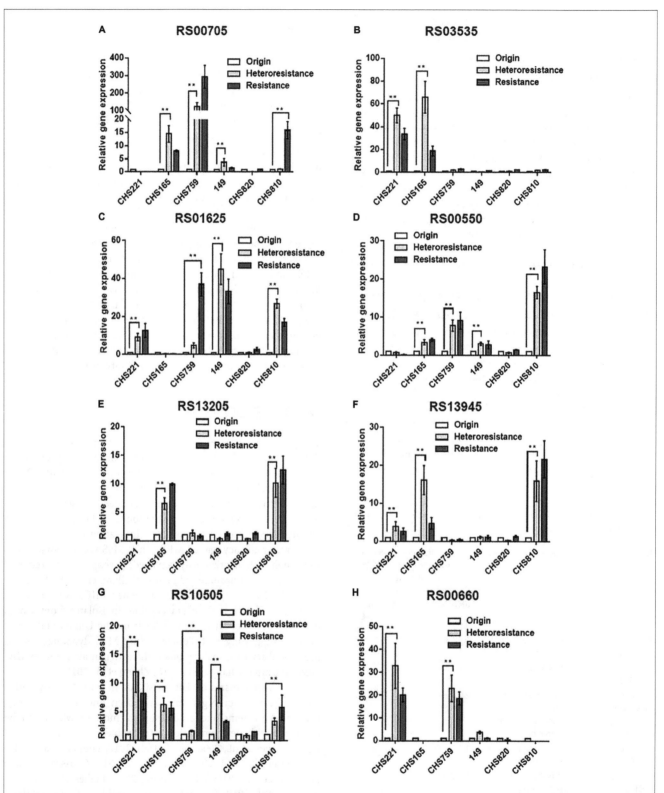

FIGURE 1 | Comparison of the relative transcription of eight candidate DEGs among parental, heteroresistant derivative, and resistant isolates. Relative expression of USA300HOU_RS00705 **(A)**, USA300HOU_RS03535 **(B)**, USA300HOU_RS01625 **(C)**, USA300HOU_RS00550 **(D)**, USA300HOU_RS13205 **(E)**, USA300HOU_RS13945 **(F)**, USA300HOU_RS10505 **(G)**, and USA300HOU_RS00660 **(H)** were demonstrated by qRT-PCR analysis. The housekeeping gene *gyrB* was used as the endogenous reference gene. The original strain was used as the reference strain (expression = 1.0). All qRT-PCRs were carried out in triplicate. $**p < 0.01$, $*p < 0.0.5$. Parental strains are identified below the X axis and the relative folds increased are shown on the Y axis. The parental, heteroresistant, and resistant isolates are described in **Table 2**.

TABLE 4 | Non-synonymous mutations of candidate proteins correlated with Omad resistance found between MS4 and MS4O8.

Gene_ID	Gene description	Amino acid mutations (non-syn) between MS4 and MS4O8
NI36_11090	30S ribosomal protein S10	D60Y
NI36_12460	FnBP	T672S, I665V
NI36_00170	RecB	R10R, I23V, I23N, H24N, H24Q, V29L, V35M

TABLE 5 | Omad and Tig MICs in *S. aureus* derivatives with overexpression of candidate genes and their impact on PAPs.

Vector	Strain	MIC (mg/L)				PAP test positivity
		Parental isolates		Derivative isolates*		
		Omad	Tig	Omad	Tig	
pRS00550	SE7	0.25	0.5	0.25	0.5	10
	CHS545	0.5	0.5	0.25	0.5	12
	CHS569	0.25	0.5	0.25	0.5	5
pRS01625	SE4	0.25	0.5	0.25	0.5	3
	SE7	0.25	0.5	0.25	0.5	5
	CHS569	0.25	0.5	0.25	0.5	9
pRS03535	SE4	0.25	0.5	0.25	0.5	0
	SE7	0.25	0.5	0.25	0.5	0
	SE13	0.25	0.5	0.25	0.5	0
	CHS545	0.5	0.25	0.5	0.25	0
	CHS569	0.25	0.25	0.25	0.25	0
ptet(K)	SE4	0.25	0.5	0.5	0.5	0
	SE7	0.25	0.5	0.25	0.5	0
	SE13	0.25	0.5	0.25	0.5	0
	CHS545	0.5	0.25	0.25	0.5	0
	CHS569	0.25	0.25	0.25	0.5	0
pRecB	SE4	0.25	–	0.25	–	–
pRecB-M	SE4	0.25	–	0.25	–	–
pFBP	SE4	0.25	0.5	0.5	1	–
pFBP-M	SE4	0.25	0.5	1	1	–

FBP-M has T672S and/or I665V mutations. RecB-M has R10R, I23V, I23N, H24N, H24Q, V29L, and/or V35M mutation. Positive PAP results are highlighted with shading.

Tet(L). Notwithstanding, Tig MICs were shown recently to be increased by a high transcriptional level of tet(M) and tet(L) in *Enterococcus faecium* (Fiedler et al., 2016). Because we observed a higher frequency of Tet-specific genes in MSSA than in MRSA from China and three isolates with MICs ≥ 1 mg/L harbored *tet*(K) in this study, we hypothesize that *tet*(K) overexpression may elevate Omad MICs, as was found in *E. coli* (Linkevicius et al., 2016). Our data demonstrate that *tet*(K) overexpression does not impact *S. aureus* susceptibility to Omad *in vitro*, and thus indicate that Omad can overcome the Tet(K)-mediated resistance in *S. aureus*.

Prior epidemiological data have revealed ST239 and ST59 to be predominant MRSA STs internationally, with MSSA ST predominance being more variable across regions (Atshan et al., 2013; Leon-Sampedro et al., 2016; Recker et al., 2017). *S. aureus*

clonality of drug-resistance and virulence factors has been reported (Atshan et al., 2013; Leon-Sampedro et al., 2016; Recker et al., 2017). The present examination of the relationship of ST clonality with Omad susceptibility revealed a far higher frequency of the top-three MRSA STs with MICs ≥ 0.5 mg/L than of the top-three such MSSA STs. Although a definite relationship of ST clustering with Omad MICs has not been established, it is noteworthy that ST59-MSSA were much more likely to have Omad MICs ≥ 0.5 mg/L than were ST59-MRSA.

Heteroresistance frequency is an important harbinger of last-resort antibiotic resistance risk (Zhang et al., 2018; Zheng et al., 2018). The present findings of heteroresistance in 16.98% of MSSA and 3.75% of MRSA with Omad MICs ≥ 0.5 mg/L suggest a need to be alert to selection resistance under Omad pressure for *S. aureus*, especially in strains from China. Moreover, we observed relatively high Tig MICs for Omad heteroresistance-derived clones (2–8 mg/L), indicating a potential risk of Omad-Tig cross-resistance. Mutations affecting 30S ribosomal subunits, which have been reported to participate in Tet or Tig resistance, were not found in our heteroresistance-derived clones or clinical isolates with Omad MICs ≥ 1 mg/L, indicating that 30S ribosomal subunit mutations cannot explain Omad MIC creep and heteroresistance occurrence (Nguyen et al., 2014; Grossman, 2016; Argudin et al., 2018).

The progression of reduced Tig susceptibility in *S. aureus* has been linked with *mepR/mepA* encoded efflux pumps (Lupien et al., 2015). However, the possible role of efflux pumps and cell envelopes in Omad heteroresistance in *S. aureus* is unclear. Multiple reports have shown that protonophore efflux pump inhibitors (e.g., CCCP and PaβN) can be used to evaluate interactions between antibiotics and cell envelope components in bacteria (Klionsky et al., 2016; Bai et al., 2018; Yao et al., 2018). Here, we found that the efflux pump inhibitor PAβN and the cell envelope component inhibitor *CCCP* reduced Omad MICs of heteroresistance-derived *S. aureus* clones to as low as ≤0.03 mg/L and 0.12–1 mg/L, respectively, pointing to involvement of efflux pumps or cell envelopes in the progression of Omad heteroresistance in *S. aureus* (Klionsky et al., 2016; Bai et al., 2018). Omad MICs of isolates with Omad MICs ≥ 1 mg/L could also be reduced by CCCP and PAβN, supporting the notion that efflux pumps or cell envelopes may play an important role in reducing susceptibility to Omad. Our findings showing that overexpression of RS00550 or RS01625 can lead to Omad heteroresistance occurrence, despite having no impact on Omad MICs in the absence of Omad pressure, indicate that expression of genes can facilitate the formation of Omad resistance under antibiotic exposure. Our phylogenic analysis showed that both RS00550 and RS01625 encode efflux pump family proteins, supporting our hypothesis that efflux pump or membrane proteins contribute to Omad heteroresistance.

Crystallographic studies of the *Thermus thermophilus* 30S ribosomal subunit revealed at least one high-occupancy Tet-binding site and five other minor binding sites in 16S rRNA (Draper et al., 2014; Honeyman et al., 2015; Heidrich et al., 2016). Crystallographic studies with Tet, Tig, and Omad showed that, although they produced slightly different patterns of RNA cleavage and dimethylsulfate modification, all three antibiotics associated with the same binding site, albeit in somewhat different orientations. In several bacterial species, Tig and Omad have been shown to exhibit higher binding affinities and greater antitranslational potencies than Tet or minocycline, and 16SrRNA mutations have been shown to affect Tet binding sites in the 30S ribosomal subunit, which may confer Tet/Tig resistance (Nguyen et al., 2014; Grossman, 2016; Zheng et al., 2018). Consistent with previous reports, we found that greater numbers of 16S rRNA copies with genetic mutations were associated with higher levels Omad/Tig resistance in *S. aureus* isolates with Omad-resistance induced under Omad pressure (Nguyen et al., 2014; Grossman, 2016). This finding implicates the participation of 16SrRNA mutations in the development of the Omad resistance. Additionally, our finding of frequent 30S ribosomal protein S10 mutations in Omad-derived resistant isolates indicates that such mutations may be an important factor in Omad resistance evolution. It will be important to examine the unknown mechanism(s) underlying MIC elevation during Omad resistance evolution in *S. aureus*. In this study, NGS was performed to identify candidate genes that may be involved in Omad resistance development and FnBP was identified as a novel membrane molecule that may contribute to Omad MIC elevation. Mechanistically, we hypothesized that the overexpression of FnBP could alter the penetration potential of cell membranes.

CONCLUSION

Omad exhibited excellent *in vitro* activity against clinical *S. aureus* isolates from China and might represent a preferential choice for the treatment of *S. aureus* infections. However, we must be alert to the potential risk of Omad heteroresistance in *S. aureus*, especially in strains with MICs ≥ 0.5 mg/L. Compared with MRSA, MSSA had relatively low MICs with a more facile tendency for the occurrence of Omad heteroresistance. Omad

heteroresistance in both MSSA and MRSA could be reversed by CCCP and PaβN, indicating involvement of efflux pumps in Omad heteroresistance development in *S. aureus*. Furthermore, both RS01625 and RS00550, which encode efflux pump family proteins (a branched-chain amino acid transport system II carrier protein and an Na/Pi cotransporter family protein, respectively), were found to contribute to Omad heteroresistance. FnBP emerged as a novel molecule to be associated with Omad resistance and Omad MIC elevation in *S. aureus*. The present data contribute to understanding potential resistance mechanisms that may impact clinical applications of Omad.

AUTHOR CONTRIBUTIONS

QD and ZY initiated and designed the project. BB, ZP, and ZL performed the molecular biological experiments with bacteria. GX, XS, JZ, and ZC performed the PCRs. FZ, PL, and GX performed the bacterial culturing and MIC testing. All authors participated in the data analysis. QD, ZY, and BB wrote the manuscript incorporating comments from all authors.

FUNDING

This work was supported by grants from the National Natural Science Foundation of China (Nos. 81170370 and 81601797); Science, Technology, and Innovation Commission of Shenzhen Municipality of basic research funds (No. JCYJ20170412143551332); Shenzhen Health and Family Planning Commission (SZXJ2018027 and SZXJ2017032); Sanming Project of Medicine in Shenzhen; the Shenzhen Nanshan District Scientific Research Program of the People's Republic of China (No. 2018010, 2018011, and 2018021); and provincial medical funds of Guangdong (No. A2018163).

REFERENCES

Argudin, M. A., Roisin, S., Dodemont, M., Nonhoff, C., Deplano, A., and Denis, O. (2018). Mutations at the ribosomal S10 gene in clinical strains of *Staphylococcus aureus* with reduced susceptibility to tigecycline. *Antimicrob. Agents Chemother.* 62:e01852-17. doi: 10.1128/AAC.01852-17

Atshan, S. S., Nor Shamsudin, M., Lung, L. T., Sekawi, Z., Pei Pei, C., Karunanidhi, A., et al. (2013). Genotypically different clones of *Staphylococcus aureus* are diverse in the antimicrobial susceptibility patterns and biofilm formations. *Biomed. Res. Int.* 2013:515712. doi: 10.1155/2013/515712

Bai, B., Hu, K., Li, H., Yao, W., Li, D., Chen, Z., et al. (2018). Effect of tedizolid on clinical *Enterococcus* isolates: in vitro activity, distribution of virulence factor, resistance genes and multilocus sequence typing. *FEMS Microbiol. Lett.* 365:fnx284. doi: 10.1093/femsle/fnx284

Bal, A. M., David, M. Z., Garau, J., Gottlieb, T., Mazzei, T., Scaglione, F., et al. (2017). Future trends in the treatment of methicillin-resistant *Staphylococcus aureus* (MRSA) infection: an in-depth review of newer antibiotics active against an enduring pathogen. *J. Glob. Antimicrob. Resist.* 10, 295–303. doi: 10.1016/j.jgar.2017.05.019

Calfee, D. P. (2017). Trends in community versus health care-acquired methicillin-resistant *Staphylococcus aureus* infections. *Curr. Infect. Dis. Rep.* 19:48. doi: 10.1007/s11908-017-0605-6

Claeys, K. C., Lagnf, A. M., Hallesy, J. A., Compton, M. T., Gravelin, A. L., Davis, S. L., et al. (2016). Pneumonia caused by methicillin-resistant *Staphylococcus aureus*: does vancomycin heteroresistance matter? *Antimicrob. Agents Chemother.* 60, 1708–1716. doi: 10.1128/AAC.02388-15

Dabul, A. N. G., Avaca-Crusca, J. S., Van Tyne, D., Gilmore, M. S., and Camargo, I. (2018). Resistance in in vitro selected tigecycline-resistant methicillin-resistant *Staphylococcus aureus* sequence type 5 is driven by mutations in mepR and mepA genes. *Microb. Drug Resist.* 24, 519–526. doi: 10.1089/mdr.2017.0279

Draper, M. P., Weir, S., Macone, A., Donatelli, J., Trieber, C. A., Tanaka, S. K., et al. (2014). Mechanism of action of the novel aminomethylcycline antibiotic omadacycline. *Antimicrob. Agents Chemother.* 58, 1279–1283. doi: 10.1128/AAC.01066-13

El-Halfawy, O. M., and Valvano, M. A. (2013). Chemical communication of antibiotic resistance by a highly resistant subpopulation of bacterial cells. *PLoS One* 8:e68874. doi: 10.1371/journal.pone.0068874

El-Halfawy, O. M., and Valvano, M. A. (2015). Antimicrobial heteroresistance: an emerging field in need of clarity. *Clin. Microbiol. Rev.* 28, 191–207. doi: 10.1128/CMR.00058-14

Fiedler, S., Bender, J. K., Klare, I., Halbedel, S., Grohmann, E., Szewzyk, U., et al. (2016). Tigecycline resistance in clinical isolates of *Enterococcus faecium* is mediated by an upregulation of plasmid-encoded tetracycline determinants tet(L) and tet(M). *J. Antimicrob. Chemother.* 71, 871–881. doi: 10.1093/jac/dkv420

Grossman, T. H. (2016). Tetracycline antibiotics and resistance. *Cold Spring Harb. Perspect. Med.* 6:a025387. doi: 10.1101/cshperspect.a025387

Heidrich, C. G., Mitova, S., Schedlbauer, A., Connell, S. R., Fucini, P., Steenbergen, J. N., et al. (2016). The novel aminomethylcycline omadacycline has high specificity for the primary tetracycline-binding site on the bacterial ribosome. *Antibiotics* 5:32. doi: 10.3390/antibiotics5040032

Honeyman, L., Ismail, M., Nelson, M. L., Bhatia, B., Bowser, T. E., Chen, J., et al. (2015). Structure-activity relationship of the aminomethylcyclines and the discovery of omadacycline. *Antimicrob. Agents Chemother.* 59, 7044–7053. doi: 10.1128/AAC.01536-15

Jones, C. H., Tuckman, M., Howe, A. Y., Orlowski, M., Mullen, S., Chan, K., et al. (2006). Diagnostic PCR analysis of the occurrence of methicillin and tetracycline resistance genes among *Staphylococcus aureus* isolates from phase 3 clinical trials of tigecycline for complicated skin and skin structure infections. *Antimicrob. Agents Chemother.* 50, 505–510. doi: 10.1128/AAC.50.2.505-510.2006

Klionsky, D. J., Abdelmohsen, K., Abe, A., Abedin, M. J., Abeliovich, H., Acevedo Arozena, A., et al. (2016). Guidelines for the use and interpretation of assays for monitoring autophagy (3rd edition). *Autophagy* 12, 1–222. doi: 10.1080/15548627.2015.1100356

Leon-Sampedro, R., Novais, C., Peixe, L., Baquero, F., and Coque, T. M. (2016). Diversity and evolution of the Tn5801-tet(M)-like integrative and conjugative elements among *Enterococcus, Streptococcus,* and *Staphylococcus. Antimicrob. Agents Chemother.* 60, 1736–1746. doi: 10.1128/AAC.01864-15

Lin, Z., Cai, X., Chen, M., Ye, L., Wu, Y., Wang, X., et al. (2017). Virulence and stress responses of *Shigella* flexneri regulated by PhoP/PhoQ. *Front. Microbiol.* 8:2689. doi: 10.3389/fmicb.2017.02689

Linkevicius, M., Sandegren, L., and Andersson, D. I. (2016). Potential of tetracycline resistance proteins to evolve tigecycline resistance. *Antimicrob. Agents Chemother.* 60, 789–796. doi: 10.1128/AAC.02465-15

Lupien, A., Gingras, H., Leprohon, P., and Ouellette, M. (2015). Induced tigecycline resistance in *Streptococcus pneumoniae* mutants reveals mutations in ribosomal proteins and rRNA. *J. Antimicrob. Chemother.* 70, 2973–2980. doi: 10.1093/jac/dkv211

Macone, A. B., Caruso, B. K., Leahy, R. G., Donatelli, J., Weir, S., Draper, M. P., et al. (2014). In vitro and in vivo antibacterial activities of omadacycline, a novel aminomethylcycline. *Antimicrob. Agents Chemother.* 58, 1127–1135. doi: 10.1128/AAC.01242-13

Nguyen, F., Starosta, A. L., Arenz, S., Sohmen, D., Donhofer, A., and Wilson, D. N. (2014). Tetracycline antibiotics and resistance mechanisms. *Biol. Chem.* 395, 559–575. doi: 10.1515/hsz-2013

Noel, G. J., Draper, M. P., Hait, H., Tanaka, S. K., and Arbeit, R. D. (2012). A randomized, evaluator-blind, phase 2 study comparing the safety and efficacy of omadacycline to those of linezolid for treatment of complicated skin and skin structure infections. *Antimicrob. Agents Chemother.* 56, 5650–5654. doi: 10.1128/AAC.00948-12

Osei Sekyere, J., and Amoako, D. G. (2017). Carbonyl cyanide m-chlorophenylhydrazine (CCCP) reverses resistance to colistin, but Not to Carbapenems and tigecycline in multidrug-resistant *Enterobacteriaceae. Front. Microbiol.* 8:228. doi: 10.3389/fmicb.2017.00228

Pfaller, M. A., Huband, M. D., Rhomberg, P. R., and Flamm, R. K. (2017a). Surveillance of omadacycline activity against clinical isolates from a global collection (North America, Europe, Latin America, Asia-Western Pacific), 2010-2011. *Antimicrob. Agents Chemother.* 61:e00018-e17. doi: 10.1128/AAC.00018-17

Pfaller, M. A., Rhomberg, P. R., Huband, M. D., and Flamm, R. K. (2017b). Activities of omadacycline and comparator agents against *Staphylococcus aureus* isolates from a surveillance program conducted in North America and Europe. *Antimicrob. Agents Chemother.* 61:e02411-16. doi: 10.1128/AAC.02411-16

Recker, M., Laabei, M., Toleman, M. S., Reuter, S., Saunderson, R. B., Blane, B., et al. (2017). Clonal differences in *Staphylococcus aureus* bacteraemia-associated mortality. *Nat. Microbiol.* 2, 1381–1388. doi: 10.1038/s41564-017-0001-x

Villano, S., Steenbergen, J., and Loh, E. (2016). Omadacycline: development of a novel aminomethylcycline antibiotic for treating drug-resistant bacterial infections. *Future Microbiol.* 11, 1421–1434. doi: 10.2217/fmb-2016-0100

Wu, Y., Wang, J., Xu, T., Liu, J., Yu, W., Lou, Q., et al. (2012). The two-component signal transduction system ArlRS regulates *Staphylococcus epidermidis* biofilm formation in an ica-dependent manner. *PLoS One* 7:e40041. doi: 10.1371/journal.pone.0040041

Yao, W., Xu, G., Bai, B., Wang, H., Deng, M., Zheng, J., et al. (2018). In vitro-induced erythromycin resistance facilitates cross-resistance to the novel fluoroketolide, solithromycin, in *Staphylococcus aureus. FEMS Microbiol. Lett.* 365:fny116. doi: 10.1093/femsle/fny116

Zhang, F., Bai, B., Xu, G. J., Lin, Z. W., Li, G. Q., Chen, Z., et al. (2018). Eravacycline activity against clinical *S. aureus* isolates from China: in vitro activity, MLST profiles and heteroresistance. *BMC Microbiol.* 18:211. doi: 10.1186/s12866-018-1349-7

Zheng, J. X., Lin, Z. W., Sun, X., Lin, W. H., Chen, Z., Wu, Y., et al. (2018). Overexpression of OqxAB and MacAB efflux pumps contributes to eravacycline resistance and heteroresistance in clinical isolates of *Klebsiella pneumoniae. Emerg. Microbes Infect.* 7:139. doi: 10.1038/s41426-018-0141-y

6

Alternative Therapeutic Options to Antibiotics for the Treatment of Urinary Tract Infections

Paul Loubet[1], Jérémy Ranfaing[2], Aurélien Dinh[3], Catherine Dunyach-Remy[2],
Louis Bernard[4,5], Franck Bruyère[4,6], Jean-Philippe Lavigne[2]* and Albert Sotto[1]

[1] VBMI, INSERM U1047, Université de Montpellier, Service des Maladies Infectieuses et Tropicales, CHU Nîmes, Nîmes, France, [2] VBMI, INSERM U1047, Université de Montpellier, Service de Microbiologie et Hygiène Hospitalière, CHU Nîmes, Nîmes, France, [3] Service des Maladies Infectieuses, AP-HP Raymond-Poincaré, Garches, France, [4] PRES Centre Val de Loire, Université François Rabelais de Tours, Tours, France, [5] Service des Maladies Infectieuses, CHU Tours, Tours, France, [6] Service d'Urologie, CHU Tours, Tours, France

*Correspondence:
Jean-Philippe Lavigne
jean.philippe.lavigne@chu-nimes.fr

Urinary tract infections (UTIs) mainly caused by Uropathogenic *Escherichia coli* (UPEC), are common bacterial infections. Many individuals suffer from chronically recurring UTIs, sometimes requiring long-term prophylactic antibiotic regimens. The global emergence of multi-drug resistant uropathogens in the last decade underlines the need for alternative non-antibiotic therapeutic and preventative strategies against UTIs. The research on non-antibiotic therapeutic options in UTIs has focused on the following phases of the pathogenesis: colonization, adherence of pathogens to uroepithelial cell receptors and invasion. In this review, we discuss vaccines, small compounds, nutraceuticals, immunomodulating agents, probiotics and bacteriophages, highlighting the challenges each of these approaches face. Most of these treatments show interesting but only preliminary results. *Lactobacillus*-containing products and cranberry products in conjunction with propolis have shown the most robust results to date and appear to be the most promising new alternative to currently used antibiotics. Larger efficacy clinical trials as well as studies on the interplay between non-antibiotic therapies, uropathogens and the host immune system are warranted.

Keywords: urinary tract infection, alternative therapeutics, vaccines, nutraceuticals, immunomodulating agents, probiotics, cranberry, bacteriophages

INTRODUCTION

Urinary Tract Infections (UTIs) are frequent bacterial infections (Silverman et al., 2013) especially in women, estimated to affect more than one in every two women at least once in her lifetime (Foxman, 2014; McLellan and Hunstad, 2016). Uropathogenic *Escherichia coli* (UPEC) is the main pathogen isolated from patients with UTIs (>85%) (Flores-Meireles et al., 2015), while other Gram-negative rods (e.g., *Proteus mirabilis*, *Klebsiella pneumoniae*) and Gram-positive cocci (e.g., *Staphylococcus saprophyticus*, *Enterococcus faecalis*) are responsible for the remaining cases (Flores-Meireles et al., 2015). UTI recurrence is defined by the occurrence of more than two episodes in 6 months, or three in 12 months (Professionals, 2019). The annual incidence of UTI in women is estimated to be 30 per 1000 subjects (Laupland et al., 2007), with approximately

20–40% experiencing recurrence within 6–12 months (Ikähelmo et al., 1996; Foxman, 2014). The epidemiology of UTI changes significantly in the healthcare environment. Urethral catheterization is strongly associated with UTI, and the risk of infection increases with the length of catheterization (Suetens et al., 2018). Catheter-associated UTI (CAUTI) is the most common nosocomial infection (Suetens et al., 2018). CAUTI affects both sexes, with long-term urinary catheterization of both men and women almost invariably leading to detection of bacteria in the urine (bacteriuria). Long-term catheterization carries a daily risk of 3–7% for the development of symptomatic CAUTI (Saint et al., 2009).

The urinary tract is normally sterile, with the exception of the flora of the distal urethra which is diverse and reflects both the digestive flora, the cutaneous flora and genital flora (*Lactobacilli* in women). There are several physiological mechanisms to prevent the host from the development of an ascending infection. First, the urethra itself, which is an obstacle to the intravesical inoculation; second, the physicochemical characteristics of normal urine (osmolarity, pH, organic acid content) that makes growth of most of the bacteria colonizing the urethra difficult; third urination that eliminates most of the bacterial population; fourth the presence in the urine of glycoproteins and oligosaccharides acting as soluble receptors to capture bacteria and enhance their clearance. Finally, in case of bacterial colonization, three factors contribute to avoid the invasion of the mucous membrane (Sobel, 1997): (i) the presence of inhibitors of bacterial adhesion to the surface of urothelial cells (Tamm-Horsfall protein, mucopolysaccharides); (ii) the existence of a local bactericidal effect (independent of inflammatory response or immune response); (iii) a process of exfoliation of the infected urothelial cells. The occurrence of UTI implies either a flaw in these defense mechanisms or the development in the urethral flora of a virulent bacteria, termed uropathogenic. Only a minority of *E. coli* strains, are endowed with uropathogenicity by the production of one or more adhesins (fimbriae): (i) type 1 allowing low urinary tract colonization, (ii) type P inducing pyelonephritis by modification of ureteral peristalsis in binding to glomerulus and endothelial cells of vessel walls helping *E. coli* to cross the epithelial barrier to enter the bloodstream and causing hemagglutination of erythrocytes and by decreasing the renal filtrate flow due to the formation of dense bacterial communities within the tubular lumen (Roberts, 1991; Melican et al., 2011), and (iii) non-fimbrial adhesins such as UpaB that facilitate *E. coli* adherence to extracellular matrix proteins and colonization of the urinary tract (Paxman et al., 2019). An increased adherence of *E. coli* to uroepithelial cells is observed in patients with recurrent UTIs compared to healthy controls (Schaeffer et al., 1981). Moreover, it has been demonstrated that UPEC can invade and replicate within the bladder cells to form intracellular bacterial communities (Mulvey et al., 2001), which can be frequently found in urothelial cells in women with symptomatic UTIs (Rosen et al., 2007) and may act as a source of recurrence in women with same-strain recurrent UTIs (Beerepoot et al., 2012a). Finally, biofilm formation is a critical aspect of CAUTI (Soto et al., 2006; Beerepoot et al., 2012a). Mechanisms of recurrence in UTIs are not fully characterized.

Besides pathogen virulence factors, an impaired mucosal immune response (with urinary IgA involved in the UPEC clearance from the bladder mucosa) of the urogenital tract may have a role in the host-pathogen process (Ingersoll and Albert, 2013; Abraham and Miao, 2015).

Long-term low dose antibiotic use is currently the keystone of the preventive treatment for UTI recurrence. Indeed, prophylactic antibiotics have been shown to decrease UTI recurrence by 85% compared to patients with placebo (relative risk (RR) 0.15, 95% confidence interval (95%CI) 0.08 to 0.28) (Albert et al., 2004). Moreover, with regard to urinary tract conditions such as neurogenic bladder, it has been suggested that weekly cycling of antibiotics could be the most optimal preventative strategy (Salomon et al., 2006; Dinh et al., 2019). Indeed, this original strategy seems effective with only a limited ecological effect on native gut microbiota according to long-term follow-up (Poirier et al., 2015). However, prolonged antibiotic use often results in the emergence of multidrug-resistant organisms (Beerepoot et al., 2012b) and increases the cost of care. Consequently, the development of new therapeutic options to prevent and treat UTIs, and most particularly recurrent UTIs, are of interest.

This review aims to describe all the existing non-antibiotic treatment options in UTI (**Table 1** and **Figure 1**).

VACCINES

Vaccines have been studied to prevent recurrent UTI in the aim not to kill infectious pathogens but to protect the host against infection by priming the immune response to uropathogens. Different vaccine strategies have considered the use of both surface antigen or inactivated whole bacterium, from uropathogens, to generate protective antibodies as a preventive strategy for recurrent UTIs. An ideal vaccine will target factors critical for establishment of bladder colonization (O'Brien et al., 2016). In this way, vaccines containing O antigens (important virulence factors that are targets of both the innate and adaptive immune systems), fimbrial subunits (responsible for the attachment to host cells, the first step of UTI), α-hemolysin (a membrane-active protein exotoxin leading to serious tissue damage), siderophores and a variety of outer membrane siderophore receptors (allowing the sequestration of iron, the main source of bacterial growth) have been developed.

Current Vaccine Solutions

There are currently four available vaccines with established results from randomized control trials (RCT): Uro−Vaxom®, Urovac®, ExPEC4V and Uromune® (Aziminia et al., 2019).

– Uro−Vaxom®, also known as OM−89, is comprised of bacterial extracts from 18 UPEC strains that mediated its effect by the ability of bacterial component pathogen-associated molecular patterns to non-specifically stimulate cells of the innate immune systems (Huber et al., 2000). This effect was shown in mouse models inducing an immunological defense response within the bladder.

TABLE 1 | Non-antibiotic therapeutic options for the treatment of urinary tract infections.

Therapeutic options	References	Mechanism	Benefits	Drawbacks
Vaccine				
Targeting adhesion	(O'Hanley et al., 1985; De Ree and Van den Bosch, 1987; Riegman et al., 1988; Wizemann et al., 1999; Langermann et al., 2000; Roberts et al., 2004; Poggio et al., 2006; Habibi et al., 2016)	• Block the liaison adhesin-host cell receptor (pili vaccine) • Reduction of adhesion and protection against cystitis (FimH vaccine)	• Decrease the bacterial colonization • Protection of the bladder and the kidneys	• Heterogeneity of the proteins of the bacterial membrane
Targeting capsule	(Kaijser et al., 1983; Roberts et al., 1993; Kumar et al., 2005; Stenutz et al., 2006)		• Promising animal model results	• No human studies • Great heterogeneity in antigen used making creation of a vaccine with broad protection difficult
Targeting toxins	(O'Hanley et al., 1991; Ellis and Kuehn, 2010)	• Reduction of renal injury	• Decrease virulence	• No long-term protection
Targeting iron metabolism	(Alteri et al., 2009; Brumbaugh et al., 2013)	• Effective immunologic reaction against specific molecules	• Protection of the bladder and the kidneys • Reduce UTI recurrence	• Cannot target all UPEC strains (heterogeneity of the targets)
Small compounds				
Pillicide	(Åberg and Almqvist, 2007; Greene et al., 2014; Pinkner et al., 2006; Svensson et al., 2001)	• Prevent the formation of pili • Decrease the expression of genes related to fimbriae	• Reduce adhesion, virulence and biofilm formation of UPEC	• No in vivo experiments
Mannoside	(Cusumano et al., 2011; Klein et al., 2010)	• Diminution of bladder colonization • Orally bioavailable	• Reduction of the adhesion	• Clinical study in progress
Hydroxamic acid	(Griffith et al., 1978, 1988, 1991; Munakata et al., 1980; Bailie et al., 1986; Benini et al., 2000; Amtul et al., 2002; Xu et al., 2017)	• Prevent urine alkalization	• Prevent the formation of urinary stones • Decrease bladder inflammation	• Side effects (mutagenic power)
Phenyl phosphoramidates	(Texier-Maugein et al., 1987; Faraci et al., 1995; Morris and Stickler, 1998; Pope et al., 1998)	• Prevent urine alkalization	• Prevent the formation of urinary stones • Decrease bladder inflammation	• Poor stability
Capsule inhibitor	(Roberts, 1995, 1996; Llobet et al., 2008; Varki, 2008; Anderson et al., 2010; Goller et al., 2014)	• Reduce biofilm formation	• Affects a large proportion of UPEC strains	• Antigenicity in human • Poor bioavailability • Conflicting results
Nutraceutical				
Cranberry	(Ahuja et al., 1998; Howell et al., 2005; Freitas et al., 2006; Liu et al., 2006, 2019; AFSSA, 2007; Jepson and Craig, 2008; Pereira et al., 2011; Ermel et al., 2012; Jepson et al., 2012; Stapleton et al., 2012; Chan et al., 2013; Boonsai et al., 2014; Olczyk et al., 2014; Ulrey et al., 2014; Rafsanjany et al., 2015; Rodríguez-Pérez et al., 2016; Wojnicz et al., 2016; Pasupuleti et al., 2017; Ranfaing et al., 2018a,b; Anger et al., 2019; Bruyère et al., 2019)	• Reduction of adhesion, motility, and biofilm formation	• Impacts UPEC strains and also P. aeruginosa, P. mirabilis and E. faecalis • Could be used in prophylaxis	• Conflicting results
Hyaluronic acid	(Constantinides et al., 2004; Birder and de Groat, 2007; Cicione et al., 2014; Ciani et al., 2016; Torella et al., 2016; Goddard and Janssen, 2018)	• Reduction of adhesion	• Promising results in humans	• Only retrospective studies

(Continued)

TABLE 1 | Continued

Therapeutic options	References	Mechanism	Benefits	Drawbacks
D-mannose	(Hills et al., 2001; Klein et al., 2010; Cusumano et al., 2011; Kranjčec et al., 2014; Domenici et al., 2016)	• Reduction of adhesion	• Fast effect after oral administration	• Conflicting results
Galabiose	(Strömberg et al., 1990; Sung et al., 2001; Larsson et al., 2003)	• Reduction of adhesion	• Diminution of kidney infections	• Not enough *in vivo* results
Chinese Medical Herb and other plants	(Banu and Kumar, 2009; Gu et al., 2011; Issac Abraham et al., 2011; Tong et al., 2011; Zhao et al., 2011; Flower et al., 2015; Meng et al., 2015; Hou and Wang, 2016; Pu et al., 2016; Sharifi-Rad et al., 2016; Mazarei et al., 2017; Jaiswal et al., 2018; Mickymaray and Al Aboody, 2019)	• Reduction of adhesion	• Reduction of UTI recurrences	• Small size studies • Little safety data
Immunomodulant agents				
COX-2 inhibitor	(Bleidorn et al., 2010; Hannan et al., 2014; Moore et al., 2019)	• Reduction of inflammation linked to cystitis	• Substantial reduction of UTI recurrences	• No significant results in clinical trials
Green Tea Extract	(Hoshino et al., 1999; Arakawa et al., 2004; Cooper et al., 2005a,b; Reygaert and Jusufi, 2013; Bae et al., 2015)	• Reduction of inflammation	• Reduction of UTI recurrences	• Mechanisms of action unclear • Not proved in humans
Probiotics				
Vaginal lactobacilli	(Isolauri et al., 2001; Galdeano and Perdigón, 2006; De Vuyst and Leroy, 2007; Cribby et al., 2008; Cadieux et al., 2009; Riaz et al., 2010; Hardy et al., 2013; Kemgang et al., 2014; Di Cerbo et al., 2016; Chikindas et al., 2018; Ng et al., 2018; Koradia et al., 2019)	• Competition, reduction of adhesion and virulence	• Natural production of antimicrobial compounds • No known side effects	• Not enough *in vivo* results
E. coli 83972	(Hull et al., 2000; Darouiche et al., 2001, 2005; Dashiff et al., 2011; Roos et al., 2006; Trautner et al., 2007; Prasad et al., 2009; Sundén et al., 2010)	• Colonization of the bladder by avirulent strain	• Reduction of UPEC colonization	• Not enough inclusions in clinical studies
Predatory bacteria	(Stolp and Starr, 1963; Kadouri and O'Toole, 2005; Sockett, 2009; Dashiff et al., 2011; Shatzkes et al., 2015; Gupta et al., 2016)	• Decrease of bacterial number and biofilm formation	• Efficient against Gram-negative bacteria	• Not yet tested to treat UTIs
Bacteriophages	(Dufour et al., 2016; Sybesma et al., 2016; Leitner et al., 2017; Ferry et al., 2018; Ujmajuridze et al., 2018; Jault et al., 2019; Kuipers et al., 2019)	• Direct bacteria killing	• Interesting animal models and human case reports.	• More human studies are required

However, its use in human trials has shown conflicting results. Four placebo controlled studies (Tammen, 1990; Schulman et al., 1993; Magasi et al., 1994; Bauer et al., 2005) showed that taking one Uro-Vaxom® tablet daily for 3 months significantly reduced the number of UTIs in the treatment group, with a RR = 0.61 (95%CI 0.48–0.78) of developing a UTI in the treatment group during an observation ranging from 3 to 12 months.

However, a recent multicenter double-blind control trial of 451 patients showed no significant difference in UTI rates between Uro-Vaxom® and the placebo (Wagenlehner et al., 2015).

- Urovac® is a mucosal vaccine in the form of a vaginal suppository containing 10 different strains of heat-inactivated uropathogenic bacteria (six serotypes of *E. coli* strains, *P. vulgaris*, *Morganella morganii*, *E. faecalis* and

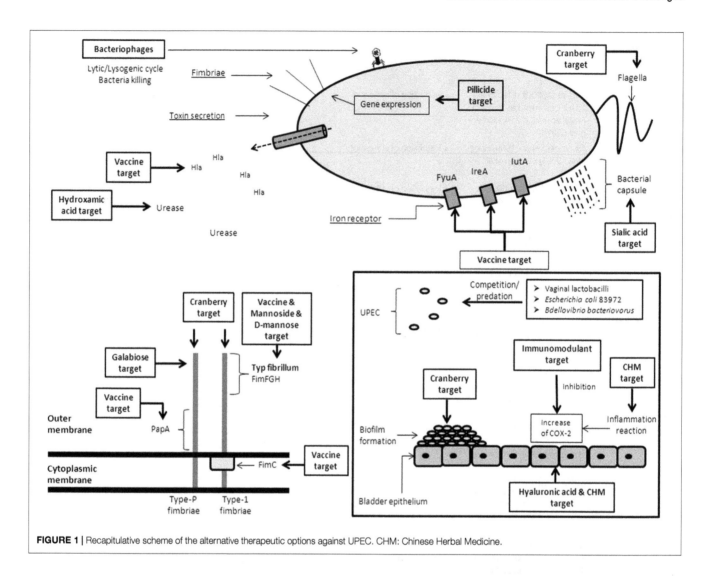

FIGURE 1 | Recapitulative scheme of the alternative therapeutic options against UPEC. CHM: Chinese Herbal Medicine.

K. pneumoniae) (Yang and Foley, 2019). The aim of this vaccine preparation was to incorporate a broader range of commonly implicated uropathogens and thus provide broad protection. Overall, Urovac® has been shown to reduce the risk of recurrence (RR 0.75, 95% CI 0.63–0.89) (Uehling et al., 1997, 2003; Hopkins et al., 2007). This effect was more pronounced in the group that received a follow-up booster vaccination (Aziminia et al., 2019).

- ExPEC4V is composed of O–antigens of four *E. coli* serotypes (O1A, O2, O6A, and O25B) delivered as a single intra-muscular injection. These serotypes are a key immune evasion strategy used by the bacterium. This vaccine has shown good safety and immunogenicity in several phase 1 and 2 trials (Hopkins et al., 2007; Huttner et al., 2017; Huttner and Gambillara, 2018; Frenck et al., 2019).
- Uromune® is a new sublingual vaccine composed of inactivated *E. coli*, *K. pneumoniae*, *Proteus vulgaris* and *E. faecalis*. This vaccine has been evaluated in three large retrospective Spanish studies and showed a 70–90% reduction of recurrence when compared to

antibiotic prophylaxis (Lorenzo-Gómez et al., 2013, 2015). A prospective observational study showed that 59 out of 75 women (78%) which received 3 months of Uromune® treatment as a sub-lingual spray once a day, had no new UTIs during both the treatment and the one year of follow-up period (Yang and Foley, 2018). Another recent lager prospective study showed that 65% of 784 women had 0 or 1 UTI after 6 months of daily sub-lingual administration of Uromune® (Ramirez Sevilla et al., 2019).

This interesting result should be confirmed in a larger study with a control group. It has to be noted that the need for a 3-month daily administration raises questions on the immunogenicity and the expected compliance to this treatment. One international multicenter phase III RCT is currently underway.

A recent meta-analysis noted that the use of vaccines appeared to reduce UTI recurrence compared to placebo. However, the heterogeneity amongst studies renders interpretation and recommendation for routine clinical use difficult at present (Prattley et al., 2020). Further randomized controlled trials are warranted to assess the efficiency and the safety of the existing vaccines against UTIs.

New Candidates

Several bacterial virulence factors involved in UTI are promising vaccine targets.

Vaccines Targeting Adhesion

Bacterial adhesion to urothelium represents a crucial step in the pathogenesis of UTIs. It permits bacteria to resist mechanical elimination by the flow of urine and bladder and increases persistence of E. coli. One large family of adhesive organelles are pili assembled by the chaperone-usher pathway (CUP) pili. These pili are critical virulence factors in a wide range of pathogenic bacteria, including E. coli. CUP pili mediate adhesion to host and environmental surfaces, facilitate invasion of host tissues, and promote interaction of bacteria with each other to form biofilms (Sauer et al., 2004). The most studied of the CUP pili are the Type 1, P, and S pili, present in UPEC and allowing the colonization of mucosal surfaces. They promote both irreversible bacterial attachment and invasion of uroepithelial cell membrane within the bladder. Interactions mediated by these adhesins can stimulate a number of host responses that can directly influence the outcome of a UTI (Mulvey, 2002). They are thus promising vaccine candidates because of the importance of this adhesion. The potential exists to develop antibodies that block the adhesin-host cell receptor interaction and thus decrease bacterial colonization (Wizemann et al., 1999).

FimH is a major determinant of the adhesive subunit of Type 1 fimbriae, which has high tropism for urinary tract receptors. It binds to mono-mannose. Lack of this compound on renal epithelia has suggested a limited role in pyelonephritis. It has been targeted as a good candidate for a vaccine because of its critical role in cystitis pathogenesis (**Figure 1**). A FimCH vaccine protected cynomolgus monkeys from cystitis (Langermann et al., 2000). Another study on mice with an intranasal and intramuscular administration also showed a protection against cystitis, but the intranasal method produced a stronger immune response (Poggio et al., 2006). In a more recent study, a recombinant protein MrpH.FimH (consisting of a combination between two adhesins, FimH from UPEC and MprH from P. mirabilis) was injected with a transurethral instillation and the authors demonstrated a high immune response and a protection against E. coli and P. mirabilis (Habibi et al., 2016).

By comparison the Type P pilus is more involved in pyelonephritis due to the presence of globoseries glycosphingolipids (the receptor of this pilus) in kidney. This P fimbria helps to cross the epithelial barrier to enter the bloodstream and can cause hemagglutination of erythrocytes (Riegman et al., 1988). Approximatively 1,000 of subunits form a P fimbria. Among them the major constituent is the protein subunit PapA, and minor subunits are PapD, PapE, PapF, and PapG. So subunit vaccines based on this pilus have been developed to block renal colonization. Attempts on using the major subunit PapA as a vaccine, although initially favorable in mice (O'Hanley et al., 1985), failed due to the poor generation

of protective antibodies most probably due to natural variation in the PapA pilus subunit (**Figure 1**; De Ree and Van den Bosch, 1987). A new vaccine based on purified PapDG protein demonstrated a good efficiency to prevent colonization of kidney on cynomolgus monkeys (Roberts et al., 2004).

Vaccines Targeting Capsule

The main role of a capsule is to cover and protect E. coli from the host immune system. It provides protection against engulfment and complement-mediated bactericidal effect in the host (Johnson, 1991). Based on this implication in virulence strategy, capsules represent a promising vaccine target. In this way, conjugate UTI vaccines against UPEC capsule and lipopolysaccharide (LPS) components have shown protection in animal models after same-strain challenge. In early studies, intraperitoneal, subcutaneous or bladder injection of O-antigen from E. coli of different serotypes (O6, O8 and K13) protected rats and rhesus monkeys from pyelonephritis (Kaijser et al., 1983; Roberts et al., 1993; Kumar et al., 2005). A considerable challenge in formulating a vaccine targeting capsule or O-antigen, the most exposed component of LPS, is the great heterogeneity of serotypes among E. coli isolates. Indeed, six different O serotypes account for only 75% of UPEC isolates (Stenutz et al., 2006), making the formulation of a broadly protective conjugate vaccine impractical. Furthermore, some capsule serotypes, such as K1 and K5, are thought to evade the host immune response by molecular mimicry, potentially making them poor vaccine candidates. No studies on these vaccines have been conducted in humans yet.

Vaccines Targeting Toxins

Several toxins secreted by UPEC play a consequential role as virulence factors in UTI. They have the ability to alter the host cell signaling cascade and modulate inflammatory responses. They also contribute to the stimulation of the host cell death and the ability to access deeper tissues. Many toxins have been reported including α-hemolysin (HlyA) or cytotoxic necrotizing factor 1 (CNF1). α-hemolysin is a pore-forming toxin, it can lyse erythrocytes, and induces the apoptosis of target host cells promoting the exfoliation of bladder epithelial cells (Johnson, 1991). CNF1 stimulates actin stress fiber formation and membrane ruffle formation resulting in the entry of E. coli into the cells. This protein interferes with polymorphonuclear phagocytosis and provokes apoptotic death of bladder epithelial cells (Asadi Karam et al., 2019). Following their importance in virulence, the toxins produced by UPEC have been used to develop vaccines to protect the bladder and kidney during a UTI. However, as they are secreted and thus removed from the bacteria, they do not make ideal vaccine candidates. Indeed, a purified α-hemolysin toxoid vaccine prevented renal injury, but not colonization, in mice after challenge with a hemolytic UPEC strain (**Figure 1**; O'Hanley et al., 1991). Of note, rather than being secreted as "naked" proteins, α-hemolysin and CNF1 are associated with outer membrane vesicles (OMVs), which bleb from the surface of Gram-negative bacteria during all stages of growth (Ellis and Kuehn, 2010). OMVs also contain adhesins, enzymes, and non-protein antigens like LPS. OMVs are intriguing vaccine candidates, and because they contain LPS and other pro-inflammatory virulence factors, they should not require adjuvants to stimulate the immune system. However, no UPEC OMV vaccines have yet been tested.

Vaccines Targeting Iron Metabolism
The acquisition of iron is crucial for bacteria life and *E. coli* uses iron for transporting and storing oxygen, DNA synthesis, electron transport and metabolism peroxides. However, the amount of iron availability is reduced in host. In response, *E. coli* produces siderophores, molecules that mediate iron uptake. Four siderophore systems have been identified such as yersiniabatin, aerobactin, enterobactin, and salmochelin (Johnson, 1991).

Some studies have targeted siderophore, heme receptors and other functional molecules involved in iron acquisition. In one study, the authors tested six iron receptors and found that the antibodies against the yersiniabatin receptor, FyuA, conferred kidney protection in mice (Brumbaugh et al., 2013). In another mouse model, instead of targeting iron receptors, the same authors targeted molecules involved in iron metabolism. Of the six candidates, two conferred a protection to the bladder (IreA and IutA) and one protected the kidneys (Hma) after an intranasal immunization (Alteri et al., 2009).

SMALL COMPOUNDS

In the current setting small compounds are low molecular weight molecules that are typically bacterial substrates or products or mimics thereof. They can act as inhibitors by binding active sites and substrate binding sites of proteins involved in pathogenicity and so impact bacterial infections.

Small Compounds Targeting Adhesion
As previously noted, one of the critical mechanisms for the pathogenesis of the uropathogenic bacteria is its adhesion to uroepithelium (Beerepoot and Geerlings, 2016), due to fimbriae (specially the Type 1 and the P-fimbriae), playing a role in both cystitis and pyelonephritis (Beerepoot and Geerlings, 2016; Muenzner et al., 2016). The very conserved structure of the adhesive organelles makes them good candidates to develop antibacterial agents (Piatek et al., 2013). The small molecules targeting adhesion can be classified into two categories: those inhibiting the capacity of adhesion of the fimbriae, and those targeting fimbriae assembly.

Pilicide
The main action of these molecules is to prevent the formation of UPEC pili by decreasing the levels of Type 1 and P piliation (Åberg and Almqvist, 2007). Pilicides are small molecules which have a ring-fused 2-pyridone backbone. Some pilicides act directly on pili assembly chaperones, through adhering to their hydrophobic substrate binding sites (Svensson et al., 2001; Pinkner et al., 2006). Others interfere with the transcription of pili genes and some cases genes involved in flagella biogenesis such as the pilicide ec240, the most potent inhibitor of Type 1 piliation and of type 1 pilus-dependent biofilm formation to date (Greene et al., 2014).

In vitro studies testing the potential of pilicides have shown promising results. These compounds decreased (i) the adhesion of UPEC strains on cells by a strong reduction (70–80%) of fimbriae density (Piatek et al., 2013), and (ii) the ability to form Type 1 pilus dependent biofilms (Pinkner et al., 2006). In a mouse study, the pilicide had a strong impact on adhesion and biofilm formation and also reduced the virulence *in vivo*. It is also interesting to note that it reduced the biofilm formation on abiotic surface (Cegelski et al., 2010).

To develop this compound into a therapeutic, further studies are needed to assess its pharmacokinetics and pharmacodynamics and to determine the concentration at which it accumulates in the bladder or other potential sites of infection.

Small Compounds Targeting Urease
Urease, an enzyme which catalyzes the hydrolysis of urea, is crucial in the pathogenesis of several uropathogenic bacteria such as *P. mirabilis*, *Klebsiella* sp., *Pseudomonas* sp. and *Staphylococcus* sp. (Mobley and Hausinger, 1989). This enzyme leads to the alkalinization of the urine and the production of struvite and carbonate apatite that make up the major component of urinary stones (Burne and Chen, 2000). These conditions lead to the inflammation of the urogenital epithelia thus increasing the risk of catheter-associated biofilm formation that may contribute to pyelonephritis (Musher et al., 1975; Jacobsen et al., 2008), mainly due to both bacterial and host cysteine protease (Xu et al., 2017).

The most studied inhibitors of urease are hydroxamic acids (Amtul et al., 2002; **Figure 1**). These molecules have a high inhibitory activity against urease, by bonding to the two nickel ions in the urease active site (Benini et al., 2000). Initially, these molecules were used to treat UTIs by preventing urine alkalization (Griffith et al., 1978, 1988). However, because of the growing evidence of side effects such as mutagenic power, they were progressively phased out (Munakata et al., 1980; Bailie et al., 1986; Griffith et al., 1991).

Through similarly interacting with nickel ions in the urease active site, the phenyl phosphoramidates were found to have the highest inhibitory activity (Faraci et al., 1995). Studies testing these molecules in an *in vitro* model (Morris and Stickler, 1998) and in a rat model (Texier-Maugein et al., 1987) found promising results. Since then, no *in vivo* studies or clinical trials have been developed, probably due to the poor hydrolytic stability of these molecules which leads to a very short half-life (Pope et al., 1998).

Other molecules that possess inhibitory activity against bacterial urease have been developed, but they are not fully adapted to treat UTIs. One of them is the quinones, a class of active compounds with a high oxidizing potency (Zaborska et al., 2002). These molecules had not been evaluated *in vivo* models due to their cytotoxic and cancerogenic properties.

Small Compounds Targeting Bacterial Capsule
Polysaccharide capsule biogenesis plays an important role in UPEC virulence. Like other pathogens, the capsule is used as a defense against opsonophagocytosis and complement-mediated killing (Roberts, 1995, 1996). The capsule is also involved in the

formation of biofilm and the formation of intracellular bacterial communities (Llobet et al., 2008; Anderson et al., 2010). Until now, the human use of small-molecule inhibitors of UPEC capsule biogenesis was not available because of their antigenicity and poor bioavailability (Varki, 2008). Nevertheless, mouse studies identified two active agents (DU003 and DU01), that caused significant bacterial death (Goller et al., 2014; **Figure 1**).

NUTRACEUTICALS

Nutraceuticals are pharmaceutical alternatives, consisting of all the foods or food products which provide medical benefits and can be delivered under medical form. They provide health benefits in addition to their basic nutritional value.

Cranberry (*Vaccinium macrocarpon*)

Cranberry (*Vaccinium macrocarpon* Ait.) is a berry that grows in North America. In recent years, the use of cranberry has increased in the prophylactic approach of recurrent UTI (Howell et al., 2005). Although, its mechanism of action is unclear, there are several possible targets of cranberry (**Figure 1**).

The main efficacy is related to the antiadherence properties of cranberry (Ahuja et al., 1998; Liu et al., 2006) due to the A-type proanthocyanidin (PAC-A) that has been shown to be an important inhibitor of Type-I fimbriae *E. coli* adhesion to uroepithelial cells. Some *in vitro* and *in vivo* studies demonstrated the capacity of the cranberry to reduce the adhesion of bacteria to the cells (Ermel et al., 2012; Rafsanjany et al., 2015; Liu et al., 2019). Cranberry has also shown convincing results on motility and biofilm formation. Indeed, it has a negative impact on the swarming of *Pseudomonas aeruginosa* and *P. mirabilis* (Chan et al., 2013) and on the biofilm formation of *E. faecalis*, *P. aeruginosa* and *E. coli* (Ulrey et al., 2014; Rodríguez-Pérez et al., 2016; Wojnicz et al., 2016).

The use of cranberry has been associated with a decrease in the incidence of UTIs, although some conflicting results have been reported in the literature. Although cranberry products have been shown to significantly reduce the incidence of UTIs at 12 months (RR 0.65, 95% CI 0.46–0.90) compared with placebo/control in women with recurrent UTIs in a Cochrane review from 2008 (Jepson and Craig, 2008), an updated review concluded that cranberry products did not show any significant reduction in the occurrence of symptomatic UTI in the same population (Jepson et al., 2012).

A placebo controlled trial, published after the last review, showed that women randomized to cranberry juice had a non-significant reduction in numbers of P-fimbriated *E. coli* in urine and in the rate of symptomatic UTIs (Stapleton et al., 2012).

Because dosage, concentration and formulation of PAC-A are not well defined, the conflicting results may be explained by the difference in PAC-A concentration between cranberry formulations (juice, beverage, tablets) in the different studies making it difficult to choose one formulation over another (Anger et al., 2019).

It must be noted that many of the products containing cranberry used in studies are only for research purposes, limiting the prophylactic application of cranberries beyond research (Stapleton et al., 2012).

Finally, a recent publication showed that the cranberry proanthocyanidins had a variable effect on a collection of *E. coli* strains that could explain the discordant results observed in the clinical studies (Ranfaing et al., 2018a).

In order to enhance the effectiveness of cranberry, combinations of cranberry and other natural products with antimicrobial properties could be used, such as propolis. Propolis is a resinous material collected by bees from plants then mixed with wax and bee enzymes (AFSSA, 2007). Propolis has antimicrobial, anti-inflammatory, anti-tumoral, immune-modulatory and anti-oxidant activities (Boonsai et al., 2014). It has been used for several years to treat gastrointestinal disorders (food supplement) (Freitas et al., 2006), to promote oral health (mouthwash) (Pereira et al., 2011) and in dermatological care (creams and ointments) (Olczyk et al., 2014; Pasupuleti et al., 2017; Ranfaing et al., 2018b). *In vitro* studies showed that propolis potentiated the effect of cranberry proanthocyanidins on adhesion, motility (swarming and swimming), biofilm formation (early formation and fully-formed biofilm), iron metabolism and stress response of UPEC (Olczyk et al., 2014; Pasupuleti et al., 2017; Ranfaing et al., 2018a,b). Moreover, this association was active in all the *E. coli* strains studied, ruling out the variable effect observed with the cranberry used alone (Ranfaing et al., 2018a).

A recent RCT versus placebo in 85 women with recurrent UTIs showed a slight reduction in the number of cystitis events in the first 3 months in the propolis and cranberry group after adjustment on water consumption (0.7 vs. 1.3, $p = 0.02$), but no difference in the mean number of infections in women with at least one infection. Of note, the mean time to onset of the first cystitis episode was significantly longer in the propolis + cranberry group (70 vs. 43 days, $p = 0.03$) and tolerance to the treatment was similar in both groups (Bruyère et al., 2019).

Hyaluronic Acid

The urinary bladder epithelium is composed of urothelial cells which carry specific sensors and properties as well as forming the first barrier to pathogens (Birder and de Groat, 2007). To maintain this capacity to fight infections, these cells produce sulfated polysaccharide glycosaminoglycan (GAG) which covers the epithelium and forms a non-specific anti-adherence factor. A major proportion of the GAG layer of the bladder is composed of hyaluronic acid (HA) and chondroitin sulfate (CS). Virulence factors (secreted by *E. coli* for example) damage the GAG layer to prepare its adhesion (Constantinides et al., 2004; **Figure 1**). One strategy for the management of UTI is based on the re-establishment of the GAG layer of the bladder epithelium with intravesical instillations of HA alone or in combination with CS. Various randomized and non-randomized studies have been performed.

A study investigated the impact of HA and CS on recurrent UTIs on 276 women (aged 18–75 years). The intravesical administration of HA and CS was given to 181 women and the standard treatment against recurrent UTIs was given to 95 women. There was a 49% reduction in the rate of recurrence (defined as one bacteriologically confirmed UTI in the year following the treatment initiation) in patients treated with HA + CS compared with standard care [adjusted OR 0.51 (95%CI 0.27–0.96)]. However, no significant difference was found when considering the number of recurrences or the median time to first recurrence (Ciani et al., 2016).

Another retrospective study in 157 women found similar results with a significant reduction in UTI recurrence and an increased time-to-recurrence between UTIs (Cicione et al., 2014).

It has to be noted that the administration protocol (different between participating centers) of weekly instillation for one month followed by monthly instillations may be a limiting factor for patients.

A synergy might exist between HA + CS and estrogen. This association has been explored in 145 postmenopausal women with mild-to-moderate urogenital atrophy and a history of recurrent UTI. Participants were divided into three groups: vaginal estrogen, oral HA, and oral HA + CS and vaginal estrogen. Oral treatments were effective in preventing recurrent UTI (number of patients with fewer than two infective episodes in the 6-month follow-up and fewer than three episodes in the 12-month follow-up), especially if administered with vaginal estrogen therapy. A slight effect on the HA alone but also a significant impact of the estrogen and the HA + CS on the recurrence of UTIs in postmenopausal women was observed (Torella et al., 2016).

Recently a meta-analysis suggested that HA ± CS decreased the rate of UTI recurrence and increased the time to recurrence (Goddard and Janssen, 2018). Moreover the authors noted the safety of HA therapy even if the intravesical instillation is more invasive than other administrations (usually *per os*). The combination therapy was more performant than the use of HA alone. It seems essential to perform a well-designed, randomized, controlled clinical trials with larger population.

D-mannose

As seen above, CUP pili are important virulence factors and represent optimal targets for antivirulence compound development. *E. coli* binds to mannosylated host cells via their mannose-binding lectin domains of FimH.

Two developments have been proposed to prevent this interaction:

- D-mannose is a monosaccharide closely related to glucose. It blocks the adhesion by high affinity binding to the FimH, thus preventing FimH from binding host mannose on urinary tract surfaces. Absorption after oral administration is fast (30 min to reach the organs) and it is eliminated via the urinary tract (Hills et al., 2001).
- The structure of the FimH adhesin bound to mannosilable proteins has been used to design mannosides, These molecules block FimH function by binding in the FimH mannose-binding pocket (Pinkner et al., 2006; Domenici et al., 2016). Mannosides are also potent inhibitors of biofilm formation *in vitro*. Some mouse models

demonstrated a decrease in bladder colonization after an oral administration of mannosides and a prevention of acute and chronic UTI (Klein et al., 2010; Cusumano et al., 2011; **Figure 1**). In this way, an exogenous intake of D-mannose competitively blocks the interaction between the bacterial fimbriae and host cells (Cusumano et al., 2011; **Figure 1**). One RCT compared the recurrence of UTIs in a group of patients taking daily nitrofurantoin to a group treated with daily D-mannose powder. The risk of recurrence was similar between groups, whilst there was a reduction of the side effects in the D-mannose group (Kranjčec et al., 2014).

Galabiose

Type P fimbriae adhere to the galabiose-like receptor via PapG (Larsson et al., 2003). As previously noted, this kind of fimbriae is essential for the pathogenesis of UTIs in helping the bacteria to reach the kidneys (Strömberg et al., 1990). Better understanding of the structure of the different variants of PapG (mostly PapG II and PapG III) might lead to drugs designed to target this adhesin (Sung et al., 2001; **Figure 1**). No *in vivo* studies on the impact of this sugar on UTIs have yet been performed. Evaluation on the most prevalent uropathogenic bacteria is essential to clearly evaluate the potential of galabiose to reduce UTI.

Vitamin C

Vitamin C (ascorbic acid) is known to possess antioxidant and antimicrobial activities. As microbial infections cause reactive oxygen species (ROS) release by phagocytes, it is helpful in the limitation of infection through deactivation of microorganism killing. ROS may also cause damage to the host cells, therefore the level of ROS released by phagocytes should be reduced directly after infection (Liu et al., 2018). Vitamin C is an essential co-enzyme in the oxidative stress pathways, capable of ROS removal. Habash et al. (1999) suggested that vitamin C decreased the adhesion and microorganisms colonization of the biomaterials used in diagnostic/treatment procedures involving the urinary tract.

Moreover, two trials have studied the use of vitamin C to prevent UTIs. In a single-blind randomized study in thirteen spinal cord injury patients randomized to placebo or 500 mg ascorbic acid four times daily, there was no clinical benefit on urinary infection from the use of ascorbic acid (Castelló et al., 1996). In a second single-blind randomized trial in 110 pregnant women, participants taking a vitamin regimen with 100 mg ascorbic acid per day for 3 months showed a reduction in symptomatic UTIs incidence from 29.1 to 12.7% compared to participants following a vitamin regimen without ascorbic acid (Ochoa-Brust et al., 2007).

To date, there is no evidence of vitamin C action in the prevention of UTI.

Chinese Herbal Medicine (CHM)

Chinese Herbal Medicine (CHM) is the ancient art of compiling complex herbal formulae usually comprising up to 15 herbs. CHM has been historically used to treat UTI. Some frequently used Chinese herbs are known to have significant diuretic, antibiotic, immune enhancing, antipyretic, anti-inflammatory and pain relieving activities. Some of these herbs have shown an *in vitro* inhibitory activity against several uropathogens, especially against *E. coli* in decreasing its adherence to bladder epithelial cells (Tong et al., 2011). In an antibacterial test against mice, it was found that Sanjin tablets (composed by five kinds of CHM) have strong bacteriostasis activity (Hou and Wang, 2016). This product is used to treat acute uncomplicated lower UTI (Meng et al., 2015) and to reduce the symptoms of chronic UTI by reducing the secretory level of some urinary cytokines (Hou and Wang, 2016). A first meta-analysis of three RCTs including 282 women suggested that CHM significantly reduced recurrent UTI rates compared to antibiotics (RR 0.28, 95%CI [0.09 to 0.82]) (Flower et al., 2015). The second one has concluded that the current evidence is insufficient to support the efficacity and safety of Sanjin tablets for acute uncomplicated lower UTI (Pu et al., 2016). Only two of these RCTs reported adverse events (Gu et al., 2011; Zhao et al., 2011). Neither found any liver or renal impairment. Further studies are needed to definitively evaluate the potential of CHM on prevention/treatment of UTI.

Other Phytochemicals

For centuries, plants have been used as alternative and traditional medicine around the world notably as therapies for infectious diseases (Banu and Kumar, 2009; Sharifi-Rad et al., 2016). Plants and their secondary metabolic derivatives are a major resource of antioxidants due to the presence of phenolic compounds including flavonoids, phenolic acids, or tannins. Different extracts from plants and spices have demonstrated anti-inflammatory, antimicrobial and diuretic activities (Mickymaray and Al Aboody, 2019). They also exhibited anti-quorum sensing and anti-biofilm potentials (Issac Abraham et al., 2011; Mazarei et al., 2017). One of the main mechanism of action is the antiadhesive action due to the formation of H-bonds between the FimH protein ligand and the plant compounds (Jaiswal et al., 2018). Future clinical trials must be done after complete pharmacokinetic/pharmacodynamic analyses.

IMMUNOMODULANT AGENTS

The innate immune system activation through the secretion of cytokines and the recruitment of macrophages and neutrophils rapidly occurs after the onset of UTI (Duell et al., 2012). Even in the absence of an effective antibiotic treatment, this immune reaction might be enough to counter the infection. In the case of the persistence of several bacterial strains in the bladder, persistent acute immune response and tissue inflammation can be observed. Moreover, multiple infections can lead to chronic inflammation that increases the risk of developing recurrent UTIs (Ferry et al., 2004; Hannan et al., 2010). There is an increase in the expression of cyclooxygenase (COX)-2 after an infection of the bladder epithelial cells by UPEC. Moreover, there is a correlation between the severity of the inflammation and the increase of COX-2 expression (Chen et al., 2011; **Figure 1**). COX-2 inhibition prevents urothelial transmigration by neutrophils and damage to the urothelial barrier and facilitates the innate

responses (Hannan et al., 2014). A double-blind RCT on 79 women with uncomplicated UTI showed equivalent symptoms at Day 4, when taking ibuprofen (200 mg t.i.d) compared to ciprofloxacin (Bleidorn et al., 2010).

A recent 2 × 2 factorial placebo RCT evaluating ibuprofen in 382 women demonstrated a substantial reduction in antibiotic use in patients taking ibuprofen without differences in terms of symptom relief or speed of recovery (Moore et al., 2019).

Plant-based immunomodulants such as Green Tea Extract (GTE) have also shown promise (Bae et al., 2015). GTE contains an array of polyphenolic compounds, especially catechins. The biological properties of catechins are antioxidant, antiangiogenesis, antiproliferative activity, and antineoplastic (Cooper et al., 2005a,b). Some *in vitro* studies showed an antibacterial impact of GTE against UPEC (Hoshino et al., 1999; Arakawa et al., 2004; Reygaert and Jusufi, 2013) and in a rat model of cystitis, catechins significantly decreased inflammation and uroepithelium edema (Noormandi and Dabaghzadeh, 2015). These results are promising even though the mechanisms of action are still unclear.

PROBIOTICS

A probiotic is a live microorganism that confers a health benefit.

Vaginal Lactobacilli

Lactobacilli are frequently dominant microorganisms in vaginal flora (Mendling, 2016). Different observations can be done: (i) they have the ability to interfere with the adherence, growth and colonization of UPEC (Falagas et al., 2006); (ii) a change in the normal vaginal flora has been shown to facilitate the recurrence of UTIs (Cribby et al., 2008); and (iii) the use of commensal bacteria (such as *Lactobacilli*) reduces the proportion of uropathogens and thus restores bacterial homeostasis (Hardy et al., 2013). Although their exact mechanisms of action are still unknown, lactobacilli strains seem to have at least three different modes of action (Ng et al., 2018; **Figure 1**):

- The first one is the bacteriostatic effect due to the direct competition of probiotics with uropathogens in terms of nutrient and attachment sites (Di Cerbo et al., 2016).
- The second is the impact of probiotics on uropathogens virulence through the ability of *Lactobacillus* byproducts (such as lactic acid and hydrogen peroxide) to downregulate the expression of virulence genes. This has been illustrated in an *in vitro* study in which *Lactobacillus* byproducts inhibited the expression of Type 1- and P-fimbriae-encoding genes in *E. coli*, disrupting adhesion and invasion capacity (Cadieux et al., 2009).
- The third is the bactericidal effect of *Lactobacillus* on uropathogens. This effect can be achieved through the production of antimicrobial peptides known as bacteriocins. These bacteriocins reduce the number of uropathogens (Chikindas et al., 2018) in a strain-specific manner (De Vuyst and Leroy, 2007). *Lactobacillus* species that produce bacteriocins against *E. coli* have been identified (Riaz et al., 2010).

Probiotics can also modulate the immune system. In addition, bacterial strains secreting "immunomodulins" and cytokines are able to reduce infection by pathogenic bacteria (Galdeano and Perdigón, 2006; Kemgang et al., 2014). *Lactobacillus* species have these anti-inflammatory and immune-regulatory actions (Isolauri et al., 2001).

A non-inferiority randomized trial compared antibiotic prophylaxis and *Lactobacillus* prophylaxis in 252 postmenopausal women with recurrent UTIs who received 12 months of prophylaxis with trimethoprim-sulfamethoxazole (TMP-SMX), 480 mg once daily or oral capsules containing 10^9 CFU of *Lactobacillus rhamnosus* GR-1 and *Lactobacillus reuteri* RC-14 twice daily (Beerepoot et al., 2012b). The *Lactobacillus* treatment did not demonstrate non- inferiority, with an average number of symptomatic UTIs during the year of follow-up of 2.9 in the antibiotic group versus 3.3 in the lactobacilli group. The benefit of Lactobacilli was that it had no impact on antibiotic resistance compared to trimethoprim-sulfamethoxazole.

A reduction in the recurrence rate of UTI with the use of lactobacilli products (pooled RR = 0.68, 95%CI 0.44 to 0.93, $p < 0.001$) (Ng et al., 2018) was underlined in a meta-analysis including 620 patients. In this study, two intravaginal suppositories (containing *Lactobacillus crispatus* CTV05, *Lactobacillus rhamnosus* GR1 and *Lactobacillus reuteri* RC14) had the highest efficacy (Ng et al., 2018).

A recent randomized, double-blind, placebo-controlled pilot study in 81 premenopausal women showed that the administration of Bio-Kult Pro-Cyan (a commercially available product containing probiotic strains (*Lactobacillus acidophilus* PXN 35, *Lactobacillus plantarum* PXN 47) and cranberry extract (36 mg/d PACs) twice-daily for 26 weeks, led to significantly lower number of recurrent UTIs compared to placebo (9.1 vs. 33.3%; $P = 0.0053$) (Koradia et al., 2019).

Bacterial Interference: *Escherichia coli* Strain 83972

The intentional colonization of the bladder with a non-virulent strain, also called bacterial interference, has been studied among patients with neurogenic bladder. *E. coli* 83972 is a clinical strain, isolated from a woman with chronic urinary colonization and which has naturally lost its capacity to develop Type 1 and Type P fimbriae. This strain has been used for prophylactic purposes to deliberately colonized the bladders with this bacterium to prevent colonization/infection by pathogenic species.

In a mouse model of UTI, *E. coli* 83972 demonstrated a better fitness than a virulent strain of UPEC. In a poor environment, like the bladder, this difference in fitness is a crucial advantage for the competition between bacteria. The 83972 strain could reduce the impact of UTIs by a monopolization of resources and space (Roos et al., 2006).

Seven clinical studies are available: three are RCT, one of which is a crossover designed study; and four are prospective cohorts (Hull et al., 2000; Darouiche et al., 2001, 2005; Dashiff et al., 2011; Trautner et al., 2007; Prasad et al., 2009; Sundén et al., 2010). Sample sizes were small and varied from 12 to 44 patients.

Clinical endpoints were the interval before first recurrence or the incidence of UTI during follow up.

Despite this heterogeneity, all studies demonstrated the ability of non-virulent strain to protect patients from UTI. One limit is the difficulty to achieve bladder colonization with the non-virulent strain (only 38% of patients in one of the RCT) (Darouiche et al., 2011).

Predatory Bacteria

Predatory bacteria are small, motile, deltaproteobacteria that are a predatory invader of other Gram-negative bacteria (**Figure 1**). They occupy an intraperiplasmic niche and kill, digest and lyse their host, the prey cell. *Bdellovibrio* and *Micavibrio* are the most studied predatory bacteria (Stolp and Starr, 1963). *Bdellovibrio bacteriovorus* uses its type IV pilus to adhere and penetrate the outer membrane (bdelopast) of its prey. Inside the bacteria, *B. bacteriovorus* modifies the membrane of its prey to allow its growth until it uses all the nutrients. This entire process takes only 2–3 h (Sockett, 2009). Several Gram-negative human pathogenic bacteria such as *E. coli*, *Klebsiella* spp. and *Pseudomonas* spp. can be targeted by these predatory bacteria (Dashiff et al., 2011). Furthermore, it has been showed *in vitro* that *B. bacteriovorus* significantly reduced the quantity of biofilm (Kadouri and O'Toole, 2005).

In vitro and mouse model studies have underlined the fact that the predatory bacteria have no negative impact on human cell lines (Gupta et al., 2016) nor on animals (Shatzkes et al., 2015). *B. dellovibrioa* is thus a potential therapeutic agent, but has not been yet applied in this way. No studies have investigated *B. bacteriovorus* to treat UTIs to date. However, these bacteria offer an exciting path for further research where *in vivo* studies should be the focus.

BACTERIOPHAGES

Bacteriophages are viruses that parasitize a bacterium by infecting it and reproducing inside it and can act as bactericidal agents. Bacteriophage therapy is currently applied in different areas of medical research. Indeed, it has been recognized as an alternative treatment in localized infections such as otitis, infected burns and osteoarticular infections (Ferry et al., 2018; Jault et al., 2019). However, its use in UTI is scarce.

One research team has studied the combination of transurethral resection of prostate with bacteriophage therapy used instead of per operative antibiotics. They first demonstrated the *in vitro* lytic activity of commercial bacteriophage cocktails on 41 *E. coli* and 9 *K. pneumoniae* strains. The lytic activity of the bacteriophage cocktails varied between 66% and 93%. They also showed the potential of bacteriophage adaptation experiments to increase the lytic activity, leading to an increase from 66 to 93% for one of the cocktails (Sybesma et al., 2016).

In an animal model, Dufour et al. (2016) showed the ability of phage to treat an *E. coli* UTI. The administration of the same bacteriophage cocktail showed a significant reduction of the bacterial load in the *E. coli* kidney infection model as well as in the *E. coli* pneumonia model, but not in an *E. coli* sepsis model.

In vivo studies were performed with a commercial preparation called Pyo bacteriophage, composed of bacteriophage lines active against a broad spectrum of uropathogenic bacteria: *S. aureus, E. coli, Streptococcus* spp. (including *Enterococcus* spp.), *P. aeruginosa*, and *Proteus spp.* in nine patients planned for transurethral resection. Bacteria load decreased in two-thirds of the patients (6/9), without any associated adverse events (Ujmajuridze et al., 2018).

One case report described the treatment of a recurrent *P. aeruginosa* UTI associated with a bilateral ureteral stent. A phage cocktail containing phages with activity against *Streptococcus pyogenes, S aureus, E. coli, P. aeruginosa, P. vulgaris,* and *P. mirabilis* was administered. After 6 days of treatment, meropenem and colistin were started for 30 days. The results showed a 10-fold reduction of bacteria load in the urine after the first 5 days of phage treatment. The bacterial load was undetectable after 2 days of subsequent antibiotic treatment. Urine samples remained sterile until 1 year after the end of the antibiotic treatment.

Another case report showed the treatment of a recurrent UTI with an ESBL-producing *K. pneumoniae* in a renal transplant patient whose infection evolved into an epididymitis. The patient was definitively cured after an oral and intravesical bacteriophage treatment of 10 days following 6-week meropenem treatment (Kuipers et al., 2019).

One randomized, double-blind trial versus placebo in patients planned for transurethral resection of the prostate with UTI is ongoing. Patients will be randomized in a 1:1:1 ratio to receive 7 days of either: (i) bacteriophage (Pyo bacteriophage) solution, (ii) placebo solution, or (iii) antibiotic treatment (Leitner et al., 2017).

More human studies are warranted to further define the role of this treatment option in UTIs.

CONCLUSION

Although prophylactic antibiotics remain the preferred preventive treatment in recurrent UTIs, the emergence of antimicrobial resistance worldwide has made the development of non-antibiotics strategies a priority. The better understanding of UTI mechanisms will help direct future research on the topic. Indeed, recent studies have revealed that infection with UPEC and a number of other Gram-negative uropathogens proceeds through dynamic intracellular and extracellular host niches during the course of acute and chronic infection.

Several targets such as uropathogenic adhesins, toxins, urease, iron metabolism and motility have been explored. Although non-antibiotic prophylactic agents appear to be well tolerated and do not seem to increase the antimicrobial resistance of the commensal flora, most of therapeutic options displayed in this review are still preliminary.

Other approaches have also been evaluated in prevention of CAUTI. In case of prolonged utilization of catheter, some techniques have been developed to prevent bacterial growth and biofilm formation. These techniques, including the devices with antimicrobial coatings such as silver, peptides, enzymes or bacteriophages, provide minimal reduction in infection incidence and will need further assessment (Percival et al., 2015; Al-Qahtani et al., 2019).

While *Lactobacillus*-containing products appear to be the most promising new alternative to currently used antibiotics, cranberry products combined with propolis would need further investigations. Studies should now be designed to investigate the interaction between non-antibiotic therapies, uropathogens and the host immune system. Importantly, clinical trials must use standardized definitions of UTI (infection versus colonization based on urinary symptoms), treatment regimens and control groups as well as an assessment of the risk/benefit ratio especially on tolerance and antibiotic resistance and an economic evaluation of the reviewed therapeutics versus prolonged antibiotic treatments. Likewise, further research is needed for vaccines, which have shown potential in initial trials.

AUTHOR CONTRIBUTIONS

PL, JR, J-PL, and AS wrote the manuscript. AD, CD-R, LB, and FB critically reviewed the manuscript. All authors contributed to the article and approved the submitted version.

FUNDING

This work was supported by CHU Nîmes (Grant Thématiques phares).

ACKNOWLEDGMENTS

PL, CD-R, AS and J-PL belong to the FHU INCh (Federation Hospitalo Universitaire Infections Chroniques, Aviesan). We thank the Nîmes University hospital for its structural, human and financial support through the award obtained by our team during the internal call for tenders Thématiques phares. We also thank Sarah Kabani for her editing assistance.

REFERENCES

Åberg, V., and Almqvist, F. (2007). Pilicides—small molecules targeting bacterial virulence. *Org. Biomol. Chem.* 5, 1827–1834. doi: 10.1039/b702397a

Abraham, S. N., and Miao, Y. (2015). The nature of immune responses to urinary tract infections. *Nat. Rev. Immunol.* 15, 655–663. doi: 10.1038/nri3887

AFSSA (2007). *Saisine n° 2007.* Available online at: https://www.anses.fr/fr/system/files/DIVE2007sa0209.pdf (accessed January 13, 2009).

Ahuja, S., Kaack, B., and Roberts, J. (1998). Loss of fimbrial adhesion with the addition of *Vaccinum macrocarpon* to the growth medium of P-fimbriated *Escherichia coli. J. Urol.* 159, 559–562. doi: 10.1016/s0022-5347(01)63983-1

Albert, X., Huertas, I., Pereiro, I., Sanfélix, J., Gosalbes, V., and Perrotta, C. (2004). Antibiotics for preventing recurrent urinary tract infection in non−pregnant women. *Cochrane Database Syst. Rev.* 3:CD001209.

Al-Qahtani, M., Safan, A., Jassim, G., and Abadla, S. (2019). Efficacy of anti-microbial catheters in preventing catheter associated urinary tract infections in hospitalized patients: a review on recent updates. *J. Infect. Public Health* 12, 760–766. doi: 10.1016/j.jiph.2019.09.009

Alteri, C. J., Hagan, E. C., Sivick, K. E., Smith, S. N., and Mobley, H. L. T. (2009). Mucosal immunization with iron receptor antigens protects against urinary tract infection. *PLoS Pathog.* 5:e1000586. doi: 10.1371/journal.ppat.1000586

Amtul, Z., Rahman, A.-U., Siddiqui, R. A., and Choudhary, M. I. (2002). Chemistry and mechanism of urease inhibition. *Curr. Med. Chem.* 9, 1323–1348. doi: 10.2174/0929867023369853

Anderson, G. G., Goller, C. C., Justice, S., Hultgren, S. J., and Seed, P. C. (2010). Polysaccharide capsule and sialic acid-mediated regulation promote biofilm-like intracellular bacterial communities during cystitis. *Infect. Immun.* 78, 963–975. doi: 10.1128/iai.00925-09

Anger, J., Lee, U., Ackerman, A. L., Chou, R., Chughtai, B., Clemens, J. Q., et al. (2019). Recurrent uncomplicated urinary tract infections in women: AUA/CUA/SUFU guideline. *J. Urol.* 202, 282–289. doi: 10.1097/ju.0000000000000296

Arakawa, H., Maeda, M., Okubo, S., and Shimamura, T. (2004). Role of hydrogen peroxide in bactericidal action of catechin. *Biol. Pharm. Bull.* 27, 277–281. doi: 10.1248/bpb.27.277

Asadi Karam, M. R., Habibi, M., and Bouzari, S. (2019). Urinary tract infection: pathogenicity, antibiotic resistance and development of effective vaccines against Uropathogenic *Escherichia coli. Mol. Immunol.* 108, 56–67. doi: 10.1016/j.molimm.2019.02.007

Aziminia, N., Hadjipavlou, M., Philippou, Y., Pandian, S. S., Malde, S., and Hammadeh, M. Y. (2019). Vaccines for the prevention of recurrent urinary tract infections: a systematic review. *BJU Int.* 123, 753–768. doi: 10.1111/bju.14606

Bae, W.-J., Ha, U.-S., Kim, S., Kim, S.-J., Hong, S.-H., Lee, J.-Y., et al. (2015). Reduction of oxidative stress may play a role in the anti-inflammatory effect of the novel herbal formulation in a rat model of hydrochloric acid-induced cystitis. *Neurourol. Urodyn.* 34, 86–91. doi: 10.1002/nau.22507

Bailie, N. C., Osborne, C. A., Leininger, J. R., Fletcher, T. F., Johnston, S. D., Ogburn, P. N., et al. (1986). Teratogenic effect of acetohydroxamic acid in clinically normal beagles. *Am. J. Vet. Res.* 47, 2604–2611.

Banu, G. S., and Kumar, G. (2009). Preliminary screening of endophytic fungi from medicinal plants in India for antimicrobial and antitumor activity. *Int. J. Pharma. Sci. Nanotechnol.* 2, 566–571.

Bauer, H. W., Alloussi, S., Egger, G., Blümlein, H.-M., Cozma, G., Schulman, C. C., et al. (2005). A long-term, multicenter, double-blind study of an *Escherichia coli* extract (OM-89) in female patients with recurrent urinary tract infections. *Eur. Urol.* 47, 542–548. doi: 10.1016/j.eururo.2004.12.009

Beerepoot, M., and Geerlings, S. (2016). Non-antibiotic prophylaxis for urinary tract infections. *Pathogens* 5:36. doi: 10.3390/pathogens5020036

Beerepoot, M. A. J., den Heijer, C. D. J., Penders, J., Prins, J. M., Stobberingh, E. E., and Geerlings, S. E. (2012a). Predictive value of *Escherichia coli* susceptibility in strains causing asymptomatic bacteriuria for women with recurrent symptomatic urinary tract infections receiving prophylaxis. *Clin. Microbiol. Infect.* 18, E84–E90.

Beerepoot, M. A. J., ter Riet, G., Nys, S., van der Wal, W. M., de Borgie, C. A. J. M., de Reijke, T. M., et al. (2012b). Lactobacilli vs antibiotics to prevent urinary tract infections: a randomized, double-blind, noninferiority trial in postmenopausal women. *Arch. Intern. Med.* 172, 704–712.

Benini, S., Rypniewski, W. R., Wilson, K. S., Miletti, S., Ciurli, S., and Mangani, S. (2000). The complex of *Bacillus pasteurii* urease with acetohydroxamate anion from X-ray data at 1.55 A resolution. *J. Biol. Inorg. Chem.* 5, 110–118. doi: 10.1007/s007750050014

Birder, L. A., and de Groat, W. C. (2007). Mechanisms of disease: involvement of the urothelium in bladder dysfunction. *Nat. Clin. Pract. Urol.* 4, 46–54. doi: 10.1038/ncpuro0672

Bleidorn, J., Gágyor, I., Kochen, M. M., Wegscheider, K., and Hummers-Pradier, E. (2010). Symptomatic treatment (ibuprofen) or antibiotics (ciprofloxacin) for uncomplicated urinary tract infection?–results of a randomized controlled pilot trial. *BMC Med.* 8:30. doi: 10.1186/1741-7015-8-30

Boonsai, P., Phuwapraisirisan, P., and Chanchao, C. (2014). Antibacterial activity of a cardanol from Thai *Apis mellifera* propolis. *Int. J. Med. Sci.* 11, 327–336. doi: 10.7150/ijms.7373

Brumbaugh, A. R., Smith, S. N., and Mobley, H. L. T. (2013). Immunization with the yersiniabactin receptor, FyuA, protects against pyelonephritis in a murine model of urinary tract infection. *Infect. Immun.* 81, 3309–3316. doi: 10.1128/iai.00470-13

Bruyère, F., Azzouzi, A. R., Lavigne, J.-P., Droupy, S., Coloby, P., Game, X., et al. (2019). A multicenter, randomized, placebo-controlled study evaluating the efficacy of a combination of propolis and cranberry (*Vaccinium macrocarpon*) (DUAB®) in preventing low urinary tract Infection recurrence in women complaining of recurrent cystitis. *Urol. Int.* 103, 41–48. doi: 10.1159/000496695

Burne, R. A., and Chen, Y. Y. M. (2000). Bacterial ureases in infectious diseases. *Microbes Infect.* 2, 533–542. doi: 10.1016/s1286-4579(00)00312-9

Cadieux, P. A., Burton, J., Devillard, E., and Reid, G. (2009). Lactobacillus by-products inhibit the growth and virulence of uropathogenic *Escherichia coli. J. Physiol. Pharmacol.* 60, 13–18.

Castelló, T., Girona, L., Gómez, M. R., Mena Mur, A., and García, L. (1996). The possible value of ascorbic acid as a prophylactic agent for urinary tract infection. *Spinal Cord.* 34, 592–593. doi: 10.1038/sc.1996.105

Cegelski, L., Pinkner, J. S., Hammer, N. D., Cusumano, C. K., Hung, S., Chorell, E., et al. (2010). Small-molecule inhibitors target *Escherichia coli* amyloid biogenesis and biofilm formation. *Natl. Inst. Health* 5, 913–919. doi: 10.1038/nchembio.242

Chan, M., Hidalgo, G., Asadishad, B., Almeida, S., Muja, N., Mohammadi, M. S., et al. (2013). Inhibition of bacterial motility and spreading via release of cranberry derived materials from silicone substrates. *Colloids Surf. B Biointerfaces* 110, 275–280. doi: 10.1016/j.colsurfb.2013.03.047

Chen, T.-C., Tsai, J.-P., Huang, H.-J., Teng, C.-C., Chien, S.-J., Kuo, H.-C., et al. (2011). Regulation of cyclooxygenase-2 expression in human bladder epithelial cells infected with type I fimbriated uropathogenic *E. coli. Cell. Microbiol.* 13, 1703–1713. doi: 10.1111/j.1462-5822.2011.01650.x

Chikindas, M. L., Weeks, R., Drider, D., Chistyakov, V. A., and Dicks, L. M. (2018). Functions and emerging applications of bacteriocins. *Curr. Opin. Biotechnol.* 49, 23–28. doi: 10.1016/j.copbio.2017.07.011

Ciani, O., Arendsen, E., Romancik, M., Lunik, R., Costantini, E., Di Biase, M., et al. (2016). Intravesical administration of combined hyaluronic acid (HA) and chondroitin sulfate (CS) for the treatment of female recurrent urinary tract infections: a European multicentre nested case-control study. *BMJ Open* 6:e009669. doi: 10.1136/bmjopen-2015-009669

Cicione, A., Cantiello, F., Ucciero, G., Salonia, A., Torella, M., De Sio, M., et al. (2014). Intravesical treatment with highly-concentrated hyaluronic acid and chondroitin sulphate in patients with recurrent urinary tract infections: results from a multicentre survey. *J. Can. Urol. Assoc.* 8, E721–E727.

Constantinides, C., Manousakas, T., Nikolopoulos, P., Stanitsas, A., Haritopoulos, K., and Giannopoulos, A. (2004). Prevention of recurrent bacterial cystitis by intravesical administration of hyaluronic acid: a pilot study. *BJU Int.* 93, 1262–1266. doi: 10.1111/j.1464-410x.2004.04850.x

Cooper, R., Morré, D. J., and Morré, D. M. (2005a). Medicinal benefits of green tea: Part I. Review of noncancer health benefits. *J. Altern. Complement. Med.* 11, 521–528. doi: 10.1089/acm.2005.11.521

Cooper, R., Morré, D. J., and Morré, D. M. (2005b). Medicinal benefits of green tea: Part II. Review of anticancer properties. *J. Altern. Complement. Med.* 11, 639–652. doi: 10.1089/acm.2005.11.639

Cribby, S., Taylor, M., and Reid, G. (2008). Vaginal microbiota and the use of probiotics. *Interdiscip. Perspect. Infect. Dis.* 2008:256490.

Cusumano, C. K., Pinkner, J. S., Han, Z., Greene, S. E., Ford, B. A., Crowley, J. R., et al. (2011). Treatment and prevention of urinary tract infection with orally active FimH inhibitors. *Sci. Transl. Med.* 3:109ra115. doi: 10.1126/scitranslmed.3003021

Darouiche, R. O., Donovan, W. H., Del Terzo, M., Thornby, J. I., Rudy, D. C., and Hull, R. A. (2001). Pilot trial of bacterial interference for preventing urinary tract infection. *Urology* 58, 339–344. doi: 10.1016/s0090-4295(01)01271-7

Darouiche, R. O., Green, B. G., Donovan, W. H., Chen, D., Schwartz, M., Merritt, J., et al. (2011). Multicenter randomized controlled trial of bacterial interference for prevention of urinary tract infection in patients with neurogenic bladder. *Urology* 78, 341–346. doi: 10.1016/j.urology.2011.03.062

Darouiche, R. O., Thornby, J. I., Stewart, C. C., Donovan, W. H., and Hull, R. A. (2005). Bacterial Interference for prevention of urinary tract infection: a prospective, randomized, placebo-controlled, double-blind pilot trial. *Clin. Infect. Dis.* 41, 1531–1534. doi: 10.1086/497272

Dashiff, A., Junka, R. A., Libera, M., and Kadouri, D. E. (2011). Predation of human pathogens by the predatory bacteria *Micavibrio aeruginosavorus* and

Bdellovibrio bacteriovorus. J. Appl. Microbiol. 110, 431–444. doi: 10.1111/j. 1365-2672.2010.04900.x

De Ree, J. M., and Van den Bosch, J. F. (1987). Serological response to the P fimbriae of uropathogenic *Escherichia coli* in pyelonephritis. *Infect. Immun.* 55, 2204–2207. doi: 10.1128/iai.55.9.2204-2207.1987

De Vuyst, L., and Leroy, F. (2007). Bacteriocins from lactic acid bacteria: production, purification, and food applications. *J. Mol. Microbiol. Biotechnol.* 13, 194–199. doi: 10.1159/000104752

Di Cerbo, A., Palmieri, B., Aponte, M., Morales-Medina, J. C., and Iannitti, T. (2016). Mechanisms and therapeutic effectiveness of lactobacilli. *J. Clin. Pathol.* 69, 187–203. doi: 10.1136/jclinpath-2015-202976

Dinh, A., Hallouin-Bernard, M. C., Davido, B., Lemaignen, A., Bouchand, F., Duran, C., et al. (2019). Weekly sequential antibioprophylaxis for recurrent UTI among patients with neurogenic bladder: a randomized controlled trial. *Clin. Infect. Dis.* ciz1207. doi: 10.1093/cid/ciz1207. [Epub ahead of print].

Domenici, L., Monti, M., Bracchi, C., Giorgini, M., Colagiovanni, V., Muzii, L., et al. (2016). D-mannose: a promising support for acute urinary tract infections in women. A pilot study. *Eur. Rev. Med. Pharmacol. Sci.* 20, 2920–2925.

Duell, B. L., Carey, A. J., Tan, C. K., Cui, X., Webb, R. I., Totsika, M., et al. (2012). Innate transcriptional networks activated in bladder in response to uropathogenic *Escherichia coli* drive diverse biological pathways and rapid synthesis of IL-10 for defense against bacterial urinary tract infection. *J. Immunol.* 188, 781–792. doi: 10.4049/jimmunol.1101231

Dufour, N., Clermont, O., La Combe, B., Messika, J., Dion, S., Khanna, V., et al. (2016). Bacteriophage LM33_P1, a fast-acting weapon against the pandemic ST131-O25b:H4 *Escherichia coli* clonal complex. *J. Antimicrob. Chemother.* 71, 3072–3080. doi: 10.1093/jac/dkw253

Ellis, T. N., and Kuehn, M. J. (2010). Virulence and immunomodulatory roles of bacterial outer membrane vesicles. *Microbiol. Mol. Biol. Rev.* 74, 81–94. doi: 10.1128/mmbr.00031-09

Ermel, G., Georgeault, S., Inisan, C., and Besnard, M. (2012). Inhibition of adhesion of uropathogenic *Escherichia coli* Bacteria to uroepithelial cells by extracts from cranberry. *J. Med. Food* 15, 126–134. doi: 10.1089/jmf.2010. 0312

Falagas, M. E., Betsi, G. I., Tokas, T., and Athanasiou, S. (2006). Probiotics for prevention of recurrent urinary tract infections in women : a review of the evidence from microbiological and clinical studies. *Drugs* 66, 1253–1261. doi: 10.2165/00003495-200666090-00007

Faraci, W. S., Yang, B. V., O'Rourke, D., and Spencer, R. W. (1995). Inhibition of *Helicobacter* pylori urease by phenyl phosphorodiamidates: mechanism of action. *Bioorg. Med. Chem.* 3, 605–610. doi: 10.1016/0968-0896(95)00043-g

Ferry, S. A., Holm, S. E., Stenlund, H., Lundholm, R., and Monsen, T. J. (2004). The natural course of uncomplicated lower urinary tract infection in women illustrated by a randomized placebo controlled study. *Scand. J. Infect. Dis.* 36, 296–301. doi: 10.1080/00365540410019642

Ferry, T., Boucher, F., Fevre, C., Perpoint, T., Chateau, J., Petitjean, C., et al. (2018). Innovations for the treatment of a complex bone and joint infection due to XDR *Pseudomonas aeruginosa* including local application of a selected cocktail of bacteriophages. *J. Antimicrob. Chemother.* 73, 2901–2903. doi: 10.1093/jac/dky263

Flores-Meireles, A., Walker, J., Caparon, M., and Hultgren, S. (2015). Urinary tract infections: epidemiology, mechanisms of infection and treatment options. *Nat. Rev. Microbiol.* 13, 269–284. doi: 10.1038/nrmicro3432

Flower, A., Wang, L.-Q., Lewith, G., Liu, J. P., and Li, Q. (2015). Chinese herbal medicine for treating recurrent urinary tract infections in women. *Cochrane Database Syst. Rev.* 2015:CD010446.

Foxman, B. (2014). Urinary tract infection syndromes: occurrence, recurrence, bacteriology, risk factors, and disease burden. *Infect. Dis. Clin. North Am.* 28, 1–13. doi: 10.1016/j.idc.2013.09.003

Freitas, S. F., Shinohara, L., Sforcin, J. M., and Guimarães, S. (2006). In vitro effects of propolis on *Giardia duodenalis* trophozoites. *Phytomedicine* 13, 170–175. doi: 10.1016/j.phymed.2004.07.008

Frenck, R. W., Ervin, J., Chu, L., Abbanat, D., Spiessens, B., Go, O., et al. (2019). Safety and immunogenicity of a vaccine for extra-intestinal pathogenic *Escherichia coli* (ESTELLA): a phase 2 randomised controlled trial. *Lancet Infect. Dis.* 19, 631–640. doi: 10.1016/s1473-3099(18)30803-x

Galdeano, C. M., and Perdigón, G. (2006). The probiotic bacterium *Lactobacillus casei* induces activation of the gut mucosal immune system through innate

immunity. *Clin. Vaccine Immunol.* 13, 219–226. doi: 10.1128/cvi.13.2.219-226. 2006

Goddard, J. C., and Janssen, D. A. W. (2018). Intravesical hyaluronic acid and chondroitin sulfate for recurrent urinary tract infections: systematic review and meta-analysis. *Int. Urogynecol. J.* 29, 933–942. doi: 10.1007/s00192-017-3508-z

Goller, C. C., Arshad, M., Noah, J. W., Ananthan, S., Evans, C. W., Nebane, N. M., et al. (2014). Lifting the mask: identification of new small molecule inhibitors of uropathogenic *Escherichia coli* group 2 capsule biogenesis. *PLoS One* 9:e96054. doi: 10.1371/journal.pone.0096054

Greene, S. E., Pinkner, J. S., Chorell, E., Dodson, K. W., Shaffer, C. L., Conover, M. S., et al. (2014). Pilicide ec240 disrupts virulence circuits in uropathogenic *Escherichia coli. mBio* 5:14.

Griffith, D. P., Gibson, J. R., Clinton, C. W., and Musher, D. M. (1978). Acetohydroxamic acid: clinical studies of a urease inhibitor in patients with staghorn renal calculi. *J. Urol.* 119, 9–15. doi: 10.1016/s0022-5347(17)57366-8

Griffith, D. P., Gleeson, M. J., Lee, H., Longuet, R., Deman, E., and Earle, N. (1991). Randomized, double-blind trial of Lithostat (acetohydroxamic acid) in the palliative treatment of infection-induced urinary calculi. *Eur. Urol.* 20, 243–247. doi: 10.1159/000471707

Griffith, D. P., Khonsari, F., Skurnick, J. H., and James, K. E. (1988). A randomized trial of acetohydroxamic acid for the treatment and prevention of infection-induced urinary stones in spinal cord injury patients. *J. Urol.* 140, 318–324. doi: 10.1016/s0022-5347(17)41592-8

Gu, X. C., Xu, Z., Chen, M., and Wang, M. (2011). Study of erding erxian docoction compared with sanjin tablet in treating recurrent urinary tract infection. *Zhongguo Zhongxiyi Jiehe Shenbing Zazhi.* 12, 623–624.

Gupta, S., Tang, C., Tran, M., and Kadouri, D. E. (2016). Effect of predatory bacteria on human cell lines. *PLoS One* 11:e0161242. doi: 10.1371/journal.pone.0161242

Habash, M. B., Van der Mei, H. C., Busscher, H. J., and Reid, G. (1999). The effect of water, ascorbic acid, and cranberry derived supplementation on human urine and uropathogen adhesion to silicone rubber. *Can. J. Microbiol.* 45, 691–694. doi: 10.1139/w99-065

Habibi, M., Asadi Karam, M. R., and Bouzari, S. (2016). Transurethral instillation with fusion protein MrpH.FimH induces protective innate immune responses against uropathogenic *Escherichia coli* and *Proteus mirabilis. APMIS* 124, 444–452. doi: 10.1111/apm.12523

Hannan, T. J., Mysorekar, I. U., Hung, C. S., Isaacson-Schmid, M. L., and Hultgren, S. J. (2010). Early severe inflammatory responses to uropathogenic *E. coli* predispose to chronic and recurrent urinary tract infection. *PLoS Pathog.* 6:e1001042. doi: 10.1371/journal.ppat.1001042

Hannan, T. J., Roberts, P. L., Riehl, T. E., van der Post, S., Binkley, J. M., Schwartz, D. J., et al. (2014). Inhibition of cyclooxygenase-2 prevents chronic and recurrent cystitis. *EBioMedicine* 1, 46–57. doi: 10.1016/j.ebiom.2014.10.011

Hardy, H., Harris, J., Lyon, E., Beal, J., and Foey, A. D. (2013). Probiotics, prebiotics and immunomodulation of gut mucosal defences: homeostasis and immunopathology. *Nutrients* 5, 1869–1912. doi: 10.3390/nu5061869

Hills, A. E., Patel, A., Boyd, P., and James, D. C. (2001). Metabolic control of recombinant monoclonal antibody N-glycosylation in GS-NS0 cells. *Biotechnol. Bioeng.* 75, 239–251. doi: 10.1002/bit.10022

Hopkins, W. J., Elkahwaji, J., Beierle, L. M., Leverson, G. E., and Uehling, D. T. (2007). Vaginal mucosal vaccine for recurrent urinary tract infections in women: results of a phase 2 clinical trial. *J. Urol.* 177, 1349–1353. doi: 10.1016/j.juro.2006.11.093

Hoshino, N., Kimura, T., Yamaji, A., and Ando, T. (1999). Damage to the cytoplasmic membrane of *Escherichia coli* by catechin-copper (II) complexes. *Free Radic. Biol. Med.* 27, 1245–1250. doi: 10.1016/s0891-5849(99)00157-4

Hou, X., and Wang, L. X. (2016). Research progress of sanjin tablets. *Eval. Anal. Drug Chin. Hosp.* 16, 1148–1151.

Howell, A. B., Reed, J. D., Krueger, C. G., Winterbottom, R., Cunningham, D. G., and Leahy, M. (2005). A-type cranberry proanthocyanidins and uropathogenic bacterial anti-adhesion activity. *Phytochemistry* 66, 2281–2291. doi: 10.1016/j.phytochem.2005.05.022

Huber, M., Ayoub, M., Pfannes, S. D., Mittenbühler, K., Weis, K., Bessler, W. G., et al. (2000). Immunostimulatory activity of the bacterial extract OM-8. *Eur. J. Med. Res.* 5, 101–109.

Hull, R., Rudy, D., Donovan, W., Svanborg, C., Wieser, I., Stewart, C., et al. (2000). Urinary tract infection prophylaxis using *Escherichia coli* 83972 in spinal cord injured patients. *J. Urol.* 163, 872–877. doi: 10.1016/s0022-5347(05)67823-8

Huttner, A., and Gambillara, V. (2018). The development and early clinical testing of the ExPEC4V conjugate vaccine against uropathogenic *Escherichia coli*. *Clin. Microbiol. Infect.* 24, 1046–1050. doi: 10.1016/j.cmi.2018.05.009

Huttner, A., Hatz, C., van den Dobbelsteen, G., Abbanat, D., Hornacek, A., Frölich, R., et al. (2017). Safety, immunogenicity, and preliminary clinical efficacy of a vaccine against extraintestinal pathogenic *Escherichia coli* in women with a history of recurrent urinary tract infection: a randomised, single-blind, placebo-controlled phase 1b trial. *Lancet Infect. Dis.* 17, 528–537. doi: 10.1016/s1473-3099(17)30108-1

Ikähelmo, R., Siitonen, A., Heiskanen, T., Kärkkäinen, U., Kuosmanen, P., Lipponen, P., et al. (1996). Recurrence of urinary tract infection in a primary care setting: analysis of a I-year follow-up of 179 women. *Clin. Infect. Dis.* 22, 91–99. doi: 10.1093/clinids/22.1.91

Ingersoll, M. A., and Albert, M. L. (2013). From infection to immunotherapy: host immune responses to bacteria at the bladder mucosa. *Mucosal Immunol.* 6, 1041–1053. doi: 10.1038/mi.2013.72

Isolauri, E., Sütas, Y., Kankaanpää, P., Arvilommi, H., and Salminen, S. (2001). Probiotics: effects on immunity. *Am. J. Clin. Nutr.* 73, 444S–450S.

Issac Abraham, S. V., Palani, A., Ramaswamy, B. R., Shunmugiah, K. P., and Arumugam, V. R. (2011). Antiquorum sensing and antibiofilm potential of *Capparis spinosa*. *Arch. Med. Res.* 42, 658–668. doi: 10.1016/j.arcmed.2011.12.002

Jacobsen, S. M., Stickler, D. J., Mobley, H. L. T., and Shirtliff, M. E. (2008). Complicated catheter-associated urinary tract infections due to *Escherichia coli* and *Proteus mirabilis*. *Clin. Microbiol. Rev.* 21, 26–59. doi: 10.1128/cmr.00019-07

Jaiswal, S. K., Sharma, N. K., Bharti, S. K., Krishnan, S., Kumar, A., Prakash, O., et al. (2018). Phytochemicals as uropathogenic *Escherichia coli* FimH antagonist: in vitro and in silico approach. *Curr. Mol. Med.* 18, 640–653. doi: 10.2174/1566524019666190104104507

Jault, P., Leclerc, T., Jennes, S., Pirnay, J. P., Que, Y.-A., Resch, G., et al. (2019). Efficacy and tolerability of a cocktail of bacteriophages to treat burn wounds infected by *Pseudomonas aeruginosa* (PhagoBurn): a randomised, controlled, double-blind phase 1/2 trial. *Lancet Infect. Dis.* 19, 35–45. doi: 10.1016/s1473-3099(18)30482-1

Jepson, R. G., and Craig, J. C. (2008). Cranberries for preventing urinary tract infections. *Cochrane Database Syst. Rev.* CD001321. doi: 10.1002/14651858.CD001321.pub4

Jepson, R. G., Williams, G., and Craig, J. C. (2012). Cranberries for preventing urinary tract infections. *Cochrane Database Syst. Rev.* 10:CD001321.

Johnson, J. R. (1991). Virulence factors in *Escherichia coli* urinary tract infection. *Clin. Microbiol. Rev.* 4, 80–128. doi: 10.1128/cmr.4.1.80

Kadouri, D., and O'Toole, G. A. (2005). Susceptibility of biofilms to *Bdellovibrio bacteriovorus* attack. *Appl. Environ. Microbiol.* 71, 4044–4051. doi: 10.1128/aem.71.7.4044-4051.2005

Kaijser, B., Larsson, P., Olling, S., and Schneerson, R. (1983). Protection against acute, ascending pyelonephritis caused by *Escherichia coli* in rats, using isolated capsular antigen conjugated to bovine serum albumin. *Infect. Immun.* 39, 142–146. doi: 10.1128/iai.39.1.142-146.1983

Kemgang, T. S., Kapila, S., Shanmugam, V. P., and Kapila, R. (2014). Cross-talk between probiotic lactobacilli and host immune system. *J. Appl. Microbiol.* 117, 303–319. doi: 10.1111/jam.12521

Klein, T., Abgottspon, D., Wittwer, M., Rabbani, S., Herold, J., Jiang, X., et al. (2010). FimH antagonists for the oral treatment of urinary tract infections: from design and synthesis to in vitro and in vivo evaluation. *J. Med. Chem.* 53, 8627–8641. doi: 10.1021/jm101011y

Koradia, P., Kapadia, S., Trivedi, Y., Chanchu, G., and Harper, A. (2019). Probiotic and cranberry supplementation for preventing recurrent uncomplicated urinary tract infections in premenopausal women: a controlled pilot study. *Exp. Rev. Anti Infect. Ther.* 17, 733–740. doi: 10.1080/14787210.2019.1664287

Kranjčec, B., Papes, D., and Altarac, S. (2014). D-mannose powder for prophylaxis of recurrent urinary tract infections in women: a randomized clinical trial. *World J. Urol.* 32, 79–84. doi: 10.1007/s00345-013-1091-6

Kuipers, S., Ruth, M. M., Mientjes, M., de Sévaux, R. G. L., and van Ingen, J. A. (2019). Dutch case report of successful treatment of chronic relapsing urinary tract infection with bacteriophages in a renal transplant patient. *Antimicrob. Agents Chemother.* 64:e01281-19.

Kumar, V., Ganguly, N., Joshi, K., Mittal, R., Harjai, K., Chhibber, S., et al. (2005). Protective efficacy and immunogenicity of *Escherichia coli* K13 diphtheria toxoid conjugate against experimental ascending pyelonephritis. *Med. Microbiol. Immunol.* 194, 211–217. doi: 10.1007/s00430-005-0241-x

Langermann, S., Möllby, R., Burlein, J. E., Palaszynski, S. R., Auguste, C. G., DeFusco, A., et al. (2000). Vaccination with FimH adhesin protects cynomolgus monkeys from colonization and infection by uropathogenic *Escherichia coli*. *J. Infect. Dis.* 181, 774–778. doi: 10.1086/315258

Larsson, A., Ohlsson, J., Dodson, K. W., Hultgren, S. J., Nilsson, U., and Kihlberg, J. (2003). Quantitative studies of the binding of the class II PapG adhesin from uropathogenic *Escherichia coli* to oligosaccharides. *Bioorg. Med. Chem.* 11, 2255–2261. doi: 10.1016/s0968-0896(03)00114-7

Laupland, K. B., Ross, T., Pitout, J. D. D., Church, D. L., and Gregson, D. B. (2007). Community-onset urinary tract infections: a population-based assessment. *Infection* 35, 150–153. doi: 10.1007/s15010-007-6180-2

Leitner, L., Sybesma, W., Chanishvili, N., Goderdzishvili, M., Chkhotua, A., Ujmajuridze, A., et al. (2017). Bacteriophages for treating urinary tract infections in patients undergoing transurethral resection of the prostate: a randomized, placebo-controlled, double-blind clinical trial. *BMC Urol.* 17:90. doi: 10.1186/s12894-017-0283-6

Liu, H., Howell, A. B., Zhang, D. J., and Khoo, C. (2019). A randomized, double-blind, placebo-controlled pilot study to assess bacterial anti-adhesive activity in human urine following consumption of a cranberry supplement. *Food Funt.* 10, 7645–7652. doi: 10.1039/c9fo01198f

Liu, Y., Black, M. A., Caron, L., and Camesano, T. A. (2006). Role of cranberry juice on molecular-scale surface characteristics and adhesion behavior of *Escherichia coli*. *Biotechnol. Bioeng.* 93, 297–305. doi: 10.1002/bit.20675

Liu, Z., Ren, Z., Zhang, J., Chuang, C. C., Kandaswamy, E., Zhou, T., et al. (2018). Role of ROS and nutritional antioxidants in human diseases. *Front. Physiol.* 9:477. doi: 10.3389/fphys.2018.00477

Llobet, E., Tomás, J. M., and Bengoechea, J. A. (2008). Capsule polysaccharide is a bacterial decoy for antimicrobial peptides. *Microbiol. Read. Engl.* 154, 3877–3886. doi: 10.1099/mic.0.2008/022301-0

Lorenzo-Gómez, M. F., Padilla-Fernández, B., García-Cenador, M. B., Virseda-Rodríguez, ÁJ., Martín-García, I., Sánchez-Escudero, A., et al. (2015). Comparison of sublingual therapeutic vaccine with antibiotics for the prophylaxis of recurrent urinary tract infections. *Front. Cell. Infect. Microbiol.* 5:50. doi: 10.3389/fcimb.2015.00050

Lorenzo-Gómez, M. F., Padilla-Fernández, B., García-Criado, F. J., Mirón-Canelo, J. A., Gil-Vicente, A., Nieto-Huertos, A., et al. (2013). Evaluation of a therapeutic vaccine for the prevention of recurrent urinary tract infections versus prophylactic treatment with antibiotics. *Int. Urogynecology J.* 24, 127–134. doi: 10.1007/s00192-012-1853-5

Magasi, P., Pánovics, J., Illés, A., and Nagy, M. (1994). Uro-Vaxom and the management of recurrent urinary tract infection in adults: a randomized multicenter double-blind trial. *Eur. Urol.* 26, 137–140. doi: 10.1159/000475363

Mazarei, F., Jooyandeh, H., Noshad, M., and Hojjati, M. (2017). Polysaccharide of caper (*Capparis spinosa* L.) Leaf: extraction optimization, antioxidant potential, and antimicrobial activity. *Int. J. Biol. Macromol.* 95, 224–231. doi: 10.1016/j.ijbiomac.2016.11.049

McLellan, L. K., and Hunstad, D. A. (2016). Urinary tract infection: pathogenesis and outlook. *Trends Mol. Med.* 22, 946–957. doi: 10.1016/j.molmed.2016.09.003

Melican, K., Sandoval, R. M., Kader, A., Josefsson, L., Tanner, G. A., Molitoris, B. A., et al. (2011). Uropathogenic *Escherichia coli* P and Type 1 fimbriae act in synergy in a living host to facilitate renal colonization leading to nephron obstruction. *PLoS Pathog.* 7:e1001298. doi: 10.1371/journal.ppat.1001298

Mendling, W. (2016). Vaginal microbiota. *Adv. Exp. Med. Biol.* 902, 83–93.

Meng, J., Zou, Z., and Lu, C. (2015). Identification and characterization of bioactive compounds targeting uropathogenic *Escherichia coli* from Sanjin tablets. *J. Chem.* 2015, 789809.

Mickymaray, S., and Al Aboody, M. S. (2019). In vitro antioxidant and bactericidal efficacy of 15 common spices: novel therapeutics for urinary tract infections? *Medicina (Kaunas)* 55:E289.

Mobley, H. L., and Hausinger, R. P. (1989). Microbial ureases: significance, regulation, and molecular characterization. *Microbiol. Rev.* 53, 85–108. doi: 10.1128/mmbr.53.1.85-108.1989

Moore, M., Trill, J., Simpson, C., Webley, F., Radford, M., Stanton, L., et al. (2019). Uva-ursi extract and ibuprofen as alternative treatments for uncomplicated urinary tract infection in women (ATAFUTI): a factorial randomized trial. *Clin. Microbiol. Infect.* 25, 973–980. doi: 10.1016/j.cmi.2019.01.011

Morris, N. S., and Stickler, D. J. (1998). The effect of urease inhibitors on the encrustation of urethral catheters. *Urol. Res.* 26, 275–279. doi: 10.1007/s002400050057

Muenzner, P., Tchoupa, A. K., Klauser, B., Brunner, T., Putze, J., Dobrindt, U., et al. (2016). Uropathogenic *E. coli* exploit CEA to promote colonization of the urogenital tract mucosa. *PLoS Pathog.* 12:e1005608. doi: 10.1371/journal.ppat.1005608

Mulvey, M. A. (2002). Adhesion and entry of uropathogenic *Escherichia coli*. *Cell. Microbiol.* 4, 257–271. doi: 10.1046/j.1462-5822.2002.00193.x

Mulvey, M. A., Schilling, J. D., and Hultgren, S. J. (2001). Establishment of a persistent *Escherichia coli* reservoir during the acute phase of a bladder infection. *Infect. Immun.* 69, 4572–4579. doi: 10.1128/iai.69.7.4572-4579.2001

Munakata, K., Mochida, H., Kondo, S., and Suzuki, Y. (1980). Mutagenicity of N-acylglycinohydroxamic acids and related compounds. *J. Pharmacobiodyn.* 3, 557–561. doi: 10.1248/bpb1978.3.557

Musher, D. M., Griffith, D. P., Yawn, D., and Rossen, R. D. (1975). Role of urease in pyelonephritis resulting from urinary tract infection with *Proteus*. *J. Infect. Dis.* 131, 177–181. doi: 10.1093/infdis/131.2.177

Ng, Q. X., Peters, C., Venkatanarayanan, N., Goh, Y. Y., Ho, C. Y. X., and Yeo, W.-S. (2018). Use of *Lactobacillus* spp. to prevent recurrent urinary tract infections in females. *Med. Hypotheses* 114, 49–54. doi: 10.1016/j.mehy.2018.03.001

Noormandi, A., and Dabaghzadeh, F. (2015). Effects of green tea on *Escherichia coli* as a uropathogen. *J. Tradit. Complement. Med.* 5, 15–20. doi: 10.1016/j.jtcme.2014.10.005

O'Brien, V. P., Hannan, T. J., Nielsen, H. V., and Hultgren, S. J. (2016). Drug and vaccine development for the treatment and prevention of urinary tract infections. *Microbiol. Spectr.* 4:10.1128/microbiolsec.UTI-0013-2012.

Ochoa-Brust, G. J., Fernández, A. R., Villanueva-Ruiz, G. J., Velasco, R., Trujillo-Hernández, B., and Vásquez, C. (2007). Daily intake of 100 mg ascorbic acid as urinary tract infection prophylactic agent during pregnancy. *Acta Obstet. Gynecol. Scand.* 86, 783–787. doi: 10.1080/00016340701223189

O'Hanley, P., Lalonde, G., and Ji, G. (1991). Alpha-hemolysin contributes to the pathogenicity of piliated digalactoside-binding *Escherichia coli* in the kidney: efficacy of an alpha-hemolysin vaccine in preventing renal injury in the BALB/c mouse model of pyelonephritis. *Infect. Immun.* 59, 1153–1161. doi: 10.1128/iai.59.3.1153-1161.1991

O'Hanley, P., Lark, D., Falkow, S., and Schoolnik, G. (1985). Molecular basis of *Escherichia coli* colonization of the upper urinary tract in BALB/c mice. *J. Clin. Invest.* 75, 347–360. doi: 10.1172/jci111707

Olczyk, P., Komosinska-Vassev, K., Wisowski, G., Mencner, L., Stojko, J., and Kozma, E. M. (2014). Propolis modulates fibronectin expression in the matrix of thermal injury. *BioMed Res. Int.* 2014:748101.

Pasupuleti, V. R., Sammugam, L., Ramesh, N., and Gan, S. H. (2017). Honey, propolis, and royal jelly: a comprehensive review of their biological actions and health benefits. *Oxid. Med. Cell. Longev.* 2017, 1–21. doi: 10.1155/2017/1259510

Paxman, J. J., Lo, A. W., Sullivan, M. J., Panjikar, S., Kuiper, M., Whitten, A. E., et al. (2019). Unique structural features of a bacterial autotransporter adhesin suggest mechanisms for interaction with host macromolecules. *Nat. Comm.* 10:1967.

Percival, S. L., Suleman, L., Vuotto, C., and Donelli, G. (2015). Healthcare-associated infections, medical devices and biofilms: risk, tolerance and control. *J. Med. Microbiol.* 64, 323–334. doi: 10.1099/jmm.0.000032

Pereira, E. M. R., da Silva, J. L. D. C., Silva, F. F., De Luca, M. P., Ferreira, E. F. E., Lorentz, T. C. M., et al. (2011). Clinical evidence of the efficacy of a mouthwash containing propolis for the control of plaque and gingivitis: a phase II study. *Evid.-based complement. Altern. Med.* 2011:750249.

Piatek, R., Zalewska-Piatek, B., Dzierzbicka, K., Makowiec, S., Pilipczuk, J., Szemiako, K., et al. (2013). Pilicides inhibit the FGL chaperone/usher assisted biogenesis of the Dr fimbrial polyadhesin from uropathogenic *Escherichia coli*. *BMC Microbiol.* 13:131. doi: 10.1186/1471-2180-13-131

Pinkner, J. S., Remaut, H., Buelens, F., Miller, E., Aberg, V., Pemberton, N., et al. (2006). Rationally designed small compounds inhibit pilus biogenesis in uropathogenic bacteria. *Proc. Natl. Acad. Sci. U.S.A.* 103, 17897–17902. doi: 10.1073/pnas.0606795103

Poggio, T. V., La Torre, J. L., and Scodeller, E. A. (2006). Intranasal immunization with a recombinant truncated FimH adhesin adjuvanted with CpG oligodeoxynucleotides protects mice against uropathogenic *Escherichia coli* challenge. *Can. J. Microbiol.* 52, 1093–1102. doi: 10.1139/w06-065

Poirier, C., Dinh, A., Salomon, J., Grall, N., Andremont, A., and Bernard, L. (2015). Antibiotic cycling prevents urinary tract infections in spinal cord injury patients and limits the emergence of multidrug resistant organism. *J. Infect.* 71, 491–493. doi: 10.1016/j.jinf.2015.06.001

Pope, A. J., Toseland, C. D., Rushant, B., Richardson, S., McVey, M., and Hills, J. (1998). Effect of potent urease inhibitor, fluorofamide, on *Helicobacter* sp. in vivo and in vitro. *Dig. Dis. Sci.* 43, 109–119.

Prasad, A., Cevallos, M. E., Riosa, S., Darouiche, R. O., and Trautner, B. W. (2009). A bacterial interference strategy for prevention of UTI in persons practicing intermittent catheterization. *Spinal Cord.* 47, 565–569. doi: 10.1038/sc.2008.166

Prattley, S., Geraghty, R., Moore, M., and Somani, B. K. (2020). Role of vaccines or recurrent urinary tract infections: a systematic review. *Eur. Urol. Focus* 6, 593–604. doi: 10.1016/j.euf.2019.11.002

Professionals, S.-O. (2019). *EAU Guidelines: Urological Infections [Internet]*. Uroweb [cité 2019 juill 9]. Available online at: https://uroweb.org/guideline/urological-infections/ (accessed July 9, 2019).

Pu, X., Zhang, L. Y., and Zhang, J. H. (2016). A systemtic review of Sanjin tablets in the treatment of simple urinary tract infection: a randomized controlled trial. *Lishizhen Med. Mat. Med. Res.* 27, 1012–1014.

Rafsanjany, N., Senker, J., Brandt, S., Dobrindt, U., and Hensel, A. (2015). In vivo consumption of cranberry exerts ex Vivo antiadhesive activity against FimH-dominated uropathogenic *Escherichia coli*: a combined in vivo, ex vivo, and in vitro study of an extract from *Vaccinium macrocarpon*. *J. Agric. Food Chem.* 63, 8804–8818. doi: 10.1021/acs.jafc.5b03030

Ramirez Sevilla, C., Gómez Lanza, E., Manzanera, J. L., Martin, J. A. R., and Sanz, M. A. B. (2019). Active immunoprophylaxis with uromune® decreases the recurrence of urinary tract infections at three and six months after treatment without relevant secondary effects. *BMC Infect. Dis.* 19:901. doi: 10.1186/s12879-019-4541-y

Ranfaing, J., Dunyach-Remy, C., Lavigne, J.-P., and Sotto, A. (2018a). Propolis potentiates the effect of cranberry (*Vaccinium macrocarpon*) in reducing the motility and the biofilm formation of uropathogenic *Escherichia coli*. *PLoS One* 13:e0202609. doi: 10.1371/journal.pone.0202609

Ranfaing, J., Dunyach-Remy, C., Louis, L., Lavigne, J.-P., and Sotto, A. (2018b). Propolis potentiates the effect of cranberry (*Vaccinium macrocarpon*) against the virulence of uropathogenic *Escherichia coli*. *Sci. Rep.* 8:10706.

Reygaert, W., and Jusufi, I. (2013). Green tea as an effective antimicrobial for urinary tract infections caused by *Escherichia coli*. *Front. Microbiol.* 4:162. doi: 10.3389/fmicb.2013.00162

Riaz, S., Kashif Nawaz, S., and Hasnain, S. (2010). Bacteriocins produced by *L. fermentum* and *L. acidophilus* can inhibit cephalosporin resistant *E. coli*. *Braz. J. Microbiol.* 41, 643–648. doi: 10.1590/s1517-83822010000300015

Riegman, N., van Die, I., Leunissen, J., Hoekstra, W., and Bergmans, H. (1988). Biogenesis of F71 and F72 fimbriae of uropathogenic *Escherichia coli*: influence of the FsoF and FstFG proteins and localization of the Fso/FstE protein. *Mol. Microbiol.* 2, 73–80. doi: 10.1111/j.1365-2958.1988.tb00008.x

Roberts, I. S. (1995). Bacterial polysaccharides in sickness and in health. *Microbiology* 141, 2023–2031. doi: 10.1099/13500872-141-9-2023

Roberts, I. S. (1996). The biochemistry and genetics of capsular polysaccharide production in bacteria. *Annu. Rev. Microbiol.* 50, 285–315. doi: 10.1146/annurev.micro.50.1.285

Roberts, J. A. (1991). Etiology and pathophysiology of pyelonephritis. *Am. J. Kidney Dis.* 17, 1–9. doi: 10.1016/s0272-6386(12)80242-3

Roberts, J. A., Kaack, M. B., Baskin, G., Chapman, M. R., Hunstad, D. A., Pinkner, J. S., et al. (2004). Antibody responses and protection from pyelonephritis following vaccination with purified *Escherichia coli* PapDG protein. *J. Urol.* 171, 1682–1685. doi: 10.1097/01.ju.0000116123.05160.43

Roberts, J. A., Kaack, M. B., Baskin, G., and Svenson, S. B. (1993). Prevention of renal scarring from pyelonephritis in nonhuman primates by vaccination with a synthetic *Escherichia coli* serotype O8 oligosaccharide-protein conjugate. *Infect. Immun.* 61, 5214–5218. doi: 10.1128/iai.61.12.5214-5218.1993

Rodríguez-Pérez, C., Quirantes-Piné, R., Uberos, J., Jiménez-Sánchez, C., Peña, A., and Segura-Carretero, A. (2016). Antibacterial activity of isolated phenolic compounds from cranberry (*Vaccinium macrocarpon*) against *Escherichia coli*. *Food Funct.* 7, 1564–1573. doi: 10.1039/c5fo01441g

Roos, V., Ulett, G. C., Schembri, M. A., and Klemm, P. (2006). The asymptomatic bacteriuria *Escherichia coli* strain 83972 outcompetes uropathogenic *E. coli* strains in human urine. *Infect. Immun.* 74, 615–624. doi: 10.1128/iai.74.1.615-624.2006

Rosen, D. A., Hooton, T. M., Stamm, W. E., Humphrey, P. A., and Hultgren, S. J. (2007). Detection of intracellular bacterial communities in human urinary tract infection. *PLoS Med.* 4:e329. doi: 10.1371/journal.pmed.0040329

Saint, S., Meddings, J. A., Calfee, D., Kowalski, C. P., and Krein, S. L. (2009). Catheter-associated urinary tract infection and the medicare rule changes. *Ann. Intern. Med.* 150, 877–884.

Salomon, J., Denys, P., Merle, C., Chartier-Kastler, E., Perronne, C., Gaillard, J.-L., et al. (2006). Prevention of urinary tract infection in spinal cord-injured patients: safety and efficacy of a weekly oral cyclic antibiotic (WOCA) programme with a 2 year follow-up—an observational prospective study. *J. Antimicrob. Chemother.* 57, 784–788. doi: 10.1093/jac/dkl010

Sauer, F. G., Remaut, H., Hultgren, S. J., and Waksman, G. (2004). Fiber assembly by the chaperone-usher pathway. *Biochim. Biophys. Acta.* 1694, 259–267. doi: 10.1016/j.bbamcr.2004.02.010

Schaeffer, A. J., Jones, J. M., and Dunn, J. K. (1981). Association of in vitro *Escherichia coli* adherence to vaginal and buccal epithelial cells with susceptibility of women to recurrent urinary-tract infections. *N. Engl. J. Med.* 304, 1062–1066. doi: 10.1056/nejm198104303041802

Schulman, C. C., Corbusier, A., Michiels, H., and Taenzer, H. J. (1993). Oral immunotherapy of recurrent urinary tract infections: a double-blind placebo-controlled multicenter study. *J. Urol.* 150, 917–921. doi: 10.1016/s0022-5347(17)35648-3

Sharifi-Rad, J., Mnayer, D., Roointan, A., Shahri, F., Ayatollahi, S. A., Sharifi-Rad, M., et al. (2016). Antibacterial activities of essential oils from Iranian medicinal plants on extended-spectrum β-lactamase-producing *Escherichia coli*. *Cell. Mol. Biol.* 62, 75–82.

Shatzkes, K., Chae, R., Tang, C., Ramirez, G. C., Mukherjee, S., Tsenova, L., et al. (2015). Examining the safety of respiratory and intravenous inoculation of *Bdellovibrio bacteriovorus* and *Micavibrio aeruginosavorus* in a mouse model. *Sci. Rep.* 5:12899.

Silverman, J. A., Schreiber, H. L. IV, Hooton, T. M., and Hultgren, S. J. (2013). From physiology to pharmacy: developments in the pathogenesis and treatment of recurrent urinary tract infections. *Curr. Urol. Rep.* 14, 448–456. doi: 10.1007/s11934-013-0354-5

Sobel, J. D. (1997). Pathogenesis of urinary tract infection. Role of host defenses. *Infect. Dis. Clin. North Am.* 11, 531–549.

Sockett, R. E. (2009). Predatory Lifestyle of *Bdellovibrio bacteriovorus*. *Annu. Rev. Microbiol.* 63, 523–539.

Soto, S. M., Smithson, A., Horcajada, J. P., Martinez, J. A., Mensa, J. P., and Vila, J. (2006). Implication of biofilm formation in the persistence of urinary tract infection caused by uropathogenic *Escherichia coli*. *Clin. Microbiol. Infect.* 12, 1034–1036. doi: 10.1111/j.1469-0691.2006.01543.x

Stapleton, A. E., Dziura, J., Hooton, T. M., Cox, M. E., Yarova-Yarovaya, Y., Chen, S., et al. (2012). Recurrent urinary tract infection and urinary *Escherichia coli* in women ingesting cranberry juice daily: a randomized controlled trial. *Mayo Clin. Proc.* 87, 143–150. doi: 10.1016/j.mayocp.2011.10.006

Stenutz, R., Weintraub, A., and Widmalm, G. (2006). The structures of *Escherichia coli* O-polysaccharide antigens. *FEMS Microbiol. Rev.* 30, 382–403.

Stolp, H., and Starr, M. P. (1963). *Bdellovibrio bacteriovorus* gen. et sp. n., a predatory, ectoparasitic, and bacteriolytic microorganism. *Antonie Van Leeuwenhoek* 29, 217–248. doi: 10.1007/bf02046064

Strömberg, N., Marklund, B. I., Lund, B., Ilver, D., Hamers, A., Gaastra, W., et al. (1990). Host-specificity of uropathogenic *Escherichia coli* depends on differences in binding specificity to Gal alpha 1-4Gal-containing isoreceptors. *EMBO J.* 9, 2001–2010. doi: 10.1002/j.1460-2075.1990.tb08328.x

Suetens, C., Latour, K., Kärki, T., Ricchizzi, E., Kinross, P., Moro, M. L., et al. (2018). Prevalence of healthcare-associated infections, estimated incidence and composite antimicrobial resistance index in acute care hospitals and long-term care facilities: results from two European point prevalence surveys, 2016 to 2017. *Euro Surveill.* 23:1800516.

Sundén, F., Håkansson, L., Ljunggren, E., and Wullt, B. (2010). *Escherichia coli* 83972 bacteriuria protects against recurrent lower urinary tract infections in patients with incomplete bladder emptying. *J. Urol.* 184, 179–185. doi: 10.1016/j.juro.2010.03.024

Sung, M. A., Fleming, K., Chen, H. A., and Matthews, S. (2001). The solution structure of PapGII from uropathogenic *Escherichia coli* and its recognition of glycolipid receptors. *EMBO Rep.* 2, 621–627. doi: 10.1093/embo-reports/kve133

Svensson, A., Larsson, A., Emtenäs, H., Hedenström, M., Fex, T., Hultgren, S. J., et al. (2001). Design and evaluation of pilicides: potential novel antibacterial agents directed against uropathogenic *Escherichia coli*. *Chembiochem* 2, 915–918. doi: 10.1002/1439-7633(20011203)2:12<915::aid-cbic915>3.0.co;2-m

Sybesma, W., Zbinden, R., Chanishvili, N., Kutateladze, M., Chkhotua, A., Ujmajuridze, A., et al. (2016). Bacteriophages as potential treatment for urinary tract infections. *Front. Microbiol.* 7:465. doi: 10.3389/fmicb.2016.00465

Tammen, H. (1990). Immunobiotherapy with Uro-vaxom in recurrent urinary tract infection. The German urinary tract infection study group. *Br. J. Urol.* 65, 6–9. doi: 10.1111/j.1464-410x.1990.tb14649.x

Texier-Maugein, J., Clerc, M., Vekris, A., and Bebear, C. (1987). *Ureaplasma urealyticum*-induced bladder stones in rats and their prevention by flurofamide and doxycycline. *Isr. J. Med. Sci.* 23, 565–567.

Tong, Y., Wu, Q., Zhao, D., Liu, Y., Cao, M., Zhang, L., et al. (2011). Effects of Chinese herbs on the hemagglutination and adhesion of *Escherichia coli* strain in vitro. *Afr. J. Tradit. Complement. Altern. Med.* 8, 82–87.

Torella, M., Del Deo, F., Grimaldi, A., Iervolino, S. A., Pezzella, M., Tammaro, C., et al. (2016). Efficacy of an orally administered combination of hyaluronic acid, chondroitin sulfate, curcumin and quercetin for the prevention of recurrent urinary tract infections in postmenopausal women. *Eur. J. Obstet. Gynecol. Reprod. Biol.* 207, 125–128. doi: 10.1016/j.ejogrb.2016.10.018

Trautner, B. W., Hull, R. A., Thornby, J. I., and Darouiche, R. O. (2007). Coating urinary catheters with an avirulent strain of *Escherichia coli* as a means to establish asymptomatic colonization. *Infect. Control Hosp. Epidemiol.* 28, 92–94. doi: 10.1086/510872

Uehling, D. T., Hopkins, W. J., Balish, E., Xing, Y., and Heisey, D. M. (1997). Vaginal mucosal immunization for recurrent urinary tract infection: phase II clinical trial. *J. Urol.* 157, 2049–2052. doi: 10.1097/00005392-199706000-00004

Uehling, D. T., Hopkins, W. J., Elkahwaji, J. E., Schmidt, D. M., and Leverson, G. E. (2003). Phase 2 clinical trial of a vaginal mucosal vaccine for urinary tract infections. *J. Urol.* 170, 867–869. doi: 10.1097/01.ju.0000075094.54767.6e

Ujmajuridze, A., Chanishvili, N., Goderdzishvili, M., Leitner, L., Mehnert, U., Chkhotua, A., et al. (2018). Adapted bacteriophages for treating urinary tract infections. *Front. Microbiol.* 9:1832. doi: 10.3389/fmicb.2018.01832

Ulrey, R. K., Barksdale, S. M., Zhou, W., and van Hoek, M. L. (2014). Cranberry proanthocyanidins have anti-biofilm properties against *Pseudomonas aeruginosa*. *BMC Complement. Altern. Med.* 14:499. doi: 10.1186/1472-6882-14-499

Varki, A. (2008). Sialic acids in human health and disease. *Trends Mol. Med.* 14, 351–360. doi: 10.1016/j.molmed.2008.06.002

Wagenlehner, F. M. E., Ballarini, S., Pilatz, A., Weidner, W., Lehr, L., and Naber, K. G. (2015). A randomized, double-blind, parallel-group, multicenter clinical study of *Escherichia coli*-Lyophilized lysate for the prophylaxis of recurrent uncomplicated urinary tract infections. *Urol. Int.* 95, 167–176. doi: 10.1159/000371894

Wizemann, T. M., Adamou, J. E., and Langermann, S. (1999). Adhesins as targets for vaccine development. *Emerg. Infect. Dis.* 5, 395–403. doi: 10.3201/eid0503.990310

Wojnicz, D., Tichaczek-Goska, D., Korzekwa, K., Kicia, M., and Hendrich, A. B. (2016). Study of the impact of cranberry extract on the virulence factors and biofilm formation by *Enterococcus faecalis* strains isolated from urinary tract infections. *Int. J. Food Sci. Nutr.* 67, 1005–1016. doi: 10.1080/09637486.2016.1211996

Xu, W., Flores-Mireles, A. L., Cusumano, Z. T., Takagi, E., Hultgren, S. J., and Caparon, M. G. (2017). Host and bacterial proteases influence biofilm formation and virulence in a murine model of enterococcal catheter-associated urinary tract infection. *NPJ Biofilms Microbiomes.* 3:28.

Yang, B., and Foley, S. (2018). First experience in the UK of treating women with recurrent urinary tract infections with the bacterial vaccine Uromune®. *BJU Int.* 121, 289–292. doi: 10.1111/bju.14067

Yang, B., and Foley, S. (2019). Urinary tract infection vaccines – the 'burning' issue. *BJU Int.* 123, 743–744. doi: 10.1111/bju.14678

Zaborska, W., Kot, M., and Superata, K. (2002). Inhibition of jack bean urease by 1,4-benzoquinone and 2,5-dimethyl-1,4-benzoquinone. Evaluation of the inhibition mechanism. *J. Enzyme Inhib. Med. Chem.* 17, 247–253. doi: 10.1080/1475636021000011670

Zhao, K., Liu, B., Wei, W., Ma, Q., Zhao, W., and Zhang, S. (2011). Clinical study of clearing liver fire, removing dampness, strengthening spleen and tonifying kidney methods in treating middle-aged and old woman with chronic urinary tract infection. *Int. J. Tradit. Chin. Med.* 33, 976–978.

7

Hospital-Associated Multidrug-Resistant MRSA Lineages are Trophic to the Ocular Surface and Cause Severe Microbial Keratitis

Paulo J. M. Bispo [1,2], *Lawson Ung* [1,2], *James Chodosh* [1,2] *and Michael S. Gilmore* [1,2,3*]

[1] *Department of Ophthalmology, Massachusetts Eye and Ear, Harvard Medical School, Boston, MA, United States,*
[2] *Infectious Disease Institute, Harvard Medical School, Boston, MA, United States,* [3] *Department of Microbiology and Immunobiology, Harvard Medical School, Boston, MA, United States*

Correspondence:
Michael S. Gilmore
michael_gilmore@meei.harvard.edu

Methicillin-resistant *Staphylococcus aureus* (MRSA) is a common cause of severe and difficult to treat ocular infection. In this study, the population structure of 68 ocular MRSA isolates collected at Massachusetts Eye and Ear between January 2014 and June 2016 was assessed. By using a combination of multilocus sequence typing (MLST) analysis, SCC*mec* typing and detection of the panton-valentine leukocidin (PVL) gene, we found that the population structure of ocular MRSA is composed of lineages with community and hospital origins. As determined by eBURST analysis of MLST data, the ocular MRSA population consisted of 14 different sequence types (STs) that grouped within two predominant clonal complexes: CC8 (47.0%) and CC5 (41.2%). Most CC8 strains were ST8, harbored type IV SCC*mec* and were positive for the PVL-toxin (93.7%). The CC5 group was divided between strains carrying SCC*mec* type II (71.4%) and SCC*mec* type IV (28.6%). Remaining isolates grouped in 6 different clonal complexes with 3 isolates in CC6 and the other clonal complexes being represented by a single isolate. Interestingly, major MRSA CC5 and CC8 lineages were isolated from discrete ocular niches. Orbital and preseptal abscess/cellulitis were predominantly caused by CC8-SCC*mec* IV PVL-positive strains. In contrast, infections of the cornea, conjunctiva and lacrimal system were associated with the MDR CC5 lineage, particularly as causes of severe infectious keratitis. This niche specialization of MRSA is consistent with a model where CC8-SCC*mec* IV PVL-positive strains are better adapted to cause infections of the keratinized and soft adnexal eye tissues, whereas MDR CC5 appear to have greater ability in overcoming innate defense mechanisms of the wet epithelium of the ocular surface.

Keywords: MRSA, Ocular infection, Molecular Epidemiology, Tissue tropism, biogeography of infections

INTRODUCTION

Antimicrobial resistance in human infections has reached alarming levels and has become one of the major public health threats of the twenty first Century (1). Methicillin-resistant *Staphylococcus aureus* (MRSA) remains a leading cause of antibiotic-resistant infections at many anatomical sites (2, 3). MRSA initially were confined to the hospital environment, but in the mid 1990s began to proliferate in the community (4), and are now leading causes of antibiotic-resistant infections in both settings (5). In US, strains within lineages that constitute clonal complex 5 (CC), notably the USA100 clone, are most commonly hospital-associated (5). USA300, a representative of CC8, has emerged as the most prevalent CA-MRSA clone in the US (5, 6). USA300 has also invaded the hospital setting where it is now a common cause of MRSA infections in American hospitals (7).

Ocular infections caused by MRSA have become increasingly common in the last two decades (8–11). These infections have been associated with serious ocular damage and permanent vision loss (12, 13), including bilateral blindness (14). Despite the growing importance of MRSA in ophthalmology, little is known about the population structure of MRSA causing the most common eye infections, or the microbial and host features that dictate this structure. The eye has extensive defenses for protection of vital structures from constant environmental exposure. These include mechanical barriers (e.g., lids, lashes), a polarized wet epithelium, a secreted tear film containing immunoglobulins and various other antimicrobial factors, mucins (secreted MUC5AC and shed epithelial cell surface-associated transmembrane mucins MUC1, MUC4, and MUC16), and cells of the innate immune system (15–17).

This unique environment of the ocular wet mucosa and its components are expected to act as selective forces that can shape the spatial distribution of microorganisms colonizing and infecting this ocular niche. The study of these ecological and geographical forces, as classically applied in ecology to study the biogeography of life in the natural world can now be combined with refined genetic and genomic epidemiology data to advance our understanding of community structures and distribution of microbes in different body sites (18, 19). We previously reported the genomic characteristics of a divergent cluster of unencapsulated *Streptococcus pneumoniae* strains that are uniquely tropic and adapted to the conjunctiva (20). These strains carry a set of genes that are absent or substantially different from those encoded within the genomes of encapsulated respiratory strains, which appear to be important for the pathogenesis of epidemic conjunctivitis. We have demonstrated that a unified model of microbial biogeography that incorporates classic ecological principles to explain community assemblage and dynamics can be applied to the understanding of this radical bifurcation in phylogeny and niche subspecialization of the unencapsulated *S. pneumoniae* conjunctivitis cluster (21). Because MRSA now rank among leading causes of a variety of ocular infections, to gain insight into particular features of importance in the pathogenesis of infection, it was of interest to determine the microscale biogeography of MRSA eye infections, whether dominant genetic lineages were associated with all sites of infection, or if there was evidence of a tissue tropism that would drive a specific population structure. We report that the population structure of ocular MRSA strains isolated at Massachusetts Eye and Ear (MEE) is dominated by the two major clonal complexes that cause infections at other body sites, but exhibit a distinct distribution in the types of infection they cause.

METHODS

Bacterial Strains

Protocols for obtaining bacterial isolates collected for infection diagnosis were approved by the MEE Institutional Review Board (IRB). Since this study only included discarded bacterial isolates that were frozen in our pathogen repository, written informed consent was waived by the MEE IRB. In total, 68 consecutive MRSA isolates recovered from January 2014 to June 2016 were analyzed for this study. For patients from whom multiple isolates from the same eye were obtained for infection diagnosis within a period of 6 months, only the first isolate was included. Specimens were obtained by the attending ophthalmologist or resident physician following institutional guidelines and submitted to the clinical laboratory for processing. Suspected *S. aureus* colonies were routinely identified using a combination of phenotypic methods including detection of coagulase and protein A by latex agglutination, followed by confirmation of species and antimicrobial susceptibility testing using the MicroScan Walkaway 40 Plus System (Beckman Coulter, Brea, CA). Isolates were stored at −80°C in Microbank™ cryopreservative tubes (ProLab Diagnostics). Frozen isolates were cultured twice on blood agar before further testing.

Clinical Data Collection and Statistical Analyses

Demographic data and risk factors for MRSA infection were collected using the IRB-approved Research Electronic Data Capture (REDCap) tool, hosted by MEE and Harvard Medical School (22). General demographic data included age, sex and ethnicity. Ocular comorbidities, including any ophthalmic surgical history, ocular surface disease, eyelid disease, lacrimal system dysfunction, atopy, contact lens use and trauma were collected (see **Table 2** legend for full definitions). Patient systemic comorbidities and previous healthcare exposures were also captured. To identify possible healthcare exposures which may potentiate selective pressures for antibiotic-resistant infection, we identified these following groups in our data: patients residing in nursing homes and/or residential facilities; those requiring chronic ambulatory care such as renal replacement therapy (dialysis) and hospital-based infusions; and patients who had either inpatient hospital admission and/or day admission for eye surgery within the preceding 3 prior to developing an MRSA infection. For patients with MRSA keratitis, we recorded the presenting features of the ulcers according to an institution-wide clinical algorithm which mandates the collection of corneal cultures for lesions meeting any of the following criteria: ≥1+ cells in the anterior chamber; ≥2 mm infiltrate and/or the presence of ≥2 satellite lesions; or infiltrate located ≤3 mm from the corneal center (23). Simple 2 by 2 tests of proportion (Fischer's exact test) were used to compare CC5 and CC8 groups according to collected categorical variables, while age was compared using the non-parametric Wilcoxon rank-sum test.

Antimicrobial Susceptibility Testing

In vitro susceptibility to ciprofloxacin (Fluka), ofloxacin, levofloxacin (TCI America), moxifloxacin, and besifloxacin

(Sigma-Aldrich) was performed by broth microdilution methods according to the Clinical and Laboratory Standards Institute (CLSI) (24). Quality control was performed by testing the *S. aureus* ATCC 29213 control strain. The interpretative criteria for each antimicrobial agent tested were those published by CLSI (25).

DNA Extraction

DNA extraction was performed using Chelex 100 molecular biology resin (Bio-Rad) as previously described (26). Purified genomic DNA was diluted 1:10, and was assessed for purity and DNA concentration using a Synergy 2 Multi-Mode Plate Reader and Take3 software system (BioTek).

SCC*mec* Typing

PCR-based genotyping of the chromosomal cassette recombinase (*ccr*) and *mec* complexes comprising the SCC*mec* was determined by a combination of multiplex PCR designed to classify the *mec* complex and *ccr* complex using a previously published protocol (27). For each multiplex PCR assay, reference MRSA strains for SCC*mec* types II (USA100) and IV (USA800), provided by the Network of Antimicrobial Resistance in *Staphylococcus aureus* (NARSA) were included. SCC*mec* was considered nontypeable if *mec* and/or *ccr* complex gave no amplification results, if the isolate carried more than one *ccr* or *mec* complex, or if there was a *mec*/*ccr* complex combination not previously described.

PVL Detection

The presence or absence of the Panton-Valentine Leukocidin (PVL) toxin gene was determined by PCR amplification of the *LukS-PV-lukF-PV* genes as previously described (28). Reference MRSA strains (provided by NARSA) USA300 and USA100 served as positive and negative controls, respectively.

MLST

Multilocus sequence typing (MLST) was performed for all MRSA isolates using a scheme based on the sequencing of internal fragments of seven *S. aureus* housekeeping genes (*arcC, aroE, glpF, gmk, pta, tpi,* and *yqiL*). The PCR products were purified (QIAquick PCR purification kit; Qiagen), and both strands were sequenced by Genewiz Incorporated (South Plainfield, NJ). The sequences obtained were edited using Geneious R8 and sequence types (STs) were assigned using the *S. aureus* MLST database (https://pubmlst.org/saureus/). Clonal complexes (CC) were determined using the go eBURST algorithm (http://www.phyloviz.net/goeburst/).

Statistics

Descriptive statistics were calculated using SPSS software (version 25, IBM, Armonk, New York), and proportions were compared by χ^2 or Fisher exact test, as appropriate. A *P* value of <0.05 was considered statistically significant.

RESULTS

A total of 75 MRSA were identified from 281 *S. aureus* recovered from ocular sites at MEE from January 2014 to June 2016 (overall

rate of 26.7%). The proportion of ocular MRSA isolates did not change considerably in 2014 (25.9%) compared to 2015 (22.3%), but was substantially higher during the sampling period of 2016 (37.7%). Of those, 7 MRSA were obtained from second cultures of the same patient eye, and were excluded from further study. The remaining 68 non-duplicate MRSA isolates were then analyzed. Sites of infection from which MRSA were isolated included orbital and preseptal abscess/cellulitis (*n* = 27), keratitis (*n* = 14), conjunctivitis (*n* = 9), lacrimal system infection (*n* = 8), eyelid margin infections (*n* = 4), endophthalmitis (*n* = 2), and miscellaneous (*n* = 4).

Two Major Clonal Complexes Dominate the Ocular MRSA Population

Despite the clinical importance of MRSA, much remains to be learned about the pathogenesis of infection at different anatomical sites on and around the eye. Because the tissues of the eye and adnexa differ widely in host defenses (e.g., wet epithelium vs. keratinized epithelium and soft tissues), it was of interest to know whether some MRSA lineages were enriched in pathogenic features that select for one MRSA lineage over another. By using a combination of multilocus sequence typing analysis, SCC*mec* typing and detection of the PVL-toxin encoding gene, we found that the population structure of ocular MRSA is diverse, but dominated by the CC5 and CC8 lineages associated with infection at other anatomical sites (4, 5). As determined by eBURST analysis of MLST data (**Figure 1**), 14 different sequence types (STs) were identified, with most belonging to clonal clusters CC8 (47.0%, *n* = 32) and CC5 (41.2%, *n* = 28). The clonal cluster CC6 encompassed 3 strains (4.4%), and 5 strains represented single sequence types. Most CC8 strains (93.7%, *n* = 30) were ST8, harbored a SCC*mec* type IV and were positive for the PVL-toxin, common features of the USA300 strain. The CC5 group could be divided into those carrying a SCC*mec* type II (71.4%, *n* = 20), which includes isolates with the characteristics of the USA100 clone, and (28.6%, *n* = 8) SCC*mec* type IV, typical of the USA800 clone (**Table 1**).

Age at presentation ranged from 2 to 102 years (median 53.08) with CC5-infected patients being significantly older (median age, 68.05 vs. 35.9, *p* < 0.001) (**Table 2**). CC5-infected patients were more frequently subjected to eye surgery (66.7 vs. 16.7%, *p* <0.001), especially cataract surgery with implantation of intraocular lenses (44.4 vs. 10%, *p* = 0.006). Healthcare exposure was more common among patients infected with CC5 strains, including higher rates of topical antibiotic use at presentation (55.6 vs. 10.0%, *p* < 0.001) and prior to presentation (48.5 vs. 16.7%, *p* = 0.02). There was also a higher proportion of patients known to require non-acute clinical care and/or residents of aged care facilities in the CC5 group (22.2 vs. 3.3%, *p* = 0.05).

Distribution of MRSA Lineages Across Different Ocular Niches

Although *S. aureus* causes a wide range of human infections, patterns of association of distinct genotypes have been noted with

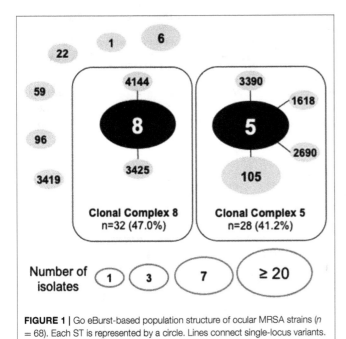

FIGURE 1 | Go eBurst-based population structure of ocular MRSA strains (*n* = 68). Each ST is represented by a circle. Lines connect single-locus variants. The black circles represent clonal complex founders. Circles not connected represent singleton STs in this particular population structure.

TABLE 1 | SCC*mec* typing and PVL detection according to the clonal complex.

Clonal complex (No.)	SCC*mec* typing		No. PVL positive
	Type	No. (% of total)	
CC8 (32)	IV	31 (45.6)	30
	V	1 (1.5)	1
CC5 (28)	II	20 (29.4)	–
	IV	8 (11.7)	–
CC6 (3)	IV	3 (4.4)	–
CC1 (1)	IV	1 (1.5)	1
CC15 (1)	II	1 (1.5)	1
CC22 (1)	IV	1 (1.5)	1
CC59 (1)	IV	1 (1.5)	1
CC96 (1)	NT	1 (1.5)	–

specific types of infection (29–32). The most well documented example is community-acquired skin and soft-tissue infection (SSTI) in the US, where a large majority of cases are caused by the CC8/USA300 lineage (29, 32). In agreement, ocular SSTIs including mainly orbital and preseptal abscess/cellulitis were found in this study to be caused mainly by CC8 SCC*mec* IV PVL-positive strains, characteristics of the USA300 clone ($p < 0.001$; **Table 3**). Interestingly, infections of the wet epithelial tissues of the ocular surface were substantially enriched in the CC5 lineage, which was particularly pronounced for infectious keratitis cases ($p < 0.001$; **Table 3**). Keratitis patients frequently presented with potentially sight-threatening corneal ulcers (85.7%) according to the 1,2,3 rule (23) for categorization of the severity of bacterial keratitis (**Table 5**).

TABLE 2 | Demographic and clinicopathologic data for patients with culture-positive MRSA ocular infections at MEE, 2014–2016 (*n* = 58).[a]

Patient characteristics	MRSA clonal group		P value
	CC5 (*n* = 27)	CC8 (*n* = 30)	
DEMOGRAPHIC DATA			
Age (years, median)	68.05	35.4	**< 0.001**
Gender			
Male	6 (22.2)	13 (43.4)	0.16
Female	21 (77.8)	17 (56.7)	
Ethnicity			
Caucasian	22 (81.5)	23 (76.7)	0.75
Non-Caucasian	5 (18.5)	7 (23.3)	
OCULAR HISTORY			
History of contact lens wear	8 (29.6)	5 (16.7)	0.35
History of eye trauma	3 (11.1)	4 (13.3)	1
Prior eye surgery	18 (66.7)	5 (16.7)	**< 0.001**
Previous intraocular lens insertion	12 (44.4)	3 (10.0)	**0.006**
Ocular surface disease*	9 (33.3)	5 (16.7)	0.22
Dry eye syndrome	4 (14.8)	4 (13.3)	1
Atopic eye disease	1 (3.7)	1 (3.3)	1
Lid disease**	9 (33.3)	6 (20.0)	0.37
Lacrimal system dysfunction***	5 (18.5)	5 (16.7)	1
Glaucoma	6 (22.2)	1 (3.3)	**0.05**
Glaucoma drainage device	1 (3.7)	0 (0)	0.47
HEALTHCARE EXPOSURES			
Use of topical antibiotic at presentation	15 (55.6)	3 (10.0)	**< 0.001**
Use of topical antibiotic within the last week preceding presentation	13 (48.5)	5 (16.7)	**0.02**
Use of topical steroids at presentation	11 (40.7)	5 (16.7)	0.08
Use of topical steroids within the last week preceding presentation	10 (37.0)	5 (16.7)	0.13
Known inpatient hospital admission in the last 3 months	4 (14.8)	3 (10.0)	0.7
Admission for eye surgery in the last 3 months‡	5 (18.5)	2 (6.7)	0.24
Non-acute clinical care‡‡	6 (22.22)	1 (3.3)	**0.05**
Healthcare worker‡‡‡	4 (14.8)	5 (16.7)	1

[a]*Out of 68 isolates included, 66 patient records were reviewed. One patient had two separate MRSA episodes (caused by different clones) and for one patient the record was not available.*

**includes corneal degenerative disease, bullous keratopathy, exposure keratopathy, dry eye syndrome, atopy, Stevens-Johnson syndrome and toxic epidermal necrolysis.*
***including blepharitis, trichiasis, floppy eyelid syndrome, ectropion and entropion, and lagophthalmos.*
****including dacryocystitis and dacryoadenitis.*
‡*including day-only procedures and overnight stays.*
‡‡*includes long-term care residents, nursing home care, chronic ambulatory care.*
‡‡‡*includes professions in close working contact with patients (e.g., nursing and allied health).*
Bold values are represent statistically significant.

CC5 Strains Preferentially Associated With Infection of the Wet Epithelial Ocular Surface Are Multidrug Resistant

To compare rates of antibiotic resistance among ocular MRSA of various lineages and from the different ocular sites, we tested the sensitivities of all isolates to a panel of clinically relevant antibiotics using an automated microbiology system (MicroScan WalkAway). Overall, moderate to high rates of resistance to erythromycin (88.2%), levofloxacin (54.4%), and clindamycin (42.6%) was found among this MRSA collection. Resistance to gentamycin (2.9%) and tetracycline (1.5%) was rare (**Figure 2B**). Stratified analysis by clonal complex showed that CC5 strains are significantly more likely to be multidrug resistant (resistance to ≥3 non-beta-lactam antimicrobial classes) than CC8 strains (78.8 vs. 6.1%; $p < 0.0001$; **Figure 2A**). Ocular CC5-SCC*mec* II strains, which include isolates resembling the hospital-adapted clone USA100, were all resistant to erythromycin, clindamycin and levofloxacin (**Figure 2B**). CC5-SCC*mec* IV strains, including isolates with the characteristics of the USA800 clone, were frequently resistant to erythromycin (62.5%), levofloxacin (62.5%), and clindamycin (25.0%). While CC5 strains were frequently resistant to ≥3 non-beta-lactam antibiotics, CC8 isolates were usually resistant to only one antibiotic class in addition to beta-lactams, most often to the macrolide erythromycin (**Figures 2A,B**).

Because topical fluoroquinolone is widely used for empirical treatment of ocular infection, we assessed the *in vitro* susceptibility of the main ocular MRSA clonal complexes for the most commonly used fluoroquinolones (**Table 4**). The minimum inhibitory concentrations (MICs) for these agents were determined by reference broth microdilution (24, 25). CC5 isolates were in general highly resistant to the older fluoroquinolones ciprofloxacin, ofloxacin and levofloxacin. All canonical CC5-SCC*mec* II strains were resistant to oxifloxacin, levofloxacin, ofloxacin and ciprofloxacin with MIC_{90} values >256 μg/mL. Among CC5-SCC*mec* IV strains, the MIC_{90} values ranged from 64 μg/mL for moxifloxacin to >256 μg/mL for levofloxacin, ofloxacin and ciprofloxacin (% of non-susceptible = 62.5% for the 3 drugs). Remarkably, many CC5 isolates were also highly resistant to the newer 8-methoxyfluoroquinolone moxifloxacin (MIC_{90} 64 μg/mL, 62.5% non-susceptible for CC5-SCC*mec* IV; MIC_{90} 32μg/mL, 100% non-susceptible for CC5-SCC*mec* II).

DISCUSSION

The population structure of *S. aureus* isolates from human infections is highly diverse (33). However, only a small proportion of these lineages have become successful MRSA clones that are now widely disseminated in both community and hospital settings (5). These epidemic lineages cause a variety of human infections, with some showing strong tropisms for specific body niches (29–32).

The eye has developed unique mechanisms to protect its delicate and exceptionally important structures against constant external disturbance (15–17). Because of this, we postulated that the uniqueness of this environment could be a driving force shaping the population structure of ocular MRSA infections, in a similar manner as reported for *Streptococcus pneumoniae* (20). To begin testing this hypothesis, we selected a collection of consecutive and non-duplicate MRSA strains prospectively isolated from a variety of eye infections, representing two major

TABLE 3 | Distribution of the main ocular MRSA clones across different infections.

Eye infection	Total no. of cases	No. of eyes infected by			Fisher's test (CC5 vs. CC8)
		CC5	CC8	Others	
Abscess/Cellulitis	27	1	22	4	**e<0.001**
Keratitis	14	12	1	1	**<0.001**
Conjunctivitis	9	6	2	1	0.1300
Lacrimal system	8	5	2	1	0.2349
Eyelids	4	–	4	–	–
Endopthalmitis	2	2	–	–	–
Miscellaneous	4	2	1	1	–

Bold values are represent statistically significant.

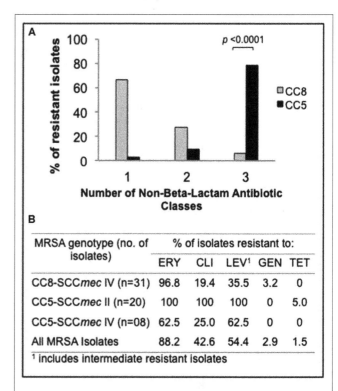

FIGURE 2 | Antimicrobial susceptibility profile of the main ocular MRSA clonal complexes. **(A)** Frequency (%) of CC5 and CC8 strains resistant to additional non-beta-lactam antibiotic classes. **(B)** Resistance rates for common antibiotics representing 5 different classes. Statistical significance was determined using Fisher's exact test.

and distinct localizations: (i) the ocular surface and (ii) the ocular adnexal soft tissues. We found that the ocular MRSA population was dominated by two major clonal complexes that are also common causes of MRSA infections in other body sites: CC8 (47.0%) and CC5 (41.2%). The distribution of lineages within these clonal complexes followed a pattern of enrichment that was split into the main ocular niches tested, with preseptal and orbital abscess/cellulitis being predominantly associated to CC8, while ocular surface infections were frequently caused by CC5 strains, with a significant enrichment in keratitis (**Table 3**).

TABLE 4 | *In vitro* susceptibility profile for topically used fluorquinolones among ocular MRSA isolates according to the clonal group.

Antimicrobial agent	CC8-SCC*mec* IV (*n* = 31)		CC5-SCC*mec* II (*n* = 20)		CC5-SCC*mec* IV (*n* = 08)	
	MIC_{90}	%NS[a]	MIC_{90}	%NS[a]	MIC_{90}	%NS[a]
Moxifloxacin	2	35.5	32	100	64	62.5
Levofloxacin	8	35.5	>256	100	>256	62.5
Ofloxacin	16	38.7	>256	100	>256	62.5
Ciprofloxacin	32	42.0	>256	100	>256	62.5

[a]includes intermediate resistant isolates.

TABLE 5 | Molecular typing and antimicrobial resistances of MRSA keratitis cases.

Patient	Year	Sequence type	Clonal complex	SCC*mec* type	PVL	Resembles clonal lineage	Antimicrobial resistances	Number of 1, 2, 3 criteria met on presentation*	Topical ATBs at time of culture
1	2014	ST5	CC5	II	Negative	USA100	OXA, CLIN, ERY, CIP, LEV, OFLX, MOX	3	Vigamox
2	2014	ST105	CC5	II	Negative	SLV of ST5	OXA, CLIN, ERY, CIP, LEV, OFLX, MOX	3	None
3	2014	ST5	CC5	IV	Negative	USA800	OXA	1	UKN
4	2014	ST5	CC5	II	Negative	USA100	OXA, CLIN, ERY, CIP, LEV, OFLX, MOX	0	None
5	2014	ST5	CC5	II	Negative	USA100	OXA, CLIN, ERY, CIP, LEV, OFLX, MOX	2	UKN
6	2015	ST5	CC5	IV	Negative	USA800	OXA, CLIN, ERY, CIP, LEV, OFLX, MOX	2	Polytrim + Erythromycin
7	2015	ST5	CC5	II	Negative	USA100	OXA, CLIN, ERY, CIP, LEV, OFLX, MOX	1	UKN
8	2015	ST5	CC5	II	Negative	USA100	OXA, CLIN, ERY, CIP, LEV, OFLX, MOX	3	None
9	2015	ST96	CC96	NT	Negative	NA	OXA, ERY	3	None
10	2015	ST8	CC8	IV	Positive	USA300	OXA, CLIN, ERY, CIP, LEV, OFLX, MOX	2	None
11	2015	ST105	CC5	II	Negative	SLV of ST5	OXA, CLIN, ERY, CIP, LEV, OFLX, MOX	2	Eythromycin and Ofloxacin
12	2016	ST5	CC5	II	Negative	USA100	OXA, CLIN, ERY, CIP, LEV, OFLX, MOX	0	Vigamox + Tobramycin
13	2016	ST3390	CC5	II	Negative	SLV of ST5	OXA, CLIN, ERY, CIP, LEV, OFLX, MOX	3	Vigamox
14	2016	ST5	CC5	II	Negative	USA100	OXA, CLIN, ERY, CIP, LEV, OFLX, MOX	3	None

*The "1, 2, 3-Rule," originally conceived by Vital et al. (23), was formally implemented across MEE on July 1, 2015 as a means of identifying patients at greatest risk of developing sight-threatening complications. It is composed of three simple features on clinical examination, and the presence of any of these warrants the collection of corneal cultures and treatment with topical fortified antibiotics. These rules are: ≥1+ anterior chamber cells; ≥2 mm infiltrate and/or ≥2 satellite lesions; edge of lesion within 3mm of the corneal center.

The basis for the discernable tropism of CC5 strains for the ocular surface is unknown, but viewed in light of the findings of others, we can develop a testable model. Strains grouped within CC5, notably the USA100 and USA800, are well established as major causes of healthcare-related infections in the US (5). CC5 strains are often replete with acquired antibiotic resistances (34, 35), and were implicated in the first 12 cases of frank vancomycin resistant *S. aureus* stemming from independent acquisitions of the *van*A gene from *Enterococcus* spp. (36). Despite their hospital association, CC5-MRSA strains also occur in the community, potentially bridged by long-term

care facilities. The nasal reservoir of MRSA of long-term care facility residents mirrors the molecular epidemiology of US hospitals, with CC5-related strains being predominant (37). Data from national surveillance programs show that CC5 lineages USA100 and USA800 are now widely disseminated in the community, even among noninstitutionalized individuals with no known risk factors for nasal colonization with these hospital-adapted clones (38). Although CC5 strains are frequently found among carriers in the community, they are only occasionally associated with community-acquired infection (32). In our population, despite the community origins of the patients in which ocular infections occurred, CC5 strains predominated as causes of infection of the wet epithelial surface of the eye. Keratitis in our series was predominantly caused by strains resembling the USA100 lineage, and mostly presented as severe and potentially sigh-threatening infections as determined the "1, 2, 3-Rule" (23). The severity of CC5-caused keratitis points toward the possible existence of virulence factors that could be particularly associated with corneal damage. In addition to carrying a variety of antimicrobial resistance genes, CC5 strains also posses a constellation of virulence genes (35). Of particular interest is the enterotoxin gene cluster (*egc*), which represents a unique group of enterotoxins with superantigen activities, and seems to be particularly enriched among CC5 strains (35), while being completely absent in CC8 strains (36, 39). Epidemiological observations have found an association of *egc*-encoded enterotoxins in the development of corneal ulcer in patients with atopic keratoconjunctivitis (40). Whether this locus is associated with exacerbation of the ocular surface inflammatory response and aggravation of the corneal damage is yet to be fully elucidated.

Empirical use of topical broad-spectrum antibiotics remains the first-line treatment for bacterial keratitis (41) and is commonly initiated with a topical newer fluoroquinolone ophthalmic solution (e.g., moxifloxacin 0.5%) (42). CC5 strains display generally higher fluoroquinolone MICs (non-susceptibility rate for moxifloxacin of 89.3%, MIC_{90} 64 μg/mL) (**Table 4**). However, CC8-SCC*mec* IV strains associated with ocular infections at other sites were also often resistant to the commonly used fourth-generation fluoroquinolone, moxifloxacin (non-susceptibility rate using systemic breakpoints of 35.5%, MIC_{90} 2 μg/mL). The influence of degrees of resistance on population structure is unclear. In light of its pharmacokinetics on the ocular surface, neither CC5 nor CC8 would be predicted to respond to topical moxifloxacin therapy. Based on pharmacokinetic data for topical moxifloxacin in the cornea of pigmented rabbits (43), we calculated PK/PD (AUC_{0-24h}/MIC_{90} ratio) indices for the main MRSA lineages examined in our study (**Figure S1**). Although the index was higher for CC8 strains compared to CC5, all the indices were far below the PK/PD target that predicts clinical efficacy as determined for systemic infections (44) and also for keratitis treated with fluoroquinolone (45). In addition, a review of the medical records of 14 patients with MRSA keratitis included in this study showed that only 4/14 had prior exposure to a fluoroquinolone (Vigamox, $n = 2$; erythromycin plus ofloxacin, $n = 1$; and Vigamox plus tobramycin, $n = 1$), with no information available for 3 patients (**Table 5**). Together, the data on prior topical antibiotic use and the calculated PK/PD indices for the ocular MRSA lineages discounts the role of direct fluoroquinolone selection as the driver of the CC5 predominant population structure associated with keratitis.

Our results are consistent with a report of 30 cases of *S. aureus* keratitis in Japan, that also found CC5 strains to be the predominant cause of MRSA-infected ulcers (46). CC8 isolates were more frequently isolated from the healthy conjunctival sac (46). Together, these findings suggest an enhanced ability of CC5 to endure selective pressures and colonize the cornea

and adjacent tissues. Lactoferrin, one the most abundant tear proteins with antimicrobial activity is inhibitory for *S. aureus*, including MRSA, but this activity varies among clinical isolates from different sites of isolation (47, 48). In one study, clinical *S. aureus* isolates causing bloodstream infections (50%) were frequently resistant to lactoferrin concentrations ≥ 20 μM, while isolates from conjunctivitis (33%) and SSTI (13%) were less often resistant (47). Since these infections are caused by distinct MRSA lineages, with CC5 strains being commonly associated to bloodstream infections (49), variations across different genotypes may contribute to increased resistance to this tear antimicrobial compound, especially among CC5. Similarly, the antimicrobial activity of phospholipase A2 (PLA_2), an enzyme that has been found to be the major tear molecule with bactericidal activity against staphylococci, varies against methicillin-susceptible and -resistant isolates, with MRSA being more resistant to its action following short incubations (50), pointing toward a variance of this enzyme in its ability to kill *S. aureus* according to the genetic background. Further, previous reports have demonstrated that *S. aureus* strains may be differently equipped to bind to and invade ocular tissues *in vitro* and in a rabbit model of conjunctivitis and keratitis (51, 52), suggesting the existence of specific sets of adhesive surface proteins that enhance *S. aureus* ability to bind and invade the ocular tissues in a strain-specific manner.

A recent study of *S. aureus* keratitis in South Florida (53) found both CC5 (40%) and CC8 (37.3%) MRSA among isolates, clearly showing that although CC5 strains are most common, CC8 strains in other circumstances are also capable of causing keratitis. Among our patients, 12 out of 14 (85.7%), were classified as potentially sight-threatening MRSA keratitis cases according to an institution-wide grading system based on the "1, 2, 3" rule (23). For these patients, corneal cultures were unequivocally positive at diagnostic levels for the pathogen. We do not yet know whether the differences between studies stem from levels of disease severity, or other factors such as association with contact lens wear. Larger studies with well-defined criteria for enrollment will be important for determining conditions that favor infection by various pathogenic, antibiotic resistant lineages of *S. aureus*.

In contrast to the wet epithelial surface of the eye, CC8 MRSA strains, typified by the USA300 lineage, predominate as causes of infections of the keratinized epithelium and eye soft tissues. Lineage enrichment has been also reported in patients with bloodstream infection with haematogenous complications (30) infective endocarditis (31) and respiratory tract infections (54). Among our patients, CC8 strains were the predominant causes of preseptal and orbital abscess/cellulitis (22 out of 27 cases), consistent with their known tropism for infecting keratinized epithelium and soft tissues (29, 32). Among the remaining abscess/cellulitis cases, only one was caused by a CC5 isolate and 3 by other lineages (**Table 3**). In the early 2000s, the USA300 clone appeared in outbreaks of community-acquired SSTIs in otherwise healthy people (55, 56). Because of its ability to rapidly spread through person-to-person contact and readily compete with commensal skin flora (56), the USA300 lineage quickly predominated as the main cause of SSTIs (29, 32), and a significant cause of severe invasive infections (6). USA300 is generally more virulent, causing infections of greater severity and associated with worse outcome compared to other MRSA clones (57, 58). The aggressiveness of USA300 type strains is thought to be associated to the carriage of a variety of virulence factors, including the pore-forming toxin PVL, which is predominantly found in CC8 strains (59), and has been linked to the ability of this strain to cause necrotizing infections (60).

Orbital and preseptal abscesses are SSTIs commonly caused by *Staphylococcus aureus* (61, 62), and MRSA rates appear to be rising (63). Severe cases have been reported, including orbital and periorbital necrotizing fasciitis (64–66), necrotizing conjunctivitis with orbital invasion (12) and orbital cellulitis with bilateral involvement that progressed to blindness (14). A prospective study (2012–2015) of children and adolescents presenting with staphylococcal periorbital and orbital cellulitis in Houston found that most of the *S. aureus* isolates in their population were methicillin-resistant (67%) and were genetically related to the USA300 clone (78%) (67). Similarly, in a series of 11 patients presenting with culture-positive MRSA infections of the eye and orbit in San Francisco, most (82%) were caused by USA300 (13). Preseptal and orbital abscess/cellulitis were among the most common manifestations in these cases, some presenting with extensive necrosis of the eyelid and orbital tissues.

Collectively, these results are consistent with various MRSA lineages being enriched for properties that enhance their ability to resist defenses and competitive pressures, and colonize and infect either the wet epithelial surface or the ocular adnexal tissues. We propose that many of the features that have allowed CC5-type MRSA to adapt and be transmitted in the hospital environment, and readily acquire antibiotic resistances, endows them with properties that enhance their ability to resist robust ocular surface defenses and infect the cornea. In a comparative analysis of the genomes of the CC5 strains that had acquired vancomycin resistance from enterococci, we identified a constellation of traits with the *S. aureus* pathogenicity island as likely involved with their ability to persist in a mixed infection and acquire resistances by horizontal gene transfer (36). These same traits may well enhance their survival despite the defenses of the wet epithelial surface. In contrast, CC8-SCC*mec* IV PVL-positive strains are already well known to have features that enhance their ability to colonize the skin and compete effectively for that niche with coagulase negative strains, including the ACME locus (68). We believe these features account for their association with infection of the keratinized surfaces of the ocular adnexa.

Direct testing of isogenic mutants will be required to identify the major contributors to pathogenesis of various anatomical sites of the eye by MRSA, and to develop new approaches for mitigating that common threat. It is important to note that these findings represent the population structure of a relatively small ocular MRSA population isolated at the Massachusetts Eye and Ear, and validation of our results using a larger bacterial collection and isolates from other locations would be warranted.

AUTHOR CONTRIBUTIONS

PB, LU, JC, and MG contributed conception and design of the study and wrote sections of the manuscript. PB and LU organized the database and performed the statistical analysis. PB wrote the first draft of the manuscript. All authors contributed to manuscript revision, read and approved the submitted version.

FUNDING

This work was supported in part by NEI grant EY024285, and the Harvard-wide Program on Antibiotic Resistance NIAID grant AI083214. Funding agencies had no role in study design, data analysis, decision to publish or preparation of the manuscript.

ACKNOWLEDGMENTS

The authors thank Rick Body, James Cadorette and other medical technologists from the Clinical Microbiology Laboratory at MEE for their support in creating a microbial repository of strains isolated from ocular and otolaryngology infections.

SUPPLEMENTARY MATERIAL

Figure S1 | PK/PD ($AUC_{0–24h}/MIC_{90}$ ratio) indices for the main MRSA clones isolated in our study. $AUC_{0–24h}$ data was derived from pharmacokinetic studies of topical moxifloxacin in the cornea of pigmented rabbits (43). Dashed line indicates the PK/PD target that predicts clinical efficacy in keratitis patients treated with topical fluoroquinolone (45).

REFERENCES

World Health Organization (WHO). *Antimicrobial Resistance: Global Report on Surveillance*. (2014).

Klein EY, Mojica N, Jiang W, Cosgrove SE, Septimus E, Morgan DJ, et al. Trends in methicillin-Resistant staphylococcus aureus hospitalizations in the united states, 2010–2014. *Clin Infect Dis*. (2017) 65:1921–3. doi: 10.1093/cid/cix640

Kourtis AP, Hatfield K, Baggs J, Mu Y, See I, Epson E, et al. Vital signs: epidemiology and recent trends in methicillin-Resistant and in methicillin-Susceptible staphylococcus aureus bloodstream infections - united states. *MMWR Morb Mortal Wkly Rep*. (2019) 68:214–9. doi: 10.15585/mmwr.mm6809e1

van Duin D, Paterson DL. Multidrug-Resistant bacteria in the community: trends and lessons learned. *Infect Dis Clin North Am*. (2016) 30:377–90. doi: 10.1016/j.idc.2016.02.004

DeLeo FR, Chambers HF. Reemergence of antibiotic-resistant staphylococcus aureus in the genomics era. *J Clin Invest*. (2009) 119:2464–74. doi: 10.1172/JCI38226

David MZ, Daum RS. Community-associated methicillin-resistant staphylococcus aureus: epidemiology and clinical consequences of an emerging epidemic. *Clin Microbiol Rev.* (2010) 23:616–87. doi: 10.1128/CMR. 00081-09

Diekema DJ, Richter SS, Heilmann KP, Dohrn CL, Riahi F, Tendolkar S, et al. Continued emergence of uSA300 methicillin-resistant staphylococcus aureus in the united states: results from a nationwide surveillance study. *Infect Control Hosp Epidemiol.* (2014) 35:285–92. doi: 10.1086/675283

Asbell PA, Colby KA, Deng S, McDonnell P, Meisler DM, Raizman MB, et al. Ocular tRUST: nationwide antimicrobial susceptibility patterns in ocular isolates. *Am J Ophthalmol.* (2008) 145:951–8. doi: 10.1016/j.ajo.2008.01.025

Asbell PA, Sahm DF, Shaw M, Draghi DC, Brown NP. Increasing prevalence of methicillin resistance in serious ocular infections caused by staphylococcus aureus in the united states: 2000 to 2005. *J Cataract Refract Surg.* (2008) 34:814–8. doi: 10.1016/j.jcrs.2008.01.016

Asbell PA, Sanfilippo CM, Pillar CM, DeCory HH, Sahm DF, Morris TW. Antibiotic resistance among ocular pathogens in the united states: five-Year results from the antibiotic resistance monitoring in ocular microorganisms (ARMOR) surveillance study. *JAMA Ophthalmol.* (2015) 133:1445–54. doi: 10.1001/jamaophthalmol.2015.3888

Cavuoto K, Zutshi D, Karp CL, Miller D, Feuer W. Update on bacterial conjunctivitis in south florida. *Ophthalmology.* (2008) 115:51–6. doi: 10.1016/j.ophtha.2007.03.076

Brown SM, Raflo GT, Fanning WL. Transconjunctival orbital invasion by methicillin-resistant staphylococcus aureus. *Arch Ophthalmol.* (2009) 127:941–2. doi: 10.1001/archophthalmol.2009.144

Rutar T, Chambers HF, Crawford JB, Perdreau-Remington F, Zwick OM, Karr M, et al. Ophthalmic manifestations of infections caused by the uSA300 clone of community-associated methicillin-resistant staphylococcus aureus. *Ophthalmology.* (2006) 113:1455–62. doi: 10.1016/j.ophtha.2006.03.031

Rutar T, Zwick OM, Cockerham KP, Horton JC. Bilateral blindness from orbital cellulitis caused by community-acquired methicillin- resistant staphylococcus aureus. *Am J Ophthalmol.* (2005) 140:740–2. doi: 10.1016/j.ajo.2005.03.076

Mantelli F, Argueso P. Functions of ocular surface mucins in health and disease. *Curr Opin Allergy Clin Immunol.* (2008) 8:477–83. doi: 10.1097/ACI.0b013e32830e6b04

McClellan KA. Mucosal defense of the outer eye. *Surv Ophthalmol.* (1997) 42:233–46. doi: 10.1016/S0039-6257(97)00090-8

Sack RA, Nunes I, Beaton A, Morris C. Host-defense mechanism of the ocular surfaces. *Biosci Rep.* (2001) 21:463–80. doi: 10.1023/A:1017943826684

Costello EK, Stagaman K, Dethlefsen L, Bohannan BJ, Relman DA. The application of ecological theory toward an understanding of the human microbiome. *Science.* (2012) 336:1255–62. doi: 10.1126/science.1224203

Martiny JB, Bohannan BJ, Brown JH, Colwell RK, Fuhrman JA, Green JL, et al. Microbial biogeography: putting microorganisms on the map. *Nat Rev Microbiol.* (2006) 4:102–12. doi: 10.1038/nrmicro1341

Valentino MD, McGuire AM, Rosch JW, Bispo PJ, Burnham C, Sanfilippo CM, et al. Unencapsulated streptococcus pneumoniae from conjunctivitis encode variant traits and belong to a distinct phylogenetic cluster. *Nat Commun.* (2014) 5:5411. doi: 10.1038/ncomms6411

Ung L, Bispo PJM, Bryan NC, Andre C, Chodosh J, Gilmore MS. The best of all worlds: streptococcus pneumoniae conjunctivitis through the lens of community ecology and microbial biogeography. *Microorganisms.* (2019) 8:46. doi: 10.3390/microorganisms8010046

Harris PA, Taylor R, Thielke R, Payne J, Gonzalez N, Conde JG. Research electronic data capture (REDCap)–a metadata-driven methodology and workflow process for providing translational research informatics support. *J Biomed Inform.* (2009) 42:377–81. doi: 10.1016/j.jbi.2008.08.010

Vital MC, Belloso M, Prager TC, Lanier JD. Classifying the severity of corneal ulcers by using the "1, 2, 3" rule. *Cornea.* (2007) 26:16–20. doi: 10.1097/ICO.0b013e31802b2e47

Clinical and Laboratory Standard Institute. *Methods for Dilution Antimicrobial Susceptibility Tests for Bacteria That Grow Aerobically; Approved Standard-Ninth Edition.* CLSI document M07-A9. Wayne, PA: Clinical and Laboratory Standard Institutes. (2012).

Clinical and Laboratory Standard Institute. *Performance Standards for Antimicrobial Susceptibility Testing. 28th ed.* CLSI supplement M100. Wayne, PA: Clinical and Laboratory Standards Institute (2018).

Bispo P, Höfling-Lima A, Pignatari A. Characerization of ocular methicillin-resistant staphylococcs epidermidis isolates belonging predominantly to

clonal complex 2 subcluster iI. *J Clin Microbiol.* (2014) 52:1412–7. doi: 10.1128/JCM.03098-13

Kondo Y, Ito T, Ma X, Watanabe S, Kreiswirth B, Etienne J, et al. Combination of multiplex pCRs for staphylococcal cassette chromosome mec type assignment: rapid identification system for mec, ccr, and major differences in junkyard regions. *Antimicro Agents Chem.* (2007) 51:264–74. doi: 10.1128/AAC.00165-06

David MZ, Boyle-Vavra S, Zychowski DL, Daum RS. Methicillin- susceptible staphylococcus aureus as a predominantly healthcare-associated pathogen: a possible reversal of roles? *PLoS ONE.* (2011) 6:e18217. doi: 10.1371/journal.pone.0018217

Albrecht VS, Limbago BM, Moran GJ, Krishnadasan A, Gorwitz RJ, McDougal LK, et al. Staphylococcus aureus colonization and strain type at various body sites among patients with a closed abscess and uninfected controls at US Emergency Departments. *J Clin Microbiol.* (2015) 53:3478–84. doi: 10.1128/JCM.01371-15

Fowler VG, Jr, Nelson CL, McIntyre LM, Kreiswirth BN, Monk A, Archer GL, et al. Potential associations between hematogenous complications and bacterial genotype in staphylococcus aureus infection. *J Infect Dis.* (2007) 196:738–47. doi: 10.1086/520088

Nienaber JJ, Sharma Kuinkel BK, Clarke-Pearson M, Lamlertthon S, Park L, Rude TH, et al. Methicillin-susceptible staphylococcus aureus endocarditis isolates are associated with clonal complex 30 genotype and a distinct repertoire of enterotoxins and adhesins. *J Infect Dis.* (2011) 204:704–13. doi: 10.1093/infdis/jir389

Talan DA, Krishnadasan A, Gorwitz RJ, Fosheim GE, Limbago B, Albrecht V, et al. Comparison of staphylococcus aureus from skin and soft-tissue infections in uS emergency department patients, 2004 and 2008. *Clin Infect Dis.* (2011) 53:144–9. doi: 10.1093/cid/cir308

Wurster JI, Bispo PJM, Van Tyne D, Cadorette JJ, Boody R, Gilmore MS. Staphylococcus aureus from ocular and otolaryngology infections are frequently resistant to clinically important antibiotics and are associated with lineages of community and hospital origins. *PLoS ONE.* (2018) 13:e0208518. doi: 10.1371/journal.pone.0208518

Aanensen DM, Feil EJ, Holden MT, Dordel J, Yeats CA, Fedosejev A, et al. Whole-Genome sequencing for routine pathogen surveillance in public health: a population snapshot of invasive staphylococcus aureus in europe. *MBio.* (2016) 7:16. doi: 10.1128/mBio.00444-16

Monecke S, Coombs G, Shore AC, Coleman DC, Akpaka P, Borg M, et al. A field guide to pandemic, epidemic and sporadic clones of methicillin-resistant staphylococcus aureus. *PLoS ONE.* (2011) 6:e17936. doi: 10.1371/journal.pone.0017936

Kos VN, Desjardins CA, Griggs A, Cerqueira G, Van Tonder A, Holden MT, et al. Comparative genomics of vancomycin-resistant staphylococcus aureus strains and their positions within the clade most commonly associated with methicillin-resistant S. aureus hospital-acquired infection in the United States. *MBio.* (2012) 3:12. doi: 10.1128/mBio.00112-12

Hudson LO, Reynolds C, Spratt BG, Enright MC, Quan V, Kim D, et al. Diversity of methicillin-resistant staphylococcus aureus strains isolated from residents of 26 nursing homes in orange county, california. *J Clin Microbiol.* (2013) 51:3788–95. doi: 10.1128/JCM.01708-13

Tenover FC, McAllister S, Fosheim G, McDougal LK, Carey RB, Limbago B, et al. Characterization of staphylococcus aureus isolates from nasal cultures collected from individuals in the united states in 2001 to 2004. *J Clin Microbiol.* (2008) 46:2837–41. doi: 10.1128/JCM.00480-08

van Belkum A, Melles DC, Snijders SV, van Leeuwen WB, Wertheim HF, Nouwen JL, et al. Clonal distribution and differential occurrence of the enterotoxin gene cluster, egc, in carriage- versus bacteremia-associated isolates of *Staphylococcus aureus. J Clin Microbiol.* (2006) 44:1555–7. doi: 10.1128/JCM.44.4.1555-1557.2006

Fujishima H, Okada N, Dogru M, Baba F, Tomita M, Abe J, et al. The role of staphylococcal enterotoxin in atopic keratoconjunctivitis and corneal ulceration. *Allergy.* (2012) 67:799–803. doi: 10.1111/j.1398-9995.2012.02818.x

Austin A, Lietman T, Rose-Nussbaumer J. Update on the management of infectious keratitis. *Ophthalmology.* (2017) 124:1678–89. doi: 10.1016/j.ophtha.2017.05.012

Hsu HY, Nacke R, Song JC, Yoo SH, Alfonso EC, Israel HA. Community opinions in the management of corneal ulcers and ophthalmic antibiotics: a survey of 4 states. *Eye Contact Lens.* (2010) 36:195–200. doi: 10.1097/ICL.0b013e3181e3ef45

Proksch JW, Ward KW. Ocular pharmacokinetics/pharmacodynamics of besifloxacin, moxifloxacin, and gatifloxacin following topical administration to pigmented rabbits. *J Ocul Pharmacol Ther.* (2010) 26:449–58. doi: 10.1089/jop.2010.0054

Segreti J, Jones RN, Bertino JS, Jr. Challenges in assessing microbial susceptibility and predicting clinical response to newer- generation fluoroquinolones. *J Ocul Pharmacol Ther.* (2012) 28:3–11. doi: 10.1089/jop.2011.0072

Wilhelmus KR. Evaluation and prediction of fluoroquinolone pharmacodynamics in bacterial keratitis. *J Ocul Pharmacol Ther.* (2003) 19:493–9. doi: 10.1089/108076803322473042

Hayashi S, Suzuki T, Yamaguchi S, Inoue T, Ohashi Y. Genotypic characterization of *Staphylococcus aureus* isolates from cases of keratitis and healthy conjunctival sacs. *Cornea.* (2014) 33:72–6. doi: 10.1097/ICO.0b013e3182a4810f

Aguila A, Herrera AG, Morrison D, Cosgrove B, Perojo A, Montesinos I, et al. Bacteriostatic activity of human lactoferrin against staphylococcus aureus is a function of its iron-binding properties and is not influenced by antibiotic resistance. *FEMS Immunol Med Microbiol.* (2001) 31:145–52. doi: 10.1111/j.1574-695X.2001.tb00511.x

Chen PW, Jheng TT, Shyu CL, Mao FC. Synergistic antibacterial efficacies of the combination of bovine lactoferrin or its hydrolysate with probiotic secretion in curbing the growth of meticillin-resistant staphylococcus aureus. *J Med Microbiol.* (2013) 62(Pt 12):1845–51. doi: 10.1099/jmm.0.052639-0

Chua T, Moore CL, Perri MB, Donabedian SM, Masch W, Vager D, et al. Molecular epidemiology of methicillin-resistant staphylococcus aureus bloodstream isolates in urban detroit. *J Clin Microbiol.* (2008) 46:2345–52. doi: 10.1128/JCM.00154-08

Qu XD, Lehrer RI. Secretory phospholipase a2 is the principal bactericide for staphylococci and other gram-positive bacteria in human tears. *Infect Immun.* (1998) 66:2791–7. doi: 10.1128/IAI.66.6.2791-2797.1998

McCormick CC, Caballero AR, Balzli CL, Tang A, Weeks A, O'Callaghan RJ. Diverse virulence of staphylococcus aureus strains for the conjunctiva. *Curr Eye Res.* (2011) 36:14–20. doi: 10.3109/02713683.2010.523194

Tang A, Balzli CL, Caballero AR, McCormick CC, Taylor SD, O'Callaghan RJ. Staphylococcus aureus infection of the rabbit cornea following topical administration. *Curr Eye Res.* (2012) 37:1075–83. doi: 10.3109/02713683.2012.716485

Peterson JC, Durkee H, Miller D, Maestre-Mesa J, Arboleda A, Aguilar MC, et al. Molecular epidemiology and resistance profiles among healthcare- and community-associated staphylococcus aureus keratitis isolates. *Infect Drug Resist.* (2019) 12:831–43. doi: 10.2147/IDR.S190245

Booth MC, Pence LM, Mahasreshti P, Callegan MC, Gilmore MS. Clonal associations among staphylococcus aureus isolates from various sites of infection. *Infect Immun.* (2001) 69:345–52. doi: 10.1128/IAI.69.1.345-352.2001

Begier EM, Frenette K, Barrett NL, Mshar P, Petit S, Boxrud DJ, et al. A high-morbidity outbreak of methicillin-resistant staphylococcus aureus among players on a college football team, facilitated by cosmetic body shaving and turf burns. *Clin Infect Dis.* (2004) 39:1446–53. doi: 10.1086/425313

Kazakova SV, Hageman JC, Matava M, Srinivasan A, Phelan L, Garfinkel B, et al. A clone of methicillin-resistant staphylococcus aureus among professional football players. *N Engl J Med.* (2005) 352:468–75. doi: 10.1056/NEJMoa042859

Kempker RR, Farley MM, Ladson JL, Satola S, Ray SM. Association of methicillin-resistant staphylococcus aureus (MRSA) uSA300 genotype with mortality in mRSA bacteremia. *J Infect.* (2010) 61:372–81. doi: 10.1016/j.jinf.2010.09.021

Kreisel KM, Stine OC, Johnson JK, Perencevich EN, Shardell MD, Lesse AJ, et al. USA300 methicillin-resistant staphylococcus aureus bacteremia and the risk of severe sepsis: is uSA300 methicillin-resistant staphylococcus aureus associated with more severe infections? *Diagn Microbiol Infect Dis.* (2011) 70:285–90. doi: 10.1016/j.diagmicrobio.2011.03.010

Brown ML, O'Hara FP, Close NM, Mera RM, Miller LA, Suaya JA, et al. Prevalence and sequence variation of panton-valentine leukocidin in methicillin-resistant and methicillin-susceptible staphylococcus aureus strains in the united states. *J Clin Microbiol.* (2012) 50:86–90. doi: 10.1128/JCM.05564-11

Chi CY, Lin CC, Liao IC, Yao YC, Shen FC, Liu CC, et al. Panton- Valentine leukocidin facilitates the escape of staphylococcus aureus from human keratinocyte endosomes and induces apoptosis. *J Infect Dis.* (2014) 209:224–35. doi: 10.1093/infdis/jit445

Carniciu AL, Chou J, Leskov I, Freitag SK. Clinical presentation and bacteriology of eyebrow infections: the massachusetts eye and ear infirmary experience (2008-2015). *Ophthalmic Plast Reconstr Surg.* (2017) 33:372–5. doi: 10.1097/IOP.0000000000000797

McKinley SH, Yen MT, Miller AM, Yen KG. Microbiology of pediatric orbital cellulitis. *Am J Ophthalmol.* (2007) 144:497–501. doi: 10.1016/j.ajo.2007.04.049

Amato M, Pershing S, Walvick M, Tanaka S. Trends in ophthalmic manifestations of methicillin-resistant staphylococcus aureus (MRSA) in a northern california pediatric population. *J AAPOS.* (2013) 17:243–7. doi: 10.1016/j.jaapos.2012.12.151

Gurdal C, Bilkan H, Sarac O, Seven E, Yenidunya MO, Kutluhan A, et al. Periorbital necrotizing fasciitis caused by community-associated methicillin- resistant staphylococcus aureus periorbital necrotizing fasciitis. *Orbit.* (2010) 29:348–50. doi: 10.3109/01676831003697509

Shield DR, Servat J, Paul S, Turbin RE, Moreau A, de la Garza A, et al. Periocular necrotizing fasciitis causing blindness. *JAMA Ophthalmol.* (2013) 131:1225–7. doi: 10.1001/jamaophthalmol.2013.4816

Singam NV, Rusia D, Prakash R. An eye popping case of orbital necrotizing fasciitis treated with antibiotics, surgery, and hyperbaric oxygen therapy. *Am J Case Rep.* (2017) 18:329–33. doi: 10.12659/AJCR.902535

Foster CE, Yarotsky E, Mason EO, Kaplan SL, Hulten KG. Molecular characterization of staphylococcus aureus isolates from children with periorbital or orbital cellulitis. *J Pediatric Infect Dis Soc.* (2018) 7:205–9. doi: 10.1093/jpids/pix036

Planet PJ, LaRussa SJ, Dana A, Smith H, Xu A, Ryan C, et al. Emergence of the epidemic methicillin-resistant staphylococcus aureus strain uSA300 coincides with horizontal transfer of the arginine catabolic mobile element and speG-mediated adaptations for survival on skin. *MBio.* (2013) 4:e00889-13. doi: 10.1128/mBio.00889-13

8

Constructing and Characterizing Bacteriophage Libraries for Phage Therapy of Human Infections

Shelley B. Gibson[1], Sabrina I. Green[1], Carmen Gu Liu[1], Keiko C. Salazar[1], Justin R. Clark[1], Austen L. Terwilliger[1], Heidi B. Kaplan[2], Anthony W. Maresso[1]*, Barbara W. Trautner[1,3,4]* and Robert F. Ramig[1]*

[1] Department of Molecular Virology and Microbiology, Baylor College of Medicine, Houston, TX, United States, [2] Department of Microbiology and Molecular Genetics, McGovern Medical School, University of Texas Health Science Center at Houston, Houston, TX, United States, [3] Center for Innovations in Quality, Effectiveness and Safety, Michael E. DeBakey VA Medical Center, Houston, TX, United States, [4] Department of Medicine, Baylor College of Medicine, Houston, TX, United States

*Correspondence:
Anthony W. Maresso
maresso@bcm.edu
Barbara W. Trautner
trautner@bcm.edu
Robert F. Ramig
rramig@bcm.edu

Phage therapy requires libraries of well-characterized phages. Here we describe the generation of phage libraries for three target species: *Escherichia coli*, *Pseudomonas aeruginosa,* and *Enterobacter cloacae*. The basic phage characteristics on the isolation host, sequence analysis, growth properties, and host range and virulence on a number of contemporary clinical isolates are presented. This information is required before phages can be added to a phage library for potential human use or sharing between laboratories for use in compassionate use protocols in humans under eIND (emergency investigational new drug). Clinical scenarios in which these phages can potentially be used are discussed. The phages presented here are currently being characterized in animal models and are available for eINDs.

Keywords: phage libraries, phage therapy, host range, phage characteristics, killing spectrum, human infection

INTRODUCTION

The crisis in clinical care imposed by the increasing resistance of bacterial infections to antibiotics threatens to return clinical practice to the pre-antibiotic era (Boucher et al., 2009; Centers for Disease Control [CDC], 2013; Bassetti et al., 2017; World Health Organization [WHO], 2017). The situation is particularly acute for infections caused by Gram-negative pathogens for which few new antibiotics are in the pipeline. The bacterial "mutagenic tetrasect" (mutation, transformation, transduction, and conjugation) is responsible for the rapid evolution of bacteria and suggests that bacteria are so flexible in their ability to adapt that production of antibiotics by pharmaceutical companies, will never be able to keep up with the evolution of resistance against that drug. Fortunately, a natural alternative to conventional chemical antibiotics (Ghosh et al., 2018; Stearns, 2019) exists in the form of bacteriophages (phages). Thus, phages can evolve to efficiently target specific bacteria and have been used to treat complex drug-resistant bacterial infections in a procedure termed phage therapy (Ghosh et al., 2018).

Although phage therapy has great potential as a treatment for antibiotic resistant infections, it is not without problems. Phage have a similar mutation rate to bacteria; the organisms reproduce so rapidly that the high numbers lead to very large mutant populations on which selection can operate to enrich selected phenotypes. Host range expansion by evolution and selection has been achieved (Burrowes, 2011; Mapes et al., 2016; Burrowes et al., 2019) and is extremely rapid (unpublished data). In addition, phage ecologists have estimated the total number of phages on Earth to be greater than 10^{31} (Suttle, 2005). This suggests that the environment is a plentiful resource for new phages; indeed, environmental phages to drug-resistant and pandemic *Escherichia coli* that have excellent efficacy in animal models of infection have been discovered, characterized, and tested in as short a time period as 14 days (Green et al., 2017).

Phages were discovered over a century ago, and phage therapy has a long history (Debarbieux et al., 2018; Gelman et al., 2018). However, the advent of chemical antibiotics led to virtual abandonment of phage therapy in most of the world, whereas in the countries of Eastern Europe phage therapy was continuously pursued (Chanishvili, 2016; Myelnikov, 2018). As the development of antibiotic resistance has grown, the interest in phage has been rekindled (Kutter et al., 2015). Studies with compassionate use investigational new drug (IND) have generated considerable excitement for use of phage therapy in human subjects (Wright et al., 2009; Schooley et al., 2017; Chan et al., 2018; Aslam et al., 2019). Recently the application of phage therapy to human infections was reviewed (El Haddad et al., 2018), and the majority of the studies analyzed showed efficacy (87%) and safety (67%), however only a few of the studies examined the development of phage-resistant bacteria during therapy. Bacteria become resistant to phage infection (phage-resistant) (Labrie et al., 2010), through mutational changes just as they become antibiotic-resistant upon treatment with antibiotics. The problem of phage-resistance is often overcome by [i] the use of single broad host range phages, [ii] phages for which development of phage-resistance carries high bacterial fitness costs (Chan et al., 2016; unpublished data), or [iii] mixtures (cocktails) of phages (generally recognizing different bacterial surface receptors). Others have argued that phage resistance is not a problem in phage therapy because phage resistant bacteria often have fitness defects and new environmental phages active on the resistant host can be isolated (Ormala and Jalasvuori, 2013). Indeed it is likely that phages capable of infecting a resistant host can be isolated from the environment or evolved in the laboratory (Mapes et al., 2016, unpublished data). However, these operations are time consuming and best avoided. In addition, not all phage resistant hosts were found to have fitness defects, so that they could persist in the patient (Wei et al., 2010, our unpublished data).

The development of phages for use against human infections has been described as following two pipelines (Pirnay et al., 2011). The *"prêt à porter"* (ready-to-wear) is a method, in which a medicinal product of a single broad host range phage is developed and undergoes safety and efficacy testing. This is time consuming and costly but yields products that can be licensed by regulatory agencies. In contrast, in the *"sur-mesure"* (custom made) method many phages are isolated and characterized and can be combined as appropriate to treat the infection. This method is flexible, inexpensive, and can rapidly

respond to infections with phage- or antibiotic- resistant bacteria. However, *sur-mesure* approaches cannot currently be licensed, but therapeutic use of phage produced through this approach is under active discussion (Debarbieux et al., 2016; Pirnay et al., 2018). We have chosen the latter approach in which [i] libraries of well-characterized phages are generated and stored, [ii] as the clinical laboratory is assessing the antibiotic-resistance of the bacterial isolate (~48 h), it is also tested for sensitivity to phages from the library (<48 h), [iii] phages to which the clinical isolate is sensitive are selected for mono-phage-therapy or used to construct cocktails containing several individual phages. Two therapeutic options are available: the patient can be treated with the phage alone, or phage plus antibiotic.

Here, we describe the preparation of well-characterized libraries of *E. coli*-specific, *Pseudomonas aeruginosa*-specific, and *Enterobacter cloacae*-specific phages for use in a *sur-mesure* approach to phage therapy, which will ultimately result in a therapeutic that is personalized to the specific infection of the individual patient. We provide information on the phages including: descriptions of their sources, their efficacy against a panel of clinical strains, some basic infection characteristics (burst size and absorption rates), and their DNA sequence and annotation to determine if they harbor lysogenic, antibiotic resistance or toxin genes and their morphologic description; providing the means to select high quality phage(s) for use in therapy. Also described are the clinical scenarios for which these phage libraries have been developed, as their proposed use shaped the development of the libraries.

MATERIALS AND METHODS

Bacterial Strains

The laboratory strains used were *E. coli* (MG1655) and *P. aeruginosa* (PAO1 and BWT111). A collection of 13 *E. coli* ST131 strains (see **Supplementary Figures S1–S3**) was obtained from Dr. Jim Johnson (University of Minnesota). Two strains of *E. cloacae* were isolated from a phage therapy candidate with an infected hip prosthesis. One isolate was from a wound swab and other from the fluid exudate of the wound (collected at different times). De-identified clinical isolates of *E. coli*, *P. aeruginosa*, and *E. cloacae* and their antibiotic susceptibility data were obtained from the clinical microbiology laboratory at the Houston Veterans Administration Hospital or Baylor St. Luke's Hospital. Collection of de-identified clinical isolates was approved by the Baylor College of Medicine Institutional Review Board (IRB). An isolated colony of each clinical isolate was streaked on LB agar and grown overnight. A single colony from the LB plate was grown overnight in LB medium, diluted 1:10 into LB medium containing 15% glycerol, and frozen at −80°C. In cases where clinical isolates appeared to be mixed, the desired species was isolated from differential plates.

Phages

Four *P. aeruginosa*-specific phages φKMV, φPA2, φPaer4, and φE2005-24-39 (hereafter called φE2005) were previously described (Mapes et al., 2016). These were the only *Pseudomonas* wild type phages used in this work. All *E. coli*-specific and *E. cloacae* phages used here were isolated from environmental samples (see **Figures 1**, **4A,B**, **7** for source species) by plaque assay. Fecal samples were suspended to ~50% (w/v) in PBS, shaken, and centrifuged to remove debris. The supernatant was filtered through a 0.22 micron filter, and 0.1 ml was plated with 0.8% LB top agar containing 100 μl of an overnight culture of the desired isolation strain. After overnight incubation, well-isolated

Properties of *E. Coli* Phages

Feature	*E. Coli* Phage							
	φHP3	φEC1	φCF2	φES12	φES17	φES19	φES21	φES26
Phage Characteristics								
Source Species	Goose, & Duck	Dog	Chicken	Human	Human	Human	Human	Human
Source Location	Herman Park	E. Chew Dog Park	Rescue Farm	Raw* Sewage	Raw* Sewage	Raw* Sewage	Raw* Sewage	Raw* Sewage
Isolation Date	03/23/15	03/23/15		02/06/18	02/06/18	02/06/18	02/06/18	02/06/18
Isolation Strain	MG1655±	MG1655±	CP9[†]	JJ2050[†]	JJ2547[†]	DS104[#]	DS110[#]	DS182[#]
Plaque Size (mm)	0.5mm	0.5mm	1-2mm	0.5mm	0.5-1.0mm	0.5mm + halo	0.5mm + halo	0.5mm + halo
Plaque Morph.	Clear	Clear	Clear	Clear	Clear	Clear	Clear	Clear
Plate Stock (PFU/ml)=	3.00×10^9	4.20×10^9		7.40×10^8	9.80×10^9	2.00×10^9	9.20×10^9	2.00×10^7
CsCl Purified (PFU/ml)	1.90×10^{12}	5.80×10^{11}	2.4×10^{10}	2.85×10^{11}	4.85×10^{11}	3.10×10^{11}	1.80×10^{11}	1.43×10^{11}
EM Morphology	Myovirus	Myovirus	Myovirus	Myovirus	Podovirus	Myovirus	Myovirus	Myovirus
Sequence								
(Accession No.)	KY608976	KY608965	KY608966	MN508614	MN508615	MN508616	MN508617	MN508618
Genome (BP)	168,188	170,254	53,242	166,373	75,134	167,088	167.096	166,950
G + C (%)	35.4	37.6	45.9	35.37%	42.12	35.39	35.38	35.39%
ORFs	274	275	74	267	120	263	264	268
tRNAs	11	2	0	9	1	11	11	9
Toxin/Virulence Genes	None	None	None	None	None	None	None	None
Lysogeny Cassettes	None	None	None	None	None	None	None	None
Abx-Resistance Genes	None	None	None	None	None	None	None	None
Closest Relative	pSs-1	SHSML-52.1	BP63	slur07	PhiEco32	vB_Eco_HY01	vB_Eco_HY01	RB14
Genus	Tequatrovirus	Tequatrovirus	Unclassified	T4-like	PhiEco32-like	T4-like	T4-like	T4-like
Growth Properties								
Adsorption Constant (mL/min)	5.63×10^{-9}	5.94×10^{-9}	3.29×10^{-9}	3.49×10^{-9}	2.72×10^{-9}	6.48×10^{-9}	7.07×10^{-9}	1.68×10^{-9}
% Adsorbed (10 min)	98	61	65	93	32	96	90	16
Latent Period (Min)	22.5	22.0	40.0	26.0	33.0	28.5	23.0	25.0
Burst Size (PFU/cell)	60	57.4	>10	9.6	38.7	11	41	80.7
Summary of Phage Killing Spectra – No. Lysed/No. Tested (% Lysed) see next three pages for details								
ST131 Strains[†] (N-13)								
(EOP > 0.1)	4/13 (31%)	2/13 (15%)	1/13 (8%)	7/13 (54%)	8/13 (62%)	7/13 (54%)	7/13 (54%)	7/13 (54%)
(EOP > 0.001)	9/13 (69%)	5/13 (38%)	4/13 (31%)	7/13 (54%)	9/13 (69%)	7/13 (54%)	9/13 (69%)	7/13 (54%)
Clinical Isolates[#] (N=76)								
(EOP > 0.1)	39/76 (51%)	3/76 (4%)	8/76 (11%)	42/76 (55%)	34/76 (48%)	39/76 (51%)	43/76 (57%)	43/76 (57%)
(EOP > 0.001)	58/76 (76%)	6/76 (8%)	12/76 (16%)	44/76 (58%)	37/76 (49%)	42/76 (55%)	44/76 (58%)	45/76 (58%)
Total Strains (N-89)								
(EOP > 0.1)	43/89 (48%)	5/89 (6%)	8/89 (9%)	42/89 (47%)	34/89 (38%)	41/89 (46%)	43/89 (48%)	43/89 (48%)
(EOP > 0.001)	58/89 (65%)	6/89 (7%)	13/89 (15%)	44/89 (49%)	37/89 (42%)	42/89 (47%)	46/89 (52%)	45/89 (51%)

* Municipal Sewage Plant, Houston, Tx.
± *E. coli* K12 lab strain
[†] *E. coli* ST131 strains (ExPEC) from Jim Johnson
[#] *E. coli* clinical isolates from Houston VA Hospital
= Representative purified or plate stock

FIGURE 1 | Summary of characterization of *Escherichia coli* phages. The characteristics, DNA sequences, growth properties and a summary of phage killing spectra are presented for each phage.

plaques were picked into 1.0 ml phage storage buffer (Mapes et al., 2016), allowed to sit overnight for phage diffusion at 4°C, and 0.5 ml of suspended phage was used to prepare plate stocks using the isolation strain as host. Plate stocks were harvested and stored at 4°C.

Host Range Determination/Efficiency of Killing (Virulence)

To determine phage host range a spot titration protocol was used that allowed us to determine both host range and relative phage killing (EOP). Five microliters of serial 10-fold dilutions of a CsCl purified phage stock (10^{10}–10^{12} pfu/ml) were spotted on freshly seeded lawns of control, isolation, or clinical strains. The host range and titer were determined by formation of individual plaques within the area of the spot at terminal dilution. This avoided false positives by determining host range at dilutions where phenomena such as lysis from without (Abedon, 2011) or complementation between defective phages would not be expected. Phage virulence was determined as the efficiency of plating (EOP) (Mirzaei and Nilsson, 2015). EOP was calculated by dividing the titer of the phage at the terminal dilution on the test strain by the titer of the same phage on its isolation strain. On this basis, phages were classified as highly virulent ($0.1 < EOP > 1.00$), moderately virulent ($0.001 < EOP < 0.099$), avirulent but active ($EOP < 0.001$), or avirulent (no plaques detected – see **Figures 2, 5, 8**).

Host Range Expansion (HRE)

Pseudomonas aeruginosa-specific phages were subjected to the HRE protocol as described (Burrowes, 2011; Mapes et al., 2016; Burrowes et al., 2019). Briefly, in a 96 well plate, different host strains were placed in each of the eight rows at a dilution of 1:1000 of overnight culture. Serial 10-fold dilutions of phage (a single phage or a phage mixture) were placed in the 12 columns and the plate was incubated (37°C) with shaking (225 RPM) for 18 h. Following incubation, for each bacterial strain (row) the supernatant from the well with complete lysis and the adjacent well with higher phage dilution (partial lysis) were combined, into a single tube with the corresponding complete and partial lysis wells of the other bacterial strains. The pooled lysate was treated with CHCl$_3$ and filtered through a 0.22 micron filter. The filtered lysate was the yield of the 1st cycle of HRE. This filtered lysate was serially diluted 10-fold, and the experiment was repeated using the pooled lysate as the phage and the same bacterial strains as host for cycle 2. The HRE was repeated up to 30 cycles, and yielded a mixture of phages that had replicated on at least one of the host bacterial strains. The heterogeneous mixture of phages in the lysate from any cycle of HRE can be assayed for plaque formers on a host refractory to the parental phage(s), plaques purified, and phage stocks with expanded host range produced (Mapes et al., 2016). The HRE protocol was also successfully applied to *E. coli*-specific phages (data not shown).

The HRE protocol exposes the lysate (including mutants) that arose during a cycle to new bacteria (unevolved) of the strains used in the previous cycle. Some of the mutations may allow phages to infect and replicate on bacterial strains that were previously refractory to phage, thus amplifying the mutant that contained the host range expanding mutation.

DNA Sequencing and Annotation of Phage Genomes

CsCl purified phages were submitted to the Center for Metagenomics and Microbiome Research at Baylor College of Medicine for DNA extraction, sequencing and assembly as described previously (Green et al., 2017). Briefly, DNA samples were constructed into Illumina paired-end libraries. The libraries had an average final size of 660 bp (including adapter and barcode sequences) and were pooled in equimolar amounts to achieve a final concentration of 10 nM. The library templates were prepared for sequencing on the Illumina MiSeq. After sequencing, the.bcl files were processed through Illumina's analysis software (CASAVA), which demultiplexes pooled samples and generates sequence reads and base-call confidence values (qualities). The average raw yield per sample was 802 Mbp. For analysis, the adapter sequences were removed, and the sequence was then assembled using SPAdes v3.5.0 (Bankevich et al., 2012) on careful mode, retaining only contigs longer than 1,000 bp and with an average coverage of 1000x or greater. This generated 1–2 contigs per sample, with an average of 74% of the original reads mapping with 100% identity to the final contigs. Genomes were analyzed using both PATRIC's comprehensive genome analysis service (Wattam et al., 2017) and EDGE Bioinformatic software (Li et al., 2017). Gene calling and genome annotation was performed using PROKKA (version 1.13) (Lo and Chain, 2014), RAST (Zerbino and Birney, 2008; Bankevich et al., 2012), GLIMMER3 (version 3.02) (Peng et al., 2010), and GeneMarkS (version 4.28) (Peng et al., 2012). **Figures 1, 4A,B, 7** show ORF predictions from the RAST pipeline and tRNA predictions from ARAGORN (version 1.2.36) (Seemann, 2014). ORFs were searched for virulence and antibiotic resistance genes by using BLAST (Aziz et al., 2008) to compare assembled genomes against the Virulence Factor Database (VFDB) (McNair et al., 2018), the PATRIC virulence factor database (Delcher et al., 2007), the Antibiotic Resistance Gene Database (ARDB) (Besemer, 2001) and the Comprehensive Antibiotic Resistance Database (CARD) (Laslett, 2004). ShortBRED (version 0.9.4M) (Johnson et al., 2008) was used for targeted searches of ORFs for genes in the VFDB, CARD, and the Resfam antibiotic resistance gene database (Chen et al., 2016). Genus was inferred from closest sequenced relatives identified by using BWA-Mem (version 0.7.9) (Mao et al., 2015) to aligning contigs to NCBI's RefSeq database and by ORF homology using PHAge Search Tool Enhanced Release (PHASTER) (Liu and Pop, 2009). Phage lifestyles were determined by classifying the genomes using PHACTs (McArthur et al., 2013), using PHASTER to predict integrases and attachment sites, and by parsing all versions of the annotated genome for "integrase." No virulence genes of known toxicity (viral or bacterial) or genes involved in lysogeny were detected. Thus it appears the phages examined here are devoid of any known lysogenic or toxic elements that would preclude their use in phage therapy.

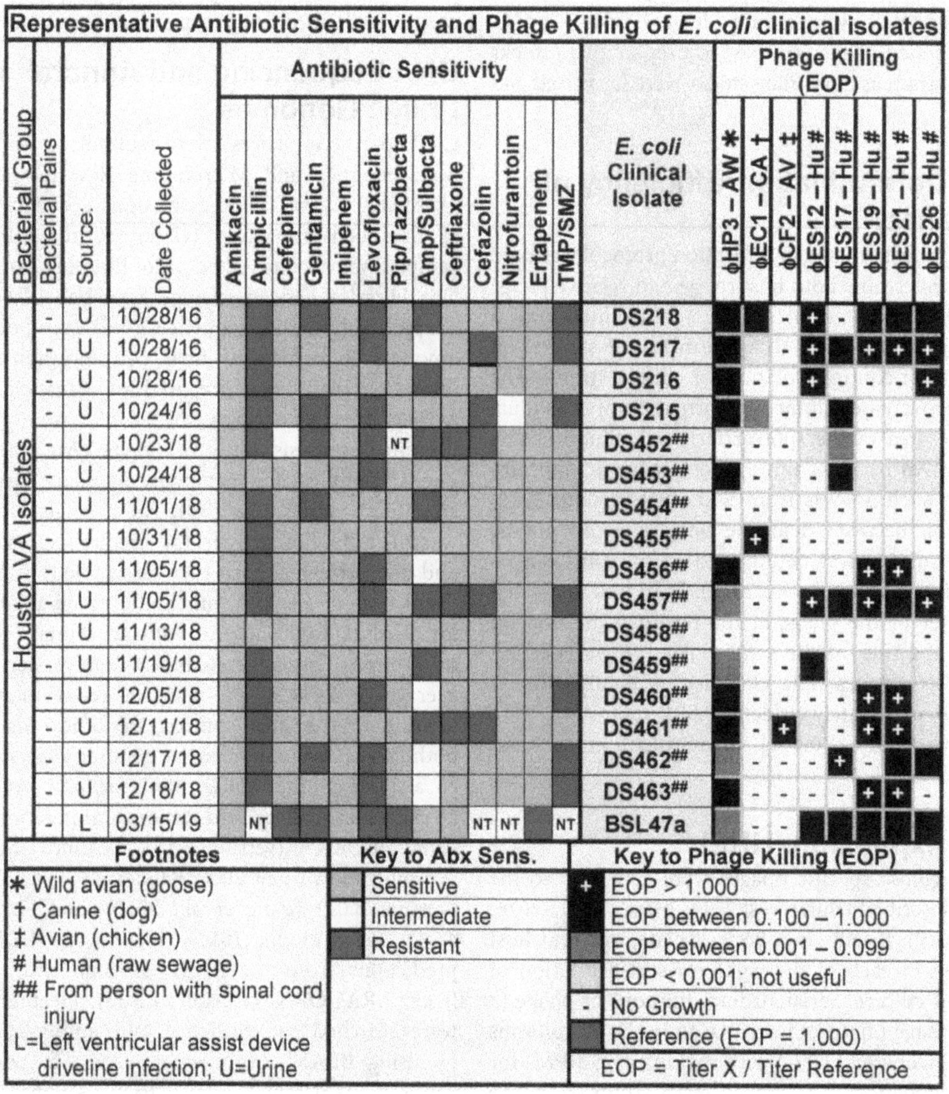

Representative Antibiotic Sensitivity and Phage Killing of *E. coli* clinical isolates

The figure presents a color-coded matrix with the following structure.

Left-hand columns: Bacterial Group, Bacterial Pairs, Source, Date Collected.

Antibiotic Sensitivity (color-coded columns): Amikacin, Ampicillin, Cefepime, Gentamicin, Imipenem, Levofloxacin, Pip/Tazobacta, Amp/Sulbacta, Ceftriaxone, Cefazolin, Nitrofurantoin, Ertapenem, TMP/SMZ.

E. coli Clinical Isolate column.

Phage Killing (EOP) (color-coded columns): φHP3 – AW *, φEC1 – CA †, φCF2 – AV ‡, φES12 – Hu #, φES17 – Hu #, φES19 – Hu #, φES21 – Hu #, φES26 – Hu #.

Bacterial Group: Houston VA Isolates.

Source	Date Collected	E. coli Clinical Isolate
U	10/28/16	DS218
U	10/28/16	DS217
U	10/28/16	DS216
U	10/24/16	DS215
U	10/23/18	DS452##
U	10/24/18	DS453##
U	11/01/18	DS454##
U	10/31/18	DS455##
U	11/05/18	DS456##
U	11/05/18	DS457##
U	11/13/18	DS458##
U	11/19/18	DS459##
U	12/05/18	DS460##
U	12/11/18	DS461##
U	12/17/18	DS462##
U	12/18/18	DS463##
L	03/15/19	BSL47a

Cells marked "NT" indicate not tested.

Footnotes
* Wild avian (goose)
† Canine (dog)
‡ Avian (chicken)
# Human (raw sewage)
From person with spinal cord injury
L=Left ventricular assist device driveline infection; U=Urine

Key to Abx Sens.
- Sensitive
- Intermediate
- Resistant

Key to Phage Killing (EOP)
- + EOP > 1.000
- EOP between 0.100 – 1.000
- EOP between 0.001 – 0.099
- EOP < 0.001; not useful
- - No Growth
- Reference (EOP = 1.000)
- EOP = Titer X / Titer Reference

FIGURE 2 | Representative data for antibiotic sensitivity and phage killing (EOP) of clinical isolates of *E. coli*. Shown are the properties of the *E. coli* clinical isolates on the left, including: source, date of isolation and antibiotic sensitivity data (VITEK2). On the right are shown the killing spectra of the phages on the individual *E. coli* clinical isolates. The keys to antibiotic sensitivity and phage killing (EOP) are shown at the bottom of the figure.

Phage Growth Parameters

The percentage of phage adsorbed in 10 min and the adsorption constant were determined for each phage on its isolation strain. Burst size and latent period (one-step growth curves) were also determined for each phage on its isolation strain (Kropinski, 2009, 2018).

RESULTS

Escherichia coli Phages

E. coli Phage Isolation

Our primary target for *E. coli* phage isolation was extraintestinal pathogenic *E. coli* (ExPEC) of the pandemic sequence type 131 (ST131). ExPEC are commonly associated with bacteremia and urinary tract infections, and the ST131 lineage is characterized by multi-drug resistance and its high frequency of isolation over the past 10 years. Interestingly, a rapid screen of common laboratory *E. coli*-specific phages (T2, T4, T6, T7, λ^vir) revealed that none of them formed plaques on the ST131 strains tested. As a result we began to isolate phages from the environment, concentrating on avian and canine species which are known reservoirs for *E. coli* ST131 (Johnson et al., 2001, 2017). Our first phage isolates were from mixed goose/duck feces collected at a local park (φHP3), canine feces from a dog park (φEC1) and chicken feces from a rehabilitation farm (φCF2). We subsequently isolated phages from raw sewage collected at a local sewage treatment plant (φES series; see **Figure 1**). All phages were plaque-purified three times prior to use.

E. coli Phage Characteristics

The phage characteristics are summarized in **Figure 1**. The phages varied in plaque size, but plaques tended to be small and clear. Some produced halos around the plaques, suggesting enzymatic activity on the surrounding cells. Regardless of the small plaque sizes, reasonable titer plate stocks were obtained, and all phages could be CsCl purified to about 10^{11} pfu/ml. Adsorption curves revealed that the phages ranged widely in adsorption (16–98%). For all the E. coli phages, one-step growth curves revealed the latent period was in the range of 22–40 min and burst sizes ranged from 9.6 to 80.7 pfu/cell. Sequence analysis revealed genome sizes ranging from (53,242 to 170,254 bp) with variable G + C content. The number of encoded ORFs and tRNAs identified was also variable. Notably, none of the sequences contained features that would preclude their use in phage therapy, such as genes to establish and maintain lysogeny, produce toxins or virulence factors, or confer antibiotic resistance (Merabishvili et al., 2018; Hyman, 2019). All of the E. coli phages had myovirus morphology except for φES17 which was a podovirus with an elongated head. Phage ES17 also contained, at marginal statistical significance, an integrase gene when examined with PHACTs and PHASTER software. When colonies were isolated in the presence of excess φES17, no phages were isolated following growth of those colonies in the presence of mitomycin C (data not shown). We concluded that φES17 is a lytic phage, lacking an integrase.

Host Range of E. coli Phages

The host ranges of the phages was determined as described in Section "Materials and Methods" by spot testing serial 10-fold phage dilutions on the isolation strain and on other laboratory and clinical isolates. The virulence of the phage was determined by comparing the titer on a test strain with the titer on the isolation strain (EOP = titer test/titer isolation). Phages with EOP > 0.1 were considered highly virulent and most useful. Phages with EOP in the range of 0.001–0.099, were considered moderately virulent and may be useful if high titers can be produced. **Figure 2** shows the host range and virulence results for eight E. coli phages on a representative selection of E. coli clinical isolates. A complete determination of host range and virulence on (1) characterized ST131 strains, (2) a collection of paired clinical isolates from two sites (urine and blood) collected from the same patient on the same day, and (3) a set of clinical isolates collected between November 2015 and December 2018 is shown (**Supplementary Figures S1–S3**).

At least one of the E. coli phage isolates was able to kill each member of the ST131 collection, except for E. coli strain JJ1886 (**Supplementary Figures S1–S3**). For individual phages, 8–62% of ST131 strains were killed at EOP > 0.1 and 31–69% were killed at EOPs in the range of 0.001–0.099 (**Supplementary Figures S1–S3**). A cocktail of as few as two E. coli phages (φHP3 and φES17) was capable of killing 12/13 (92%) of ST131 strains (**Supplementary Figures S1–S3**).

Among the 76 E. coli clinical isolates (24 paired blood and urine isolates from the same patient on the same day; 40 single clinical isolates, mostly from patients with UTI; and 12 clinical isolates from urine of catheterized spinal cord injured [SCI]

patients) the eight E. coli phages killed from 4 to 57% at an EOP > 0.1. If EOPs between 0.001 and 0.099 (moderately virulent) were included very little increase in the number of clinical isolates killed was observed, except for φHP3 where the number killed was increased by 50% (**Figure 1**). For the 24 paired blood and urine isolates, a cocktail of as few as three of the E. coli phages (φCF2, φES12, and φES17) could be assembled that killed them all at EOP > 0.1. Among the 40 clinical isolates primarily of urinary origin, cocktails (φHP3, φES17, and φES19) capable of killing 35/40 (88%) of the isolates at EOP > 0.1 could be made. Among 12 isolates originating from SCI patients, a cocktail of four phages (φHP3, φEC1, φES12, and φES17) could be made that killed 9/12 (75%) E. coli strains at EOP > 0.1. Among all 76 of the E. coli clinical isolates, we noted no correlation between killing at high efficiency and date of isolation (November 2015–December 2018) or antibiotic-sensitivity phenotype. A summary of the antibiotic sensitivity and phage killing of the 89 total E. coli isolates examined is shown in **Figure 3**. Although none of the individual phages killed more than 50–55% of the 76 bacterial strains at high efficiency, a three phage cocktail increased the high efficiency killing to nearly 90% (**Figure 3**).

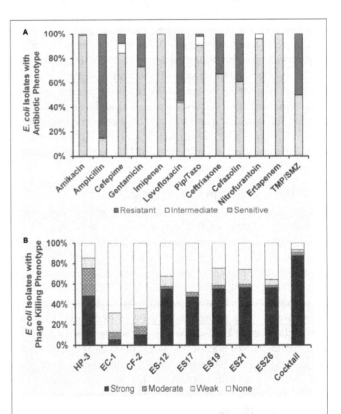

FIGURE 3 | Antibiotic Sensitivities and Phage Killing Phenotypes of E. coli Clinical Isolates (N = 89). **(A)** Antibiotic sensitvities using cut off values used in the microbiology lab at the Houston VA Hospital. **(B)** The phage killing phenotypes were based on EOP. Strong killers, EOP > 0.1; Moderate Killers, 0.099 > EOP > 0.001; Weak Killers, EOP < 0.00099 but positive; None, no growth. Strong and moderate killers have EOP high enough to be useful in phage therapy. The phage cocktail consisted of equal titers of phages: φHP-3, φES-12, and φES17. Pip/Tazo, piperacillin/tazobactam; TMP/SMX, trimethoprim/sulfamethoxazole.

Pseudomonas aeruginosa Phages

Origin of *P. aeruginosa* Phages

Four *P. aeruginosa*-specific phages previously isolated and used by other laboratories were used here: φKMV (Lavigne et al., 2003; Chibeu et al., 2009), φPA2 (ATCC 14203-B1; McVay et al., 2007), φPaer4 (Fu et al., 2010), and φE2005 (Liao et al., 2012). All four phages as a mixture, or single phages, were used in the host range expansion protocol (HRE) as described (Mapes et al., 2016; see section "Materials and Methods"). The HRE protocol generates phage mutants able to infect and replicate on bacterial strains that were previously resistant to the phage (i.e., broadening their host range). The four parental phages subjected to HRE as a mixture lysed 38% of 16 bacterial strains (development strains) used. After 30 cycles of HRE 75% of the 16 development strains were lysed by the phage mixture. When 10 strains different from those used in the HRE process (test strains) were tested 100% of them were lysed by the phage mixture resulting from 30 HRE cycles (Mapes et al., 2016). During this directed evolution process all phages present are mixed, so that at any cycle the lysate is a heterogeneous mixture of phages. Individual plaques were picked after 20 and 30 cycles of HRE and plaque purified after plating on the desired host. For example, *P. aeruginosa* strain DS38 one of the development strains, was not lysed by the parental phage mixture. The heterogeneous phage mixture from HRE cycle 30 formed plaques on strain DS38 indicating that it contained phages with the host range expanded to DS38. Purified phage clones were generated on strain DS38 from 108 plaques picked from the 30 cycle lysate containing the heterogeneous mixture phages. Among the 108 phage clones that all lysed DS38, there were 30 different killing spectra when they were tested against the 16 development and 10 test strains (Mapes et al., 2016). Similarly, φKMV was subjected to five cycles of HRE, and was found have expanded host range phages in the lysate of cycle 5.

P. aeruginosa Phage Characteristics

The characteristics of parental and host range expanded phages are shown in **Figures 4A,B**. The characteristics of the phages were variable and similar to those seen for *E. coli* phages (**Figure 1**). Importantly, DNA sequencing revealed that each of the phages derived from the HRE of the four phage mixture represented only mutants of one of the parental phages. This result indicated that recombination between parental phages did not contribute to expansion of host range in the progeny examined. Thus, the morphology of the HRE-derived clones was not determined but assumed to be like that of the parental phage (**Figures 4A,B**). Sequencing also revealed that none of the phages contained genes that would be detrimental to their use in phage therapy. The growth properties of the HRE-derived phages were also similar to the parental phages.

Host Range of *P. aeruginosa* Phages

Host range and virulence of *P. aeruginosa* phages on representative *P. aeruginosa* clinical isolates is shown in **Figure 5**. Characterization of the host range and virulence on the complete set of *P. aeruginosa* clinical isolates tested is shown in the supplementary information (**Supplementary Figures S4, S5**). Compared to the parental phages, the HRE-derived phages had expanded host range when tested against the development strains. They lysed, 19–69% of those strains compared to 12–31% for the parental phages. Likewise the HRE-derived phages had expanded host range when tested against the test strains; they lysed 20–90% of test strains compared to 1–10% for the parental phages (**Supplementary Figures S4, S5**). The parental and HRE-derived phages were then tested against a collection of 64 clinical isolates, which were mostly isolated from patient urine samples that were obtained between November 2015 and August 2017, and displayed a spectrum of antibiotic resistances. Examination of the killing activity (**Supplementary Figures S4, S5**) revealed the HRE-derived phages had expanded host range relative to the parental phages, although many of the phages were expanded at EOP < 0.001, an EOP too low to be useful. It is possible that additional rounds of HRE on some the clinical isolates could generate phage with an EOP in a useful range (EOP > 0.001). Greater numbers of HRE cycles led to greater expansion of host range in the isolated phage clones (**Figures 5, 6** and **Supplementary Figures S4, S5**), both at highly efficient killing (EOP > 0.1) and at useful levels of killing (EOP > 0.001). This was observed for both HRE using four parental phages (compare 20 and 30 cycles) and for 5 cycles of HRE using a single parental phage φKMV (**Figure 5** and **Supplementary Figures S4, S5**).

Figure 6 summarizes the antibiotic sensitivity and phage killing phenotypes of the phages on the 64 total *P. aeruginosa* clinical isolates examined. The increase in useful killing with cycles of the HRE protocol and with mixing of cocktails is shown in **Figure 6B**.

The lack of recombination in HRE-derived phages observed here, contrasts with the contribution of recombination reported by others (Burrowes et al., 2019). In retrospect, this finding is not surprising, since the four phages used were distant phylogenetically, making homology-driven recombination unlikely. The HRE-derived phage sequences contained mutations spread randomly across the genome, but all of them had mutations in the tail fiber gene as would be expected if the host range expansion was based on tail fiber-bacterial receptor interactions. In addition, the sequence analysis revealed no genes that would preclude the use of the HRE-derived phages in phage therapy. Thus, the HRE-derived *P. aeruginosa* phages are classified as variants of the parental phage to which they corresponded (**Figures 4A,B**).

Enterobacter cloacae Phages

E. cloacae Phage Isolation

Enterobacter cloacae phages were isolated from raw sewage collected on two different days by plaquing on a phage therapy candidate's isolates (**Figure 7**).

E. cloacae Phage Characteristics

Sequence analysis of the phages revealed that the four phages were similar and T4-like (**Figure 7**). The growth properties of the *E. cloacae* phages were somewhat variable but had parameters within expected values (**Figure 7**). The *E. cloacae* phages contained no genes that would preclude their use in phage therapy (**Figure 7**).

E. cloacae Phage Host Range and Virulence

The antibiotic sensitivity and phage killing phenotypes of four phages on *E. cloacae* clinical isolates are shown in **Figure 8**. The phages were strong killers, especially for *E. cloacae* isolates from LVAD infections where the original source of the infection may have been the skin. Only one phage strongly killed *E. cloacae* isolates from UTI. More isolates from various sites must be examined to determine if site of origin of the bacteria affects the efficacy of phage killing. **Figure 9**, a summary of antibiotic sensitivity and phage killing of the isolates examined, shows > 70% of strains killed by all individual phages and only a small gain in killing by a cocktail composed of two phages when compared to the best single phage.

A

Properties of *P. aeruginosa* Phages

Feature	φKMV	φPa2	φPaer4	φE2005-24-39	4φC20-Clone 2	4φC20-Clone 5	4φC20-Clone 7	4φC20-Clone 9
Phage Characteristics:								
Source Species	?	?	?	Human	--	--	--	--
Source	Pond Water Moscow	ATCC 14203-B1	CDC	Sewage Dekalb, GA	Lab-HRE	Lab-HRE	Lab-HRE	Lab-HRE
Isolation Date	2003 [1]	?	?	2005 [2]	10/18/12	10/18/12	10/18/12	10/18/12
Isolation Strain	PAO1=	PAO1r≈	Psa Strain Paer4	Psa Strain E2005-A	PAO1	PAO1	PAO1	PAO1
Plaque Size (mm)	4-5 mm + wide Halo	3-4 mm	2-3 mm	~1 mm	1.5mm	2.5mm	3.0mm	1.0mm
Plaque Morph.	Clear+Halo	Clear	Clear	Clear	Clear	Clear	Clear	Clear
Plate Stock (PFU/ml)*	4.8×10^9	2.1×10^{10}	1.2×10^{10}	5.7×10^8	4.0×10^8	2.0×10^{10}	1.8×10^{11}	1.4×10^8
CsCl Purified (PFU/ml)*	6.0×10^{12}	6.6×10^{12}	2.4×10^{11}	1.1×10^{12}	2.0×10^{11}	2.0×10^{11}	2.0×10^{10}	2.0×10^{11}
EM Morphology	Podovirus	Podovirus	Podovirus	Myovirus	Podovirus^	Podovirus^	Podovirus^	Podovirus^
Sequence								
Accession No.	AJ505558	NC027345	MN508619	MN508620	ND	MN 553583	MN553584	MN553585
Genome (BP)	42,351	73,008	45,319	66,285	ND	72,601	72,474	42,232
G + C (%)	62.3%	54.9%	52.49%	55.25%	ND	54.89%	54.89%	62.25%
ORFs	49	91	70	97	ND	92	90	58
tRNAs	0	0	3	0	ND	0	0	0
Toxin/Virulence Genes	None	None	None	None	ND	None	None	None
Lysogeny Cassettes	None	None	None	None	ND	None	None	None
Abx-Resistance Genes	None	None	None	None	ND	None	None	None
Closest Relative	ΦKMV	ΦPa2	DL54	vB_Pae_PS44	ND	ΦPa2	ΦPa2	ΦKMV
Genus	ΦKMV-like	Lit1-like	Luz24-like	Pbunalike	ND	Lit1-like	Lit1-like	ΦKMV-like
Growth Properties								
Adsorption Const. (mL/min) [4]	4.07×10^{-10}	2.00×10^{-9}	8.01×10^{-9}	2.30×10^{-9}	2.18×10^{-9}	1.22×10^{-10}	6.28×10^{-10}	3.37×10^{-10}
% Adsorbed (10 min)	3.2%	63.3%	43.8%	84.9%	16.4%	13%	9%	22.4%
Latent Period [5]	32 min	41 min	30 min	36 min	28 min	44 min	40 min	22 min
Burst Size	184	25	17.9	102	100	127	153	198
Summary of Phage Killing Spectra – # Lysed/# Tested (% lysed)								
HRE Development and Test Strains – EOP>0.1 only								
Develop. Strains N = 16	2/16† (13%)	5/16 (31%)	2/16 (13%)	2/16 (13%)	3/16 (19%)	7/16 (44%)	7/16 (44%)	3/16 (19%)
Test strains N = 10	1/10† (10%)	0/10 (0%)	1/10 (10%)	1/10 (10%)	2/10 (20%)	2/10 (20%)	2/10 (20%)	0/10 (0%)
Clinical Isolates (N=64)								
(EOP > 0.1)	3/64# (5%)	1/64 (2%)	7/64 (11%)	15/64 (23%)	0/64 (0%)	11/64 (17%)	13/64 (20%)	1/64 (2%)
Mean (EOP>0.1)	Parental φ: 10% Strains Killed				20 HRE cycle φ clones: 10% Strains Killed			
(EOP > 0.001)	7/64# (11%)	13/64 (20%)	13/64 (20%)	21/64 (33%)	6/64 (9%)	19/64 (29%)	19/64 (30%)	15/64 (23%)
Mean (EOP>0.001)	Parental φ: 21% Strains Killed				20 HRE cycle φ clones: 23% Strains Killed			

= *P. aeruginosa* lab strain
† No. killed/No. tested *P. aeruginosa* strains used for host range expansion (HRE)
# No. killed/No. tested *P. aeruginosa* clinical isolates tested
* Representative purified or plate stock
Parental Phages were φKMV, φPa2, φPaer4, φE2005-24-29. Other phages are clones from Host Range Expansion (HRE).

FIGURE 4 | Continued

B	Properties of *P. aeruginosa* Phages							
	P. aeruginosa Phage							
Feature	φKMVC⁵-(121)-Clone 4a	φKMVC⁵-(121)-Clone 13	φKMVC⁵-(111)-Clone 4	φKMVC⁵-(111)-Clone 12	4φC³⁰-DS38-Clone 39	4φC³⁰-DS38-Clone 57	4φC³⁰-DS38-Clone 54	4φC³⁰-DS38-Clone 20
Phage Characteristics;								
Source Species	--	--	--	--	--	--	--	--
Source	Lab-HRE	Lab-HRE	Lab-HRE	Lab-HRE	Lab-HRE	Lab-HRE	Lab-HRE	Lab-HRE
Isolation Date	2014	2014	2014	2014	2015	2015	2015	2015
Isolation Strain	PAO1	PAO1	BWT111	BWT111	DS38	DS38	DS38	DS38
Plaque Size (mm)	~3mm	~3mm	~3mm	~2mm	~2mm	~2mm	~2mm	~2mm
Plaque Morph.	Clear+Halo	Clear+Halo	Clear+Halo	Clear	Clear+halo	Clear+halo	Clear+halo	Clear+halo
Plate Stock (PFU/ml)	1.6×10^{10}	3.0×10^{10}	2.6×10^{10}	9.0×19^{9}	1.7×10^{9}	1.4×10^{8}	1.1×10^{9}	1.8×10^{9}
CsCl Purified (PFU/ml)⁎	2.6×10^{12}	6.0×10^{12}	2.0×10^{12}	2.0×10^{12}	1.7×10^{10}	1.9×10^{9}	1.6×10^{9}	4.6×10^{9}
EM Morphology	Podovirus^	Podovirus^	Podovirus^	Podovirus^	ND	ND	ND	ND
Sequence								
Accession No.	MN553587	MN553589	MN553586	MN553588	ND	ND	ND	ND
Genome (BP)	42,231	42,231	45,446	42,432	ND	ND	ND	ND
G + C (%)	62.23	62.25	52.48	62.24	ND	ND	ND	ND
ORFs	59	58	71	59	ND	ND	ND	ND
tRNAs	0	0	3	0	ND	ND	ND	ND
Toxin/Virulence Genes	None	None	None	None	ND	ND	ND	ND
Lysogeny Cassettes	None	None	None	None	ND	ND	ND	ND
Abx-Resistance Genes	None	None	None	None	ND	ND	ND	ND
Closest Relative	ΦKMV	ΦKMV	DL54	ΦKMV	ND	ND	ND	ND
Genus	ΦKMV-like	ΦKMV-like	Luz24-like	ΦKMV-like	ND	ND	ND	ND
Growth Properties								
Adsorption Const. (mL/min) [4]	9.41×10^{-10}	5.54×10^{-10}	1.08×10^{-9}	1.05×10^{-9}	7.30×10^{-10}	1.30×10^{-9}	1.83×10^{-9}	1.64×10^{-9}
% Adsorbed (10 min)	50.7%	34.5%	63.3%	49.6%	51.4%	71.7%	87.9%	84.8%
Latent Period [5]	18 min	22 min	28 min	18 min	48 min	40 min	30 min	32 min
Burst Size	42	7	100	17.6	72	109	63.9	94.0
Summary of Phage Killing Spectra – # Lysed/# Tested (% lysed)								
HRE Development and Test Strains – EOP>0.1 only								
Develop. Strains N = 16	4/16† (25%)	9/16 (56%)	11/16 (69%)	8/16 (50%)	10/16 (63%)	10/16 (63%)	10/16 (63%)	8/16 (50%)
Test strains N = 10	2/10† (20%)	4/10 (40%)	9/10 (90%)	3/10 (30%)	2/10 (20%)	5/10 (50%)	6/10 (60%)	2/10 (20%)
Clinical Isolates (N=64)								
(EOP > 0.1)	1/64 (2%)	5/64 (8%)	6/64 (9%)	18/64 (28%)	15/64 (23%)	19/64 (30%)	26/64 (41%)	28/64 (44%)
Mean (EOP>0.1)	5 HRE cycle φ clones: 12% Strains Killed				30 HRE cycle φ clones: 34% Strains Killed			
(EOP > 0.001)	7/64 (11%)	12/64 (19%)	12/64 (19%)	26/64 (41%)	20/64 (31%)	38/64 (59%)	37/64 (58%)	37/64 (58%)
Mean (EOP>0.001)	5 HRE cycle φ clones: 22% Strains Killed				30 HRE cycle φ clones: Strains Killed 52%			

⁼ *P. aeruginosa* lab strain
† No. killed/No. tested *P. aeruginosa* strains used for host range expansion (HRE)
⁎ No. killed/No. tested *P. aeruginosa* clinical isolates tested
⁎ Representative purified or plate stock
Parental Phages were φKMV, φPa2, φPaer4, φE2005-24-29. Other phages are clones from Host Range Expansion (HRE).

FIGURE 4 | (A,B) Summary of characterization of *Pseudomonas aeruginosa* phages. The characteristics, DNA sequences, growth properties and a summary of phage killing spectra are presented for each phage.

DISCUSSION

This study presents a *"sur mesure"* approach to phage therapy (Pirnay et al., 2011). Here phage libraries were constructed, characterized, and prepared for use in preclinical or clinical situations. Specifically, we plan to concurrently test clinical isolates against phages from the appropriate library to identify phages for mono- or cocktail-based therapy while they are being characterized in the clinical microbiology laboratory. It will then be the physician's choice to treat the patient with phage alone, antimicrobials alone or the combination of the two. A broader interpretation of the *"sur mesure"* approach is to develop a phage library using the full spectrum of bacterial strains available in the clinical microbiology laboratory of a specific medical facility, so that the shelf-ready phage strains or cocktails can reasonably be expected to cover multidrug-resistant organisms that cause infections in patients in that facility. These libraries can be tested in the clinical laboratory of the hospital,

Representative Antibiotic Sensitivity and Phage Killing Spectra of *P. aeruginosa* Strains

Clinical Source of Isolates	Anatomic Source[†]	Date Collected	Antibiotic Sensitivity							*Pseudomonas aeruginosa* Clinical Isolate	Phage and Killing (EOP)															
												Parental*				Host Range Expanded#											
			Amikacin	Cefepime	Pip/Tazobactam	Gentamicin	Imipenem	Levofloxacin	Ceftazidime		φKMV	φPA2	φPaer4	φE2005	4φ-C20-(PAO1)-Clone 2	4φ-C20-(PAO1)-Clone 5	4φ-C20-(PAO1)-Clone 7	4φ-C20-(PAO1)-Clone 9	φKMV-C5-(PAO1)-Clone 4a	φKMV-C5-(PAO1)-Clone 13	φKMV-C5-(BWT111)-Clone 4	φKMV-C5-(PAO1)-Clone 12	4φ-C30-(DS38)-Clone 20	4φ-C30-(DS38)-Clone 39	4φ-C30-(DS38)-Clone 54	4φ-C30-(DS38)-Clone 57
Houston VA Hospital	U	01/25/17								DS330-1																
	U	01/26/17								DS331																
	U	02/22/17								DS345																
	U	02/26/17								DS350																
	U	03/02/17								DS352																
	U	03/08/17								DS356																
	U	03/05/17								DS357																
	U	03/17/17								DS358																
	U	03/15/17								DS360																
	U	03/20/17								DS362																
	U	03/20/17								DS363																
	Sp	03/16/17								DS364																
	U	07/03/17								DS370																
	Sy	06/29/17								DS371																
	U	06/27/17								DS372																
	U	07/03/17								DS373																

Footnotes	Key to Antibiotic Sensitivity		Key to Phage Killing (EOP)	
[†] Isolate Source: U=urine; B=blood; Sp=sputum, S=stone, Sy=synovial, L=LVAD driveline	Sensitive		+	EOP > 1.0000
* Parental Phages for (HRE)	Intermediate			EOP between 0.100 – 1.000
# Phage clones generated by HRE	Resistant			EOP between 0.001 – 0.099
4φ -mixture of 4 parentals in HRE	NT Not Tested			EOP < 0.001; not useful
φKMV - from KMV alone HRE			-	No Growth
Cˣˣ: Number of cycles of HRE				Reference (EOP = 1.000)
(XXX): isolation strain of phage clone			EOP = Titer X / Titer Reference	

FIGURE 5 | Representative data for antibiotic sensitivity and phage killing (EOP) of clinical isolates of *P. aeruginosa*. Shown are the properties of the *P. aeruginosa* clinical isolates on the left, including: source, date of isolation and antibiotic sensitivity data (VITEK2). On the right are shown the killing spectra of the phages on the individual *P. aeruginosa* clinical isolates. The keys to antibiotic sensitivity and phage killing (EOP) are shown at the bottom of the figure.

or the hospital can send isolates for phage susceptibility testing to basic science laboratories that agree to participate, such as those associated with educational institutions (Center for Phage Technology, Texas A&M University, United States; The Tailored Antimicrobials and Innovative Laboratories for Phage Research [tialφr], Baylor College of Medicine, Houston, TX, United States), government laboratories (The Biological Defense Research Directorate of the Naval Medical Research Center, United States; The Eliava Institute, Tbilisi, Georgia; The Phage Therapy Unit, The Hirzfeld Institute, Poland; Center for Innovative Phage Applications and Therapeutics [IPATH], UCSD, San Diego, CA, United States), or industry partners (AmpliPhi Biosciences; Adaptive Phage Therapeutics). For example, we are prospectively collecting bacterial strains from the urine of all hospitalized patients with SCI at our Veterans Affairs Hospital, so that we can create phage libraries to treat any bacterial pathogens causing urosepsis among those SCI patients. Similarly, at the Baylor-St.

Luke's hospital we are collecting all bacterial strains causing infections of left-ventricular assist device (LVAD) drivelines. In both situations our goal is to create a phage library that is able to treat infections caused by the most antibiotic resistant bacteria in that specific clinical setting. While creating phage libraries for many species seems like an attainable goal, it is likely to be more difficult for some species. Phages against *Staphylococcus aureus* are infrequently isolated from environmental samples (Mattila et al., 2015; Latz et al., 2016) and identification of phages active against *Clostridium difficile* required induction of lysogens (Hargreaves et al., 2015). Thus, construction of large libraries of phage will depend on the target bacterial species.

Despite the near certainly that phage-resistant bacteria will emerge during therapy, we envision multiple clinical scenarios in which even a single well-timed dose of phage, in addition to standard antibiotics, may be life saving. For example, rapid initiation of effective antimicrobial therapy is essential to

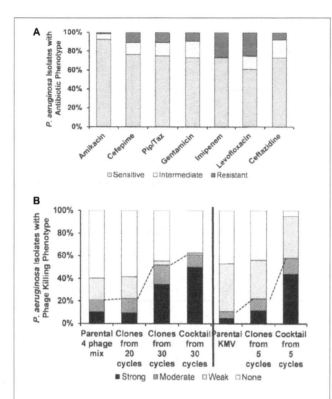

FIGURE 6 | Antibiotic Sensitivities and Phage Killing Phenotypes of *P. aeruginosa* Clinical Isolates (N = 64). **(A)** Antibiotic sensitivities based on cut off values used in the microbiology lab at the Houston VA Hospital. **(B)** The phage killing phenotypes were based on EOP. Strong killers, EOP > 0.1; Moderate Killers, 0.099 > EOP > 0.001; Weak Killers, EOP < 0.00099 but positive; None, no growth. Strong and moderate killers have EOP high enough to be useful in phage therapy (dotted lines indicate useful levels of killing). The 30 cycle 4 phage cocktail: consisted of equal titers of the following host range expanded phages: $4\phi C$-C^{30}-(DS38)-Clone 20, $4\phi C$-C^{30}-(DS38)-Clone 39, $4\phi C$-C^{30}-(DS38)-Clone 54, and $4\phi C$-C^{30}-(DS38)-Clone 57. The "5 cycle KMV cocktail" consisted of clones: ϕKMV-C^5-(PAO1)-Clone 4a, ϕKMV-C^5-(PAO1)-Clone 13, ϕKMV-C^5-(PAO1)-Clone 12, and ϕKMV-C^5-(BWT111)-Clone 4. Pip/Taz, piperacillin/tazobactam.

preventing clinical deterioration in sepsis (Kalil et al., 2017). Many patients are at high risk for sepsis caused by antibiotic resistant organisms, by virtue of prior healthcare exposures and/or known colonization with multidrug-resistant organisms. When such high-risk patients present with sepsis, a few early doses of a broad-spectrum phage cocktail used empirically, together with empiric antibiotics could act as a safety net, ensuring adequate coverage of the causative organisms, until the microbiology lab can identify the organism and determine its antibiotic sensitivities. In this scenario a "*sur mesure*" phage cocktail developed against the full panel of multidrug-resistant organisms isolated in the clinical microbiology laboratory of that specific institution would be used for initial treatment together with empiric antibiotics. Another example of a clinical scenario in which a single dose of phage might be very useful would be to temporarily sterilize a patient's urine prior to an invasive urologic procedure. Phage cocktails mixed specifically for the organisms found in standard pre-procedure urine cultures at a given institution would offer a more targeted approach than our

current approach, which involves wiping out the bladder and much of the bowel flora with broad spectrum antibiotics.

In contrast, treatment of biofilm infections, such as those that cause life-threatening LVAD infections, would likely require a longer course of phage therapy, in part because of the longer clinical time frame given the chronicity of LVAD infections. New phage cocktails could be mixed to address phage-resistant bacterial pathogens that might develop during the course of therapy. Alternatively, treating these biofilm infections with phage and antibiotics simultaneously may allow for synergy, particularly if the phage is able to restore antibiotic susceptibility in the infecting pathogen (Comeau et al., 2007; Ryan et al., 2012; Chaudhry et al., 2017). This approach of re-mixing *sur-mesure* phage cocktails and using them together with an antibiotic to which the infecting organism is resistant was successful in treating a patient with disseminated *Acinetobacter* infection (Schooley et al., 2017).

To achieve these clinical goals, we have demonstrated that unmanipulated phages isolated from the environment on *E. coli* ST131, are capable of lysing as many as 58% of a collection of 76 *E. coli* clinical isolates. Cocktails of as few as three of the individual phages ($\phi HP3$, $\phi ES12$, and $\phi ES17$) were capable of lysing 92% of the 76 clinical isolates. These results indicate that environmental samples provide good reservoirs of phages capable of being used against *E. coli*, and that highly effective cocktails can be generated from them. In all cases the cocktails tested were highly effective against clinical isolates, killing at EOP > 0.1. The highly effective killing of the phages and the high titers obtained in the CsCl-purified preparations indicates that these phages should be useful in clinical therapy where a concentrated dose could be administered without fear of generating a septic response due to the presence of contaminating endotoxin (**Figures 1**, **4A,B**, **7**). Similar broad coverage was found for *E. cloacae* phages. In addition, we demonstrated that laboratory isolates of *P. aeruginosa*-specific phages can evolve to expand their host ranges to *P. aeruginosa* clinical isolates. A mixture of four parental phages subjected to 20 or 30 cycles of host range expansion was capable of killing 2–44% of the 64 clinical isolates tested, whereas the uncycled parental phages could lyse only 2–23% of the clinical isolates. However, cocktails containing as few as three individual HRE-derived phages were capable of killing 52 of the 64 clinical isolates tested (81%) (**Figure 6**). Additional cycles of HRE using the 12 clinical isolates not killed by any of the phages at useable EOP (>0.001), seems likely to further expand the host range among those isolates.

In addition to phage isolation for *E. coli*-, *P. aeruginosa*-, and *E. cloacae*-specific phage collections, a number of parameters were characterized that can be useful in choosing phages for phage therapy, making new phage isolates, and general work with the phages (Abedon, 2017). Our "phage master lists" (**Figures 1**, **4A,B**, **7**) contain information on the source of the phages, morphology, growth properties, DNA sequence, and host range much like a Physician's Desk Reference provides useful parameters for chemical antibiotics. The DNA sequence analyses and morphologies of the phages are important to establish the relationship of the individual phage to other phages in the databases (Weber-Dabrowska et al., 2016;

Properties of *Enterobacter cloacae* Phages

Feature	E. cloacae Phage			
	φEC-W1	φEC-W2	φEC-F1	φEC-F2
Phage Characteristics				
Source Species	Human	Human	Human	Human
Source Location (Houston)	Raw Sewage	Raw Sewage	Raw Sewage	Raw Sewage
Isolation Date	03/25/19	03/27/19	03/25/19	03/27/19
Isolation Strain	E.c –W*	E.c –W*	E.c –F*	E.c –F*
Plaque Size (mm)	1.0-1.5	1.0-1.5	1.0-1.5	1.0-1.5
Plaque Morph.	Clear	Clear	Clear	Clear
Plate Stock (PFU/ml)^	1.2×10^{10}	4.2×10^{10}	5.6×10^{9}	1.0×10^{10}
CsCl Purified (PFU/ml)^	2.2×10^{11}	7.2×10^{11}	1.0×10^{11}	8.6×10^{12}
EM Morphology	Myovirus	Myovirus	Myovirus	Myovirus
Sequence				
(Accession No.)	MN 508621	MN 508622	MN 508623	MN 508624
Genome (BP)	178,607	176,610	178,147	178,307
G + C (%)	44.79%	44.72%	44.74	44.73
ORFs	283	275	277	278
tRNAs	2	1	2	2
Toxin/Virulence Genes	None	None	None	None
Lysogeny Genes	None	None	None	None
Abx-Resistance Genes	None	None	None	None
Closest Relative	Margaery	vB_CsaM_GAP161	vB_CsaM_GAP161	vB_CsaM_GAP161
Genus	T4-like	T4-like	T4-like	T4-like
Growth Properties				
Adsorption Constant (mL/min)	9.52×10^{-7}	7.31×10^{-8}	4.51×10^{-7}	2.74×10^{-7}
% Adsorbed (10 min)	99.0	34.6	83.7	72..0
Latent Period (Min)	21	24	25	20
Burst Size (PFU/cell)	15.7	20.4	33.5	18.6
Summary of Phage Killing Spectra – No. Lysed/No. Tested (% Lysed)				
E.cl. SCI• isolates[†] (N=2)				
(EOP > 0.1)	1/2 (50%)	0/2 (0%)	0/2 (0%)	0/2 (0%)
(EOP > 0.001)	1/2 (50%)	0/2 (0%)	0/2 (0%)	0/2 (0%)
E.cl. LVAD[††] isolates[#] (N=10)				
(EOP > 0.1)	9/10 (90%)	9/10 (90%)	9/10 (90%)	8/10 (80%)
(EOP > 0.001)	0/10 (0%)	0/10 (0)%)	1/10 (10%)	2/10 (80%)
Total Strains (N=14)				
(EOP > 0.1)	12/14 (86%)	11/14 (78%)	12/14 (86%)	12/14 (86%)
(EOP > 0.001)	1/14 (7%)	0/14 (0%)	1/14 (7%)	2/14 (14%)

* *Enterobacter cloacae* isolated from a hip prosthesis.
    E.c.-W = isolate from wound
    E.c.-F = isolate from wound fluid (different date)
[†] *Enterobacter cloacae* isolated from spinal cord injured patient urine (Houston VA Hospital)
[#] *Enterobacter cloacae* isolated from left ventricular assist device driveline infection
    (Houston St. Luke's Hospital)
^ Titer of representative preparation
• SCI = from patient with spinal cord injury
[††] LVAD = left ventricular assist device driveline

FIGURE 7 | Summary of characterization of *Enterobacter cloacae* phages. The characteristics, DNA sequences, growth properties and a summary of phage killing spectra are presented for each phage.

Casey et al., 2018). In addition, DNA sequence analysis provides important information on the properties of the phage genome, ensuring that phages can be used as therapeutic agents because they do not encode genes to establish and maintain lysogeny, toxins, virulence factors, or antibiotic resistance. The data on adsorption constant, adsorption rate, latent period, and burst size all represent parameters that can affect the success of phage therapy (Weber-Dabrowska et al., 2016). Finally, in our determinations of phage host range we examined EOP, a parameter that allows one to determine the relative killing power of a phage on a test strain compared to its killing power on the isolation strain. EOP has been shown to be an excellent method for estimating phage virulence on a given bacterial strain. Simple spot tests of high titer phage were found to overestimate

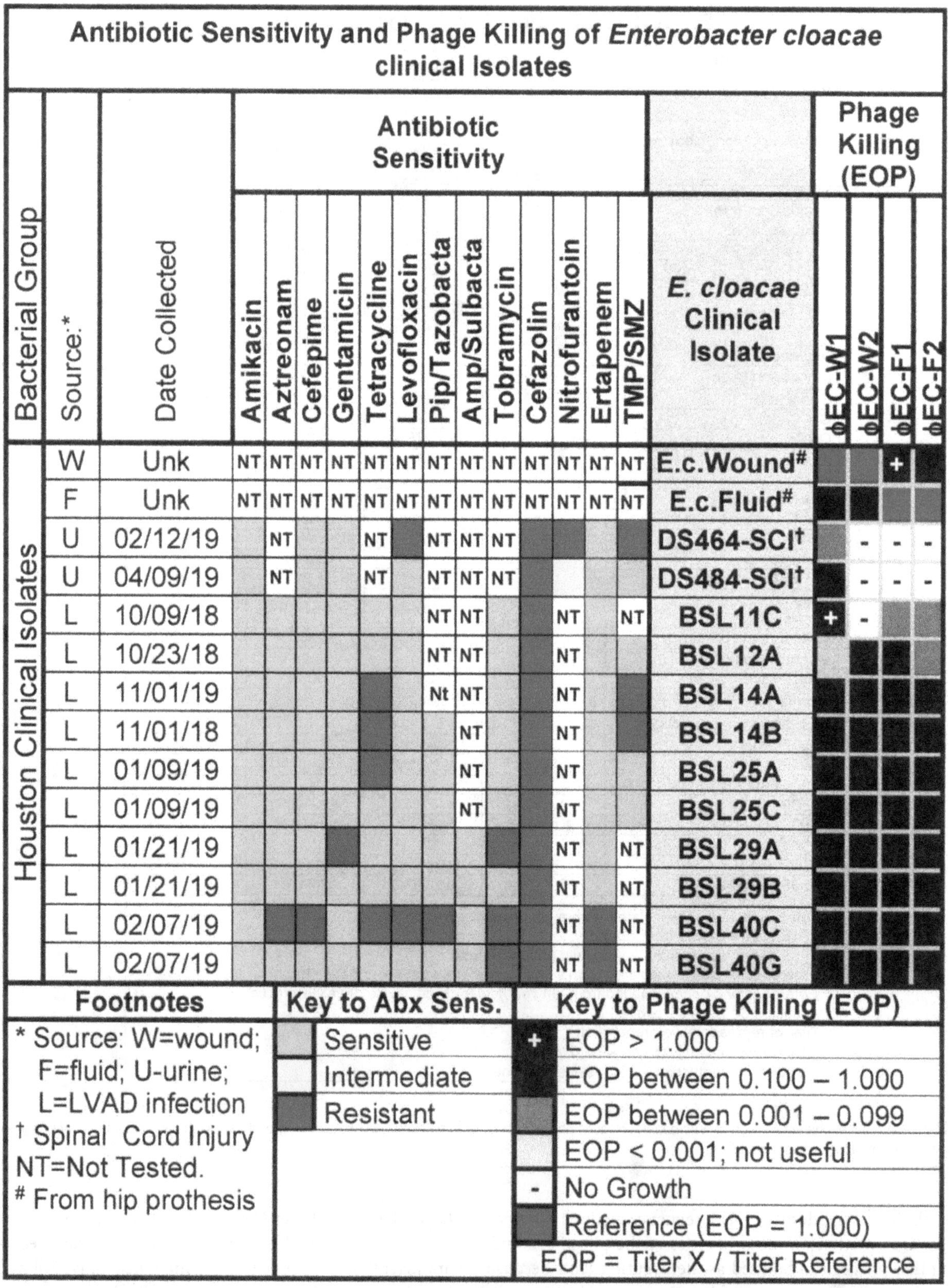

Antibiotic Sensitivity and Phage Killing of *Enterobacter cloacae* clinical Isolates

Bacterial Group	Source*	Date Collected	Amikacin	Aztreonam	Cefepime	Gentamicin	Tetracycline	Levofloxacin	Pip/Tazobacta	Amp/Sulbacta	Tobramycin	Cefazolin	Nitrofurantoin	Ertapenem	TMP/SMZ	*E. cloacae* Clinical Isolate	φEC-W1	φEC-W2	φEC-F1	φEC-F2
Houston Clinical Isolates	W	Unk	NT	NT	NT	NT	NT	NT	NT	NT	NT	NT	NT	NT	NT	E.c.Wound#			+	
	F	Unk	NT	NT	NT	NT	NT	NT	NT	NT	NT	NT	NT	NT	NT	E.c.Fluid#				
	U	02/12/19		NT			NT		NT	NT	NT					DS464-SCI†		-	-	-
	U	04/09/19		NT			NT		NT	NT	NT					DS484-SCI†		-	-	-
	L	10/09/18						NT	NT			NT		NT		BSL11C	+	-		
	L	10/23/18						NT	NT			NT				BSL12A				
	L	11/01/19						Nt	NT			NT				BSL14A				
	L	11/01/18							NT			NT				BSL14B				
	L	01/09/19							NT			NT				BSL25A				
	L	01/09/19							NT			NT				BSL25C				
	L	01/21/19											NT		NT	BSL29A				
	L	01/21/19											NT		NT	BSL29B				
	L	02/07/19											NT		NT	BSL40C				
	L	02/07/19											NT		NT	BSL40G				

Footnotes	Key to Abx Sens.	Key to Phage Killing (EOP)
* Source: W=wound; F=fluid; U-urine; L=LVAD infection † Spinal Cord Injury NT=Not Tested. # From hip prothesis	Sensitive Intermediate Resistant	+ EOP > 1.000 EOP between 0.100 – 1.000 EOP between 0.001 – 0.099 EOP < 0.001; not useful - No Growth Reference (EOP = 1.000) EOP = Titer X / Titer Reference

FIGURE 8 | Representative data for antibiotic sensitivity and phage killing (EOP) of clinical isolates of *E. cloacae*. Shown are the properties of the *E. cloacae* clinical isolates on the left, including: source, date of isolation and antibiotic sensitivity data (VITEK2). On the right are shown the killing spectra of the phages on the individual *E. cloacae* clinical isolates. The keys to antibiotic sensitivity and phage killing (EOP) are shown at the bottom of the figure.

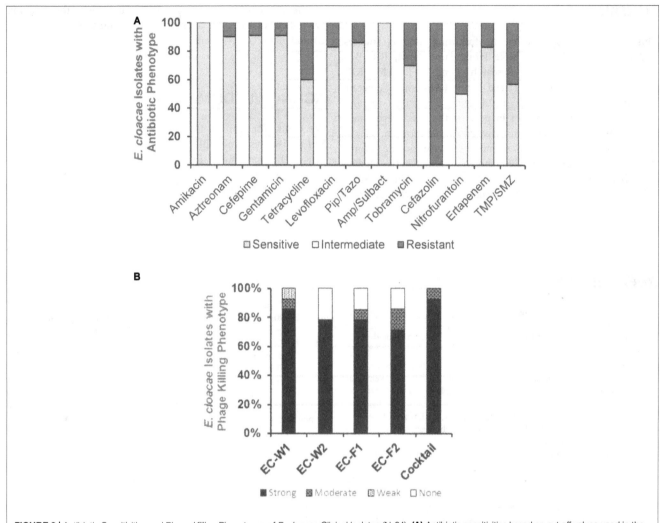

FIGURE 9 | Antibiotic Sensitivities and Phage Killing Phenotypes of *E. cloacae* Clinical Isolates (N-64). **(A)** Antibiotic sensitivities based on cut off values used in the microbiology lab at the Houston VA Hospital. **(B)** The phage killing phenotypes were based on EOP. Strong killers, EOP > 0.1; Moderate Killers, 0.099 > EOP > 0.001; Weak Killers, EOP < 0.00099 but positive; None, no growth. The cocktail was consisted of equal titers of φEC-W1 and φEC-W2. Pip/Taz, piperacillin/tazobactam; TMA/SMZ, trimethoprim/sulfamethoxazole.

both the virulence and the host range of a phage (Mirzaei and Nilsson, 2015). Indeed, we have shown that phage virulence and bacterial susceptibility to the phage determined *in vitro* allowed us to predict the outcome of therapy *in vivo* (Green et al., 2017). While bacterial receptors for the phages were not identified here, that information is important for the rational mixing of phage cocktails. We are in the process of identifying receptors for phages in our libraries, and have identified the receptor for φHP3 as lipopolysaccharide in the *E. coli* JJ2528 host (unpublished data). Having all these parameters at hand aids in the selection of a phage for monotherapy, or a mixture of phages for cocktail therapy. Cesium chloride purified stocks of all phages described here exist and their endotoxin content has been reduced below clinically permissible levels, so that they can quickly be put to use. Our *E. coli*, *P. aeruginosa*, and *E. cloacae* phage libraries are now ready for rigorous *in vivo* studies in animal models of urinary tract infections and LVAD infections, as well as available for compassionate use protocols in humans.

ETHICS STATEMENT

The collection of de-identified clinical isolates was approved by the Baylor College of Medicine Institutional Review Board (IRB).

AUTHOR CONTRIBUTIONS

AM, RR, HK, and BT conceived the experiments and guided their performance. SBG, SIG, CL, JC, AT, and KS performed the experiments and analyzed the results. BT arranged for collection of clinical isolates and corresponding antibiotic sensitivity data. RR wrote the manuscript with editing from BT, HK, and AM. All authors contributed to manuscript revision, read and approved the submitted version.

FUNDING

This work was supported by the following funding sources: 1R21AI121545 (RR), The Mike Hogg Fund (AM, RR, BT), The MacDonald General Research Fund (BT, AM, RR), Baylor College of Medicine seed funds (AM), and Veterans Administration RR&D I01 RX002595 (BT). The research reported here was supported in part by the U.S. Department of Veterans Affairs, Veterans Health Administration, Health Services Research and Development Service at the Center for Innovations in Quality, Effectiveness and Safety, Michael E. DeBakey VA Medical Center, Houston, TX, United States (CIN 13-413). The views expressed in this article are those of the authors and do not necessarily reflect the position or policy of the Department of Veterans Affairs or the United States Government.

ACKNOWLEDGMENTS

We thank Jim Johnson for providing well-characterized *E. coli* ST131 isolates from his collection. Laura Dillon and Dr. Faisal Cheema assisted in collecting clinical isolates from the hospital. Dr. Jason Kaelber and Kara Schoenemann performed electron microscopy.

REFERENCES

Abedon, S. T. (2011). Lysis from without. *Bacteriophage* 1, 46–49. doi: 10.4161/bact.1.1.13980

Abedon, S. T. (2017). Information phage therapy research should report. *Pharmaceuticals* 10:42. doi: 10.3390/ph10020043

Aslam, S., Pretorius, V., Lehman, S. M., Morales, S., and Schooley, R. T. (2019). Novel bacteriophage therapy for treatment of left ventricular assist device infection. *J. Heart Lung Transplant.* 38, 475–476. doi: 10.1016/j.healun.2019.01.001

Aziz, R. K., Bartels, D., Best, A. A., DeJongh, M., Disz, T., Edwards, R. A., et al. (2008). The RAST server: rapid annotations using subsystems technology. *BMC Genomics* 9:75. doi: 10.1186/1471-2164-9-75

Bankevich, A., Nurk, S., Antipov, D., Gurevich, A. A., Dvorkin, M., Kulikov, A. S., et al. (2012). SPAdes: a new genome assembly algorithm and its applications to single-cell sequencing. *J. Comput. Biol.* 19, 455–477. doi: 10.1089/cmb.2012.0021

Bassetti, M., Poulacou, G., Ruppe, E., Bouza, E., Van Hal, S. J., and Brink, A. (2017). Antimicrobial resistance in the next 30 years, humankind, bugs and drugs; a visionary approach. *Intensive Care Med.* 43, 1464–1475. doi: 10.1007/s00134-017-4878-x

Besemer, J. (2001). GeneMarkS: a self-training method for prediction of gene starts in microbial genomes. Implications for finding sequence motifs in regulatory regions. *Nucleic Acids Res.* 29, 2607–2618. doi: 10.1093/nar/29.12.2607

Boucher, H. W., Talbot, G. H., Bradley, J. S., Edwards, J. E., Gilbert, D., Rice, L. B., et al. (2009). Bad bugs, no drugs; no ESKAPE: an update from the infectious diseases society of America. *Clin. Infect. Dis.* 48, 1–12. doi: 10.1086/595011

Burrowes, B. (2011). *Analysis of the Appelman protocol for the Generation of Therapeutic Bacteriophages.* Ph.D. thesis, Texas Tech Health Sciences center, Lubbock, TX.

Burrowes, B. H., Molineux, I. J., and Fralick, J. A. (2019). Directed in vitro evolution of therapeutic bacteriophages: the Appelmans protocol. *Viruses* 11:241. doi: 10.3390/v11030241

Casey, E., van Sinderen, D., and Mahoney, J. (2018). In vitro characteristics of phages to guide 'real life' phage therapy suitability. *Viruses* 10:163. doi: 10.3390/v10040163

Centers for Disease Control [CDC] (2013). *Antibiotic Resistance Threats in the United States.* Available at: https://www.cdc.gov/drugresistance/pdf/ar-threats-2013-508.pdf (accessed May 10, 2018).

Chan, B. K., Sistrom, M., Wertz, J. E., Kortright, K. E., Narayan, D., and Turner, P. E. (2016). Phage selection restores antibiotic sensitivity in MDR *Pseudomonas aeruginosa. Sci. Rep.* 6:26717. doi: 10.1038/srep26717

Chan, B. K., Turner, P. E., Kim, S., Mojibian, H. R., Elefteriades, J. A., and Narayan, D. (2018). Phage treatment of an aortic graft infected with *Pseudomonas aeruginosa. Evol. Med. Public Health* 2018, 60–66. doi: 10.1093/emph/eoy005

Chanishvili, N. (2016). Phages as therapeutic and prophylactic means: summary of the soviet and post-soviet experience. *Curr. Drug Deliv.* 13, 309–323. doi: 10.2174/1567201813013160520193946

Chaudhry, W. N., Concepcion-Acevedo, J., Park, T., Andleeb, S., Bull, J. J., and Levin, B. R. (2017). Synergy and order effects of antibiotics and phages in killing *Pseudomonas aeruginosa* biofilms. *PLoS One* 12:e0168615. doi: 10.1371/journal.pone.0168615

Chen, L., Zheng, D., Liu, B., Yang, J., and Jin, Q. (2016). VFDB 2016: hierarchical and refined dataset for big data analysis—10 years on. *Nucleic Acids Res.* 44, D694–D697. doi: 10.1093/nar/gkv1239

Chibeu, A., Ceyssens, P. J., Hertveldt, K., Volkaert, G., Cornelis, P., Matthujs, S., et al. (2009). The adsorption of *Pseudomonas aeruginosa* bacteriophage phiKMV is dependent on expression regulation of type IV pili genes. *FEMS Microbiol. Lett.* 296, 210–218. doi: 10.1111/j.1574-6968.2009.01640.x

Comeau, A. M., Tetart, F., Trojet, S. N., Prere, M. F., and Krisch, H. M. (2007). Phage-antibiotic synergy (PAS): beta-lactam and quinolone antibiotics stimulate virulent phage growth. *PLoS One* 2:e799. doi: 10.1371/journal.pone.0000799

Debarbieux, L., Forterre, P., Krupovic, M., Kutateladze, M., and Prangishvili, D. (2018). Centennial celebration of bacteriophage research. *Res. Microbiol.* 169, 479–480. doi: 10.1016/j.resmic.2018.10.001

Debarbieux, L., Pirnay, J. P., Verbeken, G., De Vos, D., Merabishvili, M., Huys, I., et al. (2016). A bacteriophage journey at the european medicines agency. *FEMS Microtiol. Lett.* 363:fnv225. doi: 10.1093/femsle/fnv225

Delcher, A. L., Bratke, K. A., Powers, E. C., and Salzberg, S. L. (2007). Identifying bacterial genes and endosymbiont DNA with Glimmer. *Bioinformatics* 23, 673–679. doi: 10.1093/bioinformatics/btm009

El Haddad, L., Harb, C. P., Gebara, M. A., Stibuch, M. A., and Chemaly, R. F. (2018). A systematic and critical review of phage therapy against multi-drug resistant ESKAPE organisms in humans. *Clin. Infect. Dis.* 69, 167–178. doi: 10.1093/cid/ciy947

Fu, W., Forster, T., Mayer, O., Curtin, J. J., Lehman, S. M., and Donlan, R. M. (2010). Bacteriophage cocktail for the prevention of biofilm formation by *Pseudomonas aeruginosa* on catheters in an in vitro model system. *Antimicrob. Agents Chemother.* 54, 397–404. doi: 10.1128/AAC.00669-09

Gelman, D., Eisenkraft, A., Chanishvili, N., Nachman, D., Coppenhagem, G. S., and Hazan, R. (2018). The history and promising future of phage therapy in the military service. *J. Trauma Acute Care Surg.* 85(1S Suppl. 2), S18–S126. doi: 10.1097/TA.0000000000001809

Ghosh, C., Sarkar, P., Issa, R., and Haldar, J. (2018). Alternatives to conventional antibiotics in the era of antimicrobial resistance. *Trends Microbiol.* 27, 323–338. doi: 10.1016/j.tim.2018.12.010

Green, S. L., Kaelber, J. T., Ma, L., Trautner, B. W., Ramig, R. F., and Maresso, A. W. (2017). Bacteriophages from ExPEC reservoirs kill pandemic multidrug-resistant strains of clonal group ST131 in animal models of bacteremia. *Sci. Rep.* 7:46151. doi: 10.1038/srep46151

Hargreaves, K. R., Otieno, J. R., Thanki, A., Blades, M. J., Millard, A. D., Browne, H. P., et al. (2015). As clear as mud? determining the diversity and prevalence of prophages in the draft genomes of estuarine isolates of *Clostridium difficile*. *Genome Biol. Evol.* 7, 1842–1855. doi: 10.1093/gbe/evv094

Hyman, P. (2019). Phages for phage therapy: isolation, characterization, and host range breadth. *Pharmaceuticals* 12:35. doi: 10.3390/ph12010035

Johnson, J. R., Porter, S. B., Johnston, B., Thuras, P., Clock, S., Crupain, M., et al. (2017). Extraintestinal pathogenic and antimicrobial-resistant *Escherichia coli*, including sequence type 131 (ST131), from retail chicken breasts in the United States in 2013. *Appl. Environ. Microbiol.* 83:e02956-16. doi: 10.1128/AEM.02956-16

Johnson, J. R., Stell, A. L., and Delavari, P. (2001). Canine fees as reservoir of extraintestinal pathogenic *Escherichia coli*. *Infect. Immun.* 69, 1306–1314. doi: 10.1128/IAI.69.3.1306-1314.2001

Johnson, M., Zaretskaya, I., Raytselis, Y., Merezhuk, Y., McGinnis, S., and Madden, T. L. (2008). NCBI BLAST: a better web interface. *Nucleic Acids Res.* 36, W5–W9. doi: 10.1093/nar/gkn201

Kalil, A. C., Johnson, D. W., Lisco, S. J., and Sun, J. (2017). Early goal-directed therapy for sepsis: a novel solution for discordant survival outcomes in clinical trials. *Crit. Care Med.* 45, 607–614. doi: 10.1097/CCM.0000000000002235

Kropinski, A. M. (2009). "Measurement of the rate of attachment of bacteriophage to cells," in *Bacteriophages, Methods and Protocols, Volume 1: Isolation, Characterization, and Interactions*, eds M. R. J. Clokie, and A. M. Kropinski, (New York, NY: Humana Press), doi: 10.1007/978-1-60327-164-6-15

Kropinski, A. M. (2018). "Practical advice on the one-step growth curve," in *Bacteriophages, Methods and Protocols*, eds M. R. J. Clokie, A. Kropinski, and R. Lavigne, (New York, NY: Humana Press), doi: 10.1007/978-1-4939-7343-9-3

Kutter, E. M., Kuhl, S. J., and Abedon, S. T. (2015). Re-establishing a place for phage therapy in western medicine. *Future Microbiol.* 10, 685–688. doi: 10.4161/bact.1.2.15845

Labrie, S. J., Samson, J. E., and Moineau, S. (2010). Bacteriophage resistance mechanisms. *Nat. Rev. Microbiol.* 8, 317–327. doi: 10.1038/nrmicro2315

Laslett, D. (2004). ARAGORN, a program to detect tRNA genes and tmRNA genes in nucleotide sequences. *Nucleic Acids Res.* 32, 11–16. doi: 10.1093/nar/gkh152

Latz, S., Wahida, A., Arif, A., Hafner, H., Hoss, M., Ritter, K., et al. (2016). Preliminary survey of local bacteriophages with lytic activity agains multi-drug resistant bacteria. *J. Basic Microbiol.* 56, 1117–1123. doi: 10.1002/jobm.201600108

Lavigne, R., Burkal'tseva, M. V., Robben, J., Sykilinda, N. N., Kurochkina, L. P., Grymonprez, B., et al. (2003). The genome of bacteriophage phiKMV, a T7-like virus infecting *Pseudomonas aeruginosa*. *Virology* 312, 49–59. doi: 10.1016/S0042-6822(03)00123-5

Li, P.-E., Lo, C.-C., Anderson, J. J., Davenport, K. W., Bishop-Lilly, K. A., Xu, Y., et al. (2017). Enabling the democratization of the genomics revolution with a fully integrated web-based bioinformatics platform. *Nucleic Acids Res.* 45, 67–80. doi: 10.1093/nar/gkw1027

Liao, K. S., Lehman, S. M., Tweardy, D. J., Donlan, R. M., and Trautner, B. W. (2012). Bacteriophages are synergistic with bacterial interference for the prevention of *Pseudomonas aeruginosa* biofilm formation on urinary catheters. *J. Appl. Microbiol.* 113, 1530–1539. doi: 10.1111/j.1365-2672.2012.05432.x

Liu, B., and Pop, M. (2009). ARDB–Antibiotic Resistance Genes Database. *Nucleic Acids Res.* 37, D443–D447. doi: 10.1093/nar/gkn656

Lo, C.-C., and Chain, P. S. G. (2014). Rapid evaluation and quality control of next generation sequencing data with FaQCs. *BMC Bioinformatics* 15:366. doi: 10.1186/s12859-014-0366-362

Mao, C., Abraham, D., Wattam, A. R., Wilson, M. J., Shukla, M., Yoo, H. S., et al. (2015). Curation, integration and visualization of bacterial virulence factors in PATRIC. *Bioinformatics* 31, 252–258. doi: 10.1093/bioinformatics/btu631

Mapes, A. C., Trautner, B. W., Liao, K. S., and Ramig, R. F. (2016). Development of expanded host range phage active on multidrug-resistant *Pseudomonas aeruginosa*. *Bacteriophage* 6:e1096995. doi: 10.1080/21597081.2015.1096995

Mattila, S., Ruotsalainen, P., and Jalasvuori, M. (2015). On-Demand isolation of bacteriophages against drug-resistant bacteria for personalized phage therapy. *Front. Microbiol.* 6:1271. doi: 10.3389/fmicb.2015.01271

McArthur, A. G., Waglechner, N., Nizam, F., Yan, A., Azad, M. A., Baylay, A. J., et al. (2013). The comprehensive antibiotic resistance database. *Antimicrob Agents Chemother.* 57, 3348–3357. doi: 10.1128/AAC.00419-413

McNair, K., Aziz, R. K., Pusch, G. D., Overbeek, R., Dutilh, B. E., and Edwards, R. (2018). Phage genome annotation using the RAST pipeline. *Methods Mol. Biol.* 1681, 231–238. doi: 10.1007/978-1-4939-7343-9-17

McVay, C. S., Velasquez, M., and Fralick, J. A. (2007). Phage therapy of *Pseudomonas aeruginosa* infection in a mouse burn model. *Antimicrob. Agents Chemother.* 51, 1934–1938. doi: 10.1128/AAC.01028-06

Merabishvili, M., Pirnay, J.-P., and De Vos, D. (2018). Guidelines to compose an ideal bacteriophage cocktail. *Methods Mol. Biol.* 1693, 99–110. doi: 10.1007/978-1-4939-7395-8-9

Mirzaei, M. K., and Nilsson, A. S. (2015). Isolation of phages for phage therapy: a comparison of spot tests and efficiency of plating analyses for determination of host range and efficacy. *PLoS One* 10:e0118557. doi: 10.1371/journal.pone.0118557

Myelnikov, D. (2018). An alternative cure: the adoption and survival of phage therapy in the USSR, 1922-1955. *J. Hist. Med. Allied Sci.* 73, 385–411. doi: 10.1093/jhmas/jry024

Ormala, A. M., and Jalasvuori, M. (2013). Phage therapy: should bacterial resistance to phages be a concern, even in the long run? *Bacteriophage* 3:e24219. doi: 10.4161/bact.24219

Peng, Y., Leung, H. C. M., Yiu, S. M., and Chin, F. Y. L. (2010). IDBA – a practical iterative de bruijn graph de novo assembler. *Lecture Notes Comput. Sci.* 426–440. doi: 10.1007/978-3-642-12683-3-28

Peng, Y., Leung, H. C. M., Yiu, S. M., and Chin, F. Y. L. (2012). IDBA-UD: a de novo assembler for single-cell and metagenomic sequencing data with highly uneven depth. *Bioinformatics* 28, 1420–1428. doi: 10.1093/bioinformatics/bts174

Pirnay, J. P., De Vos, D., Verbeken, G., Merabishvili, M., Chanishvili, N., Vaneechoutte, M., et al. (2011). The phage therapy paradigm: Prêt à Porter or Sur-mesure? *Pharm. Res.* 28, 934–937. doi: 10.1007/s11095-010-0313-5

Pirnay, J. P., Merabishvili, M., Van Raemdonck, H., De Vos, D., and Verbeken, G. (2018). Phage production in compliance with regulatory requirements. *Meth. Mol. Biol.* 1693, 233–252. doi: 10.1007/978-1-4939-7395-8-18

Ryan, E. M., Alkawareek, M. Y., Donnelly, R. F., and Gilmore, B. F. (2012). Synergistic phage-antibiotic combinations for the control of *Escherichia coli* biofilms in vitro. *Immunol. Med. Microbiol.* 65, 395–398. doi: 10.1111/j.1574-695X.2012.00977.x

Schooley, R. T., Biswas, B., Gill, J. J., Hernandez-Morales, A., Lancaster, J., Lessor, L., et al. (2017). Development and use of personalized bacteriophage-based therapeutic cocktails to treat a patient with a disseminated resistant *Acinetobacter baumannii* infection. *Antimicrob. Agents Chemother.* 61:e00954-17. doi: 10.1128/AAC.00954-17

Seemann, T. (2014). Prokka: rapid prokaryotic genome annotation. *Bioinformatics* 30, 2068–2069. doi: 10.1093/bioinformatics/btu153

Stearns, S. C. (2019). Frontiers in molecular evolutionary medicine. *J. Mol. Evol.* [Epub ahead of print].

Suttle, C. A. (2005). Viruses in the sea. *Nature* 437, 356–361. doi: 10.1038/nature04160

Wattam, A. R., Davis, J. J., Assaf, R., Boisvert, S., Brettin, T., Bun, C., et al. (2017). Improvements to PATRIC, the all-bacterial bioinformatics database and analysis resource center. *Nucleic Acids Res.* 45, D535–D542. doi: 10.1093/nar/gkw1017

Weber-Dabrowska, B., Jonczyk-Matysiak, E., Zaczek, M., Loocka, M., Lusiak-Szelachowska, M., and Gorski, A. (2016). Phage procurement for therapeutic purposes. *Front. Microbiol.* 12:2016. doi: 10.3389/fmicb.2016.01177

Wei, Y., Ocampo, P., and Levin, B. R. (2010). An experimental study of the population and evolutionary dynamics of *Vibrio cholerae* O1 and the bacteriophage JSF4. *Proc. Biol. Sci.* 277, 3247–3254. doi: 10.1098/rspb.2010.0651

World Health Organization [WHO] (2017). *Global Priority List of Antibiotic-Resistant Bacteria to Guide Research, Discovery, and Development of New Antibiotics*. Available at: https://www.who.int/medicines/publications/global-priority-list-antibiotic-resistant-bacteria/en/ (accessed May 10, 2018).

Wright, A., Hawkins, C. H., Anggard, E. E., and Harper, D. R. (2009). A controlled clinical trial of a therapeutic bacteriophage preparation in chronic otitis due to antibiotic-resistant *Pseudomonas aeruginosa*; a preliminary report of efficacy. *Clin. Otolaryngol.* 34, 349–357. doi: 10.1111/j.1749-4486.2009.01973.x

Zerbino, D. R., and Birney, E. (2008). Velvet: algorithms for de novo short read assembly using de Bruijn graphs. *Genome Res.* 18, 821–829. doi: 10.1101/gr.074492.107

9

Extended-Spectrum Beta-Lactamase-Producing *Escherichia coli* in Drinking Water Samples from a Forcibly Displaced, Densely Populated Community Setting in Bangladesh

Zahid Hayat Mahmud[1]*, Mir Himayet Kabir[1], Sobur Ali[1], M. Moniruzzaman[1], Khan Mohammad Imran[1], Tanvir Noor Nafiz[1], Md. Shafiqul Islam[1], Arif Hussain[1], Syed Adnan Ibna Hakim[2], Martin Worth[2], Dilruba Ahmed[1], Dara Johnston[2] and Niyaz Ahmed[1]

[1] International Centre for Diarrhoeal Disease Research, Dhaka, Bangladesh, [2] WASH Division, UNICEF Bangladesh, Dhaka, Bangladesh

*Correspondence:
Zahid Hayat Mahmud
zhmahmud@icddrb.org

Introduction: Community-acquired infections due to extended-spectrum beta-lactamase (ESBL) producing *Escherichia coli* are rising worldwide, resulting in increased morbidity, mortality, and healthcare costs, especially where poor sanitation and inadequate hygienic practices are very common.

Objective: This study was conducted to investigate the prevalence and characterization of multidrug-resistant (MDR) and ESBL-producing *E. coli* in drinking water samples collected from Rohingya camps, Bangladesh.

Methods: A total of 384 *E. coli* isolates were analyzed in this study, of which 203 were from household or point-of-use (POU) water samples, and 181 were from source water samples. The isolates were tested for virulence genes, ESBL-producing genes, antimicrobial susceptibility by VITEK 2 assay, plasmid profiling, and conjugal transfer of AMR genes.

Results: Of the 384 *E. coli* isolates tested, 17% (66/384) were found to be ESBL producers. The abundance of ESBL-producers in source water contaminated with *E. coli* was observed to be 14% (27/181), whereas, 19% (39/203) ESBL producers was found in household POU water samples contaminated with *E. coli*. We detected 71% (47/66) ESBL-*E. coli* to be MDR. Among these 47 MDR isolates, 20 were resistant to three classes, and 27 were resistant to four different classes of antibiotics. Sixty-four percent (42/66) of the ESBL producing *E. coli* carried 1 to 7 plasmids ranging from 1 to 103 MDa. Only large plasmids with antibiotic resistance properties were found transferrable via conjugation. Moreover, around 7% (29/384) of *E. coli* isolates harbored at least one of 10 virulence factors belonging to different *E. coli* pathotypes.

Conclusions: The findings of this study suggest that the drinking water samples analyzed herein could serve as an important source for exposure and dissemination of MDR, ESBL-producing and pathogenic *E. coli* lineages, which therewith pose a health risk to the displaced Rohingya people residing in the densely populated camps of Bangladesh.

Keywords: ESBL-producing *E. coli*, multidrug-resistant, drinking water, Rohingya camps, Bangladesh

INTRODUCTION

Extended-spectrum beta-lactamase (ESBL)-producing *E. coli* have been recognized as a major multidrug-resistant bacteria implicated in serious hospital and community-acquired infections worldwide, especially in places where poor sanitation, and inadequate hygienic practices are very common (1–4). Infections caused by MDR-*E. coli* incur huge medical costs and limit treatment options (5–7).

Multidrug-resistant *E. coli* has been detected in different ecological niches in the community and environment (8, 9). For instance, ESBLs and New Delhi Metallo beta-lactamase 1 (NDM-1) producing *E. coli* were detected in drinking water and retail meat, respectively (10, 11). In Bangladesh, ESBL producing-*E. coli* were reported from drinking water as well as from river water samples (12, 13). Though *E. coli* has had a significant role in water microbiology as an indicator of fecal pollution, it is of greater public health concern when these *E. coli* isolates turn out to be multidrug-resistant pathogens (14). Detection of ESBL-producing *E. coli* in drinking water samples is important to recognize the risk of transmission of antimicrobial resistance (AMR) and gastrointestinal diseases. Transmission of ESBL-encoding genes among bacteria is often plasmid-mediated (15), and aquatic environments provide ideal settings for horizontal transfer of AMR genes encoded on various forms of mobile genetic elements (16).

Though the majority of *E. coli* are typically innocuous, some *E. coli* variants are virulent and may inflict varying severity of enteric infections. Currently, there are six different *E. coli* pathotypes that have been documented to cause intestinal infections, they include, enterotoxigenic *E. coli* (ETEC), enteroinvasive *E. coli* (EIEC), enteropathogenic *E. coli* (EPEC), shiga toxin-producing *E. coli* (STEC), enteroaggregative *E. coli* (EAEC), and diffusely adhering *E. coli* (DAEC) (17). In Bangladesh, following rotavirus, the second most leading cause of diarrheal infections are caused by pathogenic *E. coli* (18). Several virulence genes such as *st, lt* (ETEC); *bfp, eae* (EPEC); *aat, aai* (EAEC) are associated with diarrheagenic *E. coli* pathotypes (19), which can be used to detect these pathotypes using PCR based gene amplification. Watery diarrhea is caused by the secretion of heat-labile (LT) and/or heat-stable (ST) enterotoxins from ETEC. Shiga toxin (Stx) expression is the unique feature of EHEC where systemic absorption of this toxin leads to possibly life-threatening complications. Multiple putative virulence factors expression for typical EAEC strains, containing the aggregative adherence fimbriae (AAF), dispersin, the dispersin translocator Aat, and the Aai type VI secretion system directs to adherence and triggering

diarrhea. EPEC adhesion is associated with attaching and effacing adhesion and intestinal colonization, which also include bundle-forming pili (BFP), EspA filaments and intimin (19, 20).

The contaminated drinking water was found to be responsible for a number of waterborne gastroenteritis outbreaks due to diarrheagenic *E. coli* (21–23). Therefore, it is pertinent to analyze the prevalence and properties of ESBL-*E. coli* from drinking waters in community settings, particularly, from human habitations that are projected to pose exceptionally high risks of waterborne diseases due to overcrowding, scarcity of safe drinking water, and unhygienic living conditions. In Bangladesh, the displaced Rohingya people are one such community with a population of ~1.16 million who are living in 32 congested camps in a challenging hilly landscape of Cox's Bazar district (290,000 persons per square kilometer). This displacement, of a large population are facing compounding problems, particularly related to water, sanitation, hygiene and health care (24–27). Water from hand-pumped tube wells is the primary water supply for the people in Rohingya camps. Around 6057 water points and 50087 emergency latrines have been built (during the study in 2018). Moreover, in the absence of efficient community sanitation, insufficient sewage disposal, and treatment facilities, the risks of transmission of enteric pathogens become extremely high, and the community as a whole face serious public health concerns (28–30).

In our previous study, we analyzed source water (tubewell) samples, as well as POU drinking water samples, from Rohingya camps and found 10.5% source water and 34.7% POU water samples were contaminated with *E. coli*, which could cause waterborne diseases in the camps (26). An outbreak of ESBL-producing *E. coli* might create a medical emergency in a large congested habitation like Rohingya camps because of limited treatment options. The AMR surveillance, especially with regard to ESBL-producing *E. coli* has never been carried out in these camps. Therefore, this study aims to determine the prevalence of ESBL-producing, MDR, and virulent *E. coli* in drinking water samples. Furthermore, plasmid profiling and horizontal transfer of resistant gene analyses of isolated ESBL-producing *E. coli* will provide important insights in understanding the dissemination of resistance determinants.

MATERIALS AND METHODS

Bacterial Isolates

We employed drinking water samples from Rohingya camps collected in our previous study to culture *E. coli* isolates (26). From a total of 2512 *E. coli* contaminated water samples, 421 water samples were randomly selected for the present study. One random *E. coli* isolate was taken as a representative from each sample, which was further tested using the API-20E test kit (Biomerieux SA, Marcy-I'Etoile, France), and 384 API-20E confirmed *E. coli* were stored at −70°C in 30% LB glycerol-broth for downstream analysis. Out of 384 *E. coli* isolates, 203 isolates were from the household water samples and 181 from source water samples. In brief, for each sample, 100 ml water was filtered through a 0.22 μm membrane filter (Sartorius Stedim, Goettingen, Germany), the membrane filter paper was then firmly laid on the mTEC agar plate. Later, the culture plate was incubated for 2 h at 35 ± 0.5°C, followed by further incubation for 22 ± 2 h at 44.5 ± 0.2°C. After incubation, red to magenta-colored colonies, typical of *E. coli* colony was picked and subcultured on MacConkey agar plate and incubated at 35 ± 2°C for 18 h to 24 h. After incubation, the characteristics of dark pink colonies typical of *E. coli* were obtained and confirmed using API-20E kit.

Isolation and Confirmation of ESBL-Producing and Carbapenem-Resistant *E. coli* Using Chromagar

All 384 confirmed *E. coli* isolates were cultured on CHROMagar ESBL and CHROMagar KPC media at 37°C for 18–24 h. The production of extended-spectrum beta-lactamases and carbapenemase was confirmed by observing the growth and characteristic colony morphology on respective culture media. Dark pink to reddish colonies on CHROMagar ESBL plate indicate ESBL producing *E. coli* whereas pink to reddish colonies on CHROMagar KPC media suggest carbapenem-resistant *E. coli*.

Confirmation of *E. coli* by VITEK 2

ESBL positive *E. coli* isolated from the ESBL CHROMagar plate were further confirmed by the VITEK 2 system (bioMérieux, Marcy I'Etoile, France) using VITEK 2 GN ID card. *Enterobacter hormacchii* (ATCC-700323) was used as a positive control for the identification in this system. For VITEK 2 assays, pure isolates were streaked on MacConkey agar plates and incubated at 35°C overnight. One to three isolated colonies were selected from each MacConkey agar plate and suspended in saline for preparation of inoculum to obtain an absorbency of ~0.5 McFarland Units before being subjected to VITEK 2 analysis.

Detection of Diarrheagenic and ExPEC Associated Virulence Genes

Several virulence genes such as *st, lt* (ETEC); *bfp, eae* (EPEC); *aat, aai* (EAEC) are associated with diarrheagenic *E. coli* pathotypes (19) are used to detect the pathotypes using PCR based gene amplification. In the present study, PCR based screening of diarrheagenic virulence genes was carried out for all 384 *E. coli* isolates. Gene-specific primers entailing heat-labile (*lt*), heat-stable (*st*), attaching and effacing (*eae*), anti-aggregation protein transporter (*aat*), bundle forming pilus (*bfp*) and aggR-activated island (*aaiC*) were used to detect the respective genes employing a multiplex PCR setup (31–34). The boiling lysis method was used

to obtain the DNA template (35). A 3 μl template DNA was taken for a 25 μl PCR reaction containing 12.5 μl of 2X GoTaq G2 Green Master Mix (Promega, USA) with 0.44 μl of eae primer, the primers lt, st, aaiC, aat, bfp were taken in 0.4 μl volume each. The PCR was carried out at standard cycling conditions with an annealing temperature of 57°C for 20 s. A separate PCR was performed for Shiga toxin genes (*stx1* and *stx2*), which was described previously (36, 37). PCR for invasion plasmid antigen H (*ipaH*) and the invasion associated locus (*ial*) was performed according to the procedure described elsewhere (38–41). Primer details are tabulated in **Supplementary Table 1**.

To examine the presence of seven ExPEC associated virulence factors, we performed two multiplex PCRs on 55 non diarrheagenic ESBL-*E. coli* isolates (42). Among these, the first one was done to screen the presence of *kpsMII* (group II capsule), *papA* (pilus-associated protein A), *sfaS* (S-fimbrial adhesine), and *focG* (F1C fmbriae protein) genes; whereas the second multiplex was performed to detect *hlyD* (haemolysin D), *afa* (afmbrial adhesine), and *iutA* genes (aerobactin siderophore ferric receptor protein).

Antibiotic Susceptibility by VITEK 2

Antibiotic susceptibility testing (AST) was performed using VITEK 2 system with VITEK 2 cards (AST-N280) for 19 antimicrobial agents according to the CLSI guidelines and manufacturer's recommendations; two additional antimicrobial agents (cefixime and ceftazidime) were also incorporated. *E. coli* ATCC 25922, susceptible to all drugs, was used for AST in each VITEK testing step as quality control. The 21 antibiotics tested included amikacin, amoxicillin/clavulanic acid, ampicillin, cefepime, cefixime, cefoperazone/sulbactam, ceftazidime, ceftriaxone, cefuroxime, cefuroxime axetil, ciprofloxacin, colistin, ertapenem, gentamicin, imipenem, meropenem, nalidixic acid, nitrofurantoin, piperacillin, tigecycline, and trimethoprim/sulfamethoxazole. Minimum inhibitory concentrations (MIC) were determined, and the isolates were classified into resistant, intermediate and susceptible as per CLSI criteria. The raw MIC data from the VITEK 2 assay are shown in **Supplementary Table 2**.

Detection of ESBL, Quinolone, and Carbapenemase Resistance Genes by PCR

All CHROMagar confirmed ESBL-producing *E. coli* isolates were screened for molecular determinants of ESBL and carbapenem resistance comprising of *bla*SHV, *bla*TEM, *bla*CTX-M-15 and all CTX-M-groups (*bla*CTX-M-1-group, *bla*CTX-M-2-group, *bla*CTX-M-8-group, *bla*CTX-M-9-group) including, *bla*OXA-1-group, *bla*OXA-47, and *bla*NDM-1 were screened (34, 43–48). The gene *bla*CMY-2 encoding for AmpC β-lactamase was also screened by PCR as per a published protocol (12, 49). Besides, all 66 isolates were tested for the three *qnr* (quinolone) resistance genes; *qnrA*, *qnrB*, and *qnrS* according to the methods described by others (50–52).

Plasmid Profiling and Conjugal Transfer

Plasmids from ESBL-*E. coli* isolates were extracted employing the Kado alkaline lysis method (53) and visualized after separation in low percent agarose gel (0.7%) electrophoresis. The size of extracted plasmids was determined comparing with size standard plasmids ran alongside. The following plasmids were used as size standards; Sa (23 MDa), RP4 (34 MDa), R1 (62 MDa), pDK9 (140 MDa), and *E. coli* V517 plasmids (1.4, 1.8, 2.0, 2.6, 3.4, 3.7, 4.8, and 35.8 MDa) (54). ESBL-producing *E. coli* were used as donors, and the sodium azide resistant strain *E. coli*-J53 was employed as a recipient for conjugation using broth mating assays at 30°C for 19 ± 1 h. Transconjugants obtained were plated on MacConkey plates prepared with cefotaxime (20 μg/L) and sodium azide (100 mg/L), transconjugants were selected observing their growth and colony morphology. Transconjugants were analyzed for antibiotic susceptibility tests using VITEK 2 assay, plasmid profiling and presence of ESBL genes (53).

Phylogenetic Analysis

As per the method described by Clermont and colleagues, the distribution of phylogenetic groups among ESBL- *E. coli* isolates was determined by performing multiplex PCRs after DNA extraction by boiling lysis (55).

RESULTS

ESBL-Positive but Carbapenem Sensitive *E. coli* Recovered From Drinking Water

To screen for ESBL-producing *E. coli*, 384 isolates were cultured on ESBL CHROMagar. The typical growth of pink colonies on the CHROMagar plate was considered as ESBL positive *E. coli*. Of the 384 isolates tested, 17.2% (*n* = 66) were found to be ESBL-producing *E. coli* (**Table 1**). About 15% (27/181), and 19% (39/203) ESBL producing *E. coli* originated from *E. coli* contaminated source water and POU water samples, respectively. Further, the ESBL producing *E. coli* was investigated for carbapenem resistance on CHROMagar KPC media, and none of the isolates was able to grow on CHROMagar KPC media. Therefore, we did not detect any carbapenem-resistance in our collection of ESBL-*E. coli* isolates.

High Prevalence of MDR in ESBL-Producing *E. coli*

Antimicrobial susceptibility of 66 ESBL-*E. coli* isolates (**Supplementary Table 3**) were tested against 21 different antibiotics (**Supplementary Table 4**) using VITEK 2 assay. All 66 CHROMagar confirmed ESBL positive *E. coli* isolates demonstrated resistance against ampicillin, ceftriaxone, ceftazidime, cefixime, cefuroxime, and cefuroxime axetil (**Figure 1**). About 70% (46/66) of the isolates were found to be resistant to nalidixic acid, 37.9% (25/66) isolates were resistant to trimethoprim/sulfamethoxazole, whereas 22.7% (15/66) and 19.7% (13/66) isolates were resistant for cefepime and ciprofloxacin, respectively. However, no resistance was detected in any of the tested strains to the antibiotics used of aminoglycosides (amikacin and gentamicin), cefoperazone/sulbactam, glycylcycline, carbapenem, and polymyxins groups. It was found that 71% (47/66) of *E. coli* isolates were MDR that were resistant to at least three classes of antibiotics. Among the 47 MDR isolates, 20 were resistant

to three different classes, and 27 were resistant to four different classes of antibiotics.

bla$_{CTX-M-1}$ Group Is the Predominant ESBL Gene Detected

The presence of molecular determinants of ESBLs was tested on all ESBL-producing *E. coli* isolates. Out of the 66 ESBL-*E. coli* isolates, 59% (39/66) isolates harbored both bla$_{CTX-M-1}$ group and bla$_{CTX-M-15}$ gene. However, 4.5% (3/66) isolates harbored either bla$_{CTX-M-1group}$ or bla$_{CTX-M-15}$ gene. The bla$_{TEM}$ β-lactamase gene was present in 35% (23/66) of isolates, and none of the isolates harbored other β-lactamase genes such as bla$_{SHV}$, bla$_{CTX-M-2}$-group, bla$_{CTX-M-8}$-group, and bla$_{CTX-M-9}$-group. The two genes, bla$_{OXA-1}$-group and bla$_{OXA-47}$ were screened among 66 ESBL- *E. coli* isolates, but none of the isolates was found to be positive. In addition, the New Delhi metallo-β-lactamase gene, bla$_{NDM-1}$ as well as plasmid-mediated ampC-type β-lactamase gene the bla$_{CMY-2}$ was not present in any of the isolates. The quinolone resistance gene; *qnrS*, and *qnrB* were found in 34% (22/66) and 5% (3/66) of the ESBL-*E. coli* isolates, respectively (**Figure 2**, **Supplementary Table 5**).

Distribution of *E. coli* Pathotypes

Screening for the presence of virulence factors demonstrated that 7% (29/384) of *E. coli* isolates were positive for at least one virulence factor out of the 10 *E. coli* pathotype-specific virulence genes tested. Ten isolates were positive for only *aaiC* gene and five isolates were positive for both *aaiC* and *aat*; whereas four isolates were positive for both *bfp* and *eae* genes. Heat labile (*lt*) gene was present in 7 isolates, whereas the heat stable (*st*) gene was found in 2 isolates and a single isolate was found positive for *stx1*. None of the isolates was positive for *ipaH* and *iaa* genes. Among the 29 pathogenic *E. coli* isolates detected; 52% (15/29) were EAEC, 31% (9/29) were ETEC, 14% (4/29) were EPEC and 4% (1/29) were EHEC (**Figure 3**).

When the ExPEC virulence genes were screened only three out of the seven virulence factors were detected that comprised of *KpsMII*, *sfaS*, and *iutA* genes, their prevalence rates were, 21.8% (12/55), 5.4% (3/55), and 16.4% (9/55), respectively. Most of isolates (12/18) harboring ExPEC genes were affiliated to phylogenetic group D. However, out of the 55 isolates tested, only 6 isolates qualify as ExPEC as per the inclusion criteria (strains harboring at least two ExPEC associated virulence factors) 5 out of these 6 isolates were from phylogroup D.

The potential pathogenic (diarrheagenic and ExPEC) *E. coli* isolates showed high resistance rates 83% (39/47) to ampicillin, followed by 74% (35/47) to nalidixic acid, 68% (32/47) to cefuroxime, cefuroxime axetil, 61% (29/47) to cefixime, ceftazidime, and 51% (24/47) to sulfonamides. Out of 29 pathogenic *E. coli* 11 were found to be ESBL producing in this study (**Table 2**). Of note, all the pathogenic isolates detected were found to be susceptible to carbapenems, aminoglycosides (amikacin and gentamicin), and polymyxin.

TABLE 1 | Antibiotic resistance pattern, presence of antibiotic resistance genes and plasmid patterns of ESBL-producing *Escherichia coli* isolated from water sample.

Serial no	Isolates ID	Antibiotic resistance Pattern[a]	Presence of antibiotic resistant genes	Plasmid size in MDa
1	05095B	Amp, Cro, Cxm, Cfa, Caz, Cfm, NA	$bla_{CTX-M-1}$, $bla_{CTX-M-15}$, bla_{TEM}, *qnr*S	75, 54, 4.5, 2.8, 2.6, 2
2	09036H2	Amp, Cro, Cxm, Cfa, Caz, Cfm, NA	$bla_{CTX-M-1}$, $bla_{CTX-M-15}$, *qnr*S	No plasmid
3	34022A	Amp, Fep, Cro, Cxm, Cfa, NA, Sxt, Caz, Cfm	$bla_{CTX-M-1}$, $bla_{CTX-M-15}$, bla_{TEM}	90
4	34008B	Amp, Fep, Cro, Cxm, Cfa, Caz, Cfm	$bla_{CTX-M-1}$, $bla_{CTX-M-15}$, *qnr*S	No plasmid
5	34012H2	Amp, Fep, Cro, Cxm, Cfa, NA, Caz, Cfm		No plasmid
6	05080H2	Amp, Fep, Cro, Cxm, Cfa, Cip, NA, Sxt, Caz, Cfm	$bla_{CTX-M-1}$, bla_{TEM}	No plasmid
7	11023H2	Amp, Cro, Cxm, Cfa, Caz, Cfm	$bla_{CTX-M-1}$, $bla_{CTX-M-15}$, *qnr*S	No plasmid
8	34022H1	Amp, Cro, Cxm, Cfa, NA, Caz, Cfm	$bla_{CTX-M-1}$, $bla_{CTX-M-15}$	94
9	5375B	Amp, Cro, Cxm, Cfa, NA, Tzp, Caz, Cfm	$bla_{CTX-M-1}$, $bla_{CTX-M-15}$, bla_{TEM}, *qnr*S	22
10	5095H2	Amc, Amp, Cro, Cxm, Cfa, NA, Caz, Cfm	$bla_{CTX-M-1}$, $bla_{CTX-M-15}$, *qnr*S	3.1, 2.04, 1.9
11	1109H1	Amp, Cro, Cxm, Cfa, Caz, Cfm	$bla_{CTX-M-1}$, $bla_{CTX-M-15}$, *qnr*S	6.5, 4.6, 4.3, 3.4, 2.7
12	8E756H2	Amp, Cro, Cxm, Cfa, Cip, NA, Caz, Cfm	$bla_{CTX-M-1}$, $bla_{CTX-M-15}$	77, 56, 6.5, 4.6, 4.3, 3.4, 2.8
13	9125B	Amc, Amp, Cro, Cxm, Cfa, Sxt, Caz, Cfm	bla_{TEM}	85, 57, 49, 37
14	8E285B	Amc, Amp, Cro, Cxm, Cfa, Caz, Cfm	$bla_{CTX-M-1}$	No plasmid
15	11269H1	Amp, Cro, Cxm, Cfa, Cip, NA, Caz, Cfm		29, 2.5
16	9736H2	Amc, Amp, Cro, Cxm, Cfa, Cip, NA, Tzp, Caz, Cfm		37, 3.3
17	11597A	Amp, Cro, Cxm, Cfa, NA, Sxt, Caz, Cfm	$bla_{CTX-M-1}$, $bla_{CTX-M-15}$	68
18	11611H1	Amp, Cro, Cxm, Cfa, NA, Sxt, Caz, Cfm	$bla_{CTX-M-1}$, $bla_{CTX-M-15}$	65
19	04584H2	Amp, Cro, Cxm, Cfa, Caz, Cfm	$bla_{CTX-M-1}$, $bla_{CTX-M-15}$, *qnr*S	No plasmid
20	8W645H2	Amp, Cro, Cxm, Cfa, Caz, Cfm	$bla_{CTX-M-1}$, $bla_{CTX-M-15}$, *qnr*S	No plasmid
21	8W390H1	Amp, Cro, Cxm, Cfa, Caz, Cfm	$bla_{CTX-M-1}$, $bla_{CTX-M-15}$, *qnr*S	42, 3.2, 2.6
22	8W803H2	Amp, Cro, Cxm, Cfa, NA, Sxt, Caz, Cfm	$bla_{CTX-M-1}$, $bla_{CTX-M-15}$	103, 4.9, 2.9, 2.6
23	8W454H1	Amp, Fep, Cro, Cxm, Cfa, Cip, NA, Sxt, Caz, Cfm	$bla_{CTX-M-1}$, $bla_{CTX-M-15}$	No plasmid
24	18544A	Amp, Cro, Cxm, Cfa, NA, Fd, Caz, Cfm		No plasmid
25	18162H2	Amp, Cro, Cxm, Cfa, NA, Fd, Caz, Cfm		No plasmid
26	18544B	Amp, Cro, Cxm, Cfa, NA, Fd, Caz, Cfm		No plasmid
27	12224H1	Amp, Cro, Cxm, Cfa, NA, Caz, Cfm	$bla_{CTX-M-1}$, $bla_{CTX-M-15}$, *qnr*S	97, 39, 2
28	11448B	Amp, Cro, Cxm, Cfa, Caz, Cfm	*qnr*B	34, 2.3
29	9441H2	Amp, Cro, Cxm, Cfa, NA, Caz, Cfm	$bla_{CTX-M-1}$, $bla_{CTX-M-15}$	No plasmid
30	1E181H2	Amp, Fep, Cro, Cxm, Cfa, NA, Sxt, Caz, Cfm	$bla_{CTX-M-1}$, $bla_{CTX-M-15}$	67, 52
31	2W242H2	Amp, Cro, Cxm, Cfa, Cip, NA, Sxt, Caz, Cfm	$bla_{CTX-M-1}$, $bla_{CTX-M-15}$, bla_{TEM}	63, 6.4
32	2W246A	Amp, Cro, Cxm, Cfa, NA, Sxt, Caz, Cfm	$bla_{CTX-M-1}$, $bla_{CTX-M-15}$, bla_{TEM}	89, 4.4
33	1E365B	Amp, Cro, Cxm, Cfa, Caz, Cfm	$bla_{CTX-M-1}$, $bla_{CTX-M-15}$, *qnr*S	55
34	1E07H2	Amp, Cro, Cxm, Cfa, Caz, Cfm	bla_{TEM},	71, 33, 30
35	2W150H2	Amp, Cro, Cxm, Cfa, Caz, Cfm	bla_{TEM}	No plasmid
36	2W047H2	Amp, Cro, Cxm, Cfa, NA, Caz, Cfm	$bla_{CTX-M-1}$, $bla_{CTX-M-15}$, bla_{TEM}, *qnr*S	42, 8.3
37	2W246B	Amp, Cro, Cxm, Cfa, NA, Caz, Cfm	$bla_{CTX-M-1}$, $bla_{CTX-M-15}$, *qnr*S	92, 74, 55
38	1E391A	Amp, Cro, Cxm, Cfa, Caz, Cfm	$bla_{CTX-M-15}$, *qnr*S	92, 74, 56
39	1E424H2	Amp, Fep, Cro, Cxm, Cfa, Caz, Cfm	$bla_{CTX-M-1}$, $bla_{CTX-M-15}$, *qnr*S	53
40	2E218H1	Amp, Cro, Cxm, Cfa, Caz, Cfm		No plasmid
41	2E219A	Amp, Cro, Cxm, Cfa, Caz, Cfm	*qnr*S	83
42	2E179H2	Amp, Fep, Cro, Cxm, Cfa, NA, Caz, Cfm	$bla_{CTX-M-1}$, $bla_{CTX-M-15}$, bla_{TEM}	No plasmid

(Continued)

TABLE 1 | Continued

Serial no	Isolates ID	Antibiotic resistance pattern[a]	Presence of antibiotic resistant genes	Plasmid size in MDa
43	2E0280B	Amp, Fep, Cro, Cxm, Cfa, NA, Caz, Cfm	$bla_{CTX-M-1}$, $bla_{CTX-M-15}$, bla_{TEM}	No plasmid
44	1E345A	Amc, Amp, Cro, Cxm, Cfa, Cip, NA,Tzp, Sxt, Caz, Cfm	bla_{TEM}	32, 1.9
45	1E370H2	Amp, Cro, Cxm, Cfa, Cip, NA, Fd, Tzp, Sxt, Caz, Cfm	$bla_{CTX-M-1}$, $bla_{CTX-M-15}$, bla_{TEM}	81, 19, 7.6
46	2W241H2	Amp, Cro, Cxm, Cfa, NA, Sxt, Caz, Cfm	$bla_{CTX-M-1}$, $bla_{CTX-M-15}$, bla_{TEM}	4.2
47	2W146H2	Amp, Cro, Cxm, Cfa, NA, Sxt, Caz, Cfm	$bla_{CTX-M-1}$, $bla_{CTX-M-15}$, bla_{TEM}	No plasmid
48	1E336H2	Amp, Cro, Cxm, Cfa, NA, Sxt, Caz, Cfm	$bla_{CTX-M-15}$, bla_{TEM}	No plasmid
49	1E414A	Amp, Cro, Cxm, Cfa, NA, Sxt, Caz, Cfm	$qnrB$	74, 45, 36, 3.5
50	1E586A	Amp, Cro, Cxm, Cfa, NA, Caz, Cfm	bla_{TEM}	No plasmid
51	11512H2	Amp, Fep, Cro, Cxm, Cfa, Caz, Cfm	$bla_{CTX-M-1}$, $bla_{CTX-M-15}$, $qnrS$	56, 44.7, 4.4, 3.8
52	18433H2	Amp, Cro, Cxm, Cfa, NA, Sxt, Caz, Cfm	$bla_{CTX-M-1}$, $bla_{CTX-M-15}$, $qnrS$	52, 42.7, 4.3,3.6
53	1E286H2	Amc, Amp, Cro, Cxm, Cfa, Cip, NA, Sxt, Caz, Cfm	bla_{TEM}	No plasmid
54	C-2WH4	Amp, Cro, Cxm, Cfa, Caz, Cfm		91, 37
55	18441A	Amp, Fep, Cro, Cxm, Cfa, Cip, NA, Sxt, Caz, Cfm	$bla_{CTX-M-1}$, $bla_{CTX-M-15}$, $qnrS$	81
56	1E499H1	Amp, Cro, Cxm, Cfa, NA, Caz, Cfm	$bla_{CTX-M-15}$, $qnrS$	2.8, 1.9
57	07137A	Amp, Cro, Cxm, Cfa, Cip, NA, Sxt, Caz, Cfm	$bla_{CTX-M-1}$, $bla_{CTX-M-15}$	84, 2.2, 1.7
58	34034B	Amp, Fep, Cro, Cxm, Cfa, NA, Sxt, Caz, Cfm	$bla_{CTX-M-1}$, $bla_{CTX-M-15}$, bla_{TEM}	82
59	410H2	Amp, Cro, Cxm, Cfa, Caz, Cfm	$bla_{CTX-M-1}$, $bla_{CTX-M-15}$, $qnrS$	No plasmid
60	192B	Amp,Cro, Cxm, Cfa, NA, Caz, Cfm		No plasmid
61	2W147H2	Amp, Cro, Cxm, Cfa, Caz, Cfm	$qnrB$	56,37, 2.8, 2.5, 2
62	2W158B	Amp, Cro, Cxm, Cfa, Cip, NA, Sxt, Caz, Cfm	$bla_{CTX-M-1}$, $bla_{CTX-M-15}$	49, 4.1, 1.9, 1.4
63	2W160H2	Amp, Cro, Cxm, Cfa, Cip, NA, Caz, Cfm	bla_{TEM}, $qnrS$	No plasmid
64	266B	Amp, Fep Cro, Cxm, Cfa, NA, Sxt, Caz, Cfm	$bla_{CTX-M-1}$, $bla_{CTX-M-15}$	49, 4, 1.9, 1.4
65	31029B	Amp, Fep, Cro, Cxm, Cfa, NA, Sxt, Caz, Cfm	$bla_{CTX-M-1}$, bla_{TEM}	84
66	35001H1	Amp, Fep, Cro, Cxm, Cfa, NA, Sxt, Caz, Cfm	bla_{TEM}	75, 54, 4.5, 2.8, 2.6, 2

[a]Ak, Amikacin; Amc, Amoxicillin/Clavulanic Acid; Amp, Ampicillin; Fep, Cefepime; Scf, Cefoperazone/Sulbactam; Cro, Ceftriaxone; Cxm, Cefuroxime; Cfa, Cefuroxime Axetil; Cip, Ciprofloxacin; Cl, Colistin; Etp, Ertapenem; Cn, Gentamicin; Imp, Imipenem; Men, Meropenem; NA, Nalidixic Acid; Fd, Nitrofurantoin; Tzp, Piperacillin-Tazobactam; Tgc, Tigecycline; Sxt, Sulphamethoxazoletrimethoprim; Cfm, Cefixime; Caz, Ceftazidime.

Phylogrouping

Among the ESBL-*E. coli* isolates, all phylogenetic groups were represented except for phylogroup F. The predominant phylogenetic group identified was B1 (23/66; 34.8%), followed by D (22/66; 33.3%), E (17/66; 25.7%), B2 and C (2/66; each 3%). Among the 47 multidrug resistant ESBL-*E. coli* (20/47) were of phylogroup D followed by A (13/47), B1 (12/47), C (2/47). Majority of isolates carrying diarrheagenic virulence genes were from B1(14/29; 48%) followed by A(6/29; 20.6%), B2, C, and unknown groups (2/29; each 7%) (**Figure 4**).

Plasmid Analysis of ESBL-Producing *E. coli*

Plasmid profiling and conjugation analysis were performed to see whether the antibiotic-resistance genes of the 66 ESBL producing isolates were plasmid-mediated and can they be horizontally transferred. Plasmid number and size were determined using conventional lysis and agarose gel electrophoresis. About 63% ($n = 42$) isolates carried 1 to 7 plasmids ranging in size from

~1 to 103 MDa (**Figure 5**), and the distribution of plasmids was heterogeneous (**Table 1**). Further, the plasmid containing isolates that showed the ESBL phenotype were tested for their ability to transfer the ESBL determinant by conjugation experiments. Nine isolates were able to transfer the cefotaxime resistance marker to a susceptible *E. coli* recipient with transfer rates ranging from 4.75×10^{-6} to 1.19×10^{-4} per donor cell (**Table 3**). Large plasmids (30–103 MDa) were transferred to the sodium azide resistant *E. coli*-J53 recipient. Whereas, the smaller plasmids (<30 MDa) were not seen to be transferred during conjugation. Among the nine donor isolates, two were able to transfer two plasmids each whereas seven isolates transferred single plasmids (**Table 3**).

DISCUSSION

In our previous study, we investigated the occurrence of *E. coli* and fecal coliforms in source and household drinking water samples in Rohingya camps, wherein 10.5% tubewell water and

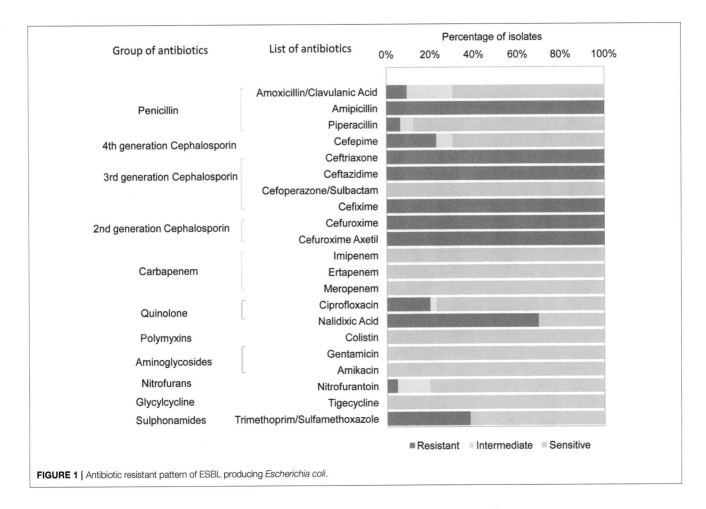

FIGURE 1 | Antibiotic resistant pattern of ESBL producing *Escherichia coli*.

34.7% POU water samples were found to be contaminated with *E. coli* (26). In the current study, the ESBL-producing *E. coli* isolates from the contaminated drinking water samples of our previous study were characterized concerning antimicrobial susceptibility, dissemination of drug resistance, and pathogenic potential to comprehend the extent of public health threat due to the exposure of contaminated drinking water in Rohingya camps of Bangladesh.

ESBL-producing *E. coli* has been increasingly reported globally, it is not only restricted to clinical settings but also recovered from environmental niches like livestock, wildlife and particularly water (56–58). The pandemic spread of ESBL-producing Gram-negative bacteria is a serious health concern. Human habitation and the surrounding environment in Bangladesh are reportedly contaminated by antimicrobial-resistant bacteria (59, 60). Reports emanating from developing countries like Bangladesh indicated a high prevalence of ESBL-producing *E. coli* in hospital and community drinking water samples (34, 61).

In the current study, we detected 17.2% (66/384) ESBL-producing *E. coli*, of which 71% (47/66) was multidrug-resistant. The high prevalence of multidrug-resistant *E. coli* among the ESBL-producing isolates implies that not only β-lactam antibiotics but resistance to other classes of antibiotics is being

co-selected. In Bangladesh, cephalosporins and penicillins are the most commonly used antibiotics (62), which explain why all the 66 ESBL-producing isolates are found to be resistant to both the classes of antibiotics. Besides, the majority of ESBL-producing isolates were found to be resistant to the quinolone class of antibiotics (46 to nalidixic acid). This may reflect the overuse and misuse of antibiotics (63) as these drugs are often sold and distributed over the counter (64). The uncontrolled and unregulated use of antibiotics severely limits the therapeutic options as well as aids the rapid dissemination of resistance in such overpopulated Rohingya camps.

We found ESBL-producing *E. coli* isolates are 100% susceptible to the antibiotics tested of carbapenem, aminoglycoside (amikacin and gentamicin), glycylcycline, and polymyxin groups. This finding was similar to a study in Jordan, where all the *E. coli* isolates from drinking water were sensitive to carpapenem and glycylcycline (65). There might be several factors responsible for susceptibility, such as these drugs are rarely prescribed in Bangladesh (64) and are not readily available in the hard to reach hilly terrain like Rohingya camps.

In this study, most of the isolates were positive for *bla*CTX–M–1 group and *bla*CTX–M–15, genes that concur the previous reports from Bangladesh (59, 60, 66). All *bla*CTX–M–1

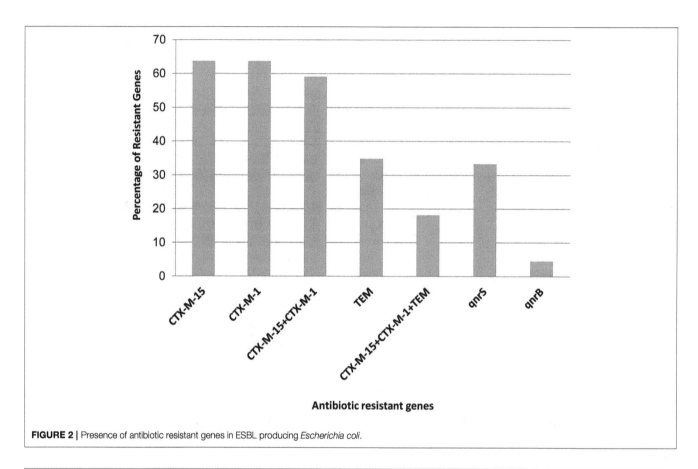

FIGURE 2 | Presence of antibiotic resistant genes in ESBL producing *Escherichia coli*.

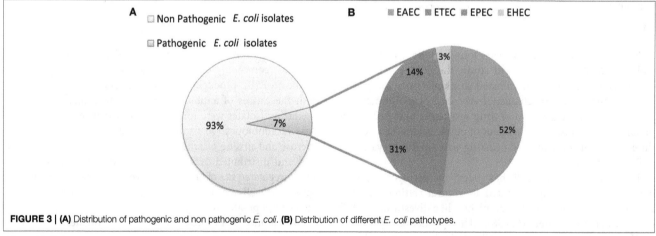

FIGURE 3 | **(A)** Distribution of pathogenic and non pathogenic *E. coli*. **(B)** Distribution of different *E. coli* pathotypes.

group, $bla_{CTX-M-15}$ and bla_{TEM} ESBL-positive *E. coli* isolates showed MDR phenotype ranging from 3 to 4 classes of antibiotics. Similar to our observation, a previous study from Bangladesh showed a high prevalence of CTX-M-15 in ESBL-producing *E. coli* cultured from drinking water samples from different households (34). The CTX-M group of beta-lactamases are a group of rapidly emerging ESBL genes globally, which has been predominantly detected in *E. coli* and *Klebsiella* spp. (56, 67–70). The NDM-1 producing bacteria have been reported in clinical isolates from Bangladesh (71), but in the current study, no NDM-1-producing *E. coli* was detected in the water samples.

The gene *qnrB* has been recognized in various enterobacterial species, such as *E. coli* and *Klebsiella* spp. (72–74). Plasmid-mediated quinolone resistance is intervened by the genes (qnr) encoding proteins that protect DNA gyrase and topoisomerase IV against quinolone compounds (75). Among the nonclinical sources, *qnr* gene was reported in *E. coli* isolated from swine, livestock and poultry (76, 77). In the present study, 25 isolates harbored plasmid-mediated *qnr* genes comprising of 22 isolates positive for *qnrS* and 3 isolates for *qnrB* genes. Isolates harboring *qnrS* gene also demonstrated co-existence of $bla_{CTX-M-15}$ and $bla_{CTX-M-1}$ group gene. Additionally, they were resistant to a

TABLE 2 | ESBL-producing pathogenic *E. coli*.

Serial no.	Isolates ID	Antibiotic resistance pattern	ESBL genes	Virulent genes	Pathotypes
1	34012H2	Amp, Fep, Cro, Cxm, Cfa, NA, Caz, Cfm		*st*	ETEC
2	05080H2	Amp, Fep, Cro, Cxm, Cfa, Cip, NA, Sxt, Caz, Cfm	*bla* CTX−M−1, *bla* TEM	*aaiC*	EAEC
3	8E285B	Amc, Amp, Cro, Cxm, Cfa, Caz, Cfm	*bla* CTX−M−1	*aaiC*	EAEC
4	8W454H1	Amp, Fep, Cro, Cxm, Cfa, Cip, NA, Sxt, Caz, Cfm	*bla* CTX−M−1, *bla* CTX−M−15	*aaiC, aat*	EAEC
5	18544A	Amp, Cro, Cxm, Cfa, NA, Fd, Caz, Cfm		*aaiC*	EAEC
6	18162H2	Amp, Cro, Cxm, Cfa, NA, Fd, Caz, Cfm		*aaiC*	EAEC
7	18544B	Amp, Cro, Cxm, Cfa, NA, Fd, Caz, Cfm		*aaiC*	EAEC
8	1E181H2	Amp, Fep, Cro, Cxm, Cfa, NA, Sxt, Caz, Cfm	*bla* CTX−M−1, *bla* CTX−M−15	*aaiC*	EAEC
9	1E370H2	Amp, Cro, Cxm, Cfa, Cip, NA, Fd, Tzp, Sxt, Caz, Cfm	*bla* CTX−M−1, *bla* CTX−M−15, *bla* TEM	*aaiC*	EAEC
10	2W241H2	Amp, Cro, Cxm, Cfa, NA, Sxt, Caz, Cfm	*bla* CTX−M−1, *bla* CTX−M−15, *bla* TEM	*aaiC, aat*	EAEC
11	192B	Amp,Cro, Cxm, Cfa, NA, Caz, Cfm		*aaiC*	EAEC

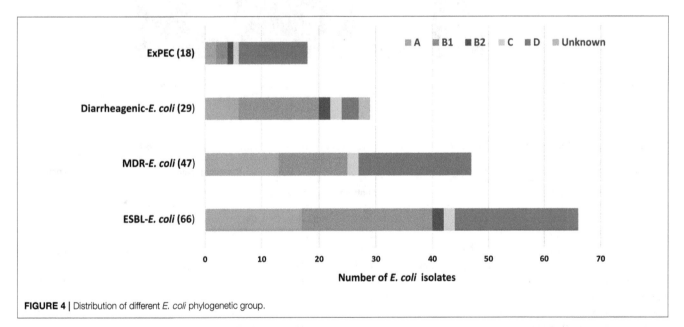

FIGURE 4 | Distribution of different *E. coli* phylogenetic group.

range of 7–11 antibiotics, including ciprofloxacin and nalidixic acid. In contrast, all isolates containing *qnrS* gene also harbored the two ESBL genes, $bla_{CTX-M-1group}$ and $bla_{CTX-M-15}$; they were resistant to 8 different antibiotics; most interestingly, they were susceptible to ciprofloxacin. Hence, the presence of *qnrS* gene alone may not be indicative of the isolate being resistant to fluoroquinolones as also been observed in a previous study (78).

Using PCR for virulence genes, 29 (7%) was found to be pathogenic out of 384 isolates from drinking water. The most prevalent pathotype was EAEC, accountable for 52% of the pathogenic isolates; followed by ETEC, EPEC, and EHEC responsible for 31, 14, and 4% of the pathogenic isolates, respectively. In addition to the diarrheagenic *E. coli* around 22% of *E. coli* isolates were at least positive for 1 ExPEC associated virulence genes, moreover 11% (6/55) of the isolates were dectected to be potential ExPEC strains. This indicates that the drinking water samples present potential risk of disease epidemic particularly, the diarreaheal disease, this assumes more importants as in this particular setting where the dirinking water is not treated before consumption. Though the reservoir for

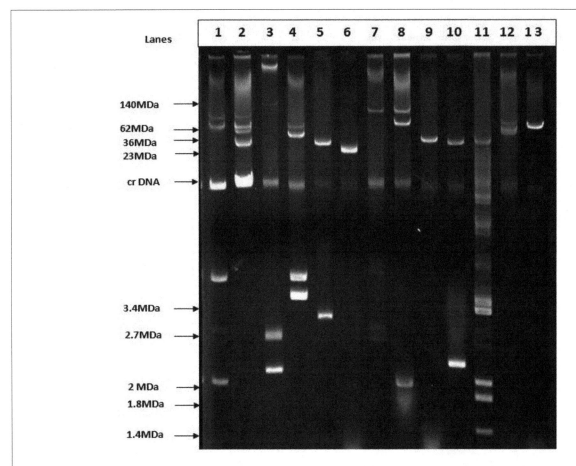

FIGURE 5 | Agarose gel electrophoresis of plasmid DNA showing the patterns among the ESBL positive isolates. Lane-3: *E. coli* strain pDK9 (140, 105, 2.7, 2.1 MDa), Lane-6: V517 (23MDa), Lane-9:RP4 (36MDa), Lane-11: V517 (35.8, 3.4,3.7, 2,1.8,1.4), Lane-13: R1 (62MDa), Lane-1,2,4,5,7,8,10, and 12 are ESBL positive *E. coli*. The molecular weight of the markers is shown in the picture.

TABLE 3 | Results of conjugation assays between antibiotic resistant *E. coli* isolates obtained from water samples and the recipient *E. coli* J53 strain.

Isolates ID	Parent Strains		Transconjugants		Transfer Rate
	Resistant pattern	Plasmid pattern	Resistant pattern	Plasmid pattern	
9125B	Amc, Amp, Cro, Cxm, Cfa, Sxt, Caz, Cfm	85, 57, 49, 37	Amc, Amp, Cxm, Cfa	57	3.33×10^{-5}
8W390H1	Amp, Cro, Cxm, Cfa, Caz, Cfm	42, 3.2, 2.6	Amp, Cro, Cxm, Cfa, Caz, Cfm	42	3.37×10^{-6}
8W803H2	Amp, Cro, Cxm, Cfa, NA, Sxt, Caz, Cfm	103, 4.9, 2.9, 2.6	Amp,Cro, Cxm, Cfa, NA, Caz, Cfm	103	1.8×10^{-5}
8W454H1	Amp, Fep, Cro, Cxm, Cfa, Cip, NA, Sxt, Caz, Cfm	82, 44, 37	Amp, Fep, Cro, Cxm, Cfa, Sxt, Caz, Cfm	44	1.57×10^{-6}
12224H1	Amp, Cro, Cxm, Cfa, NA, Caz, Cfm	97, 39, 2	Amp, Cro, Cxm, Cfa, Caz, Cfm	39	3.6×10^{-4}
1E07H2	Amp, Cro, Cxm, Cfa Caz, Cfm	71, 33, 30	Amp, Cro, Cxm, Cfa, Caz, Cfm	33, 30	5.26×10^{-5}
1E391A	Amp, Cro, Cxm, Cfa, Caz, Cfm	92, 74, 56	Amp, Cro, Cxm, Cfa, Caz, Cfm	56	5.17×10^{-6}
C-2WH4	Amp, Cro, Cxm, Cfa, Caz, Cfm	91, 37	Amp, Cro, Cxm, Cfa, Caz, Cfm	91	1.19×10^{-4}
2W147H2	Amp, Cro, Cxm, Cfa, Caz, Cfm	56,37, 2.8, 2.5, 2	Amp, Cro, Cxm, Cfa, Caz, Cfm	56, 37	4.75×10^{-6}

EAEC is still unclear, it is generally considered to be human (79–81). The transmission of EAEC is often described as waterborne or foodborne; therefore, it is assumed to be transmitted by the fecal-oral route (82). The presence of ETEC in drinking water and environmental water has been reported previously in Bangladesh; viability after long term water incubation and capacity of biofilm formation might imply that the water is

an important transmission route of ETEC (83–85). From the 29 pathogenic isolates, 11 were found to be ESBL positive and surprisingly, 10 of them were of EAEC pathotype. In recent studies of Iran and China, a high prevalence of ESBL in EAEC was also reported (86, 87). The alarming rate of ESBL-producing EAEC isolates recommends strict infection control policies to prevent additional spreading of the virulent and resistant EAEC strains. All phylogenetic groups were represented in the E. coli isolates indicating that they were not homogenous in their population structure instead they belonged to diverse phylogenetic backgrounds, mainly the phylogenetic groups that are associated with commensal (group B1) as well as pathogenic and antimicrobial resistant E. coli lineages (group D) were detected. The presence of ESBL producing E. coli among the phylogenetic group D strains represents major public health risks due to the spread of such strains via drinking water.

In this study, 64% of the isolates were observed to harbor plasmids ranging from 1 to 103 MDa and a negligible similarity of plasmids pattern among the isolates inferred their clonal diversity due to heterogenous people of diverse geographical origin. Conjugation experiments are important to understand the transfer potential of plasmids conferring extended-spectrum-β-lactamase resistance. It is reported that only plasmids above 35 MDa contain and transfer antibiotic resistance genes via conjugation (18, 88), and In line with other studies, we have also observed plasmid-mediated transfer of antibiotic resistance genes (18, 88). Conjugative plasmids, carrying cefotaxime resistance phenotype among different isolates, ranged from 42 to 103 MDa in size. These findings imply that horizontal gene transfer might worsen the existing antibiotic resistance scenario by speeding up the spread of antimicrobial resistance (AMR) within heterogeneous bacterial communities in environment (89).

Lack of proper sanitation and hygiene in a densely-populated area like Rohingya camps (26) might play a key role in the development and dissemination of AMR. Open defecation with poor personal hygiene, poor community sanitation and lack of controlled antibiotic usage has been reported to exacerbate the transmission of AMR infections (90). A previous study in four middle-income countries, Brazil, Indonesia, India, and Nigeria showed that improvement in water quality and sanitation alone could lead to reduction in antibiotic usage (90). The contamination of drinking water with ESBL-producing E. coli, as observed in this study could be due to poor sanitation and hygiene, including, open defecation, inappropriate fecal sludge management, etc. This study has shown that the environmental E. coli pose public health threat by being carriers of ESBL-genes. Moreover, these ESBL-producing E. coli were harboring virulence factors corresponding to major E. coli pathotypes. Limitations of this study include lack of genetic fingerprinting analysis of the antibiotic-resistant E. coli from drinking water, lack of exhaustive antimicrobial resistance gene, and extraintestinal pathogenic E. coli (ExPEC) virulence gene screening.

In conclusion, the findings of this study suggest that the drinking water samples analyzed herein could serve as an important source for exposure and dissemination of MDR, ESBL-producing and pathogenic E. coli variants, which also pose a health risk to the displaced Rohingya population residing in the densely populated camps in Cox's Bazar. Based on the results of this work we recommend that the policymakers should make considerable efforts in implementing strong infection control strategies by focusing on providing good quality water and ensuring water quality monitoring programs in the Rohingya camps.

ETHICS STATEMENT

The Ethical Review Committee of International Centre for Diarrhoeal Disease Research, Bangladesh has approved the study.

AUTHOR CONTRIBUTIONS

ZM, MI, SH, MW, KI, DJ, and NA planed and organized the study. ZM, MI, SA, MK, MM, TN, SH, MW, DJ, DA, and NA were involved to implement the study. ZM, SA, MK, KI, DA, and NA carried out laboratory work. ZM, MM, MI, SH, DA, and NA were involved to interpret the data. ZM, MK, SA, MM, MI, and NA had a major contribution in writing the manuscript. All authors contributed in proofreading the manuscript.

FUNDING

This research study was funded by United Nations International Children's Emergency Fund (unicef), grant number BCO/PCA/2017/035-2018/001. International Centre for Diarrhoeal Disease Research, Bangladesh (icddr,b) acknowledges with gratitude the commitment of unicef to its research efforts. icddr,b is also grateful to the Government of Bangladesh, Canada, Sweden and the UK for providing core/unrestricted support. The authors are grateful to Frederic Geser of unicef Bangaldesh for his constructive input and cooperation during the study. The authors are also grateful to Department of Public Health Engineering (DPHE) Cox's Bazar and unicef Cox's Bazar, Bangladesh for their valuable guidance and cooperation during the study.

REFERENCES

Aruna K, Mobashshera T. Prevalence of extended spectrum beta-lactamase production among uropathogens in south Mumbai and its antibiogram pattern. *EXCLI J.* (2012) 11:363–72.

Hussain A, Shaik S, Ranjan A, Nandanwar N, Tiwari SK, Majid M, et al. Risk of transmission of antimicrobial resistant *Escherichia coli* from commercial broiler and free-range retail chicken in India. *Front Microbiol.* (2017) 8:2120. doi: 10.3389/fmicb.2017.02120

Hussain A, Shaik S, Ranjan A, Suresh A, Sarker N, Semmler T, et al. Genomic and functional characterization of poultry *Escherichia coli* from India revealed diverse Extended-spectrum β-lactamase-producing lineages with shared virulence profiles. *Front Microbiol.* (2019) 10:2766. doi: 10.3389/fmicb.2019.02766

Pitout JDD, Nordmann P, Laupland KB, Poirel L. Emergence of Enterobacteriaceae producing extended-spectrum beta-lactamases (ESBLs) in the community. *J Antimicrob Chemother.* (2005) 56:52–9. doi: 10.1093/jac/dki166

Cantón R, Akóva M, Carmeli Y, Giske CG, Glupczynski Y, Gniadkowski M, et al. Rapid evolution and spread of carbapenemases among Enterobacteriaceae in Europe. *Clin Microbiol Infect.* (2012) 18:413–31. doi: 10.1111/j.1469-0691.2012.03821.x

Harris PNA, Tambyah PA, Paterson DL. β-lactam and β-lactamase inhibitor combinations in the treatment of extended-spectrum β-lactamase producing Enterobacteriaceae: time for a reappraisal in the era of few antibiotic options? *Lancet Infect Dis.* (2015) 15:475–85. doi: 10.1016/S1473-3099(14)70950-8

Paterson DL, Bonomo RA. Extended-spectrum beta-lactamases: a clinical update. *Clin Microbiol Rev.* (2005) 18:657–86. doi: 10.1128/CMR.18.4.657-686.2005

Muñoz-Miguel J, Roig-Sena J, Saa-Casal A, Salvador-Aguilá M, Bediaga-Collado A. Multidrug-resistant *E. coli* in the community: assessment and proposal of a feasible indicator. *Eur J Public Health.* (2018) 28:cky213.709. doi: 10.1093/eurpub/cky212.709

Odonkor ST, Addo KK. Prevalence of multidrug-resistant *Escherichia coli* isolated from drinking water sources. *Int J Microbiol.* (2018) 2018:7204013. doi: 10.1155/2018/7204013

Overdevest I, Willemsen I, Rijnsburger M, Eustace A, Xu L, Hawkey P, et al. Extended-spectrum β-lactamase genes of Escherichia coli in chicken meat and humans, The Netherlands. *Emerg Infect Dis.* (2011) 17:1216. doi: 10.3201/eid1707.110209

Walsh TR, Weeks J, Livermore DM, Toleman MA. Dissemination of NDM-1 positive bacteria in the New Delhi environment and its implications for human health: an environmental point prevalence study. *Lancet Infect Dis.* (2011) 11:355–62. doi: 10.1016/S1473-3099(11)70059-7

Islam MA, Talukdar PK, Hoque A, Huq M, Nabi A, Ahmed D, et al. Emergence of multidrug-resistant NDM-1-producing Gram-negative bacteria in Bangladesh. *Eur J Clin Microbiol Infect Dis.* (2012) 31:2593–600. doi: 10.1007/s10096-012-1601-2

Rashid M, Rakib MM, Hasan B. Antimicrobial-resistant and ESBL-producing *Escherichia coli* in different ecological niches in Bangladesh. *Infect Ecol Epidemiol.* (2015) 5:26712. doi: 10.3402/iee.v5.26712

Hunter PR. Drinking water and diarrhoeal disease due to *Escherichia coli. J Water Health.* (2003) 1:65–72. doi: 10.2166/wh.2003.0008

Sirot D. Extended-spectrum plasmid-mediated beta-lactamases. *J Antimicrob Chemother.* (1995) 36:19–34. doi: 10.1093/jac/36.suppl_A.19

Taylor NGH, Verner-Jeffreys DW, Baker-Austin C. Aquatic systems: maintaining, mixing and mobilising antimicrobial resistance? *Trends Ecol Evol.* (2011) 26:278–84. doi: 10.1016/j.tree.2011.03.004

Levine MM. *Escherichia coli* that cause diarrhea: enterotoxigenic, enteropathogenic, enteroinvasive, enterohemorrhagic, and enteroadherent. *J Infect Dis.* (1987) 155:377–89. doi: 10.1093/infdis/155.3.377

Talukder KA, Islam Z, Dutta DK, Islam MA, Khajanchi BK, Azmi IJ, et al. Antibiotic resistance and genetic diversity of Shigella sonnei isolated from patients with diarrhoea between 1999 and 2003 in Bangladesh. *J Med Microbiol.* (2006) 55:1257–63. doi: 10.1099/jmm.0.46641-0

Nataro JP, Kaper JB. Diarrheagenic escherichia coli. *Clin Microbiol Rev.* (1998) 11:142–201. doi: 10.1128/CMR.11.1.142

Kaper JB, Nataro JP, Mobley HLT. Pathogenic *Escherichia coli. Nat Rev Microbiol.* (2004) 2:123–40. doi: 10.1038/nrmicro818

Coleman BL, Louie M, Salvadori MI, McEwen SA, Neumann N, Sibley K, et al. Contamination of Canadian private drinking water sources with antimicrobial resistant *Escherichia coli. Water Res.* (2013) 47:3026–36. doi: 10.1016/j.watres.2013.03.008

Park J, Kim JS, Kim S, Shin E, Oh K-H, Kim Y, et al. A waterborne outbreak of multiple diarrhoeagenic *Escherichia coli* infections associated with drinking water at a school camp. *Int J Infect Dis.* (2018) 66:45–50. doi: 10.1016/j.ijid.2017.09.021

Swerdlow DL, Woodruff BA, Brady RC, Griffin PM, Tippen S, Donnell HDJ, et al. A waterborne outbreak in Missouri of *Escherichia coli* O157:H7 associated with bloody diarrhea and death. *Ann Intern Med.* (1992) 117:812–9. doi: 10.7326/0003-4819-117-10-812

Chan EYY, Chiu CP, Chan GKW. Medical and health risks associated with

communicable diseases of Rohingya refugees in Bangladesh 2017. *Int J Infect Dis.* (2018) 68:39–43. doi: 10.1016/j.ijid.2018.01.001

Islam MM, Nuzhath T. Health risks of Rohingya refugee population in Bangladesh: a call for global attention. *J Glob Health.* (2018) 8:20309. doi: 10.7189/jogh.08.020309

Mahmud ZH, Islam MS, Imran KM, Ibna Hakim SA, Worth M, Ahmed A, et al. Occurrence of *Escherichia coli* and faecal coliforms in drinking water at source and household point-of-use in Rohingya camps, Bangladesh. *Gut Pathog.* (2019) 11:52. doi: 10.1186/s13099-019-0333-6

Rahman MR. Rohingya Crisis–Health issues. *Delta Med Coll J.* (2018) 6:1–3. doi: 10.3329/dmcj.v6i1.35960

Finley R, Glass-Kaastra SK, Hutchinson J, Patrick DM, Weiss K, Conly J. Declines in outpatient antimicrobial use in Canada (1995–2010). *PLoS ONE.* (2013) 8:e76398. doi: 10.1371/journal.pone.0076398

Levy S. *The Antibiotic Paradox: How Misuse of Antibiotics Destroys Their Curative Powers* (Perseus Cambridge, 2002).

WHO. *Antimicrobial Resistance: Global Report on Surveillance.* World Health Organization (2014).

Mohamed JA, DuPont HL, Jiang Z-D, Flores J, Carlin LG, Belkind- Gerson J, et al. A single-nucleotide polymorphism in the gene encoding osteoprotegerin, an anti-inflammatory protein produced in response to infection with diarrheagenic *Escherichia coli*, is associated with an increased risk of nonsecretory bacterial diarrhea in North Ame. *J Infect Dis.* (2009) 199:477–85. doi: 10.1086/596319

Nguyen TV, Le Van P, Le Huy C, Gia KN, Weintraub A. Detection and characterization of diarrheagenic *Escherichia coli* from young children in Hanoi, Vietnam. *J Clin Microbiol.* (2005) 43:755–60. doi: 10.1128/JCM.43.2.755-760.2005

Oswald E, Schmidt H, Morabito S, Karch H, Marches O, Caprioli A. Typing of intimin genes in human and animal enterohemorrhagic and enteropathogenic Escherichia coli: characterization of a new intimin variant. *Infect Immun.* (2000) 68:64–71. doi: 10.1128/IAI.68.1.64-71.2000

Talukdar PK, Rahman M, Rahman M, Nabi A, Islam Z, Hoque MM, et al. Antimicrobial resistance, virulence factors and genetic diversity of *Escherichia coli* isolates from household water supply in Dhaka, Bangladesh. *PLoS ONE.* (2013) 8:e61090. doi: 10.1371/journal.pone.0061090

Mahmud ZH, Shirazi FF, Hossainey MRH, Islam MI, Ahmed MA, Nafiz TN, et al. Presence of virulence factors and antibiotic resistance among *Escherichia coli* strains isolated from human pit sludge. *J Infect Dev Ctries.* (2019) 13:195–203. doi: 10.3855/jidc.10768

Heuvelink AE, Van de Kar N, Meis J, Monnens LAH, Melchers WJG. Characterization of verocytotoxin-producing *Escherichia coli* O157 isolates from patients with haemolytic uraemic syndrome in Western Europe. *Epidemiol Infect.* (1995) 115:1–3. doi: 10.1017/S0950268800058064

Islam MA, Heuvelink AE, De Boer E, Sturm PD, Beumer RR, Zwietering MH, et al. Shiga toxin-producing Escherichia coli isolated from patients with diarrhoea in Bangladesh. *J Med Microbiol.* (2007) 56:380–5. doi: 10.1099/jmm.0.46916-0

Frankel G, Giron JA, Valmassoi J, Schoolnik GK. Multi-gene amplification: simultaneous detection of three virulence genes in diarrheal stool. *Mol Microbiol.* (1989) 3:1729–34. doi: 10.1111/j.1365-2958.1989. tb00158.x

Lüscher D, Altwegg M. Detection of shigellae, enteroinvasive and enterotoxigenic Escherichia coli using the polymerase chain reaction (PCR) in patients returning from tropical countries. *Mol Cell Probes.* (1994) 8:285–90. doi: 10.1006/mcpr.1994.1040

Talukder KA, Islam MA, Khajanchi BK, Dutta DK, Islam Z, Safa A, et al. Temporal shifts in the dominance of serotypes of Shigella dysenteriae from 1999 to 2002 in Dhaka, Bangladesh. *J Clin Microbiol.* (2003) 41:5053–8. doi: 10.1128/JCM.41.11.5053-5058.2003

Thong KL, Hoe SLL, Puthucheary SD, Yasin RM. Detection of virulence genes in Malaysian Shigella species by multiplex PCR assay. *BMC Infect Dis.* (2005) 5:8. doi: 10.1186/1471-2334-5-8

Johnson JR, Kuskowski MA, Smith K, O'Bryan TT, Tatini S. Antimicrobial-resistant and extraintestinal pathogenic Escherichia coli in retail foods. *J Infect Dis.* (2005) 191:1040–9. doi: 10.1086/428451

Ahmed AM, Motoi Y, Sato M, Maruyama A, Watanabe H, Fukumoto Y, et al. Zoo animals as reservoirs of gram-negative bacteria harboring integrons and antimicrobial resistance genes. *Appl Environ Microbiol.* (2007) 73:6686–90. doi: 10.1128/AEM.01054-07

Guessennd N, Bremont S, Gbonon V, Kacou-Ndouba A, Ekaza E, Lambert T, et al. Qnr-type quinolone resistance in extended-spectrum beta-lactamase producing enterobacteria in Abidjan, Ivory Coast. *Pathol Biol.* (2008) 56:439– 46. doi: 10.1016/j.patbio.2008.07.025

Jouini A, Vinué L, Slama K, Ben SY, Klibi N, Hammami S, et al. Characterization of CTX-M and SHV extended-spectrum β-lactamases and associated resistance genes in Escherichia coli strains of food samples in Tunisia. *J Antimicrob Chemother.* (2007) 60:1137–41. doi: 10.1093/jac/dkm316

Leflon-Guibout V, Jurand C, Bonacorsi S, Espinasse F, Guelfi MC, Duportail F, et al. Emergence and spread of three clonally related virulent isolates of CTX-M-15-producing *Escherichia coli* with variable resistance to aminoglycosides and tetracycline in a French geriatric hospital. *Antimicrob Agents Chemother.* (2004) 48:3736–42. doi: 10.1128/AAC.48.10.3736-3742.2004

Muzaheed YD, Adams-Haduch JM, Endimiani A, Sidjabat HE, Gaddad SM, Paterson DL. High prevalence of CTX-M-15-producing Klebsiella pneumoniae among inpatients and outpatients with urinary tract infection in Southern India. *J Antimicrob Chemother.* (2008) 61:1393. doi: 10.1093/jac/dkn109

Nordmann P, Poirel L, Carrër A, Toleman MA, Walsh TR. How to detect NDM-1 producers. *J Clin Microbiol.* (2011) 49:718–21. doi: 10.1128/JCM.01773-10

Zhao S, White DG, McDermott PF, Friedman S, English L, Ayers S, et al. Identification and expression of cephamycinasebla CMY Genes in *Escherichia coli* and Salmonella Isolates from food animals and ground meat. *Antimicrob Agents Chemother.* (2001) 45:3647–50. doi: 10.1128/AAC.45.12.3647-3650.2001

Jacoby GA, Chow N, Waites KB. Prevalence of plasmid-mediated quinolone resistance. *Antimicrob Agents Chemother.* (2003) 47:559–62. doi: 10.1128/AAC.47.2.559-562.2003

Jacoby GA, Walsh KE, Mills DM, Walker VJ, Oh H, Robicsek A, et al. qnrB, another plasmid-mediated gene for quinolone resistance. *Antimicrob Agents Chemother.* (2006) 50:1178–82. doi: 10.1128/AAC.50.4.1178-1182.2006

Pu X-Y, Pan J-C, Wang H-Q, Zhang W, Huang Z-C, Gu Y-M. Characterization of fluoroquinolone-resistant Shigella flexneri in Hangzhou area of China. *J Antimicrob Chemother.* (2009) 63:917–20. doi: 10.1093/jac/dkp087

Kado C, Liu S. Rapid procedure for detection and isolation of large and small plasmids. *J Bacteriol.* (1981) 145:1365–73. doi: 10.1128/JB.145.3.1365-1373.1981

Macrina FL, Kopecko DJ, Jones KR, Ayers DJ, McCowen SM. A multiple plasmid-containing *Escherichia coli* strain: convenient source of size reference plasmid molecules. *Plasmid.* (1978) 1:417–20. doi: 10.1016/0147-619X(78)90056-2

Clermont O, Christenson JK, Denamur E, Gordon DM. The C lermont *Escherichia coli* phylo-typing method revisited: improvement of specificity and detection of new phylo-groups. *Environ Microbiol Rep.* (2013) 5:58–65. doi: 10.1111/1758-2229.12019

Bradford PA. Extended-spectrum β-lactamases in the 21st century: characterization, epidemiology, and detection of this important resistance threat. *Clin Microbiol Rev.* (2001) 14:933–51. doi: 10.1128/CMR.14.4.933-951.2001

Ensor VM, Shahid M, Evans JT, Hawkey PM. Occurrence, prevalence and genetic environment of CTX-M β-lactamases in Enterobacteriaceae from Indian hospitals. *J Antimicrob Chemother.* (2006) 58:1260–3. doi: 10.1093/jac/dkl422

Kamruzzaman M, Shoma S, Bari SMN, Ginn AN, Wiklendt AM, Partridge SR, et al. Genetic diversity and antibiotic resistance in Escherichia coli from environmental surface water in Dhaka City, Bangladesh. *Diagn Microbiol Infect Dis.* (2013) 76:222–6. doi: 10.1016/j.diagmicrobio.2013.02.016

Hasan B, Drobni P, Drobni M, Alam M, Olsen B. Dissemination of NDM-1. *Lancet Infect Dis.* (2012) 12:99–100. doi: 10.1016/S1473-3099(11)70333-4

Hasan B, Melhus Å, Sandegren L, Alam M, Olsen B. The gull (*Chroicocephalus brunnicephalus*) as an environmental bioindicator and reservoir for antibiotic resistance on the coastlines of the Bay of Bengal. *Microb Drug Resist.* (2014) 20:466–71. doi: 10.1089/mdr.2013.0233

Rahman MM, Haq JA, Hossain MA, Sultana R, Islam F, Islam AHMS. Prevalence of extended-spectrum β-lactamase-producing *Escherichia coli* and *Klebsiella pneumoniae* in an urban hospital in Dhaka, Bangladesh. *Int J Antimicrob Agents.* (2004) 24:508–10. doi: 10.1016/j.ijantimicag.2004.05.007

Chouduri AU, Biswas M, Haque MU, Arman MSI, Uddin N, Kona N, et al. Cephalosporin-3G, highly prescribed antibiotic to outpatients in Rajshahi, Bangladesh: prescription errors, carelessness, irrational uses are the triggering causes of antibiotic resistance. *J Appl Pharm Sci.* (2018) 8:105–12. doi: 10.7324/JAPS.2018.8614

Ahmed I, Rabbi MB, Sultana S. Antibiotic resistance in Bangladesh: a systematic review. *Int J Infect Dis.* (2019) 80:54–61. doi: 10.1016/j.ijid.2018.12.017

Biswas M, Roy DN, Tajmim A, Rajib SS, Hossain M, Farzana F, et al. Prescription antibiotics for outpatients in Bangladesh: a cross-sectional health survey conducted in three cities. *Ann Clin Microbiol Antimicrob.* (2014) 13:15. doi: 10.1186/1476-0711-13-15

Swedan S, Abu Alrub H. Antimicrobial resistance, virulence factors, and pathotypes of escherichia coli isolated from drinking water sources in Jordan. *Pathogens.* (2019) 8:86. doi: 10.3390/pathogens8020086

Hasan B, Islam K, Ahsan M, Hossain Z, Rashid M, Talukder B, et al. Fecal carriage of multi-drug resistant and extended spectrum beta-lactamases producing *E. coli* in household pigeons, Bangladesh. *Vet Microbiol.* (2014) 168:221–4. doi: 10.1016/j.vetmic.2013.09.033

Bonnet R. Growing group of extended-spectrum β-lactamases: the CTX-M enzymes. *Antimicrob Agents Chemother.* (2004) 48:1–14. doi: 10.1128/AAC.48.1.1-14.2004

Doublet B, Granier SA, Robin F, Bonnet R, Fabre L, Brisabois A, et al. Novel plasmid-encoded ceftazidime-hydrolyzing CTX-M-53 extended- spectrum β-lactamase from Salmonella enterica serotypes Westhampton and Senftenberg. *Antimicrob Agents Chemother.* (2009) 53:1944–51. doi: 10.1128/AAC.01581-08

Liu W, Chen L, Li H, Duan H, Zhang Y, Liang X, et al. Novel CTX-M β-lactamase genotype distribution and spread into multiple species of Enterobacteriaceae in Changsha, Southern China. *J Antimicrob Chemother.* (2009) 63:895–900. doi: 10.1093/jac/dkp068

Radice M, Power P, Di Conza J, Gutkind G. Early dissemination of CTX-M-derived enzymes in South America. *Antimicrob Agents Chemother.* (2002) 46:602–4. doi: 10.1128/AAC.46.2.602-604.2002

Islam MA, Huq M, Nabi A, Talukdar PK, Ahmed D, Talukder KA, et al. Occurrence and characterization of multidrug-resistant New Delhi metallo-β-lactamase-1-producing bacteria isolated between 2003 and 2010 in Bangladesh. *J Med Microbiol.* (2013) 62:62–8. doi: 10.1099/jmm.0. 048066-0

Kao C-Y, Wu H-M, Lin W-H, Tseng C-C, Yan J-J, Wang M-C, et al. Plasmid-mediated quinolone resistance determinants in quinolone-resistant *Escherichia coli* isolated from patients with bacteremia in a university hospital in Taiwan, 2001-2015. *Sci Rep.* (2016) 6:32281. doi: 10.1038/srep32281

Poirel L, Cattoir V, Nordmann P. Is plasmid-mediated quinolone resistance a clinically significant problem? *Clin Microbiol Infect.* (2008) 14:295–7. doi: 10.1111/j.1469-0691.2007.01930.x

Takasu H, Suzuki S, Reungsang A, Viet PH. Fluoroquinolone (FQ) contamination does not correlate with occurrence of FQ-resistant bacteria in aquatic environments of Vietnam and Thailand. *Microbes Environ.* (2011) 26:135–43. doi: 10.1264/jsme2.me10204

Strahilevitz J, Jacoby GA, Hooper DC, Robicsek A. Plasmid-mediated quinolone resistance: a multifaceted threat. *Clin Microbiol Rev.* (2009) 22:664– 89. doi: 10.1128/CMR.00016-09

Ma J, Zeng Z, Chen Z, Xu X, Wang X, Deng Y, et al. High prevalence of plasmid-mediated quinolone resistance determinants qnr, aac (6')-Ib-cr, and qepA among ceftiofur-resistant Enterobacteriaceae isolates from companion and food-producing animals. *Antimicrob Agents Chemother.* (2009) 53:519– 24. doi: 10.1128/AAC.00886-08

Yue L, Jiang H-X, Liao X-P, Liu J-H, Li S-J, Chen X-Y, et al. Prevalence of plasmid-mediated quinolone resistance qnr genes in poultry and swine clinical isolates of *Escherichia coli*. *Vet Microbiol.* (2008) 132:414–20. doi: 10.1016/j.vetmic.2008.05.009

Cattoir V, Poirel L, Aubert C, Soussy C-J, Nordmann P. Unexpected occurrence of plasmid-mediated quinolone resistance determinants in environmental Aeromonas spp. *Emerg Infect Dis.* (2008) 14:231. doi: 10.3201/eid1402.070677

Beutin L, Martin A. Outbreak of Shiga toxin–producing Escherichia coli (STEC) O104: H4 infection in Germany causes a paradigm shift with regard to human pathogenicity of STEC strains. *J Food Prot.* (2012) 75:408–18. doi: 10.4315/0362-028X.JFP-11-452

Huppertz HI, Rutkowski S, Aleksic S, Karch H. Acute and chronic diarrhoea and abdominal colic associated with enteroaggregative *Escherichia coli* in young children living in western Europe. *Lancet.* (1997) 349:1660–2. doi: 10.1016/S0140-6736(96)12485-5

Oundo JO, Kariuki SM, Boga HI, Muli FW, Iijima Y. High incidence of enteroaggregative *Escherichia coli* among food handlers in three areas of Kenya: a possible transmission route of travelers' diarrhea. *J Travel Med.* (2008) 15:31–8. doi: 10.1111/j.1708-8305.2007.00174.x

Jiang Z-D, Greenberg D, Nataro JP, Steffen R, DuPont HL. Rate of occurrence and pathogenic effect of enteroaggregative *Escherichia coli* virulence factors

in international travelers. *J Clin Microbiol.* (2002) 40:4185– 90. doi: 10.1128/
JCM.40.11.4185-4190.2002

Ahmed D, Islam MS, Begum YA, Janzon A, Qadri F, Sjöling Å. Presence of
enterotoxigenic *Escherichia coli* in biofilms formed in water containers
in poor households coincides with epidemic seasons in D haka. *J Appl
Microbiol.* (2013) 114:1223–9. doi: 10.1111/jam.12109

Begum YA, Talukder KA, Nair GB, Qadri F, Sack RB, Svennerholm A-M.
Enterotoxigenic *Escherichia coli* isolated from surface water in urban and
rural areas of Bangladesh. *J Clin Microbiol.* (2005) 43:3582–3. doi: 10.1128/
JCM.43.7.3582-3583.2005

Lothigius Å, Janzon A, Begum Y, Sjöling Å, Qadri F, Svennerholm A, et al.
Enterotoxigenic Escherichia coli is detectable in water samples from
an endemic area by real-time PCR. *J Appl Microbiol.* (2008) 104:1128–36.
doi: 10.1111/j.1365-2672.2007.03628.x

Mansour Amin MS, Javaherizadeh H, Motamedifar M, Saki M, Veisi H, Ebrahimi
S, et al. Antibiotic resistance pattern and molecular characterization of
extended-spectrum β-lactamase producing enteroaggregative *Escherichia
coli* isolates in children from southwest Iran. *Infect Drug Resist.* (2018)
11:1097. doi: 10.2147/IDR.S167271

Zhang R, Gu D, Huang Y, Chan EW-C, Chen G-X, Chen S. Comparative genetic
characterization of Enteroaggregative *Escherichia coli* strains recovered from
clinical and non-clinical settings. *Sci Rep.* (2016) 6:24321. doi: 10.1038/
srep24321

Talukder KA, Islam MA, Dutta DK, Hassan F, Safa A, Nair GB, et al. Phenotypic
and genotypic characterization of serologically atypical strains of Shigella
flexneri type 4 isolated in Dhaka, Bangladesh. *J Clin Microbiol.* (2002)
40:2490–7. doi: 10.1128/JCM.40.7.2490-2497.2002

Dionisio F, Matic I, Radman M, Rodrigues OR, Taddei F. Plasmids spread very
fast in heterogeneous bacterial communities. *Genetics.* (2002) 162:1525–32.

O'Neill J. Tackling drug-resistant infections globally: Final report and
recommendations. 2016. *HM Gov. Welcome Trust UK* (2018).

10

Genomic Characterization of Prevalent *mcr-1*, *mcr-4* and *mcr-5 Escherichia coli* within Swine Enteric Colibacillosis in Spain

Isidro García-Meniño[1†], Dafne Díaz-Jiménez[1†], Vanesa García[1‡], María de Toro[2],
Saskia C. Flament-Simon[1], Jorge Blanco[1] and Azucena Mora[1]*

[1] *Laboratorio de Referencia de Escherichia coli, Departamento de Microbiología y Parasitología, Facultad de Veterinaria,*
Universidad de Santiago de Compostela, Lugo, Spain, [2] *Plataforma de Genómica y Bioinformática, Centro de Investigación*
Biomédica de La Rioja, Logroño, Spain

*Correspondence:
Azucena Mora
azucena.mora@usc.es

[†] *These authors have contributed*
equally to this work

Antimicrobial agents are crucial for the treatment of many bacterial diseases in pigs, however, the massive use of critically important antibiotics such as colistin, fluoroquinolones and 3rd–4th-generation cephalosporins often selects for co-resistance. Based on a comprehensive characterization of 35 colistin-resistant *Escherichia coli* from swine enteric colibacillosis, belonging to prevalent Spanish lineages, the aims of the present study were to investigate the characteristics of *E. coli* clones successfully spread in swine and to assess the correlation of the *in vitro* results with *in silico* predictions from WGS data. The resistome analysis showed six different *mcr* variants: *mcr-1.1*; *mcr-1.10*; *mcr-4.1*; *mcr-4.2*; *mcr-4.5;* and *mcr-5.1*. Additionally, $bla_{CTX-M-14}$, $bla_{CTX-M-32}$ and bla_{SHV-12} genes were present in seven genomes. PlasmidFinder revealed that *mcr-1.1* genes located mainly on IncHI2 and IncX4 types, and *mcr-4* on ColE10-like plasmids. Twenty-eight genomes showed a *gyrA* S83L substitution, and 12 of those 28 harbored double-serine mutations *gyrA* S83L and *parC* S80I, correlating with *in vitro* quinolone-resistances. Notably, 16 of the 35 *mcr*-bearing genomes showed mutations in the PmrA (S39I) and PmrB (V161G) proteins. The summative presence of mechanisms, associated with high-level of resistance to quinolones/fluoroquinolones and colistin, could be conferring adaptive advantages to prevalent pig *E. coli* lineages, such as the ST10-A (CH11-24), as presumed for ST131. SerotypeFinder allowed the H-antigen identification of *in vitro* non-mobile (HNM) isolates, revealing that 15 of the 21 HNM *E. coli* analyzed were H39. Since the H39 is associated with the most prevalent O antigens worldwide within swine colibacillosis, such as O108 and O157, it would be probably playing a role in porcine colibacillosis to be considered as a valuable subunit antigen in the formulation of a broadly protective Enterotoxigenic *E. coli* (ETEC) vaccine. Our data show common features with other European countries in relation to a prevalent clonal group (CC10), serotypes (O108:H39, O138:H10, O139:H1, O141:H4), high plasmid content within the isolates and *mcr* location, which would support global alternatives to the use of antibiotics in pigs. Here, we report for first time a rare finding so far, which is the co-occurrence of double colistin-resistance mechanisms in a significant number of *E. coli* isolates.

Keywords: *Escherichia coli*, colistin, *mcr*, ESBL, fluoroquinolones, ST10, colibacillosis, swine

INTRODUCTION

Multidrug-resistant Enterobacteriaceae, such as *Escherichia coli*, represent a threat to both human and veterinary health. *E. coli* has a great capacity to accumulate resistance genes, mostly through horizontal gene transfer. The major problematic mechanisms correspond to the acquisition of genes coding for extended-spectrum beta-lactamases (ESBL), carbapenemases, 16S rRNA methylases, plasmid-mediated quinolone resistance (PMQR) and *mcr* genes conferring resistance to polymyxins (Poirel et al., 2018).

Colistin has been widely used in Spain for the control of neonatal and post-weaning diarrhoea (PWD) in pigs caused by certain *E. coli* pathotypes: Enterotoxigenic *E. coli* (ETEC), defined by the presence of genes encoding enterotoxins (*eltA*, and/or *estA*, and/or *estB*); atypical Enteropathogenic *E. coli* (aEPEC), carriers of *eae* but negative for *bfpA* (aEPEC); Shiga toxin–producing *E. coli* (STEC), positive for stx_{2e}; STEC/ETEC, positive for both shiga toxin type 2e and enterotoxin-encoding genes (stx_e and *estB* and/or *estA*) (García-Meniño et al., 2018). PWD results in significant economic losses for the pig industry due to costs derived of treatment and handling, decreased weight gain, and mortality. These circumstances have promoted the use and abuse of antibiotics in intensive farming (Luppi, 2017; Rhouma et al., 2017). However, specific regulations have been set up in Europe due to the concern that colistin resistance could be transmitted from food-production animals to humans which makes necessary the investigation of sustainable alternatives to antimicrobials (EUROPEAN COMMISSION, 2018).

In Spain, the rates of antibiotic resistance in pig farming were recently analyzed in a collection of 499 *E. coli* isolates from 179 outbreaks of enteric colibacillosis occurred during a period of 10 years (2006–2016) (García et al., 2018; García-Meniño et al., 2018). The results revealed a prevalence of colistin-resistant *E. coli* implicated in PWD in Spanish farms as high as 76.9% within 186 ETEC, STEC and STEC/ETEC isolates. Besides, PCR and sequencing identified the presence of *mcr-4* in 102 isolates, *mcr-1* in 37 isolates and *mcr-5* in five isolates. Interestingly, almost all *mcr-4* isolates belonged to the clonal group ST10-A (CH11-24) (García et al., 2018), which was shown to be highly present (more than 50%) within the *mcr-1* diarrheagenic isolates of a second study (García-Meniño et al., 2018). Both studies reinforced other countries' findings that the pig industry is an important reservoir of colistin-resistant *E. coli*, as well as being carriers of other additional risk genes such as bla_{ESBL} genes (García et al., 2018; García-Meniño et al., 2018; Magistrali et al., 2018; Manageiro et al., 2019). Based on reported evidences (Beyrouthy et al., 2017; Gilrane et al., 2017), there is great concern about the *in vivo* acquisition of *mcr-* and bla_{ESBL}-bearing plasmids by human *E. coli* isolates following treatment with colistin, or via animal transmission through direct contact or via food chain. Particular attention is given to those named as high-risk clones of (ESBL)-producing bacteria, worldwide spread within humans and animals, including *Escherichia coli* sequence types ST10, ST131, ST405, and ST648 (Mathers et al., 2015; Sellera and Lincopan, 2019).

The aims of this study were (i) the characterization of resistances and plasmid profiles of successfully spread *mcr-1*, *mcr-4*, and *mcr-5 E. coli* in Spanish pig farming; (ii) the assessment of WGS-based approaches for the characterization of pathogenic *E. coli*, through the correlation of the *in vitro* results with *in silico* predictions using the bioinformatics tools of the Center for Genomic Epidemiology (CGE).

MATERIALS AND METHODS

E. coli Collection

Thirty-five swine *E. coli*, positive by PCR for *mcr*-genes, were fully sequenced. Specifically, the 35 *E. coli* were selected from 499 diarrheagenic isolates of different geographic areas of Spain (2006–2016) (García et al., 2018; García-Meniño et al., 2018), taking into account the results of prevalence and significant association observed between pathotypes, presence of *mcr* and certain serogroups. In brief, the serogroups O108, O138, O141, O149, O157 were found significantly associated with ETEC; serogroups O26, O49, O80, O111 with aEPEC; serogroups O138 and O141 with STEC/ETEC; serogroup O139 with STEC; and serogroups O2, O15, O26, O45, O111, O138, O141, O157 with *mcr*-positive isolates (García-Meniño et al., 2018). Therefore, the collection analyzed here included 27 ETEC isolates (of serogroups O7, O8, O15, O45, O108, O138, O141, O149, O157, ONT); four STEC (O2, O139); three STEC/ETEC (O138 and O141) and one aEPEC (O111). The 35 representative isolates were carriers of the three *mcr*-types (*mcr-1*, *mcr-4*, and *mcr-5*) detected so far in our *E. coli* collection of porcine origin. Conventional pheno- and geno-typing was performed to complete classical characterization of serotypes, phylogroups, pathotypes and resistance profiles.

Conventional Typing

The H antigen was established for motile isolates by serotyping using H1 to H56 antisera, while non-motile isolates (HNM) were analyzed by PCR to determine their flagellar genes as described elsewhere (García-Meniño et al., 2018). The phylogroup was assigned by means of the quadruplex PCR of Clermont et al. (2013). Antimicrobial susceptibility was determined by minimal inhibitory concentrations (MICs) using the MicroScan WalkAway®-automated system (Siemens Healthcare Diagnostics, Berkeley, CA, United States) according to the manufacturer's instructions for: amikacin, ampicillin-sulbactam, aztreonam, cefepime, ceftazidime, ciprofloxacin, colistin, fosfomycin, gentamicin, imipenem, levofloxacin, meropenem, minocycline, nitrofurantoin, piperacillin-tazobactam, ticarcillin, tigecycline, and tobramycin. Additionally, resistance to ampicillin, amoxicillin/clavulanate, cefazolin, cefotaxime, cefoxitin, cefuroxime, chloramphenicol, doxycycline, nalidixic acid and trimethoprim-sulfamethoxazole was determined by disk (Becton Dickinson, Sparks, MD, United States) diffusion assays. All results were interpreted according to the CLSI break points (Clinical and Laboratory Standards Institute, 2019). Genetic identification of the ESBLs was performed by PCR using the TEM, SHV, CTX-M-1 and CTX-M-9 group-specific primers followed by amplicon sequencing (García-Meniño et al., 2018).

Whole Genome Sequencing (WGS) and Sequence Analysis

The libraries for sequencing were prepared following the instructions provided by the TruSeq Illumina PCR-Free protocol. Mechanical DNA fragmentation was performed with Covaris E220, and the final quality of the libraries assessed with Fragment Analyzer (Std. Sens. NGS Fragment Analysis kit 1-6000 bp). Lastly, the libraries were sequenced in an Illumina HiSeq1500, obtaining 100–150 bp paired-end reads which were trimmed (Trim Galore 0.5.0) and filtered according to quality criteria (FastQC 0.11.7). The reconstruction of the genomes and plasmids in the genomes was carried out using the methodology PLAsmid Constellation NETwork (PLACNETw)[1] (Lanza et al., 2014). The assembled contigs, with genomic size ranging between 4.9 and 5.9 Mbp (mean size 5.5 Mbp), were analyzed using the bioinformatics tools of the Center for Genomic Epidemiology (CGE)[2] for the presence of antibiotic resistance (ResFinder V2.1.), virulence genes (VirulenceFinder v1.5.), plasmid replicon types (PlasmidFinder 1.3./PMLST 1.4.), and identification of clonotypes (CHTyper 1.0), sequence types (MLST 2.0) and serotypes (SerotypeFinder 2.0). All the CGE predictions were called applying a select threshold for identification and a minimum length of 95 and 80%, respectively. Phylogroups were predicted using the ClermonTyping tool at the iame-research center web[3]. The mcr gene location was determined using PlasmidFinder/ResFinder prediction, together with PLACNETw references, and automatic annotation with Prokka v1.13 (Seemann, 2014).

RESULTS AND DISCUSSION

The phenotypic and genotypic traits of the 35 mcr-positive E. coli of swine origin, as well as their resistome and mobilome are summarized in **Table 1**. ResFinder confirmed that all genomes were mcr carriers. Likewise, VirulenceFinder predicted the acquired virulence genes encoding for the enterotoxins (sta1, stb, itcA), for fimbriae (fedF, k88), verotoxin (stx2) and intimin (eae), correlating in all cases with the pathotype assignation previously determined by PCR (García et al., 2018; García-Meniño et al., 2018).

Serotype Identification

In most studies, there is lack of information on E. coli serotypes since serotyping is performed by very few laboratories worldwide, hindering epidemiological comparisons. Here, we not only proved that there is a very good correlation between serotyping and SerotypeFinder predictions, but also the advantage of in silico H-antigen identification for those non-mobile (HNM) isolates. It is of note that 15 of the 21 HNM isolates were predicted

[1]https://castillo.dicom.unican.es/upload/

[2]https://cge.cbs.dtu.dk/services/

[3]http://clermontyping.iame-research.center/

as H39 (**Table 1**), namely O108:H39, O157:H39 and O45:H39 (five genomes, each). Given that the H39 is associated with the most prevalent O antigens within swine colibacillosis, such as O108 and O157, as well as ONT (García-Meniño et al., 2018), it would be probably playing a role in porcine colibacillosis to be considered as a valuable subunit antigen in the formulation of a broadly protective ETEC vaccine (Roy et al., 2009). The remaining six HNM isolates showed different O:H combinations: O138:H14, ONT:H5, O8:H20, O50/O2:H32, and O182:H19. SerotypeFinder also allowed the O45-antigen determination of two non-typeable (ONT) isolates (LREC-141 and LREC-146) and O182 of LREC-172; while LREC-147, belonging to O157 serogroup (**Table 1**), was predicted as ONT, probably due to the limitation of the assembly based on Illumina short reads (100–150 bp paired-end reads here) (Wick et al., 2017).

Phylogroups, Sequence Types and Clonotypes

The phylogroups established for the 35 genomes were the common ones reported for porcine E. coli isolates (A, B1, D-E) (Shepard et al., 2012; Bosak et al., 2019). However, we found discrepancies in the assignation obtained with the quadruplex PCR of Clermont et al. (2013) in comparison with that predicted by ClermonTyping for seven isolates: phylogroup E by PCR, while phylogroup D in silico (**Table 1**).

MLST and CHTyper tools determined 12 different STs, but mostly belonging to CC10 (21 genomes) and clonotype CH11-24 (18 genomes) (**Table 1**). The predominance of CC10, and specifically ST10, is in accordance with published data on E. coli isolates of swine origin, independently of the pathogenicity or antibiotic-resistance/susceptibility status (Shepard et al., 2012; Kidsley et al., 2018; Magistrali et al., 2018).

Resistome, Plasmidome and Phenotypic Expression of Resistances

The resistome analysis revealed that 34 of the 35 genomes encoded mechanisms of antibiotic resistance for ≥three different antimicrobial categories (**Table 1**). Seven E. coli were carriers of bla_{ESBL}, namely bla_{CTX-M-14} (four genomes), bla_{CTX-M-32} (one) and bla_{SHV-12} (two). Besides, six different mcr variants were identified within the 35 E. coli: mcr-1.1 (in 18 genomes, including two mcr-4.2 carriers); mcr-1.10 (one); mcr-4.1 (one); mcr-4.2 (13 genomes, including the two mcr-1.1 carriers); mcr-4.5 (two) and mcr-5.1 (two).

PlasmidFinder revealed a high plasmid diversity based on the identified replicons, with two to seven different plasmid types per genome (**Table 1**). Within this heterogeneity, mcr-1.1 genes were found mainly on plasmids of the IncHI2 and IncX4 types (six and four of the 12 mcr-1.1 plasmid-located genes, respectively); however, mcr-1.1 was also found integrated in the chromosome of LREC-145, LREC-148, LREC-149 and LREC-164 genomes. The mcr-1.10 gene of LREC-151 was located on the chromosome, while mcr-4 and mcr-5 variants were on Col8282-like (mcr-4.1), ColE10-like (for all 13 mcr-4.2 and two mcr-4.5 carriers) and pKP13a-like (mcr-5.1) plasmids. Furthermore, we found that

TABLE 1 | Features of the 35 colistin-resistant *E. coli* genomes of swine origin based on *in silico* characterization (light columns) and on conventional typing (gray columns).

Code	Year of Isolation[1]	Serotype[2]	Phylo Group[3]	CHType[4]	ST[5] (CC)	Plasmid content Inc group (pMLST)[6]	Acquired resistances (in black) and point mutations (in blue)[7]	mcr/location[8]	Virulence genes[9]	Phenotypic resistance profile[10]	Pathotype-associated VF[11]
LREC-144	2010	O141:H4	A	11-24	5786 (10)	IncF (F30:A-:B-) IncX1 IncHI2 (ST4)	aadA1, aph(3'')-Ib, aph(6)-Id; mdf(A); sul1; tet(A), tet(B); dfrA1; **mcr-1.1**; gyrA D87G	mcr-1.1/ IncHI2	**sta1, stb, fedF,** astA, fedA, iha, iroN, iss	NAL*, SXT, MIN*, DOX, FOF, CST	STa, STb, F18
LREC-145	2014	O50/O2:H32	A	11-23	10 (10)	IncF (F89:A-:B56) IncI1 (ST80) IncI2 pO111-like	bla_TEM-1b; aadA1, aadA2, aadA24, aph(3')-Ia; cmlA1; erm(B), mdf(A); sul3; tet(A); dfrA1; **mcr-1.1**; gyrA S83L	mcr-1.1/ chromosome	**stx2,** iha	TIC, AMP, SAM, NAL, SXT, MIN, DOX*, CHL, FOF, CST	VT2e
LREC-147	2008	*ONT:H5	B1	29-38	156 (156)	IncF (F110:A-:B42) IncHI2 (ST4)	aadA1, aadA2, acc (6')-Ib3; catA1, catB3, cmlA1; acc(6')-Ib-cr; mdf(A); sul1, sul3; tet(B); dfrA1; **mcr-1.1**; gyrA S83L, gyrA D87N, parC S80I, parC E84G	mcr-1.1/ IncHI2	**stb,** astA, iss, lpfA, gad	TIC, AMP, SAM, AMC, TOB*, NAL, CIP, LVX, SXT, MIN, DOX, CHL, CST	STb
LREC-148	2013	O157:H39	A	11-24	10 (10)	IncF (F12/08:A-:B42) IncB/O/K/Z Col156-like	bla_CTX-M-14, bla_TEM-1A; mdf(A); tet(B); **mcr-1.1**; gyrA S83L; **pmrB V161G**	mcr-1.1/ chromosome	**itcA, stb, K88,** astA, cba, celB, cma, gad, iha, sepA	TIC, AMP, SAM, AMC*, CFZ, CXM, CTX, FEP, NAL*, MIN*, DOX, CST	LT, STb, K88
LREC-149	2010	O138:H10	A	27-0	100 (165)	IncF (F110/108:A-:B42) IncI1 (STunknown) IncI2 IncQ1	bla_TEM-1b; aadA1, aac(3)-IIa; mdf(A); tet(A); dfrA1; **mcr-1.1**	mcr-1.1/ chromosome	**itcA, stb, K88,** astA, capU, iha	TIC, AMP, SAM, AMC, GEN, TOB, NAL*, CIP, MIN*, DOX, NIT, CST	LT, STb, K88
LREC-164	2009	O111:H9	B1	4-24	29 (29)	IncHI2 (STunknown) IncX1 Col8282-like	aadA1, aadA2, aph(3')-Ib, aph(6)-Id; catA1, cmlA1; mdf(A); sul1, sul3; dfrA1; tet(A); **mcr-1.1**; gyrA S83L	mcr-1.1/ chromosome	**eae,** espA, espB, espF, espJ, tccP, tir, cif, efa1, astA, celB, iha, lpfA, nleA, nleB	TIC, NAL, SXT, DOX*, CHL, CST	Eae-β1
LREC-165	2006	O8:H20	A	7-0	398 (398)	IncF (F2:A-:B71) IncHI2 (ST4) IncI2 IncY	aadA1, aadA2; catA1, cmlA1; mdf(A); sul3; tet(A); **mcr-1.1**	mcr-1.1/ ND	**stb,** astA, capU, gad	DOX*, CHL, CST	STb

(Continued)

TABLE 1 | Continued

Code	Year of Isolation[1]	Serotype[2]	Phylo Group[3]	CHType[4]	ST[5] (CC)	Plasmid content Inc group (pMLST)[6]	Acquired resistances (in black) and point mutations (in blue)[7]	mcr/location[8]	Virulence genes[9]	Phenotypic resistance profile[10]	Pathotype-associated VF[11]
LREC-166	2010	O7:H4	A	11-27	93 (168)	IncF (F2:A-:B-) IncHI2 (STunknown) IncN (ST1) IncX1	bla_SHV-12, bla_TEM-1B; aph(3')-IIa, aph(3')-Ib, aph(6)-Id; catA1; mdf(A); sul3; **mcr-1.1**	mcr-1.1/ ND (plasmid localization)	**stb**, astA, iss	TIC, AMP, SAM, CFZ, CXM, CTX, CAZ, ATM, CHL, CST	STb
LREC-167	2007	O141:H4	A	11-24	7323 (10)	IncF (F30:A-:B-) IncI2 IncX1 IncX4	bla_CTX-M-14, bla_TEM-1A; aadA2, aph(3')-Ib, aph(6)-Id; catA1; erm(B), mdf(A); sul1; tet(B); **mcr-1.1** gyrA S83L; *pmrA S39I*	mcr-1.1/ ND (plasmid localization)	**sta1, stb, fedF**, fedA, gad, iha, iroN, iss	TIC, AMP, AMC*, CFZ, CXM, CTX, FEP, NAL, MIN*, DOX, CHL, CST	STa, F18
LREC-169	2015	O141:H4	A	11-24	7323 (10)	IncF (F30:A-:B-) IncHI2 (ST4) IncI1 (STunknown) IncN (ST1) IncQ1 IncX1	bla_TEM-1B; aac(3)-IV, aadA1, aadA2, aph(3')-Ia, aph(3')-Ib, aph(6)-Id; floR; qnrS1; mdf(A), inu(F); sul1; sul2; tet(A); dfrA1; **mcr-1.1** gyrA S83L, parC S80R; *pmrA S39I*	mcr-1.1/ IncHI2	**sta1, stb, fedF**, fedA, gad, iss	TIC, AMP, GEN*, NAL, CIP, LVX, SXT, CHL, CST	STa, STb, F18
LREC-170	2015	O139:H1	*D	2-54	1	IncF (F14:A-:B-) IncX1 IncX4	mdf(A); **mcr-1.1**	mcr-1.1/ IncX4	**stx2, fedF**, eilA, fedA, gad, lpfA	TIC, AMP, SXT, MIN*, DOX, CST	VT2e, F18
LREC-171	2008	O138:H14	*D	28-65	42	IncF (F111:A-:B42) IncX1 IncX4	bla_TEM-1B; aadA1, aph(3')-Ia, aph(3')-Ib, aph(6)-Id; mdf(A); sul1; tet(B); **mcr-1.1** gyrA S83L, gyrA D87Y, parC S80R	mcr-1.1/ ND	**itcA, sta1, stb, fedF**, air, astA, cba, cma, fedA, gad, lpfA, iss	TIC, AMP, SAM, AMC*, NAL, CIP, LVX, MIN, DOX, CST	LT, STa, STb, F18
LREC-172	2014	O182:H19	A	11-94	10 (10)	IncF (F4:A-:B56*) IncB/O/K/Z IncHI2 (ST4)	bla_CTX-M-14; aadA1; catA1; mdf(A); sul1; tet(A); dfrA1; **mcr-1.1** gyrA S83L	mcr-1.1/ IncHI2	**sta1, stb, fedF**, capU, etpD, gad, iha	TIC, AMP, SAM, CFZ, CXM, CTX, FEP, GEN*, TOB*, ATM, NAL, CIP, LVX, SXT, DOX*, CHL, CST	STa, STb, F18
LREC-174	2010	O15:H45	*D	4-331	118	IncHI2 (ST4) IncX4 ColE10-like	bla_TEM-1B; aadA1, aadA2; catA1, cmlA1; mdf(A); sul3; **mcr-1.1**	mcr-1.1/ IncX4	**stb**, air, astA, eilA, gad	TIC, AMP, SAM, GEN, TOB, NAL, MIN, DOX*, CHL, CST	STb
LREC-175	2009	O45:H45	E	550-400	4247	IncF (F72/2:A-:B71) IncX4 Col156-like ColE10-like	mdf(A); **mcr-1.1** gyrA S83L	mcr-1.1/ IncX4	**stb**, air, astA, celB, eilA, gad	NAL, NIT*, CST	STb

(Continued)

TABLE 1 | Continued

Code	Year of Isolation[1]	Serotype[2]	Phylo Group[3]	CHType[4]	ST[5] (CC)	Plasmid content Inc group (pMLST)[6]	Acquired resistances (in black) and point mutations (in blue)[7]	mcr/location[8]	Virulence genes[9]	Phenotypic resistance profile[10]	Pathotype-associated VF[11]
LREC-178	2009	O141:H4	A	11-24	10 (10)	IncF (F30:A-:B-) IncHl2 (ST9*) IncI1 (STunknown) IncX1 IncX4	bla_TEM-1B; aadA1, aadA2; cmlA1; mdf(A), mph(B); sul3; dfrA1; **mcr-1.1** gyrA D87G; **pmrB V161G**	mcr-1.1/ IncX4	**sta1, stb, stx2, fedF,** cma, fedA, iha	TIC, AMP, GEN, TOB*, SXT, CHL, CST	STa, STb, VT2e, F18
LREC-151	2013	O139:H1	*D	2-54	1	IncI1 (STunknown) IncX1	aph(3')-Ia; mdf(A); **mcr-1.10** gyrA S83L	mcr-1.10/ chromosome	**stx2, fedF,** eilA, fedA, gad, lpfA	NAL*, CST	VT2e, F18
LREC-136	2012	O149:H10	A	27-0	100 (165)	IncF (F108:A-:B54) IncI1 (STunknown) IncR Col8282-like	bla_TEM-1B; aadA1, aadA2; aph(3')-Ia; cmlA1; mdf(A); sul3; **mcr-4.1** gyrA S83L	mcr-4.1/ Col8282	**sta1, stb,** astA, capU, iha	TIC, AMP, SAM, AMC, NAL, DOX*, CHL, CST	LT, STa, STb, K88
LREC-131	2011	O108:<u>H39</u>	A	11-24	10 (10)	IncF (F111:A-:B42) IncI1 (ST3) IncI2 Col156-like ColE10-like	bla_SHV-12; aadA2, aph(3')-Ia; cmlA1; mdf(A); sul3; tet(B); dfrA12; **mcr-4.2** gyrA S83L, gyrA D87G, parC S80I	mcr-4.2/ ColE10	**itcA, sta1, fedF,** celB, fedA, iha	TIC, AMP, CFZ, CXM, CTX, CAZ, ATM, NAL, CIP, LVX, SXT, MIN*, DOX, CHL, CST	LT, STa, F18
LREC-132	2016	O108:<u>H39</u>	A	11-24	10 (10)	IncF (F111:A-:B42) IncHl2 (ST9) IncI1 (ST48) IncI2 ColE10-like	bla_TEM-1B; aac(3)-IIa, aac(3)-IV, aadA1, aph(3')-Ia, aph(3'')-Ib, aph(4)-Ia; catA1; mdf(A), mph(B); sul1; tet(B); dfrA1; **mcr-4.2** gyrA S83L, gyrA D87G, parC S80I; **pmrB V161G**	mcr-4.2/ ColE10	**itcA, sta1, stb, fedF,** astA, cma, gad, iha	TIC, AMP, AMC, GEN, TOB, NAL, CIP, LVX, SXT, MIN, DOX, CHL, CST	LT, STa, STb, F18
LREC-133	2006	O138:<u>H14</u>	*D	28-41	42	IncF (F14:A-:B-) IncX1 ColE10-like	mdf(A); **mcr-4.2** gyrA S83L, parC S80R	mcr-4.2/ ColE10	**sta1, stb, stx2, fedF,** air, eilA, fedA, gad, iha, iss, lpfA	NAL, CIP, SXT, MIN, DOX, CST	Sta, STb, VT2e, F18
LREC-134	2013	O139:H1	*D	2-54	1	IncI1 (STunknown) IncX1 ColE10-like	aac(3)-IVa, aph(3')-Ib, aph(4)-Ia, aph(6)-Id; mdf(A); **mcr-4.2** gyrA D87N	mcr-4.2/ ColE10	**stx2, fedF,** eilA, fedA, gad, lpfA	GEN, TOB, CST	VT2e, F18
LREC-137	2009	O157:<u>H39</u>	A	11-24	10 (10)	IncF (F2:A-:B42) IncI2 Col156-like ColE10-like	bla_TEM-1B; aadA1; mdf(A); sul3; tet(B); dfrA1; **mcr-4.2** gyrA S83L; **pmrB V161G**	mcr-4.2/ ColE10	**itcA, stb, K88,** astA, cba, cma, gad, iha, sepA	TIC, AMP, GEN, TOB, NAL, CIP*, SXT, MIN, DOX, CHL*, CST	LT, STb, K88

(Continued)

TABLE 1 | Continued

Code	Year of Isolation[1]	Serotype[2]	Phylo Group[3]	CHType[4]	ST[5] (CC)	Plasmid content Inc group (pMLST)[6]	Acquired resistances (in black) and point mutations (in blue)[7]	mcr/location[8]	Virulence genes[9]	Phenotypic resistance profile[10]	Pathotype-associated VF[11]
LREC-138	2008	O157:H39	A	11-24	10 (10)	IncF (F2/111:A-:B42) IncI1 (ST154) IncI2 ColE10-like	aac(3)-IV, aph(3')-Ib, aph(4)-Ia, aph(6)-Id; floR; mdf(A); tet(B); **mcr-4.2** gyrA S83L, gyrA D87G, parC S80I; pmrB V161G	mcr-4.2/ColE10	**itcA, sta1, stb,** astA, cba, cma, iha	NAL, CIP, LVX, MIN*, DOX, CHL, CST	LT, STa, STb, F18
LREC-139	2009	O108:H39	A	11-24	10 (10)	IncF (F89*C2:A-:B42) IncN (ST1) IncI2 Col156-like ColE10-like	aadA2; mdf(A), inu(F); **mcr-4.2** gyrA S83L, gyrA D87N, parC S80I	mcr-4.2/ ColE10	**itcA,** astA, cellB, gad, iha	NAL, CIP, LVX, CST	LT
LREC-140	2015	O108:H39	A	11-24	10 (10)	IncF (F111:A-:B42) IncHI2 (ST9) IncI1 (ST80) IncN (ST1) IncI2 ColE10-like	blaCTX-M-32, blaTEM-1B; aac(3)-IV, aadA1, aph(3')-Ib, aph(4)-Ia; catA1; erm(B), mdf(A), mph(B); sul1; tet(B), tet(M); dfrA1; **mcr-4.2** gyrA S83L, gyrA D87G, parC S80I; pmrB V161G	mcr-4.2/ ColE10	**itcA, sta1, stb, fedF,** astA, fedF, cma, fedA, iha	TIC, AMP, CFZ, CXM, CTX, CAZ, FEP, GEN*, TOB*, ATM, NAL, CIP, LVX, SXT, MIN, DOX, CHL, CST	LT, STa, STb, F18
LREC-142	2010	O45:H39	A	11-24	10 (10)	IncF (F89*C2:A8*:B42) IncHI1 (ST2*) IncX1 Col156-like ColE10-like	blaTEM-1B; aadA1, aadA2, acc (3)-IV, aph(3')-Ia, aph(3')-Ib, aph(4)-Ia, aph(6)-Id; cmlA1, catA1; mdf(A), inu(G); sul1, sul3; tet(B); dfrA1; **mcr-4.2** gyrA S83L, gyrA D87G, parC S80I; pmrB V161G	mcr-4.2/ ColE10	**itcA, stb, K88,** astA, gad, iha	TIC, AMP, GEN*, TOB, NAL, CIP, LVX, SXT, DOX*, CHL, NIT*, CST	LT, STb, K88
LREC-143	2006	O138:H14	*D	28-41	42	IncF (F14:A8:B-) IncHI1 (ST2*) IncX1 ColE10-like	aadA1, aph(3')-Ia; mdf(A); catA1; sul1; tet(B); dfrA1; **mcr-4.2** gyrA S83L, parC S80R	mcr-4.2/ ColE10	**sta1, stb, stx2, fedF,** air, fedA, gad, iha, lpfA, iss	NAL, CIP, SXT, MIN, DOX, CHL, CST	STa, STb, VT2e, F18

(Continued)

TABLE 1 | Continued

Code	Year of Isolation[1]	Serotype[2]	Phylo Group[3]	CHType[4]	ST[5] (CC)	Plasmid content Inc group (pMLST)[6]	Acquired resistances (in black) and point mutations (in blue)[7]	mcr/location[8]	Virulence genes[9]	Phenotypic resistance profile[10]	Pathotype-associated VF[11]
LREC-156	2011	O108:H39	A	11-24	10 (10)	IncF (F111:A8*:B42) IncHI1 (ST2*) IncI1 (STunknown) IncI2 IncY Col156-like ColE10-like	bla_CTX-M-14; bla_TEM-1B; aac(3)-IV, aadA1, aadA2, aph(3')-Ia, aph(3')-Ib, aph(4)-Ia, aph(6)-Id; cmlA1, catA1; mdf(A); sul1, sul3; tet(B); dfrA1; **mcr-4.2** gyrA S83L, gyrA D87G, parC S80I; **pmrB V161G**	mcr-4.2/ ColE10	**itcA, sta1, fedF,** astA, celB, fedA, gad, iha	TIC, AMP, CFZ, CXM, CTX, FEP, GEN*, TOB, NAL, CIP, LVX, SXT, MIN, DOX, CHL, CST	LT, STa, F18
LREC-135	2008	O45:H39	A	11-24	10 (10)	IncF (F89*C2:A-:B42) IncI1 (ST202*) IncX1 ColE10	bla_TEM-1A; aac(3)-IVa, aph (3')-Ib, aph(4)-Ia, aph(6)-Id; mdf(A); **mcr-4.5** gyrA S83L, gyrA D87G, parC S80I, parE L416F; **pmrB V161G**	mcr-4.5/ ColE10	**itcA, stb, K88,** astA, iha, sepA	TIC, AMP, GEN*, TOB, NAL, CIP, LVX, CST	LT, STb, K88
LREC-146	2008	O45:H39	A	11-24	10 (10)	IncF (F89*C2:A-:B42) IncI1 (ST202*) IncX1 ColE10-like	bla_OXA-1, bla_TEM-1A; aac(3)-IV, aadA1, aph(3')-Ib, aph(4)-Ia, aph(6)-Id; floR; mdf(A); sul1, sul2; **mcr-4.5** gyrA S83L, gyrA D87G, parC S80I; **pmrB V161G**	mcr-4.5/ ColE10	**itcA, stb, K88,** astA, iha, sepA	TIC, AMP, SAM, AMC, GEN, TOB, NAL, CIP, LVX, SXT, CHL, CST	LT, STb, K88
LREC-152	2008	O157:H39	A	11-24	10 (10)	IncF (F108:A-:B42) IncI1 (ST290*) IncX1	bla_TEM-1A; aac(3)-IV, aph(3')-Ia, aph(3')-Ib, aph(4)-Ia, aph(6)-Id; mdf(A); **mcr-5.1** gyrA S83L; **pmrB V161G**	mcr-5.1/ ND (plasmid reference pKP13a)	**itcA, stb, K88,** astA, gad, iha	TIC, AMP, SAM, GEN, TOB, NAL, CST	LT, STb, K88

(Continued)

TABLE 1 | Continued

Code	Year of Isolation[1]	Serotype[2]	Phylo Group[3]	CHType[4]	ST[5] (CC)	Plasmid content Inc group (pMLST)[6]	Acquired resistances (in black) and point mutations (in blue)[7]	mcr/location[8]	Virulence genes[9]	Phenotypic resistance profile[10]	Pathotype-associated VF[11]
LREC-177	2007	O157:H39	A	11-24	10 (10)	IncF (F2/111:A-:B42) IncI2 ColI156-like	aadA1, aph(3')-Ia; mdf(A); tet(B); dfrA1; **mcr-5.1** gyrA S83L; **pmrB V161G**	mcr-5.1/ ND (plasmid reference pKP13a)	**itcA, sta1, stb, fedF;** astA, cba, celB, cma, fedA, gad, lha	NAL, SXT, MIN, DOX, CST	LT, STa, STb, F18
LREC-141	2007	O45:H39	A	11-24	10 (10)	IncF (F89*C2:A-:B42) IncHI2 (ST4) IncQ1 IncX1 ColI156-like ColE10-like	blaTEM-1A: aac(3)-IIa, aadA1, aph(3')-Ia, aph(3'')-Ib, aph(6)-Id; mdf(A); sul1, sul2, sul3; tet(A); dfrA1; **mcr-1.1, mcr-4.2** gyrA S83L, gyrA D87G, parC S80I, parE L416F; **pmrB V161G**	mcr-1.1/ IncHI2; mcr-4.2/ ColE10	**itcA, fedF;** astA, celB, fedA, iha	TIC, AMP, SAM, AMC*, GEN, TOB, NAL, CIP, LVX, SXT, DOX*, CST	LT, F18
LREC-163	2011	O45:H39	A	1	10 (10)	IncF (F89*C2:A-:B42) IncHI2 (ST4) IncX1 pO111-like ColI156-like ColE10-like	blaTEM-1B: aadA1, aadA17, aph(3')-Ib, aph(6)-Id; inu(F); mdf(A); sul1, sul3; tetA; dfrA1; **mcr-1.1, mcr-4.2** gyrA S83L, gyrA D87G, parC S80I; **pmrB V161G**	mcr-1.1/ IncHI2; mcr-4.2/ ColE10	**itcA, fedF;** astA, celB, fedA, gad, iha	TIC, AMP, SAM, AMC*, GEN, TOB*, NAL, CIP, LVX, SXT, CST	LT, F18

[1]Year of isolation of the WGS isolates recovered from pig colibacillosis. [2]Serotypes, [4]clonotypes, [5]sequence types, [6]replicon/plasmid STs, [7]acquired antimicrobial resistance genes and/or chromosomal mutations, [9]virulence genes were determined using SerotypeFinder 2.0, CHtyper 1.0, MLST 2.0, PlasmidFinder 2.0, pMLST 2.0, ResFinder 3.1 and VirulenceFinder 2.0 online tools at the Center of Genomic Epidemiology (https://cge.cbs.dtu.dk/services/), respectively; while [3]phylogroups were predicted using the ClermonTyping tool at the lame-research Center web (http://clermontyping.iame-research.center/). [2]Serotypes: underlined those antigens that were non-typeable (ONT or HNM) by conventional serotyping but determined by SerotypeFinder. *LREC-147 was solved as O157 by conventional typing. [3]Phylogroups: **"D" indicates that LREC-133, LREC-134, LREC-143, LREC-151, LREC-170, LREC-171, LREC-174 revealed discrepancies between the assignation obtained with the quadruplex PCR of Clermont et al. (2013) and the in silico assignation using ClermonTyping tool, showing phylogroup E by PCR, but phylogroup D in silico. [6]Plasmid STs: "*" indicates alleles with less than 100% but >95% identity and 100% coverage; "*" indicates alleles with multiple perfect hits found. [7]Resistome: chromosomic and plasmid mechanisms associated to colistin resistance are highlighted in bold. Genes coding for ESBLs appear underlined. Acquired resistance genes: beta-lactam: blaTEM-1B, blaTEM-1A, blaOXA-1, blaCTX-M-14, blaCTX-M-32, blaSHV-12; aminoglycosides: aac(3)-II/IV, acc(6')-Ib3, aadA, aph(3')-Ib, aph(3'')-I/IIIa, aph(4)-Ia, aph(6')-Id; phenicols: catA1, catB3, cmlA1, floR; fluoroquinolones: aac(6')-Ib-cr, qnrS1; macrolides: erm(B), inu(F), inu(G), mdf(A), mph(B); sulfonamides: sul1, sul2, sul3; tetracyclines: tet(A), tet(B), tet(M); trimethoprim: dfrA1, dfrA12. Point mutations: quinolones and fluoroquinolones: gyrA S83L: TCG-TTG, gyrA D87G: GAC-GGC, gyrA D87N: GAC-AAT, gyrA D87Y: GAC-TAT, parC S80I: AGC-ATC, parC S80R: AGC-AGG, parE E84G: GAA-GGA, parE L416F: CT-TTT; colistin: pmrB V161G: GGG-GTG, pmrA S39I: AGC-ATC. [8]The mcr gene location was determined using PlasmidFinder/ResFinder predictions, together with PLACNETw building and references (https://castillo.dicom.unican.es/upload/), and Prokka annotations. [9]Highlighted in bold, those features defining E. coli pathotypes (STEC, ETEC, EPEC). Virulence genes: itcA, coding for heat labile enterotoxin A subunit; sta1, heat stable enterotoxin ST-Ia; stb, heat stable enterotoxin II; fedF, fimbrial adhesin AC precursor; K88, K88/F4 protein subunit; air, enteroaggregative immunoglobulin repeat protein; astA, EAST-1; capU, hexosyltransferase homolog; cba, colicin B; celB, endonuclease colicin E2; cif, type III secreted effector; cma, colicin M; eae, intimin; efa1, EHEC factor for adherence; eilA, Salmonella HilA homolog; espA, type III secretions system; espB, secreted protein B; espF, type III secretions system; espJ, prophage -encoded type III secretion system effector; etpD, type II secretion protein; fedA, F107; gad, glutamate descarboxylase; iha, adherence protein; iroN, enterobactin siderophore receptor protein; iss, increased serum survival; lpfA, long polar fimbriae; nleA, non LEE encoded effector A; nleB, non-LEE encoded effector B; sepA, Shigella extracellular protein A; tccP, Tir cytoskeleton coupling protein; tir, translocated intimin receptor protein. bp, base pairs; CHType, clonotype (fumC-fimH); ST (CC), sequence type and clonal complex according to Achtman scheme; pMLST, plasmid sequence type. [10]Phenotypic resistances interpreted according to the CLSI (intermediate resistance is indicated with an asterisk *). AMC, amoxicillin/clavulanate; AMP, ampicillin; AMP/SAM, ampicillin-sulbactam; ATM, aztreonam; CAZ, ceftazidime; CHL, chloramphenicol; CIP, ciprofloxacin; CIP ciprofloxacin; CST, colistin; CTX, cefotaxime; CXM, cefuroxime; CFZ, cefazolin; DOX, doxycycline; FEP, cefepime; FOF, fosfomycin; GEN, gentamicin; LVX, levofloxacin; MI, minocycline; NAL, nalidixic acid; NIT, nitrofurantoin; SXT, trimethoprim/sulfamethoxazole; TIC, ticarcillin; TOB, tobramycin. [11]Pathotype of the isolates, established by conventional PCR, based on specific genes encoding toxins (LT, STa, STb, Stx1, Stx2, Stx2e), fimbriae (F4, F5, F6, F18, F41) and intimin (Eae).

there was no *mcr* plasmid co-occurrence in LREC-141 and LREC-163, but rather the *mcr-1.1* and *mcr-4.2* genes were located in independent plasmids (IncHI2 and ColE10-like types, respectively). The *mcr* location remained undetermined for four isolates.

Since the *mcr-1* plasmid gene was first described (Liu et al., 2016), it has been identified in members of the Enterobacteriaceae family encoded in different plasmid types, including IncI2, IncX4, IncHI1, IncHI2, IncFI, IncFII, IncP, IncK (Sun et al., 2018). Different authors corroborate that large conjugative plasmids of types IncHI2, IncX4 and IncI2 would be the maximum responsible for the dissemination of the *mcr-1* gene among *E. coli* isolates from different sources and geographical locations (Doumith et al., 2016; Li et al., 2017; Manageiro et al., 2019). To date, other *mcr* genes (2–9) have been described (Carroll et al., 2019); among them, the *mcr-4* and *mcr-5* genes appear mostly encoded in small and non-conjugative ColE-like type plasmids (Sun et al., 2018). Here we found similar results, since *mcr-1.1* genes were located mainly on IncHI2 and IncX4 types, and *mcr-4* on ColE10-like plasmids. It is of note that the *mcr-5.1* gene, predicted in LREC-152 and LREC-177, was linked to a Kp13-like plasmid (CP003996.1), location previously described by Hammerl et al. (2018) for one *mcr-5* isolate recovered from a fecal pig sample at farm. Chromosomally-encoded *mcr-1* location remains rare, however, it was described soon after the discovery of this plasmid-borne gene (Falgenhauer et al., 2016; Veldman et al., 2016). Here, we determined chromosomal location in five genomes by means of PLACNETw, and according to the predictive annotation of the *mcr*-contigs, the only common element flanking the *mcr-1* was a putative ORF, *pap2*, which is part of the Tn*6360* and encodes a Pap2 superfamily protein. Thus, Pap2 was detected in LREC-145, LREC-148, LREC-149, and LREC-164, while the IS*ApI1* element typically associated with the initial mobilization of *mcr-1*, was missing within the five contigs (Snesrud et al., 2018).

Overall, our findings are in accordance with those reported by Magistrali et al. (2018) on 13 *mcr*-positive *E. coli* isolated from swine colibacillosis in Belgium, Italy and Spain. Both studies show common features in relation to a prevalent clonal group (CC10), serotypes (O108:H39, O138:H10, O139:H1, O141:H4), and *mcr*-plasmid types. The confirmation of these similarities are of interest for the global design of alternatives to antibiotics that would curb the dissemination of specific clones in the pig farming.

The *in vitro* analysis of resistances showed that 30 of the 35 *E. coli* were multidrug-resistant (MDR) according to Magiorakos et al. (2012) definition (**Table 1**). Phenotypic results corresponded broadly to those predicted by ResFinder (**Supplementary Table S1**) as detailed below.

The quinolones/fluoroquinolones (FQ), together with polymyxins and 3rd–4th-generation cephalosporins, all are included in Category B of restricted antimicrobials in the EMA categorization, considering that the risk to public health resulting from its veterinary use needs to be mitigated by specific restriction (EMA/CVMP/CHMP, 2019). Two major mechanisms are implicated in the resistance to FQ, namely, mutations in the genes for DNA gyrase and topoisomerase IV, and decreased

intracellular drug accumulation. In addition, plasmid-mediated quinolone resistances also play a role but usually conferring low-level FQ resistance (van Duijkeren et al., 2018). Phenotypically, 17 of the 35 isolates showed resistance to both nalidixic acid and ciprofloxacin, and other eight resistance to nalidixic acid only (**Supplementary Table S1**). In the majority of cases, phenotypic results correlated with those predicted by ResFinder. Particularly, 28 of the 35 genomes carried the *gyrA* S83L substitution, with 12 of those 28 showing double-serine mutations (*gyrA* S83L and *parC* S80I). An additional substitution (*gyrA* D87N) was detected in two of the 12 *gyrA* S83L/*parC* S80I genomes. Thus, nalidixic acid resistance *in vitro* corresponded to one single substitution (*gyrA* S83L), and FQ resistance to double or triple substitutions (*gyrA* S83L/*parC* S80I/*gyrA* D87N). Plasmid-mediated quinolone resistant genes *acc(6')-Ib-cr* and *qnrS1* were also present together with chromosomal mutations in LREC-147 and LREC-169, respectively. Double-serine mutations in specific positions of the *gyrA* and *parC* genes have been reported as a dominant feature of MDR lineages within *E. coli*, *S. aureus* and *K. pneumoniae*, with favorable fitness balance linked to high levels of resistance to FQ (Fuzi et al., 2017). This finding, in 12 out of the 28 *in silico* predicted FQ-resistant could be conferring adaptive advantages to certain widely spread pig pathogenic clonal groups of *E. coli*, such as the ST10-A (CH11-24) (García et al., 2018). This hypothesis is presently assumed for ST131 and other risk clones linked to high FQ-resistance (Johnson et al., 2015; Fuzi et al., 2017).

On the other hand, colistin has been widely used for the control of enteric diseases, mainly in swine and poultry (Rhouma et al., 2016; Hammerl et al., 2018). Several mechanisms of resistance due to chromosomal mutations or acquired resistance genes have been described so far (Olaitan et al., 2014; Poirel et al., 2018). The 35 colistin-resistant *E. coli* of this study showed MIC values > 4 mg/L. As detailed above, ResFinder confirmed that all the analyzed genomes were *mcr*-carriers. In addition to the plasmid mechanism (*mcr*) of resistance, polymyxin resistance in *E. coli* can be due to genes encoding LPS-modifying enzymes, particularly to mutations in the two-component systems PmrAB and PhoPQ, or in the MgrB regulator. Quesada et al. (2015) detected two colistin-resistant *E. coli* recovered in 2011 and 2013 from the stools of two pigs, which showed mutations in PmrB V161G and PmrA S39I, reporting the finding as a rare event. Subsequently, Delannoy et al. (2017) analyzed 90 strains of *E. coli* isolated from diseased pigs: 81 were phenotypically resistant to colistin and 72 *mcr-1* carriers (including two colistin-susceptible). Although different mutations were found in the amino acid sequences of the MgrB, PhoP, PhoQ, and PmrB proteins of eight isolates, only two of them were *mcr-1* positive (but colistin-susceptible). Surprisingly, we found here the double mechanism of colistin resistance in 16 *E. coli*, harboring *mcr*-genes together with one amino acid substitution: PmrB V161G (14 genomes) or PmrA S39I (two genomes). In a recent study on Parisian inpatient fecal *E. coli* (Bourrel et al., 2019), the authors found 12.5% of colistin-resistant *E. coli* carriers among 1,217 patients; however, *mcr-1* gene was identified in only seven of 153 isolates, while 72.6% harbored mutations in the PmrA and PmrB proteins. According to the authors, their findings indicate two evolutionary paths leading to colistin resistance in human fecal *E. coli*, one corresponding to a minority of plasmid-encoded *mcr-1* isolates of animal origin, and a second corresponding to a vast majority of human isolates exhibiting chromosomally encoded mechanisms (Bourrel et al., 2019). Thus, and given the limited data regarding the co-occurrence of double resistance mechanism, it is of note that 16 of the 35 *mcr*-bearing genomes of our study showed mutations in the PmrA and PmrB proteins. Furthermore, two *E. coli* (LREC-141 and LREC-163) shown to be carriers of two different *mcr*-bearing plasmids together with PmrB V161G mutation. An explanation for this rare finding is that these isolates would be reflecting a cumulative evolution to antibiotic pressure and, as a consequence, enhancing the transmission (vertical and horizontal) of colistin resistance. In any case, further investigation is needed to evaluate the implication of chromosomal mutations and *mcr* co-occurrence regarding colistin resistance phenotype.

In this study, 22 out of the 25 isolates showing phenotypic resistance to beta-lactams (**Supplementary Table S1**), were positive in the analysis *in silico* for the presence of bla_{TEM-1} genes, alone (14 genomes), or in combination with other *bla* genes ($bla_{CTX-M-14}$, bla_{SHV-12}, $bla_{CTX-M-32}$ and bla_{OXA-1}); additionally, two genomes showed the presence of $bla_{CTX-M-14}$ and bla_{SHV-12}, respectively. With the exception of LREC-147, LREC-164, and LREC-170, which were phenotypically resistant to narrow-spectrum beta-lactamases but negative for the presence of genes, a good correlation was observed between genes predicted and resistance shown *in vitro*. It is of note that $bla_{TEM-135}$, determined in LREC-156 by conventional typing, was not identified *in silico*. Beta-lactams are the most widely used family in current clinical practice. Numerous genes in *E. coli* confer resistance to this group, being some of them, such as bla_{TEM-1} widespread in *E. coli* from animals coding for narrow-spectrum beta-lactamases that can inactivate penicillins and aminopenicillins. However, genes encoding ESBLs/AmpCs have increasingly emerged in *E. coli* from humans and animals, including food-producing animals (Cortes et al., 2010).

Thirty out of the 35 genomes showed high frequency of resistance genes to aminoglycosides, specifically encoding AAC(3)-II/IV and AAC(6)-Ib, which are the most frequently encountered acetyltransferases among *E. coli* of human and animal origins. The subclass AAC(3)-II, which is characterized by resistance to gentamicin, netilmicin, tobramycin, sisomicin, 2′-*N*-ethylnetilmicin, 6′-*N*-ethylnetilmicin and dibekacin (Shaw et al., 1993), and AAC(6′) enzymes that specify resistance to several aminoglycosides and differ in their activity against amikacin and gentamicin C1 (Ramirez and Tolmasky, 2010) seemed to correlate with the phenotypic detection of resistance to gentamicin and/or tobramycin (12 of the 17 resistant isolates) (**Supplementary Table S1**). We also detected high prevalence of genes encoding nucleotidyltransferases (*aadA*), which specify resistance to spectinomycin and streptomycin, alone or together with phosphotransferases (APHs) (Ramirez and Tolmasky, 2010), but they were not tested in the phenotypic antimicrobial susceptibility tests.

It is noteworthy that the 35 genomes of our study were carriers of *mdf(A)*. Edgar and Bibi (1997) described that cells

expressing MdfA from a multicopy plasmid are substantially more resistant to a diverse group of cationic or zwitterionic lipophilic compounds. Besides, the authors found that MdfA also confers resistance to chemically unrelated, clinically important antibiotics such as chloramphenicol, erythromycin, and certain aminoglycosides and fluoroquinolones. This capability could correlate with the *in vitro* resistance observed for some isolates to tetracyclines and aminoglycosides, in absence of other specific genes. In our collection, of the 24 isolates showing phenotypic resistance to minocycline and, or doxycycline (**Supplementary Table S1**), 20 showed carriage of *tet* genes: 12 *tet(B)*, six *tet(A)*, one *tet(A)* + *tet(B)* and one *tet(B)* + *tet(M)*. However, two *tet(A)* isolates were susceptible to those antibiotics (LREC-163, LREC-169). Additionally, *tet* genes were not detected *in silico* in four phenotypically resistant isolates. In general, *tet(A)* and *tet(B)* are the most prevalent tetracycline resistance genes in *E. coli* of animal origin, and specifically in isolates from pigs (Tang et al., 2011; Holzel et al., 2012; Jurado-Rabadan et al., 2014).

Although the use of chloramphenicol was banned in the European Union in food-producing animals in 1994, fluorinated derivative florfenicol is allowed for the treatment of bacterial infection in these animals (Schwarz et al., 2004; OIE, 2019). In the present study, all 19 chloramphenicol-resistant isolates (**Supplementary Table S1**) correlated with the presence of genes *catA1* (12 genomes), *catB3* (one genomes), *cmlA* (ten genomes) or *floR* (three genomes) detected *in silico*. Travis et al. (2006) showed that chloramphenicol resistant genes are frequently linked to other antibioresistance genes. Thus, through transformation experiments conducted with *E. coli* from pigs demonstrated that *aadA* and *sul1* were located with *catA1* on a large ETEC plasmid, and plasmids carrying *cmlA* also carried *sul3* and *aadA*. According to the authors, this linkage might partly explain the long-term persistence of chloramphenicol resistance in ETEC despite its withdrawal years ago. In our study, ResFinder also showed an association of genes *cmlA*, *sul3* and *aadA* present in the same contig (7 of the 10 genomes positive for *cmlA*), and *cmlA*/*aadA* in all cases. Additionally, *aadA* and *sul1* were located with *floR* in LREC-146.

In *E. coli* from food-producing animals, sulfonamide resistance is mediated by *sul* genes (*sul1*, *sul2*, *sul3*), widely disseminated, and frequently found together with other antimicrobial resistance genes, while *dfr* genes confer trimethoprim resistance in *E. coli* and other gram-negative bacteria (van Duijkeren et al., 2018). Within our collection, 20 of the 35 isolates were *in vitro* resistant to trimethoprim/sulfamethoxazole (**Supplementary Table S1**), and most of them correlated with the presence of *sul* + *dfrA* genes in their genomes, with the exception of LREC-133 and LREC-170 (negative for the *in silico* detection of *sul*, *dfrA* genes) and LREC-146 (in which only *sul1* and *sul2* genes were predicted). Besides, ResFinder showed that *sul1* (present in 16 genomes), *sul3* (14 genomes) and *sul2* (three genomes) were located together with *dfrA*, and other resistance genes, as mentioned previously.

The fosfomycin resistance showed *in vitro* by two isolates of the study collection, was not predicted for LREC-144 and LREC-145 (**Supplementary Table S1**) by ResFinder, which analyzes the presence of *fos* genes encoding for fosfomycin-modifying enzymes. The use of this antibiotic has been limited to the treatment of infections by Gram-positive and negative pathogens, included *E. coli*, mainly in pig and poultry farming (Poirel et al., 2018). However, phosphonic acid derivates such as fosfomycin, have been recently categorized by the EMA (EMA/CVMP/CHMP, 2019) as Category A (antimicrobial classes not currently authorized in veterinary medicine in EU).

CONCLUSION

Swine colibacillosis control has been traditionally managed through the extensive use of antibiotics. Our results are a reflection of the situation within the industrial pig farming, where global hygiene procedures and vaccinations are essential for improvement in antimicrobial stewardship. The summative presence of antibioresistances could be conferring adaptive advantages to prevalent pig *E. coli* lineages, such as the ST10-A (CH11-24). Based on the different replicons identified by PlasmidFinder (up to seven), it is of note the high plasmid diversity found within these isolates; further research is needed to know mechanisms of maintenance and advantages conferred to them.

Here, we report for first time a rare finding so far, which is the co-occurrence of double colistin-resistance mechanisms (*mcr*-genes and chromosomal mutations in the PmrA and PmrB proteins) in a significant number of *E. coli* isolates. This fact could be increasing the risk of colistin resistance-acquisition by means of food transmission. Globally, we found a very good correlation between resistances determined *in vitro* and genes predicted using CGE tools, and the same observation applies to the *E. coli* pathotype determination.

SAMN11523829 to SAMN11523863. These sequences are part of BioProject ID PRJNA540146.

AUTHOR CONTRIBUTIONS

IG-M, DD-J, and SF-S undertook the laboratory work. AM and JB conceived and designed the study. IG-M, DD-J, VG, MT, and AM performed the data analysis. IG-M, DD-J, VG, MT, JB, and AM drafted the manuscript. All authors provided critical input and approved the final version.

FUNDING

This study was supported by projects PI16/01477 from Plan Estatal de I+D+I 2013–2016, Instituto de Salud Carlos III (ISCIII), Subdirección General de Evaluación y Fomento de la Investigación, and FEDER; AGL2016-79343-R from the Agencia Estatal de Investigación (AEI, Spain) and FEDER; ED431C 2017/57 from the Consellería de Cultura, Educación e Ordenación Universitaria (Xunta de Galicia) and FEDER. IG-M and VG acknowledge the Consellería de Cultura, Educación e Ordenación Universitaria, Xunta de Galicia for their pre-doctoral and post-doctoral grants (Grant Numbers ED481A-2015/149 and ED481B-2018/018, respectively). SF-S acknowledges the FPU programme from the Secretaría General de Universidades, Ministerio de Educación, Cultura y Deporte, Gobierno de España (Grant Number FPU15/02644).

REFERENCES

Beyrouthy, R., Robin, F., Lessene, A., Lacombat, I., Dortet, L., Naas, T., et al. (2017). MCR-1 and OXA-48 in vivo acquisition in KPC-producing *Escherichia coli* after colistin treatment. *Antimicrob. Agents Chemother.* 61:e2540-16. doi: 10.1128/AAC.02540-16

Bosak, J., Hrala, M., Pirkova, V., Micenkova, L., Cizek, A., Smola, J., et al. (2019). Porcine pathogenic *Escherichia coli* strains differ from human fecal strains in occurrence of bacteriocin types. *Vet. Microbiol.* 232, 121–127. doi: 10.1016/j.vetmic.2019.04.003

Bourrel, A. S., Poirel, L., Royer, G., Darty, M., Vuillemin, X., Kieffer, N., et al. (2019). Colistin resistance in parisian inpatient faecal *Escherichia coli* as the result of two distinct evolutionary pathways. *J. Antimicrob. Chemother.* 74, 1521–1530. doi: 10.1093/jac/dkz090

Carroll, L. M., Gaballa, A., Guldimann, C., Sullivan, G., Henderson, L. O., and Wiedmann, M. (2019). Identification of novel mobilized colistin resistance gene mcr-9 in a multidrug-resistant, colistin-susceptible *Salmonella enterica* serotype Typhimurium Isolate. *MBio* 10:e853-19. doi: 10.1128/mBio.00853-19

Clermont, O., Christenson, J. K., Denamur, E., and Gordon, D. M. (2013). The Clermont *Escherichia coli* phylo-typing method revisited: improvement of specificity and detection of new phylo-groups. *Environ. Microbiol. Rep.* 5, 58–65. doi: 10.1111/1758-2229.12019

Clinical and Laboratory Standards Institute, (2019). *Performance Standars for Antimicrobial Susceptibility Testing*, 29th Edn. Wayne, PA: CLSI.

Cortes, P., Blanc, V., Mora, A., Dahbi, G., Blanco, J. E., Blanco, M., et al. (2010). Isolation and characterization of potentially pathogenic antimicrobial-resistant *Escherichia coli* strains from chicken and pig farms in Spain. *Appl. Environ. Microbiol.* 76, 2799–2805. doi: 10.1128/AEM.02421-2429

Delannoy, S., Le Devendec, L., Jouy, E., Fach, P., Drider, D., and Kempf, I. (2017). Characterization of colistin-resistant *Escherichia coli* isolated from diseased pigs in France. *Front. Microbiol.* 8:2278. doi: 10.3389/fmicb.2017.02278

Doumith, M., Godbole, G., Ashton, P., Larkin, L., Dallman, T., Day, M., et al. (2016). Detection of the plasmid-mediated mcr-1 gene conferring colistin resistance in human and food isolates of *Salmonella enterica* and *Escherichia coli* in England and Wales. *J. Antimicrob. Chemother.* 71, 2300–2305. doi: 10.1093/jac/dkw093

Edgar, R., and Bibi, E. (1997). MdfA, an *Escherichia coli* multidrug resistance protein with an extraordinarily broad spectrum of drug recognition. *J. Bacteriol.* 179, 2274–2280. doi: 10.1128/jb.179.7.2274-2280.1997

EMA/CVMP/CHMP (2019). *Answer to the Request From the European Commission for Updating the Scientific Advice on the Impact on Public Health and Animal Health of the Use of Antibiotics in Animals - Categorisation Of Antimicrobials Ema/Cvmp/Chmp/682198/2017.* London: European Medicines Agency.

EUROPEAN COMMISSION (2018). *Overview Report on Measures to Tackle Antimicrobial Resistance (Amr) Through the Prudent Use of Antimicrobials in Animals.* Brussels: European Commission.

Falgenhauer, L., Waezsada, S.-E., Gwozdzinski, K., Ghosh, H., Doijad, S., Bunk, B., et al. (2016). Chromosomal locations of *mcr-1* and *bla*CTX−M−15 in fluoroquinolone resistant *Escherichia coli* ST410. *Emerg. Infect. Dis.* 22, 1689–1691. doi: 10.3201/eid2209.160692

Fuzi, M., Szabo, D., and Csercsik, R. (2017). Double-serine fluoroquinolone resistance mutations advance major international clones and lineages of various multi-drug resistant bacteria. *Front. Microbiol.* 8:2261. doi: 10.3389/fmicb.2017.02261

García, V., García-Meniño, I., Mora, A., Flament-Simon, S. C., Díaz-Jiménez, D., Blanco, J. E., et al. (2018). Co-occurrence of *mcr-1*, *mcr-4* and *mcr-5* genes in multidrug-resistant ST10 enterotoxigenic and shiga toxin-producing *Escherichia coli* in Spain (2006-2017). *Int. J. Antimicrob. Agents.* 52, 104–108. doi: 10.1016/j.ijantimicag.2018.03.022

García-Meniño, I., García, V., Mora, A., Díaz-Jiménez, D., Flament-Simon, S. C., Alonso, M. P., et al. (2018). Swine enteric colibacillosis in Spain: pathogenic potential of *mcr-1* ST10 and ST131 *E. coli* isolates. *Front. Microbiol.* 9:2659. doi: 10.3389/fmicb.2018.02659

Gilrane, V. L., Lobo, S., Huang, W., Zhuge, J., Yin, C., Chen, D., et al. (2017). Complete genome sequence of a colistin-resistant *Escherichia coli* strain harboring mcr-1 on an IncHI2 plasmid in the United States. *Genome Announc.* 5:e1095-17. doi: 10.1128/genomeA.01095-17

Hammerl, J. A., Borowiak, M., Schmoger, S., Shamoun, D., Grobbel, M., Malorny, B., et al. (2018). mcr-5 and a novel mcr-5.2 variant in *Escherichia coli* isolates from food and food-producing animals, Germany, 2010 to 2017. *J. Antimicrob. Chemother.* 73, 1433–1435. doi: 10.1093/jac/dky020

Holzel, C. S., Harms, K. S., Bauer, J., Bauer-Unkauf, I., Hormansdorfer, S., Kampf, P., et al. (2012). Diversity of antimicrobial resistance genes and class-1-integrons in phylogenetically related porcine and human *Escherichia coli*. *Vet. Microbiol.* 160, 403–412. doi: 10.1016/j.vetmic.2012.06.010

Johnson, J. R., Johnston, B., Kuskowski, M. A., Sokurenko, E. V., and Tchesnokova, V. (2015). Intensity and mechanisms of fluoroquinolone resistance within the H30 and H30Rx subclones of *Escherichia coli* sequence type 131 compared with other fluoroquinolone-resistant *E. coli*. *Antimicrob. Agents. Chemother.* 59, 4471–4480. doi: 10.1128/AAC.00673-615

Jurado-Rabadan, S., de la Fuente, R., Ruiz-Santa-Quiteria, J. A., Orden, J. A., de Vries, L. E., and Agerso, Y. (2014). Detection and linkage to mobile genetic elements of tetracycline resistance gene tet(M) in *Escherichia coli* isolates from pigs. *BMC Vet. Res.* 10:155. doi: 10.1186/1746-6148-10-155

Kidsley, A. K., Abraham, S., Bell, J. M., ÓDea, M., Laird, T. J., Jordan, D., et al. (2018). Antimicrobial susceptibility of *Escherichia coli* and Salmonella spp. isolates from healthy pigs in Australia: results of a pilot national survey. *Front. Microbiol.* 9:1207. doi: 10.3389/fmicb.2018.01207

Lanza, V. F., de Toro, M., Pilar Garcillan-Barcia, M., Mora, A., Blanco, J., Coque, T. M., et al. (2014). Plasmid flux in *Escherichia coli* ST131 sublineages, analyzed by plasmid constellation network (PLACNET), a new method for plasmid reconstruction from whole genome sequences. *PLoS Genet.* 10:e1004766. doi: 10.1371/journal.pgen.1004766

Li, R., Xie, M., Zhang, J., Yang, Z., Liu, L., Liu, X., et al. (2017). Genetic characterization of mcr-1-bearing plasmids to depict molecular mechanisms underlying dissemination of the colistin resistance determinant. *J. Antimicrob. Chemother.* 72, 393–401. doi: 10.1093/jac/dkw411

Liu, Y. Y., Wang, Y., Walsh, T. R., Yi, L. X., Zhang, R., Spencer, J., et al. (2016). Emergence of plasmid-mediated colistin resistance mechanism MCR-1 in animals and human beings in China: a microbiological and molecular biological study. *Lancet. Infect. Dis.* 16, 161–168. doi: 10.1016/S1473-3099(15)00424-427

Luppi, A. (2017). Swine enteric colibacillosis: diagnosis, therapy and antimicrobial resistance. *Porcine Health Manag.* 3:16. doi: 10.1186/s40813-017-0063-64

Magiorakos, A. P., Srinivasan, A., Carey, R. B., Carmeli, Y., Falagas, M. E., Giske, C. G., et al. (2012). Multidrug-resistant, extensively drug-resistant and pandrug-resistant bacteria: an international expert proposal for interim standard definitions for acquired resistance. *Clin. Microbiol. Infect.* 18, 268–281. doi: 10.1111/j.1469-0691.2011.03570.x

Magistrali, C. F., Curcio, L., Luppi, A., Pezzotti, G., Orsini, S., Tofani, S., et al. (2018). Mobile colistin resistance genes in *Escherichia coli* from pigs affected by colibacillosis. *Int. J. Antimicrob. Agents.* 52, 744–746. doi: 10.1016/j.ijantimicag.2018.08.008

Manageiro, V., Clemente, L., Romao, R., Silva, C., Vieira, L., Ferreira, E., et al. (2019). IncX4 plasmid carrying the new mcr-1.9 gene variant in a CTX-M-8-producing *Escherichia coli* isolate recovered from swine. *Front. Microbiol.* 10:367. doi: 10.3389/fmicb.2019.00367

Mathers, A. J., Peirano, G., and Pitout, J. D. (2015). The role of epidemic resistance plasmids and international high-risk clones in the spread of multidrug-resistant *Enterobacteriaceae*. *Clin. Microbiol. Rev.* 28, 565–591. doi: 10.1128/CMR.00116-114

OIE (2019). *List of Antimicrobial Agents of Veterinary Importance.* Available at: https://www.oie.int/fileadmin/Home/eng/Our_scientific_expertise/docs/pdf/AMR/A_OIE_List_antimicrobials_July2019.pdf (accessed October 23, 2019).

Olaitan, A. O., Morand, S., and Rolain, J. M. (2014). Mechanisms of polymyxin resistance: acquired and intrinsic resistance in bacteria. *Front. Microbiol.* 5:643. doi: 10.3389/fmicb.2014.00643

Poirel, L., Madec, J. Y., Lupo, A., Schink, A. K., Kieffer, N., Nordmann, P., et al. (2018). Antimicrobial resistance in *Escherichia coli*. *Microbiol. Spectr.* 6:ARBA-0026-2017. doi: 10.1128/microbiolspec.ARBA-0026-2017

Quesada, A., Porrero, M. C., Tellez, S., Palomo, G., Garcia, M., and Dominguez, L. (2015). Polymorphism of genes encoding PmrAB in colistin-resistant strains of *Escherichia coli* and *Salmonella enterica* isolated from poultry and swine. *J. Antimicrob. Chemother.* 70, 71–74. doi: 10.1093/jac/dku320

Ramirez, M. S., and Tolmasky, M. E. (2010). Aminoglycoside modifying enzymes. *Drug Resist. Updat.* 13, 151–171. doi: 10.1016/j.drup.2010.08.003

Rhouma, M., Beaudry, F., Theriault, W., and Letellier, A. (2016). Colistin in pig production: chemistry, mechanism of antibacterial action, microbial resistance emergence, and one health perspectives. *Front. Microbiol.* 7:1789. doi: 10.3389/fmicb.2016.01789

Rhouma, M., Fairbrother, J. M., Beaudry, F., and Letellier, A. (2017). Post weaning diarrhea in pigs: risk factors and non-colistin-based control strategies. *Acta Vet. Scand.* 59:31. doi: 10.1186/s13028-017-0299-297

Roy, K., Hamilton, D., Ostmann, M. M., and Fleckenstein, J. M. (2009). Vaccination with EtpA glycoprotein or flagellin protects against colonization with enterotoxigenic *Escherichia coli* in a murine model. *Vaccine* 27, 4601–4608. doi: 10.1016/j.vaccine.2009.05.076

Schwarz, S., Kehrenberg, C., Doublet, B., and Cloeckaert, A. (2004). Molecular basis of bacterial resistance to chloramphenicol and florfenicol. *FEMS Microbiol. Rev.* 28, 519–542. doi: 10.1016/j.femsre.2004.04.001

Seemann, T. (2014). Prokka: rapid prokaryotic genome annotation. *Bioinformatics* 30, 2068–2069. doi: 10.1093/bioinformatics/btu153

Sellera, F. P., and Lincopan, N. (2019). Zooanthroponotic transmission of high-risk multidrug-resistant pathogens: a neglected public health issue. *J. Infect. Public Health.* 12, 294–295. doi: 10.1016/j.jiph.2018.12.013

Shaw, K. J., Rather, P. N., Hare, R. S., and Miller, G. H. (1993). Molecular genetics of aminoglycoside resistance genes and familial relationships of the aminoglycoside-modifying enzymes. *Microbiol. Rev.* 57, 138–163.

Shepard, S. M., Danzeisen, J. L., Isaacson, R. E., Seemann, T., Achtman, M., and Johnson, T. J. (2012). Genome sequences and phylogenetic analysis of K88- and F18-positive porcine enterotoxigenic *Escherichia coli*. *J. Bacteriol.* 194, 395–405. doi: 10.1128/JB.06225-6211

Snesrud, E., McGann, P., and Chandler, M. (2018). The birth and demise of the ISApl1-mcr-1-ISApl1 composite transposon: the vehicle for transferable colistin resistance. *MBio* 9, e2381-17. doi: 10.1128/mBio.02381-17

Sun, J., Zhang, H., Liu, Y. H., and Feng, Y. (2018). Towards understanding MCR-like colistin resistance. *Trends Microbiol.* 26, 794–808. doi: 10.1016/j.tim.2018.02.006

Tang, X., Tan, C., Zhang, X., Zhao, Z., Xia, X., Wu, B., et al. (2011). Antimicrobial resistances of extraintestinal pathogenic *Escherichia coli* isolates from swine in China. *Microb. Pathog.* 50, 207–212. doi: 10.1016/j.micpath.2011.01.004

Travis, R. M., Gyles, C. L., Reid-Smith, R., Poppe, C., McEwen, S. A., Friendship, R., et al. (2006). Chloramphenicol and kanamycin resistance among porcine *Escherichia coli* in Ontario. *J. Antimicrob. Chemother.* 58, 173–177. doi: 10.1093/jac/dkl207 van Duijkeren, E., Schink, A. K., Roberts, M. C., Wang, Y., and Schwarz, S. (2018). Mechanisms of bacterial resistance to antimicrobial agents. *Microbiol. Spectr.* 6, 51–82. doi: 10.1128/microbiolspec.ARBA-0019-2017

Veldman, K., van Essen-Zandbergen, A., Rapallini, M., Wit, B., Heymans, R., van Pelt, W., et al. (2016). Location of colistin resistance gene mcr-1 in *Enterobacteriaceae* from livestock and meat. *J. Antimicrob. Chemother.* 71, 2340–2342. doi: 10.1093/jac/dkw181

Wick, R. R., Judd, L. M., Gorrie, C. L., and Holt, K. E. (2017). Completing bacterial genome assemblies with multiplex MinION sequencing. *Microb. Genom.* 3:e000132. doi: 10.1099/mgen.0.000132

11

Multiple *Klebsiella pneumoniae* KPC Clones Contribute to an Extended Hospital Outbreak

Carolina Ferrari[1], Marta Corbella[1,2], Stefano Gaiarsa[1], Francesco Comandatore[3,4],
Erika Scaltriti[5], Claudio Bandi[3,6], Patrizia Cambieri[1], Piero Marone[1] and
Davide Sassera[7]*

[1] Microbiology and Virology Unit, Fondazione IRCCS Policlinico San Matteo, Pavia, Italy, [2] Biometric and Medical Statistics Unit, Fondazione IRCCS Policlinico San Matteo, Pavia, Italy, [3] Pediatric Research Center Romeo ed Enrica Invernizzi, University of Milan, Milan, Italy, [4] Department of Biomedical and Clinical Sciences "L. Sacco", University of Milan, Milan, Italy, [5] Risk Analysis and Genomic Epidemiology Unit, Istituto Zooprofilattico Sperimentale della Lombardia e dell'Emilia Romagna (IZSLER), Brescia, Italy, [6] Department of Biosciences, University of Milan, Milan, Italy, [7] Department of Biology and Biotechnology "L. Spallanzani", University of Pavia, Pavia, Italy

*Correspondence:
Davide Sassera
davide.sassera@unipv.it

The circulation of carbapenem-resistant *Klebsiella pneumoniae* (CRKP) is a significant problem worldwide. In this work we characterize the isolates and reconstruct the spread of a multi-clone epidemic event that occurred in an Intensive Care Unit in a hospital in Northern Italy. The event took place from August 2015 to May 2016 and involved 23 patients. Twelve of these patients were colonized by CRKP at the gastrointestinal level, while the other 11 were infected in various body districts. We retrospectively collected data on the inpatients and characterized a subset of the CRKP isolates using antibiotic resistance profiling and whole genome sequencing. A SNP-based phylogenetic approach was used to depict the evolutionary context of the obtained genomes, showing that 26 of the 32 isolates belong to three genome clusters, while the remaining six were classified as sporadic. The first genome cluster was composed of multi-resistant isolates of sequence type (ST) 512. Among those, two were resistant to colistin, one of which indicating the insurgence of resistance during an infection. One patient hospitalized in this period was colonized by two strains of CRKP, both carrying the *bla*KPC gene (variant KPC-3). The analysis of the genome contig containing the *bla*KPC locus indicates that the gene was not transmitted between the two isolates. The second infection cluster comprised four other genomes of ST512, while the third one (ST258) colonized 12 patients, causing five clinical infections and resulting in seven deaths. This cluster presented the highest level of antibiotic resistance, including colistin resistance in all 17 analyzed isolates. The three outbreaking clones did not present more virulence genes than the sporadic isolates and had different patterns of antibiotic resistance, however, were clearly distinct from the sporadic ones in terms of infection status, being the only ones causing overt infections.

Keywords: KPC, genomic epidemiology, MDR, *Klebsiella pneumoniae*, nosocomial outbreak, colistin resistance

INTRODUCTION

Klebsiella pneumoniae (*Kp*) is ubiquitous in the environment, part of the normal intestinal microbiota in humans and capable of colonizing the skin and nasopharynx of healthy individuals (Podschun and Ullmann, 1998; Broberg et al., 2014). *Kp* can persist on abiotic surfaces of different origin through the synthesis of biofilm, which can also make bacteria resistant to the action of antimicrobial agents (Di Martino et al., 2003). In immunocompromised or debilitated hospitalized patients with severe underlying diseases, *Kp* causes urinary tract, respiratory tract and bloodstream infections (Podschun and Ullmann, 1998) as well as other less frequent diseases, including osteomyelitis, arthritis (Ghorashi et al., 2011), and meningitis (Ko et al., 2002; Tumbarello et al., 2006; Nordmann et al., 2009). *Kp* is responsible for roughly 12% of Gram-negative infections in hospital intensive care units (ICUs) in Europe (European Centre for Disease Prevention and Control [ECDC], 2016). *Kp* invasive infections are associated with high rates of morbidity and mortality due to the high prevalence of resistance to most available antimicrobial agents (Patel et al., 2008; Borer et al., 2009). This is an emerging concern in clinical care resulting in an increase of mortality rates and costs.

The most commonly used class of antibiotics against nosocomial infections is β-lactams, which includes penicillin derivatives, cephalosporins, monobactams and the most recently developed carbapenems. Frequent use and abuse of these drugs, combined with the transmissibility of resistance determinants mediated by mobile elements (plasmids, transposons, and other integrative conjugative elements), has contributed to the spread of resistance to β-lactams by *Kp* (Mathers et al., 2015; Navon-Venezia et al., 2017). In the last 20 years, the emergence of isolates resistant to carbapenems has limited the efficacy of this last line treatment option hampering the use of this whole class of antibiotics, with few alternatives (Mathers et al., 2015; Navon-Venezia et al., 2017). One of the most common mechanism of resistance to carbapenems in *Kp* is the *K. pneumoniae* carbapenemase (KPC). This is an Ambler molecular class A serine enzyme that is able to hydrolyze a broad variety of β-lactams. KPC carbapenemases are plasmid-encoded, they have been originally associated with the *Kp* clonal group 258 (CG258) (Samuelsen et al., 2009; Breurec et al., 2013) but are not limited to it, as a number of occurrences of strains of other sequence types (ST) carrying the gene have been reported (Giakkoupi et al., 2010; Qi et al., 2010; Tzouvelekis et al., 2013; Markovska et al., 2015; Oteo et al., 2016; Villa et al., 2016; Wei et al., 2016; Aires et al., 2017). KPC-carrying *Kp* strains have recently spread worldwide, with some countries, including Italy, being heavily affected. In Italy, in 2017, 33.9% of the *Kp* nosocomial infections were caused by KPC strains (Sabbatucci et al., 2017). Most of these strains belong to the CG258, which in Italy has been shown to have been imported on four occasions, giving rise to four Italian-subclades (Gaiarsa et al., 2015). The spread of carbapenem-resistant strains has led to the resurgence of the use of colistin, previously abandoned due to its nephrotoxicity and neurotoxicity (Javan et al., 2015; Velkov et al., 2018). This has however resulted in the emergence of colistin-resistant

strains, both due to the insurgence of chromosomal mutations (Cannatelli et al., 2014; Olaitan et al., 2014) and to the acquisition of plasmid-encoded resistance genes (Di Pilato et al., 2016; Liu et al., 2016).

Whole genome sequencing (WGS) of bacterial isolates is increasingly used for epidemiological investigations (Sabat et al., 2013). The use of genomics in clinical settings as a routine tool could in the future be an important aid to the microbiologist to accurately identify and characterize outbreaks at early stages, and to identify transmission routes. However, only from the combination of typing data with clinical and demographic data the correct interpretation of the origin and evolution of an outbreak can be obtained (Van Belkum et al., 2007).

The present retrospective study analyzes a nosocomial outbreak, lasting 10 months (August 2015 – May 2016), caused by *K. pneumoniae* KPC, in an ICU and the period immediately before and after, for a total of 12 months. Thanks to the combination of genomic, microbiological and clinical data it was possible to reconstruct the epidemic event and to characterize the multiple unrelated strains that spread in mostly temporally non-overlapping periods.

THE EVENT

At the Fondazione IRCCS Policlinico San Matteo in Pavia, a 900-bed hospital in Northern Italy, cardio-respiratory patients are admitted to a specific Cardiorespiratory ICU where preoperative assessment, anesthetic treatment and intensive post-operative treatment of the patients undergoing cardiac and thoracic surgery are performed. This ICU has eight beds and is managed by 37 staff members. All ICU patients are subjected to surveillance through rectal swab at admission and once a week during the stay in the ward, to monitor for carbapenem-resistant *Enterobacteriaceae* colonization. In case of positivity, additional contact precautions are applied, which are interrupted only after three consecutive negative surveillance samples and are resumed in case of a single new positive screening swab.

Retrospectively, an increase in the number of carbapenem-resistant *Klebsiella pneumoniae* (CRKP) colonizations and infections in the ICU was observed in the period from August 2015 to May 2016. The first infection was reported on 15th August 2015. After this event, the number of infected and colonized patients gradually increased and peaked twice, in December 2015 and March 2016. When the first increase in cases was detected (December 2015), additional surveillance measures were undertaken: increase in the training of health personnel and in the use of disposable devices, more accurate daily cleaning, and increased passive surveillance. Environmental screenings were performed in the ward after the second peak in cases in March 2016, all resulting negative. No cohorting or spatial isolation of individual patients were applied. The situation returned to the norm, with no clinical infections, in June 2016 (**Figure 1**). The period from June 2015 to May 2016 was thus analyzed to understand the characteristics of the observed prolonged outbreak. A total of 426 patients were hospitalized in the ICU during that period and the procedure for rectal swab screening

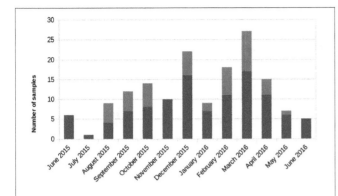

FIGURE 1 | Number of samples positive for carbapenem-resistant *Klebsiella pneumoniae* from patients hospitalized in the ICU during the August 2015 – May 2016 period. Samples positive for rectal swab screening are colored in blue; samples showing positive infection are colored in orange.

for Carbapenem-Resistant *Enterobacteriaceae* identified 23/426 CRKP-colonized patients (average age: 61.1 years; range: 27–80 years). Out of these 23 patients, 18 were negative at the admission time into the ICU. Two of the five patients (numbers 6 and 22) that were positive at admission at the ICU were previously hospitalized in other wards (respectively another ICU and Cardiac Surgery) were they became colonized. The remaining three patients (numbers 2, 4, and 7) were positive at the first swab, suggesting positivity before hospitalization. During the event 11/23 (47.8%) patients died, 2/23 (8.7%) were discharged for rehabilitation and 10/23 (43.5%) were transferred to other hospitalization facilities or hospital wards. Eleven of these 23 (47.8%) patients developed overt infections, with CRKP isolated from blood, respiratory tract, urine and wounds. Seven of the 11 infected patients died while at the ICU. The demographic and hospitalization characteristics of the 23 patients are reported in **Table 1**. During the same period, a total of eight other patients resulted infected by non-carbapenem resistant *Kp*, thus 58% of total *Kp* infections were CRKP.

MATERIALS AND METHODS

Ethics Statement

The study was designed and conducted in accordance with the Helsinki declaration and approved by the Ethics Committee of Fondazione IRCCS Policlinico San Matteo in Pavia, Italy.

Bacterial Strain Identification and Susceptibility Testing

During the entirety of the event, all surveillance rectal swabs were sent to the Microbiology and Virology Unit and were directly plated on chromID CARBA Agar (BioMérieux, Marcy-l'Étoile, France) to screen for the presence of carbapenemase-producing *Enterobacteriaceae*. In the same period, all clinical specimens (blood samples, bronchial aspirates, bronchoalveolar wash, urine samples, and wound

swabs) were all cultured in parallel on all the following media: Columbia Blood Agar with 5% sheep blood, chocolate agar, selective media or on Schaedler agar and 5% sheep blood (BioMérieux SA, Marcy-l'Étoile, France) anaerobically and incubated at 37°C overnight. Colonies suspected to be *Kp* based on morphology were identified with the MALDI Biotyper 3.1 system based on Matrix-Assisted Laser Desorption Ionization time-of-flight (MALDI-TOF) (Bruker Daltonics, Bremen, Germany).

We selected a subset of the *Kp* isolates from surveillance and clinical samples based on sample type, collection date and resistance profile, to perform additional characterization. Antibiotic susceptibility testing and minimum inhibitory concentrations (MICs) determinations were performed using the BD Phoenix 100 automated system (Becton, Dickinson and Company, Franklin Lakes, NJ, United States) and interpreted following the clinical breakpoints of the version 6.0 of the European Committee on Antimicrobial Susceptibility Testing [EUCAST] (2016)[1]. Tigecycline and carbapenems MICs were confirmed by *E*-test strips (BioMérieux, Marcy-l'Étoile, France). As recommended by European Committee on Antimicrobial Susceptibility Testing [EUCAST] (2016)[2] and the European Centre for Disease Prevention and Control [ECDC] (2016)[3], colistin MICs were confirmed performing the broth microdiluition (MIC-Strip Colistin (MERLIN Diagnostika GmbH, Germany).

DNA Extraction and Genome Sequencing

Total DNA extraction was performed for the selected isolates using the QIAamp DNA mini kit (Qiagen, Italy) according to manufacturer's instructions. DNA was sequenced using the Illumina MiSeq platform (Illumina Inc., San Diego, CA, United States), with paired-end runs of 2 × 250 bp, after Nextera XT library preparation.

Genomic Analyses

Sequencing reads were quality checked using FastQC[4] and trimmed using the Trimmomatic software (Bolger et al., 2014). SPAdes-3.10.1 (Bankevich et al., 2012) was then used to assemble the pair-end reads using the accurate setting. Multilocus sequence typing (MLST) profiles and virulence/resistance gene variants were determined *in silico* using the Kleborate tool[5]. Presence of the *mcr* gene was tested using ResFinder Version 3.1.0 (database updated to February 20, 2019) (Zankari et al., 2012). Plasmid content was characterized using PlasmidFinder Version 2.0.1 (database updated to November 20, 2018) (Carattoli et al., 2014), while the contigs containing the *bla*KPC gene were

---

[1]http://www.eucast.org/fileadmin/src/media/PDFs/EUCAST_files/Breakpoint_tables/v_6.0_Breakpoint_table.xls

[2]http://www.eucast.org/fileadmin/src/media/PDFs/EUCAST_files/General_documents/Recommendations_for_MIC_determination_of_colistin_March_2016.pdf

[3]https://ecdc.europa.eu/sites/portal/files/media/en/publications/Publications/enterobacteriaceae-risk-assessment-diseases-caused-by-antimicrobial-resistant-microorganisms-europe-june-2016.pdf

[4]www.bioinformatics.babraham.ac.uk/projects/fastqc/

[5]https://github.com/katholt/Kleborate

TABLE 1 | Table showing the hospitalization characteristics of all patients admitted to the ICU in the examined period that resulted positive to carbapenem-resistant *Klebsiella pneumoniae* at least once.

Patient number	Admission date	Discharge date	Sample number		Outcome
			Surveillance	Clinical	
1	May 24, 2015	June 17, 2015	3	0	Transfer to another hospital ward
2	June 17, 2015	June 23, 2015	2	0	Transfer to another hospital ward
3	July 31, 2015	September 16, 2015	13	1	Death
4	June 29, 2015	June 30, 2015	2	0	Transfer to another hospital ward
5	August 21, 2015	March 04, 2016	28	15	Death
6	July 11, 2015	September 18, 2015	1	1	Transfer to another hospital ward
7	October 08, 2015	October 23, 2015	3	1	Transfer to another hospital ward
8	October 14, 2015	November 17, 2015	6	2	Death
9	October 22, 2015	December 28, 2015	10	0	Death
10	October 31, 2015	December 17, 2015	7	0	Discharge for rehabilitation
11	November 24, 2015	December 03, 2015	2	0	Transfer to another hospital ward
12	November 26, 2015	December 31, 2015	9	4	Death
13	December 30, 2015	January 25, 2016	4	1	Transfer to another hospital ward
14	January 07, 2016	February 12, 2016	6	0	Death
15	January 08, 2016	May 06, 2016	17	2	Death
16	January 15, 2016	March 22, 2016	11	10	Death
17	January 22, 2016	March 21, 2016	8	0	Death
18	February 06, 2016	March 20, 2016	6	0	Death
19	February 26, 2016	April 03, 2016	6	8	Death
20	March 01, 2016	March 15,2016	3	0	Transfer to another hospital ward
21	March 31, 2016	May 25, 2016	5	1	Discharge for rehabilitation
22	April 04, 2016	April 08, 2016	1	0	Transfer to another hospital ward
23	April 11, 2016	April 26, 2016	3	0	Transfer to another hospital ward

compared using the BLASTn and the Mauve software (Darling et al., 2010) and subjected to Maximum Likelihood phylogeny using RAxML (Stamatakis, 2014) with the GAMMA substitution model, considering the Ascertainment bias and applying the Lewis correction (Lewis, 2001). The tree topology reliability was tested using 100 bootstrap replicates.

To estimate genomic variability, the obtained genome sequences were added to a selected dataset of *K. pneumoniae* genomes extracted from the PATRIC database (Wattam et al., 2016). PATRIC genomes were selected, using an in-house script, to be the closest in genomic distance to our strains. In detail, each genome was compared to all PATRIC database genomes using Mash (Ondov et al., 2016) and the 50 best hits were selected. All the obtained best hits lists were merged removing duplication, to obtain the final genomic dataset. CoreSNPs were extracted from the resulting dataset following a published method (Gaiarsa et al., 2015). Briefly, the Mauve software (Darling et al., 2010) was used to align all novel genomes and the similar PATRIC genomes to a well-characterized complete genome reference [NZ_CP006923 (DeLeo et al., 2014)]. Individual alignments were merged using a Python script to obtain a multi-alignment file, allowing to extract coreSNPs (defined as variations of a single nucleotide flanked on each side by two nucleotides conserved in all the genomes analyzed).

The distribution of the coreSNPs distances among strains was visualized using the software R Version 3.2.3

(R Core Team, 2013) and the coreSNP cut-off threshold was determined manually by looking at the graph and finding that there were two groups of genome pairs, those with less than 15 SNPs and those with more than 35 SNPs (**Figure 2**). The distribution allowed us to safely infer that two genomes could be considered as part of the same transmission cluster if their distance in number of coreSNPs was lower than the 15 SNPs threshold value. The coreSNPs alignment was used to perform a phylogenetic analysis using the software RAxML (Stamatakis, 2014) with the GAMMA substitution model, considering the Ascertainment bias and applying the Lewis correction (Lewis, 2001). The tree topology reliability was tested using 100 bootstrap replicates.

The genomes of the epidemic clusters were investigated also in order to detect possible unique genomic characteristics. A SNP based phylogeny was generated for each cluster, using the same approach as the global phylogeny, and adding to each cluster the genome not part of the cluster that resulted the closest in the global phylogeny. The phylogenies and the genomic alignments of each cluster and their outgroup were used as inputs for a recombination analysis with the software ClonalFrameML (Didelot and Wilson, 2015). Furthermore, the presence and abundance of Insertion Sequences (IS) was tested using the software ISSeeker (Adams et al., 2016) against all IS retrieved from the Issaga database (Varani et al., 2011) using "*Klebsiella*" as organism keyword (on date July 17, 2019).

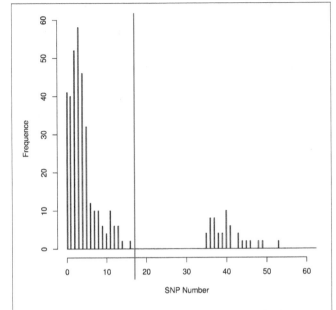

FIGURE 2 | CoreSNPs distribution between genome pairs. Pairs of genomes within a distance of 16 SNPs (SNPs threshold) were considered as part of the same transmission cluster.

RESULTS

An outbreak of CRKP occurred in the cardio-respiratory ICU from August 2015 to May 2016, involving 23 patients (12 colonized, 11 infected). In order to characterize the event, we retrieved all the CRKP strains isolated during the event and in the 2 months before. We obtained a total of 144 samples, 98/144 (68.1%) surveillance samples and 46/144 (31.9%) clinical samples (16 blood cultures, 12 bronchial aspirates, 1 bronchoalveolar wash, 8 urines, and 9 wound swabs). A total of 32/144 *K. pneumoniae* isolates, from 22 rectal swabs and 10 clinical specimens, were selected based on sample types and collection date, including at least one per each of the 23 positive patients, for antibiotic resistance characterization and genome sequencing (**Table 2**). The results of the antibiotic susceptibility tests are reported in **Supplementary Table S1** and show that all the isolates are resistant to at least one carbapenem: 32/32 to Ertapenem, 31/32 to Meropenem, 29/32 to Imipenem. Moreover, 31 isolates are resistant to aminoglycosides (25 to Amikacin, 22 to Gentamicin, 28 to Tobramycin). Twenty isolates are resistant to Fosfomycin (MICs > 64 mg/L), 20 to Colistin (MICs ranging from 4 to >64 mg/L) and three are resistant to Tigecycline (MICs > 2 mg/L). Only one strain from a surveillance sample (genome ID: 1880), resulted to be resistant to all five classes of antibiotics.

Whole-genome sequences were obtained for the 32 selected strains using Illumina technology and assembled into draft genomes after read polishing. Genomes resulted to be of good quality (average N50: 191,110; average number for contigs above 500 bp = 116; average genome size (5,671,622 bp, see **Supplementary Table S2** for complete genome characteristics).

Genomes have been submitted to EMBL and are accessible under accession PRJEB32609 (ERP115310). Genomes were characterized by calculating the MLST, detecting antibiotic resistance determinants and virulence factors (see **Supplementary Tables S3, S4** for complete results). The most prevalent ST was ST258 (*n* = 19, 59.4%), followed by ST512 (*n* = 11, 34.4%). One isolate was found to belong to ST45 (3.1%). One new ST was found, a single-locus variant (-SLV) of ST940 (genome 1998 from patient 5, now registered as ST3985). Among the 5 patients with more than one isolate sequenced, one resulted to be colonized by isolates of different STs (patients 5).

Results of the antibiotic resistance factors analysis (**Supplementary Table S3**) were grouped in 12 drug classes according to the ARG-ANNOT database (Gupta et al., 2014), with β-lactamases divided into the six Lahey classes (Bush and Jacoby, 2010). All 32 analyzed isolates carried at least one ESBL gene (3.1% CTX-M-15, 3.1% SHV-1, 87.5% SHV-11, 6.3% SHV-12) and/or inhibitor-resistant β-lactamase genes (87.5% TEM-54 and 3.1% TEM-122). All the isolates were confirmed to be resistant to carbapenems (9.4% KPC-2 and 90.6% KPC-3). Kleborate identified colistin resistance as truncation or loss of *mgrB* gene in 20 isolates (62.5%), if less than 90% of the reference gene was covered by sequencing reads. Manual analysis allowed to detect the presence of an Insertion Sequence (IS5-like) interrupting *mgrB* in two resistant isolates (1880 and 1753). The interruption due to this mobile element has been previously reported (Cannatelli et al., 2014). All the other resistant isolates, belonging to cluster 3, exhibited a frameshift mutation in *mgrB* due to a 10 nucleotide insertion in position 109 of the gene. Presence of *mcr* genes was investigated with ResFinder, but they were never detected. Colistin antibiogram and genomic data resulted to be coherent for all clones, with two exceptions, clone 1760 indicated as resistant in *Kleborate* but resulting sensitive at the microdilution test and clone 1870 resistant to the phenotypic test but not to the genomic analysis.

Results of the virulence determinants presence show that only 4/32 strains (12.5%) contained the *ybt* locus, which encodes the biosynthesis pathway of the siderophore yersiniabactin (Lam et al., 2018). None of the strains were found to harbor other siderophores (aerobactin and salmochelin were screened). All the four *ybt* positive strains were isolated from surveillance rectal swabs of different patients and were sporadic cases. Two of them (genomes 1758 and 1760) showed *ybt* allele 13, carried by integrative conjugative element: ICEKp 2. The other two isolates (genomes 1826 and 1998) showed respectively the variants: *ybt* 10 (carried by ICEKp 4) and *ybt* 4 (plasmid-borne allele). The association between the mobile genetic elements found and the allelic variants of *ybt* gene is in agreement with previous observations (Lam et al., 2018). The biosynthetic pathway for the production of the toxin colibactin, as well as the virulence factor *rmp*A/*rmp*A2 (responsible for the expression of the hypermucose-viscous phenotype) were absent from all 32 strains. Finally, using the Kleborate tool we identified three distinct K-loci. The most common K-locus was KL107 (*n* = 28, 90.3%), followed by KL106 (*n* = 2, 6.5%) and KL24 (*n* = 1, 3.2%). As expected from the literature (Shu et al., 2009), they were found to be associated with *wzi* alleles 154, 29, and 101,

TABLE 2 | Description of the 32 *Klebsiella pneumoniae* KPC isolates selected for the genomic characterization.

Genome ID	Patient number	Sample date	Sample type	Sequence type	KPC-type
1753	1	June 02, 2015	rectal swab	ST512	KPC-3
1758	2	June 23, 2015	rectal swab	ST258	KPC-2
1760	4	June 29, 2015	rectal swab	ST258	KPC-2
1826	3	August 11, 2015	rectal swab	ST45	KPC-2
1845	5	September 01, 2015	rectal swab	ST512	KPC-3
1870	5	September 14, 2015	wound swab	ST512	KPC-3
1873	5	August 31, 2015	blood	ST512	KPC-3
1880	6	September 15, 2015	rectal swab	ST512	KPC-3
1897	7	October 08, 2015	rectal swab	ST512	KPC-3
1935	8	October 26, 2015	bronchial aspirate	ST512	KPC-3
1955	9	November 10, 2015	rectal swab	ST512	KPC-3
1961	10	November 17, 2015	rectal swab	ST512	KPC-3
1987	11	December 01, 2015	rectal swab	ST258	KPC-3
1998	5	December 01, 2015	rectal swab	ST3985	KPC-3
2003	12	December 08, 2015	rectal swab	ST258	KPC-3
2018	12	December 29, 2015	bronchial aspirate	ST258	KPC-3
2066	13	January 15, 2016	bronchial aspirate	ST258	KPC-3
2079	16	January 26, 2016	rectal swab	ST258	KPC-3
2106	5	February 02, 2016	rectal swab	ST512	KPC-3
2110	14	February 02, 2016	rectal swab	ST258	KPC-3
2133	17	February 16, 2016	rectal swab	ST258	KPC-3
2137	16	February 07, 2016	blood	ST258	KPC-3
2165	19	March 01, 2016	bronchial aspirate	ST258	KPC-3
2174	19	March 14, 2016	blood	ST258	KPC-3
2176	20	March 08, 2016	rectal swab	ST258	KPC-3
2182	18	March 15, 2016	rectal swab	ST258	KPC-3
2183	15	March 15, 2016	rectal swab	ST258	KPC-3
2186	16	March 19, 2016	wound swab	ST258	KPC-3
2205	22	April 04, 2016	rectal swab	ST512	KPC-3
2218	23	April 19, 2016	rectal swab	ST258	KPC-3
2221	21	April 19, 2016	rectal swab	ST258	KPC-3
2228	21	April 24, 2016	blood	ST258	KPC-3

respectively. K-locus was not typable for one isolate (1998) (see **Supplementary Table S4** for full results).

The distribution of the coreSNPs distances among the 32 sequenced genomes was calculated and plotted to determine a threshold cut-off indicating epidemiological relatedness. A clear threshold was detected at 16 coreSNPs (**Figure 2**), allowing to determine the presence of three clades of genomes. Within each clade, all genomes have reciprocal coreSNP distances lower than the calculated threshold. A global coreSNPs maximum-likelihood phylogeny was performed, including the 32 genomes investigated in this work and 172 related genomes extracted from the PATRIC database, in order to contextualize our strains within the surrounding *Kp* diversity. The genomes with coreSNPs distance below the threshold clustered in three monophyletic clades (**Figure 3** for the cladogram, see also **Supplementary Figure S1** that shows subtrees of the three clusters) and were thus considered part of three separate outbreak clusters (green, red, and violet clusters in **Figures 3, 4**). Five of the other six genomes do not cluster with other genomes of the outbreak and are thus considered sporadic cases. The last remaining genome (2205) is the phylogenetic sister group of cluster 2, but presents a relatively high number of coreSNPs with the other genomes of the cluster (average 42 coreSNPs), and was thus considered as a separate, sporadic, case.

Comparative genomic analyses were performed within the three clades and to compare them to their nearest neighbor, showing very limited genomic variation. No recombination was detected at the origin of any of the three epidemic clades (**Supplementary Figure S2**). IS content of isolates of each of the three outbreaking clusters was compared using ISfinder. The IS content resulted to be stable within each cluster, while each cluster appears to have more ISs than the evolutionary closest sporadic isolates. Specifically, isolates of Cluster 1 have IS of families ISL3 and IS1 that are absent in the sporadic sister group. Isolates of cluster 2 present IS66 sequences, absent in the evolutionary closest sporadic isolate. Isolates of cluster 2 are also richer in ISL3 and IS6 sequences than their neighbor and those of cluster 3 are richer in IS5 and IS6. It must be noted however that the accuracy, especially quantitatively, of such an analysis on draft genomes is limited, due to the difficulties in assemblying IS sequences (**Supplementary Figure S3**).

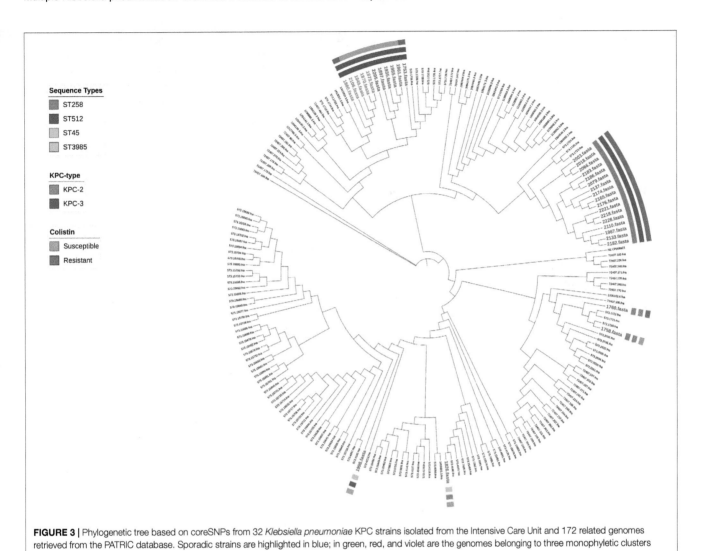

FIGURE 3 | Phylogenetic tree based on coreSNPs from 32 *Klebsiella pneumoniae* KPC strains isolated from the Intensive Care Unit and 172 related genomes retrieved from the PATRIC database. Sporadic strains are highlighted in blue; in green, red, and violet are the genomes belonging to three monophyletic clusters (distance in SNPs < 16).

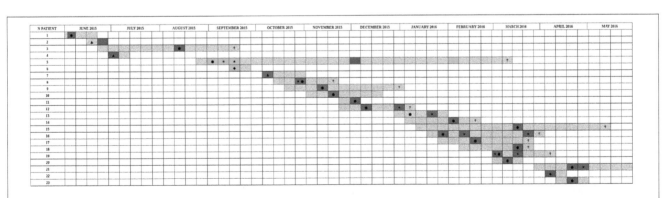

FIGURE 4 | Timeline of the presence of carbapenem-resistant *Klebsiella pneumoniae* positive patients in the ICU in the period from June 2015 to May 2016. The periods of hospitalization are colored in gray. The other colors identify the sequenced samples based on genomic characterization. The colors green, red, and violet correspond to the three clusters identified based on SNPs distance, are reported sporadic cases in blue. Samples obtained from clinical infections (not surveillance swabs) are indicated by stars. The crosses indicate patients death. Black circles indicate the first positive CRKP rectal swab for each patient, negative at the admission. Black triangles indicate the first positive CRKP rectal swab for patients already CRKP-colonized at the admission time into the hospital. Black diamonds indicated the patients that became positive in other hospital wards.

DISCUSSION

Here we present the results of the integrated characterization of the CRKP strains isolated during a 1-year period (10 months outbreak plus 2 months before) in the cardio-respiratory ICU of the San Matteo hospital in Pavia, Northern Italy. Retrospectively, starting in August 2015, we observed a strong increase in CRKP isolated from routine surveillance rectal swabs, taken from each ICU patient every week indicating a high number of colonized patients. We also observed an increase in CRKP isolations from clinical samples, indicating overt infections. This trend continued until June 2016, with a total of 23 colonized patients, among which 11 infected, prompting the investigation presented here. Antibiotic resistance characterization coupled with genome sequencing of 32 isolates from these 23 patients (**Table 2**), collected in the outbreak period and in the 2 months before, allowed the characterization of the extended outbreak. Most strains were found to belong to CG258, one of the most widespread KPC-bearing group in Italy and worldwide (Gaiarsa et al., 2015; Onori et al., 2015).

Performing a SNPs distance analysis (**Figure 1**) we found that twenty-six of the 32 isolates resulted to belong to three genome clusters (coreSNPs < 16) that appeared in the ICU, infected multiple patients, and then disappeared, with one single strain lasting for most of the event (**Figure 4**, see also **Supplementary Figure S1** for phylogenetic reconstructions of the three clusters). The remaining six genomes resulted to be unrelated and were consequently classified as sporadic isolates, as they all showed more than 35 coreSNPs with all the other analyzed genomes. This result is coherent with a recent multicenter study that proposed to set a threshold for SNPs distance in *Kp* outbreak at 21 (David et al., 2019). Interestingly, four of the six sporadic isolates represent the strains characterized in the 2 months before the outbreak (June–August 2015, see **Figure 4**), indicating that multiple strains were present in the ICU, but they were only responsible for colonization, did not cause clinical infections, nor they spread to multiple patients. The six sporadic isolates are characterized by variable levels of antibiotic resistance (number of resistance classes determined with Kleborate ranging from 3 to 11). Two of them are resistant to colistin (genomes ID: 1753, 1760). In terms of virulence, the only isolates that present yersiniabactin are four of the six sporadic isolates, all isolated from colonized, not infected, patients. Most sporadic isolates belong to the CG258 (*n* = 4), one belongs to ST45, already reported as a KPC-bearing strain in Italy (Cristina et al., 2016), and the final one to a novel ST, variant of ST940, now classified as ST3985. These sporadic isolates could be epidemiologically important, acting as a "reservoir" for the spread of the mobile element carrying *bla*KPC.

The strain responsible for the first cluster of isolations, belonging to ST512, was isolated from patient 5 from a screening sample in August 2015 and then from clinical samples in September. The patient remained colonized until his death in March. The isolates of this cluster are characterized by the resistance to 10 antibiotic classes, remaining susceptible to colistin, with two exceptions. The first one (genome ID: 1880) is

the only strain of the cluster, belonging to patient 6, which present a correspondence between phenotypic (MIC > 64 mg/L) and genotypic (loss/truncation of *mgr*B gene) colistin resistance. The other colistin-resistant strain of the cluster (genome ID: 1870) was the third of four in the temporal series isolated from patient 5 and resulted phenotypically colistin-resistant (MIC = 4 mg/L), even though no colistin-resistance mutation/gene was detected in the genome. In order to investigate the presence of other mutations potentially causing colistin resistance, the genomes of the isolates belonging to patient 5 were manually examined, detecting 2 SNPs unique to the colistin-resistant isolate. These SNPs are co-localized in an intergenic region upstream of the *pca* operon, potentially responsible for the β-ketoadipate pathway. Understanding whether these SNPs could be related to colistin resistance would require additional investigations.

One additional CRKP was isolated from patient 5 on December 1st. This isolate was unrelated to those of cluster 1, belonging to ST3985 (a novel SLV of ST940). In order to evaluate whether this strain acquired the KPC plasmid from the ST512 strain co-present in patient 5, we compared the contigs harboring the KPC gene, performing a phylogenetic analysis including contigs from isolates of cluster 1, from the ST3985, and from another sporadic isolate (1753), as control. We found that the KPC-harboring contig from the ST3985 was divergent from all identical contigs retrieved from the ST512 isolates belonging to cluster 1, but also from the sporadic control, which resulted sister group of the isolates of the cluster (**Supplementary Figure S4**).

Four isolates were grouped in cluster 2, belonging again to ST512. This clone was short-lived but was transmitted from patient 7 to three other patients in the course of 6 weeks and caused one clinical infection. The isolates of this cluster are resistant to most antibiotics, retaining susceptibility to colistin and tigecycline. Two of four isolates resulted phenotypically sensitive to aminoglycosides, while genome analysis are only in partial agreement, indicating that all four strains carry the *aph3-Ia* gene, which should confer resistance to this class of antibiotics.

The largest of the clusters is represented by 17 strains, isolated from 12 patients during 5 months, causing five clinical infections and resulting in three deaths. The isolates of this cluster are those characterized by the highest level of resistance, retaining susceptibility only to tigecycline. Genomic analysis agrees with this result indicating the presence of resistance genes against 11 antibiotic classes, one more than the two other clusters. Indeed, all the isolates of this cluster resulted resistant to colistin with phenotypic tests, and the analysis of the genome content using Kleborate highlighted a possible resistance-causing truncation in the *mgr*B gene in all 17 strains. Manual analysis allowed to detect a frameshift mutation in *mgr*B due to a ten nucleotide insertion in position 109 of the gene.

CONCLUSION

Over the course of 1 year, nine different strains of Carbapenem resistant *K. pneumoniae* were isolated in the ICU from 23 patients, 12 only colonized, 11 infected. Three strains colonized multiple patients, were the cause of all the seven clinical infections reported in the ICU in this period and were responsible for the outbreak that lasted for 10 months. The three outbreaking strains did not present more virulence genes than the six sporadic isolates, four of which were actually the only ones exhibiting yersiniabactin. In terms of antibiotic resistance, both outbreaking and sporadic strains were phenotypically resistant to most classes, a result confirmed by strong repertoires of resistance genes. A clear correlation between antibiotic resistance profiles and number of colonizations or infections is thus not clearly evident. Our results highlight the importance of the overall environmental context, possibly more than the intrinsic characteristics of a strain, in determining the spread of different CRKP isolates.

ETHICS STATEMENT

Neither ethics committee approval, nor informed consent were required as all collected data were fully anonymized, there was no contact with patients and/or their families and no interventions or changes to treatment and management were made, in accordance with institutional guidelines.

AUTHOR CONTRIBUTIONS

CF, CB, PM, and DS designed the project. MC and PC performed the microbiological analyses. ES performed the genome sequencing. CF, SG, and FC performed the bioinformatic analyses. CF, MC, and DS performed the epidemiological analyses. CF, MC, SG, and DS drafted the manuscript. CB, PM, and DS finalized the manuscript. All authors read and approved the final manuscript.

FUNDING

This research was supported by the Italian Ministry of Education, University and Research (MIUR): Dipartimenti di Eccellenza Program (2018-2022) – Department of Biology and Biotechnology "L. Spallanzani", University of Pavia to DS.

SUPPLEMENTARY MATERIAL

FIGURE S1 | Recombination analysis of Cluster 1 **(A)**, Cluster 2 **(B)** and Cluster 3 **(C)**. The analysis was performed using the software ClonalFrameML and including the evolutionary closest sporadic genome as outgroup.

FIGURE S2 | Insertion sequences (IS) content of the three epidemic clusters. The evolutionary closest sporadic genome was added as a reference, last in order in the figure for each cluster.

FIGURE S3 | Phylogenetic trees of the three genomic clusters [Cluster 1 in panel **(A)**, Cluster 2 in panel **(B)** and Cluster 3 in panel **(C)**], based on coreSNPs from the global alignment described in **Figure 1**, determined using RAxML, with 100 bootstrap, showing branch lengths and patients numbers. For each cluster, the sister group genome, as determined by the tree in **Figure 1** was used as outgroup.

FIGURE S4 | Phylogenetic comparison of the KPC-bearing contigs of the 32 isolates. The contig from isolate 1998, the ST3985 genome, is clearly distinct from the contigs from the ST512 strains belonging to Cluster 1 (1897, 1935, 1955, 1961).

TABLE S1 | Antimicrobial susceptibility profiles determined using the BD Phoenix 100 System on the 32 investigated Klebsiella pneumoniae strains.

TABLE S2 | Characteristics of the sequenced genomes.

TABLE S3 | Predicted antimicrobial susceptibility profiles determined using the Kleborate tool on 32 Klebsiella pneumoniae KPC isolates.

TABLE S4 | Factors of the 32 Klebsiella pneumoniae KPC isolates.

REFERENCES

Adams, M. D., Bishop, B., and Wright, M. S. (2016). Quantitative assessment of insertion sequence impact on bacterial genome architecture. *Microbial. Genom.* 18:e000062. doi: 10.1099/mgen.0.000062

Aires, C. A. M., Aires, da Conceição-Neto, O. C., Tavares, E., Oliveira, T. R., Dias, C. F., et al. (2017). Emergence of the plasmid-mediated mcr-1 gene in clinical KPC-2-producing *Klebsiella pneumoniae* sequence type 392 in Brazil. *Antimicrob. Agents Chemother.* 61:e00317-17. doi: 10.1128/AAC.00317-17

Bankevich, A., Nurk, S., Antipov, D., Gurevich, A. A., Dvorkin, M., Kulikov, A. S., et al. (2012). SPAdes: a new genome assembly algorithm and its applications to single-cell sequencing. *J. Comput. Biol* 19, 455–477. doi: 10.1089/cmb.2012.0021

Bolger, A. M., Lohse, M., and Usadel, B. (2014). Trimmomatic: a flexible trimmer for Illumina sequence data. *Bioinformatics* 30, 2114–2120. doi: 10.1093/bioinformatics/btu170

Borer, A., Saidel-Odes, L., Riesenberg, K., Eskira, S., Peled, N., Nativ, R., et al. (2009). Attributable mortality rate for carbapenem-resistant *Klebsiella pneumoniae* bacteremia. *Infect. Control Hosp. Epidemiol.* 30, 972–976. doi: 10.1086/605922

Breurec, S., Guessennd, N., Timinouni, M., Le, T. T. H., Cao, V., Ngandjio, A., et al. (2013). *Klebsiella pneumoniae* resistant to third-generation cephalosporins in five African and two Vietnamese major towns: multiclonal population structure with two major international clonal groups CG15 and CG258. *Clin. Microbiol. Infect.* 19, 349–355. doi: 10.1111/j.1469-0691.2012.03805.x

Broberg, C. A., Palacios, M., and Miller, V. L. (2014). *Klebsiella*: a long way to go towards understanding this enigmatic jet-setter. *F1000prime Rep.* 6:64. doi: 10.12703/P6-64

Bush, K., and Jacoby, G. A. (2010). Updated functional classification of β-lactamases. *Antimicrob. Agents Chemother.* 54, 969–976. doi: 10.1128/AAC.01009-09

Cannatelli, A., Giani, T., D'Andrea, M. M., Di Pilato, V., Arena, F., Conte, V., et al. (2014). *MgrB* inactivation is a common mechanism of colistin resistance in KPC-producing *Klebsiella pneumoniae* of clinical origin. *Antimicrob. Agents Chemother.* 58, 5696–5703. doi: 10.1128/AAC.03110-14

Carattoli, A., Zankari, E., García-Fernandez, A., Larsen, M. V., Lund, O., Villa, L., et al. (2014). In silico detection and typing of plasmids using PlasmidFinder and plasmid multilocus sequence typing. *Antimicrob. Agents Chemother.* 58, 3895–3903. doi: 10.1128/AAC.02412-14

Cristina, M. L., Sartini, M., Ottria, G., Schinca, E., Cenderello, N., Crisalli, M. P., et al. (2016). Epidemiology and biomolecular characterization of carbapenem-resistant *Klebsiella pneumoniae* in an Italian hospital. *J. Prev. Med. Hyg.* 57, E149–E156.

Darling, A. E., Mau, B., and Perna, N. T. (2010). progressiveMauve: multiple genome alignment with gene gain, loss and rearrangement. *PLoS One* 5:e11147. doi: 10.1371/journal.pone.0011147

David, S., Reuter, S., Harris, S. R., Glasner, C., Feltwell, T., Argimon, S., et al. (2019). Epidemic of carbapenem-resistant *Klebsiella pneumoniae* in Europe is driven by nosocomial spread. *Nat. Microbiol.* 4, 1919–1929. doi: 10.1038/s41564-019-0492-8

DeLeo, F. R., Chen, L., Porcella, S. F., Martens, C. A., Kobayashi, S. D., Porter, A. R., et al. (2014). Molecular dissection of the evolution of carbapenem-resistant multilocus sequence type 258 *Klebsiella pneumoniae*. *Proc. Natl. Acad. Sci. U.S.A.* 111, 4988–4993. doi: 10.1073/pnas.1321364111

Di Martino, P., Cafferini, N., Joly, B., and Darfeuille-Michaud, A. (2003). *Klebsiella pneumoniae* type 3 pili facilitate adherence and biofilm formation on abiotic surfaces. *Res. Microbiol.* 154, 9–16. doi: 10.1016/S0923-2508(02)0 0004-9

Di Pilato, V., Arena, F., Tascini, C., Cannatelli, A., De Angelis, L. H., Fortunato, S., et al. (2016). mcr-1.2, a new mcr variant carried on a transferable plasmid from a colistin-resistant KPC carbapenemase-producing *Klebsiella pneumoniae* strain of sequence type 512. *Antimicrob. Agents Chemother.* 60, 5612–5615. doi: 10.1128/AAC.01075-16

Didelot, X., and Wilson, D. (2015). ClonalFrameML: efficient inference of recombination in whole bacterial genomes. *PLoS Comput. Biol.* 11:e1004041. doi: 10.1371/journal.pcbi.1004041

European Centre for Disease Prevention and Control [ECDC], (2016). *Plasmid-Mediated Colistin Resistance in Enterobacteriaceae*. Solna Municipality: ECDC.

European Committee on Antimicrobial Susceptibility Testing [EUCAST] (2016). *Recommendations for MIC Determination of Colistin (Polymyxin E) as Recommended by the Joint CLSI-EUCAST Polymyxin Breakpoints Working Group*. Växjö: European Committee on Antimicrobial Susceptibility Testing.

Gaiarsa, S., Comandatore, F., Gaibani, P., Corbella, M., Dalla Valle, C., Epis, S., et al. (2015). Genomic epidemiology of *Klebsiella pneumoniae* in Italy and novel insights into the origin and global evolution of its resistance to carbapenem antibiotics. *Antimicrob. Agents Chemother.* 59, 389–396. doi: 10.1128/AAC. 04224-14

Ghorashi, Z., Nezami, N., Hoseinpour-feizi, H., Ghorashi, S., and Tabrizi, J. S. (2011). Arthritis, osteomyelitis, septicemia and meningitis caused by *Klebsiella* in a low-birth-weight newborn: a case report. *J. Med. Case Rep.* 5:241. doi: 10.1186/1752-1947-5-241

Giakkoupi, P., Papagiannitsis, C. C., Miriagou, V., Pappa, O., Polemis, M., Tryfinopoulou, K., et al. (2010). An update of the evolving epidemic of bla KPC-2-carrying *Klebsiella pneumoniae* in Greece (2009–10). *J. Antimicrob. Chemother.* 66, 1510–1513. doi: 10.1093/jac/dkr166

Gupta, S. K., Padmanabhan, B. R., Diene, S. M., Lopez-Rojas, R., Kempf, M., Landraud, L., et al. (2014). ARG-ANNOT, a new bioinformatic tool to discover antibiotic resistance genes in bacterial genomes. *Antimicrob. Agents Chemother.* 58, 212–220. doi: 10.1128/AAC.01310-13

Javan, A. O., Shokouhi, S., and Sahraei, Z. (2015). A review on colistin nephrotoxicity. *Eur. J. Clin. Pharmacol.* 71, 801–810. doi: 10.1007/s00228-015-1865-4

Ko, W. C., Paterson, D. L., Sagnimeni, A. J., Hansen, D. S., Von Gottberg, A., Mohapatra, S., et al. (2002). Community-acquired *Klebsiella pneumoniae* bacteremia: global differences in clinical patterns. *Emerg. Infect. Dis.* 8, 160–166. doi: 10.3201/eid0802.010025

Lam, M. M., Wick, R. R., Wyres, K. L., Gorrie, C. L., Judd, L. M., Jenney, A. W., et al. (2018). Genetic diversity, mobilisation and spread of the yersiniabactin-encoding mobile element ICEKp in *Klebsiella pneumoniae* populations. *Microb. Genom.* 4:9. doi: 10.1099/mgen.0.000196

Lewis, P. O. (2001). A likelihood approach to estimating phylogeny from discrete morphological character data. *Syst. Biol.* 50, 913–925. doi: 10.1080/106351501753462876

Liu, Y. Y., Wang, Y., Walsh, T. R., Yi, L. X., Zhang, R., Spencer, J., et al. (2016). Emergence of plasmid-mediated colistin resistance mechanism MCR-1 in animals and human beings in China: a microbiological and molecular biological study. *Lancet Infect. Dis.* 16, 161–168. doi: 10.1016/S1473-3099(15)00424-7

Markovska, R., Stoeva, T., Schneider, I., Boyanova, L., Popova, V., Dacheva, D., et al. (2015). Clonal dissemination of multilocus sequence type ST 15 KPC-2-producing *Klebsiella pneumoniae* in Bulgaria. *APMIS* 123, 887–894. doi: 10. 1111/apm.12433

Mathers, A. J., Peirano, G., and Pitout, J. D. D. (2015). The role of epidemic resistance plasmids and international high-risk clones in the spread of multidrug-resistant *Enterobacteriaceae*. *Clin. Microbiol. Rev.* 28, 565–591. doi: 10.1128/CMR.00116-14

Navon-Venezia, S., Kondratyeva, K., and Carattoli, A. (2017). *Klebsiella pneumoniae*: a major worldwide source and shuttle for antibiotic resistance. *FEMS Microbiol. Rev.* 41, 252–275. doi: 10.1093/femsre/fux013

Nordmann, P., Cuzon, G., and Naas, T. (2009). The real threat of *Klebsiella pneumoniae* carbapenemase-producing bacteria. *Lancet Infect. Dis.* 9, 228–236. doi: 10.1016/S1473-3099(09)70054-4

Olaitan, A. O., Morand, S., and Rolain, J. M. (2014). Mechanisms of polymyxin resistance: acquired and intrinsic resistance in bacteria. *Front. Microbiol.* 5:643. doi: 10.3389/fmicb.2014.00643

Ondov, B. D., Treangen, T. J., Melsted, P., Mallonee, A. B., Bergman, N. H., Koren, S., et al. (2016). Mash: fast genome and metagenome distance estimation using MinHash. *Genome Biol.* 17:132. doi: 10.1186/s13059-016-0997-x

Onori, R., Gaiarsa, S., Comandatore, F., Pongolini, S., Brisse, S., Colombo, A., et al. (2015). Tracking nosocomial *Klebsiella pneumoniae* infections and outbreaks by whole-genome analysis: small-scale Italian scenario within a single hospital. *J. Clin. Microbiol.* 53, 2861–2868. doi: 10.1128/JCM.00545-15

Oteo, J., Pérez-Vázquez, M., Bautista, V., Ortega, A., Zamarrón, P., Saez, D., et al. (2016). The spread of KPC-producing *Enterobacteriaceae* in Spain: WGS analysis of the emerging high-risk clones of *Klebsiella pneumoniae* ST11/KPC-2, ST101/KPC-2 and ST512/KPC-3. *J. Antimicrob. Chemother.* 71, 3392–3399. doi: 10.1093/jac/dkw321

Patel, G., Huprikar, S., Factor, S. H., Jenkins, S. G., and Calfee, D. P. (2008). Outcomes of carbapenem-resistant *Klebsiella pneumoniae* infection and the impact of antimicrobial and adjunctive therapies. *Infect. Control Hosp. Epidemiol.* 29, 1099–1106. doi: 10.1086/592412

Podschun, R., and Ullmann, U. (1998). *Klebsiella* spp. as nosocomial pathogens: epidemiology, taxonomy, typing methods, and pathogenicity factors. *Clin. Microbiol. Rev.* 11, 589–603. doi: 10.1128/CMR.11.4.589

Qi, Y., Wei, Z., Ji, S., Du, X., Shen, P., and Yu, Y. (2010). ST11, the dominant clone of KPC-producing *Klebsiella pneumoniae* in China. *J. Antimicrob. Chemother.* 66, 307–312. doi: 10.1093/jac/dkq431

R Core Team, (2013). *R: A Language and Environment for Statistical Computing*. Vienna: R Foundation for Statistical Computing.

Sabat, A. J., Budimir, A., Nashev, D., Sá-Leão, R., Van Dijl, J. M., Laurent, F., et al. (2013). Overview of molecular typing methods for outbreak detection and epidemiological surveillance. *Eurosurveillance* 18:20380.

Sabbatucci, M., Iacchini, S., Iannazzo, C., Farfusola, C., Marella, A. M., Bizzotti, V., et al. (2017). *Sorveglianza nazionale delle batteriemie da enterobatteri produttori di carbapenemasi. Rapporto 2013–2016*. Rapporti ISTISAN 2017. Rome: Istituto Superiore di Sanità.

Samuelsen, Ø., Naseer, U., Tofteland, S., Skutlaberg, D. H., Onken, A., Hjetland, R., et al. (2009). Emergence of clonally related *Klebsiella pneumoniae* isolates of sequence type 258 producing plasmid-mediated KPC carbapenemase in Norway and Sweden. *J. Antimicrob. Chemother.* 63, 654–658. doi: 10.1093/jac/ dkp018

Shu, H. Y., Fung, C. P., Liu, Y. M., Wu, K. M., Chen, Y. T., Li, L. H., et al. (2009). Genetic diversity of capsular polysaccharide biosynthesis in *Klebsiella pneumoniae* clinical isolates. *Microbiology* 155, 4170–4183. doi: 10.1099/mic.0. 029017-0

Stamatakis, A. (2014). RAxML version 8: a tool for phylogenetic analysis and post-analysis of large phylogenies. *Bioinformatics* 30, 1312–1313. doi: 10.1093/ bioinformatics/btu033

Tumbarello, M., Spanu, T., Sanguinetti, M., Citton, R., Montuori, E., Leone, F., et al. (2006). Bloodstream infections caused by extended-spectrum-β-lactamase-producing *Klebsiella pneumoniae*: risk factors, molecular epidemiology, and clinical outcome. *Antimicrob. Agents Chemother.* 50, 498–504. doi: 10.1128/ AAC.50.2.498-504.2006

Tzouvelekis, L. S., Miriagou, V., Kotsakis, S. D., Spyridopoulou, K., Athanasiou, E., Karagouni, E., et al. (2013). KPC-producing, multidrug-resistant *Klebsiella pneumoniae* sequence type 258 as a typical opportunistic pathogen. *Antimicrob. Agents Chemother.* 57, 5144–5146. doi: 10.1128/AAC.01052-13

Van Belkum, A., Tassios, P. T., Dijkshoorn, L., Haeggman, S., Cookson, B., Fry, N. K., et al. (2007). Guidelines for the validation and application of typing methods for use in bacterial epidemiology. *Clin. Microbiol. Infect.* 13, 1–46. doi: 10.1111/j.1469-0691.2007.01786.x

Varani, A. M., Siguier, P., Gourbeyre, E., Charneau, V., and Chandler, M. (2011). ISsaga is an ensemble of web-based methods for high throughput identification and semi-automatic annotation of insertion sequences in prokaryotic genomes. *Genome Biol.* 12:R30. doi: 10.1186/gb-2011-12-3-r30

Velkov, T., Dai, C., Ciccotosto, G. D., Cappai, R., Hoyer, D., and Li, J. (2018). Polymyxins for CNS infections: pharmacology and neurotoxicity. *Pharmacol. Ther.* 181, 85–90. doi: 10.1016/j.pharmthera.2017.07.012

Villa, L., Feudi, C., Fortini, D., Iacono, M., Bonura, C., Endimiani, A., et al. (2016). Complete genome sequence of KPC-3-and CTX-M-15-producing *Klebsiella pneumoniae* sequence type 307. *Genome Announc.* 4:e00213-16. doi: 10.1128/genomeA.00213-16

Wattam, A. R., Davis, J. J., Assaf, R., Boisvert, S., Brettin, T., Bun, C., et al. (2016). Improvements to PATRIC, the all-bacterial bioinformatics database and analysis resource center. *Nucleic Acids Res.* 45, D535–D542. doi: 10.1093/nar/gkw1017

Wei, D. D., Wan, L. G., Deng, Q., and Liu, Y. (2016). Emergence of KPC-producing *Klebsiella pneumoniae* hypervirulent clone of capsular serotype K1 that belongs to sequence type 11 in Mainland China. *Diagn. Microbiol. Infect. Dis.* 85, 192–194. doi: 10.1016/j.diagmicrobio.2015.03.012

Zankari, E., Hasman, H., Cosentino, S., Vestergaard, M., Rasmussen, S., Lund, O., et al. (2012). Identification of acquired antimicrobial resistance genes. *J. Antimicrob. Chemother.* 67, 2640–2644. doi: 10.1093/jac/dks261

12

Molecular Mechanisms and Epidemiology of Fosfomycin Resistance in *Staphylococcus aureus* Isolated from Patients at a Teaching Hospital in China

Wenya Xu[1], Tao Chen[1], Huihui Wang[1], Weiliang Zeng[2], Qing Wu[1], Kaihang Yu[2], Ye Xu[1], Xiucai Zhang[1] and Tieli Zhou[1]*

[1] Department of Clinical Laboratory, The First Affiliated Hospital of Wenzhou Medical University, Wenzhou, China, [2] School of Laboratory Medicine and Life Science, Wenzhou Medical University, Wenzhou, China

*Correspondence:
Tieli Zhou
wyztli@163.com

Staphylococcus aureus is a major cause of hospital- and community-acquired infections placing a significant burden on the healthcare system. With the widespread of multidrug-resistant bacteria and the lack of effective antibacterial drugs, fosfomycin has gradually attracted attention as an "old drug." Thus, investigating the resistance mechanisms and epidemiology of fosfomycin-resistant *S. aureus* is an urgent requirement. In order to investigate the mechanisms of resistance, 11 fosfomycin-resistant *S. aureus* isolates were analyzed by PCR and sequencing. The genes, including *fosA*, *fosB*, *fosC*, *fosD*, *fosX*, and *tet38*, as well as mutations in *murA*, *glpT*, and *uhpT* were identified. Quantitative real-time PCR (qRT-PCR) was conducted to evaluate the expression of the target enzyme gene *murA* and the efflux pump gene *tet38* under the selection pressure of fosfomycin. Furthermore, multilocus sequence typing (MLST) identified a novel sequence type (ST 5708) of *S. aureus* strains. However, none of the resistant strains carried *fosA*, *fosB*, *fosC*, *fosD*, and *fosX* genes in the current study, and 12 distinct mutations were detected in the *uhpT* (3), *glpT* (4), and *murA* (5) genes. qRT-PCR revealed an elevated expression of the *tet38* gene when exposed to increasing concentration of fosfomycin among 8 fosfomycin-resistant *S. aureus* strains and reference strain ATCC 29213. MLST analysis categorized the 11 strains into 9 STs. Thus, the mutations in the *uhpT*, *glpT*, and *murA* genes might be the primary mechanisms underlying fosfomycin resistance, and the overexpression of efflux pump gene *tet38* may play a major role in the fosfomycin resistance in these isolates.

Keywords: fosfomycin, *Staphylococcus aureus*, resistance mechanism, mutation, *tet38*

INTRODUCTION

Staphylococcus aureus is a kind of facultative anaerobe pathogenic Gram-positive coccus with strong resistance and tolerance to harsh environments (Wang et al., 2020). At present, *S. aureus* has become a significant pathogen of nosocomial infections, such as deep-seated skin and soft tissue infections (SSTI), endocarditis, and other life-threatening severe infections (Mehraj et al., 2016). In recent years, with the widespread use of antibiotics, the emergence of multidrug-resistant (MDR) *S. aureus* has become a major concern (Gatadi et al., 2019). In addition, the lack of effective clinical treatments against MDR *S. aureus* has rekindled the interest of clinicians in fosfomycin. It is an antimicrobial agent that was discovered in *Streptomyces* sp. It exhibits broad-spectrum activity against both Gram-positive and Gram-negative bacteria by inhibiting the peptidoglycan synthesis pathway, which is essential for the synthesis of the cell walls (Shorr et al., 2017). However, the number of fosfomycin-resistant *S. aureus* strains is increasing rapidly (Etienne et al., 1991).

Several mechanisms of fosfomycin resistance have been proposed, including the plasmid-encoded fosfomycin-modifying enzymes (FosA, FosB, FosC, FosD, and FosX) and the acquisition of chromosomal mutations (Nakaminami et al., 2008; Liu et al., 2017; Silver, 2017). Mutations in the MurA target enzyme and transporters (GlpT and UhpT) have been shown to be responsible for fosfomycin resistance (Michalopoulos et al., 2011). Additionally, the overexpression of target enzymes, MurA and Tet38 efflux pump, also contributes to fosfomycin resistance in *S. aureus* (Truong-Bolduc et al., 2018). Notably, there are no reports yet suggesting that fosfomycin can stimulate the expression of the efflux pump gene and mediate drug resistance. However, a few studies on *S. aureus* have described the drug sensitivity and resistance mechanism of fosfomycin in *S. aureus*, although they are not fully understood.

In the present study, we focus on the mutations of the target enzyme MurA, which catalyzes the initial step in the biosynthesis of peptidoglycan and transporters (GlpT and UhpT), as well as the overexpression of *murA* and *tet38* efflux pump in 11 fosfomycin-resistant *S. aureus*. In addition, a strong correlation was established between fosfomycin resistance and efflux pump gene *tet38* overexpression that has not been reported previously. The results of quantitative real-time PCR (qRT-PCR) indicated that the Tet38 efflux pump plays a vital role in fosfomycin resistance by pumping out the drug.

MATERIALS AND METHODS

Bacterial Strains

In 2018, a total of 200 *S. aureus* isolates were obtained from the First Affiliated Hospital of Wenzhou Medical University, a comprehensive teaching hospital in China. The bacteria were identified by matrix-assisted laser desorption/ionization time of flight mass spectrometry (MALDI-TOF MS; BioMérieux, Lyons, France). *S. aureus* ATCC 29213 (American Type Tissue Culture Collection, Manassas, VA, United States) was used as an endogenous control strain in antimicrobial susceptibility testing experiments. The study and consent procedure were approved by the Ethics Committee of the hospital.

Antimicrobial Susceptibility Testing

The minimum inhibitory concentration (MIC) of fosfomycin for each clinical strain was determined using the agar dilution method, wherein the media were supplemented with glucose-6-phosphate (25 mg/L), according to the recommendations of the Clinical and Laboratory Standards Institute [CLSI], 2018 (Ushanov et al., 2020). The data were interpreted according to the European Committee on Antimicrobial Susceptibility Testing criteria (available at http://www.eucast.org/clinical_breakpoints/) (susceptible, ≤ 32 mg/L; resistant, ≥ 64 mg/L), and the fosfomycin-resistant isolates were selected for further investigation. In addition, the MICs of fosfomycin-resistant *S. aureus* to other classes of antibiotics, including oxacillin, erythromycin, ciprofloxacin, levofloxacin, gentamicin, rifampicin, linezolid, vancomycin, and teicoplanin, were detected using the broth microdilution method.

Detection of Fosfomycin-Resistant Genes

The DNA of fosfomycin-resistant and fosfomycin-susceptible *S. aureus* isolates was extracted using a Biospin Bacterial Genomic DNA Extraction Kit (Bioflux, Tokyo, Japan) and was utilized as the template for PCR amplification of the *fosA*, *fosB*, *fosC*, *fosD*, *fosX*, *glpT*, *uhpT*, *murA*, and *tet38* genes; the primers are listed in **Table 1**. The PCR products were sequenced by Beijing Genomics Institute Technology Co., Ltd. (Shanghai, China), and the sequences were aligned by BLAST on the NCBI platform[1]. The PCR products of *uhpT*, *glpT*, and *murA* were sequenced to scan for mutations.

Fosfomycin Treatment and Total RNA Isolation

Actively growing *S. aureus* specimens were treated with increasing concentrations of fosfomycin (1/8 MIC, 1/4 MIC, and 1/2 MIC) for 2 h, after which the cells were harvested, and total RNA was extracted using a Bacterial RNA Miniprep Kit (Biomiga, Shanghai, China) according to the manufacturer's instructions. Then, 1000 ng RNA was used as the template for reverse transcription using a RevertAid First Strand cDNA Synthesis Kit (Thermo Scientific, Waltham, MA, United States) to obtain cDNA.

Quantitative Real-Time PCR (qRT-PCR)

qPCR was performed on a CFX-96 Touch[TM] Real-Time PCR system (Bio-Rad, Hercules, CA, United States) using TB Green Premix Ex Taq II (Tli RNase H Plus) (2×) (Takara, Japan), specific primers (**Table 1**), and 100 ng cDNA as the template. Cycling conditions were as follows: 95°C for 30 s, followed by 40 cycles of 95°C for 5 s and 60°C for 20 s. A melting curve was performed after each run (raising the temperature by 0.5°C/s, from 65 to 95°C). Each sample was run in triplicate, and the means of the Ct values were used for analysis. The relative expression levels of *tet38* and *murA* genes were normalized to the *gmk* reference gene (Chen and Hooper, 2018). The quantification of the target genes was analyzed using the comparative threshold cycle $2^{-\Delta\Delta Ct}$ method. All experiments

---

[1]http://blast.ncbi.nlm.nih.gov/Blast.cgi

TABLE 1 | Primers used in this study.

Gene	Primer sequences (5′→3′)	Product size (bp)	References
PCR primers			
fosA	F:GCTGCACGCCCGCTGGAATA	217	Chen et al., 2014
	R:CGACGCCCCCTCGCTTTTGT		
fosB	F:CAGAGATATTTTAGGGGCTGACA	312	Chen et al., 2014
	R:CTCAATCTATCTTCTAAACTTCCTG		
fosC	F:GGGTTACATGCCCTTGCTCA	354	Chen et al., 2014
	R:AACCCGCACAACGACAGATG		
fosD	F: AACTCTAACTTGTGTCCGTCAG	220	Liu et al., 2017
	R: GTGGCTTATGGGTTGCGTTA		
fosX	F: ATGATCAGTCATATGACATTTATCG	243	Zhang et al., 2020
	R: ATTTAGCCCCTTGTCGATAACG		
murA	F:GCCCTTGAAAGAATGGTTCGT	1600*	NC_002745.2**
	R:GTTACAATACTCGACGCAGGT		
glpT	F:TGAATAAAACAGCAGGGCAA	1699*	NC_002745.2**
	R:CACAGCTAGTATGTATAACGAC		
uhpT	F:TGTGTTTATGTTCAGTATTTTGGA	1571*	NC_002745.2**
	R:TCTTTCATCTCTTCACGCAC		
tet38	F:GCGGATACAACAGCGAGTGA	1353	Truong-Bolduc et al., 2005
	R:TCGACGCACCTAATGGGAAT		
qRT-PCR primers			
gmk	F:ACTAGGGATGCGTTTGAAGC	122	Chen and Hooper, 2018
	R:TCATGACCTTCGTCCATTGT		
tet38	F:TGACAGGTGTGGCTATTGGT	112	Chen and Hooper, 2018
	R:TTGCCTGGGAAATTTAATGC		
murA	F:TGTGCACCTTGCAATTGACT	102	G et al., 2019
	R:CCGTTTTATGCATGTTGCAG		

*PCR product including surrounding sequences adjacent to the target gene. **GenBank-EMBL-DDBL accession number.

were repeated in triplicate independently. The relative expression of the mRNA of the target gene was normalized to that of *S. aureus* ATCC 29213.

Multilocus Sequence Typing (MLST)

Isolates were screened using a previously described method to detect the following seven housekeeping genes: carbamate kinase (*arcC*), shikimate dehydrogenase (*aroE*), glycerol kinase (*glp*), guanylate kinase (*gmk*), phosphate acetyltransferase (*pta*), triosephosphate isomerase (*tpi*), and acetyl coenzyme A acetyltransferase (*yqiL*) (Enright and Spratt, 1999). The sequences of the PCR products were compared with those available from the MLST website[2] for *S. aureus*. Also, the allelic number was determined for each sequence.

Planktonic Growth Assay

The planktonic growth rates of 8 *tet38*-overexpressed *S. aureus* isolates were determined as described previously (Wijesinghe et al., 2019), with some modifications. Briefly, 8 *tet38*-overexpressed isolates and ATCC 29213 standard cell suspensions were prepared by adjusting the turbidity of suspension to 0.5 McFarland standard in sterile saline. Then, 200 μL of each suspension was inoculated in 20 mL sterile LB

broth containing fosfomycin in 0, 1/8 MIC, 1/4 MIC, and 1/2 MIC, respectively, for growth at 37°C and 180 rpm for 24 h. The growth rate of the planktonic bacteria was determined by measuring the optical density (OD) of the suspension in each well of the 96-well plate at 600 nm at 2-h intervals for 24 h using a microtiter plate reader (BioTek, United States). The growth curve was generated in triplicate for each experiment. ATCC 29213 served as the control strain.

Statistical Analysis

The relative expression of *murA* and *tet38* was compared using Student's *t*-test, and P-value < 0.05 was considered to be statistically significant.

RESULTS

Susceptibility to Fosfomycin and Other Types of Antibiotics

The susceptibility to fosfomycin of 200 *S. aureus* isolates was determined by the agar dilution method using glucose-6-phosphate (25 mg/L). The results showed that 5.5% (11/200) of the isolates were resistant to fosfomycin. Also, resistance to other antibiotics was determined (**Table 2**); 81.8% (9/11) of the

[2]http://www.mlst.net

TABLE 2 | Characteristics and resistance spectrum of fosfomycin-resistant *S. aureus* strains.

Isolates	ST type	FOM	OXA	ERY	CIP	LVX	GEN	RIF	LNZ	VAN	TEC
JP3187	5	256^R	>128^R	32^R	>256^R	32^R	4	<0.03	2	2	4
JP3189	4539	64^R	>128^R	64^R	64^R	32^R	16^R	>16^R	1	1	4
JP3212	5	256^R	>128^R	64^R	128^R	32^R	4	<0.03	2	2	8
JP3235	5708	64^R	>128^R	1	128^R	32^R	64^R	>16^R	2	1	4
JP3244	7	128^R	0.5	64^R	0.25	0.25	<0.125	<0.03	2	1	0.5
JP3505	4739	512^R	0.5	1	2	1	<0.125	<0.03	4	2	0.5
JP3535	5	64^R	>128^R	16^R	128^R	16^R	0.25	<0.03	4	1	2
JP3539	59	64^R	8^R	64^R	0.5	0.25	0.25	<0.03	4	2	1
JP3589	1	64^R	0.25	64^R	2	1	2	<0.03	2	2	1
JP3592	239	256^R	>128^R	64^R	128^R	64^R	<0.125	>8^R	4	1	1
JP3600	965	64^R	0.5	64^R	4^R	1	0.5	<0.03	2	2	2

FOM, fosfomycin; OXA, oxacillin; ERY, erythromycin; CIP, ciprofloxacin; LVX, levofloxacin; GEN, gentamicin; RIF, rifampicin; LNZ, linezolid; VAN, vancomycin; TEC, teicoplanin. Superscript "R" indicates resistance.

TABLE 3 | Characteristics and amino acid substitutions in fosfomycin-resistant and fosfomycin-sensitive *S. aureus*.

Strains	Type	tet38	fos					Amino acid substitution		
			fosA	fosB	fosC	fosD	fosX	uhpT	glpT	murA
JP3187	R	+	–	–	–	–	–	None	TypeA$_{glpT}$	TypeI$_{murA}$
JP3189	R	+	–	–	–	–	–	None	None	TypeC$_{murA}$
JP3212	R	+	–	–	–	–	–	TypeA$_{uhpT}$	None	TypeI$_{murA}$
JP3235	R	+	–	–	–	–	–	None	None	TypeI$_{murA}$ TypeC$_{murA}$
JP3244	R	+	–	–	–	–	–	None	None	TypeI$_{murA}$ TypeC$_{murA}$
JP3505	R	+	–	–	–	–	–	None	TypeI$_{glpT}$	TypeA$_{murA}$ TypeI$_{murA}$
JP3535	R	+	–	–	–	–	–	None	TypeI$_{glpT}$ TypeB$_{glpT}$	TypeI$_{murA}$
JP3539	R	+	–	–	–	–	–	None	TypeA$_{glpT}$ TypeI$_{glpT}$	TypeI$_{murA}$ TypeII$_{murA}$
JP3589	R	+	–	–	–	–	–	None	None	TypeI$_{murA}$ TypeB$_{murA}$
JP3592	R	+	–	–	–	–	–	None	None	TypeI$_{murA}$ TypeC$_{murA}$
JP3600	R	+	–	–	–	–	–	TypeII$_{uhpT}$	TypeI$_{glpT}$	TypeI$_{murA}$
JP3200	S	+	–	–	–	–	–	None	None	None
JP3203	S	+	–	–	–	–	–	TypeI$_{uhpT}$	None	None
JP3277	S	+	–	–	–	–	–	None	None	None
JP3230	S	+	–	–	–	–	–	None	None	None
JP3240	S	+	–	–	–	–	–	TypeII$_{uhpT}$	TypeI$_{glpT}$ TypeII$_{glpT}$	None
JP3245	S	+	–	–	–	–	–	None	None	None
JP3502	S	+	–	–	–	–	–	None	None	TypeI$_{murA}$ TypeII$_{murA}$
JP3512	S	+	–	–	–	–	–	None	None	None
JP3518	S	+	–	–	–	–	–	None	None	TypeI$_{murA}$
JP3520	S	+	–	–	–	–	–	None	TypeI$_{glpT}$	TypeI$_{murA}$
JP3522	S	+	–	–	–	–	–	None	None	TypeI$_{murA}$

+, carries the corresponding gene; –, does not carry the corresponding gene; None: nonsense mutation; TypeA$_{uhpT}$: T1369 G; TypeI$_{uhpT}$: G1364A; TypeII$_{uhpT}$: T1368G; TypeA$_{glpT}$: C299T; TypeB$_{glpT}$: G1064A; TypeI$_{glpT}$: G583A; TypeII$_{glpT}$: T829G; TypeA$_{murA}$: G187A; TypeB$_{murA}$: G349T; TypeC$_{murA}$: G770A; TypeI$_{murA}$: C371G; TypeII$_{murA}$: A873T.

isolates displayed resistance to erythromycin, while 72.7% (8/11) belonged to MDR *S. aureus*.

Molecular Mechanisms of Fosfomycin-Resistant Isolates

Strains carrying the *fosA*, *fosB*, *fosC*, *fosD*, or *fosX* gene were not found in the current study (**Table 3**). Based on the classification method of Fu et al. (2015) we named the sense mutations as TypeA, TypeB, and TypeC according to

the amino acid sequence, and the nonsense mutations were named as TypeI, TypeII, and TypeIII; the subscripts represent different genes (Fu et al., 2015). Three distinct mutations were detected in the *uhpT* gene of the 11 fosfomycin-resistant *S. aureus* isolates and the corresponding sensitive strains. Mutation TypeA$_{uhpT}$, found in JP3212, resulted in an amino acid substitution at position 457 (Leu457Val) of UhpT. Conversely, the other two mutations (TypeI–II$_{uhpT}$), which resulted in distinct amino acid substitutions within the UhpT protein, were identified in fosfomycin-sensitive isolates, although one mutation

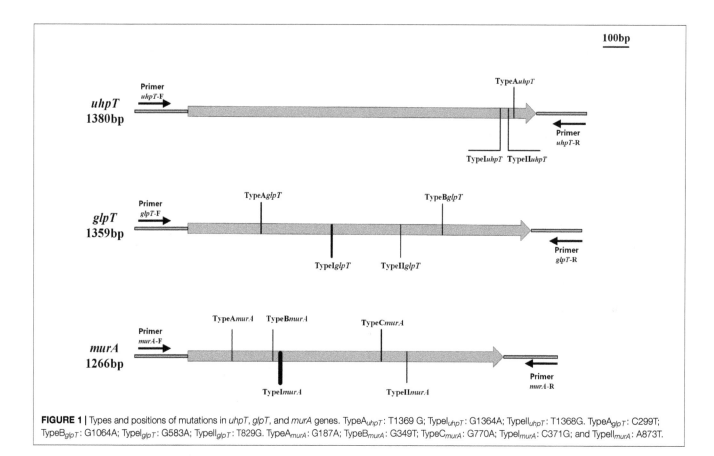

FIGURE 1 | Types and positions of mutations in *uhpT*, *glpT*, and *murA* genes. TypeA$_{uhpT}$: T1369 G; TypeI$_{uhpT}$: G1364A; TypeII$_{uhpT}$: T1368G. TypeA$_{glpT}$: C299T; TypeB$_{glpT}$: G1064A; TypeI$_{glpT}$: G583A; TypeII$_{glpT}$: T829G. TypeA$_{murA}$: G187A; TypeB$_{murA}$: G349T; TypeC$_{murA}$: G770A; TypeI$_{murA}$: C371G; and TypeII$_{murA}$: A873T.

(TypeII$_{uhpT}$) was also found in fosfomycin-resistant *S. aureus* (**Figure 1** and **Table 3**).

Moreover, four different mutations were detected in the *glpT* gene (TypeA–B$_{glpT}$ and TypeI–II$_{glpT}$). Notably, TypeB$_{glpT}$, found in the fosfomycin-resistant isolates JP3535, produced a premature stop codon within the *glpT* coding sequence at position 355 (Trp335Ter), thereby resulting in truncated proteins. In addition, TypeII$_{glpT}$ was detected only in the fosfomycin-sensitive isolates (**Figure 1** and **Table 3**).

Of the 11 fosfomycin-resistant isolates, 6 contained one of the three different mutations (TypeA–C$_{murA}$) in the *murA* gene. TypeA–C$_{murA}$, which resulted in distinct amino acid substitutions within the MurA protein at positions 63 (Ala63Thr), 117 (Gly117Trp), and 257 (Gly257Asp), could only be found in fosfomycin-resistant isolates, and two mutations (TypeI–II$_{murA}$) could be found in both fosfomycin-resistant and fosfomycin-susceptible *S. aureus* (**Figure 1** and **Table 3**). Moreover, only one sense mutation was present in each fosfomycin-resistant *S. aureus* isolate.

Expression Analysis of *murA* and *tet38*

qRT-PCR revealed significant differences in the expression of *murA* between resistant and susceptible groups of *S. aureus* as compared with *S. aureus* ATCC 29213 ($P < 0.05$) (**Table 4**). The data showed that the average expression level of *murA* gene decreased by 0.7-fold in fosfomycin-resistant and fosfomycin-susceptible *S. aureus* isolates. In addition, compared with the

fosfomycin-susceptible *S. aureus*, the expression of *murA* in the resistance isolates was not significantly higher.

However, the results (**Table 4**) indicated that compared with that in ATCC29213 and susceptible isolates, the expression level of efflux pump gene *tet38* in JP3212, JP3535, JP359, and JP3600 was elevated. Notably, the level of the *tet38* gene in JP3212, JP3535, JP3592, and JP3600 was altered markedly (21.60-, 2.74-, 143.36-, and 24.59-fold) as compared with that in ATCC29213 (**Table 4**).

Exposure to Fosfomycin Resulted in Increased Expression of *tet38* Efflux Pump Genes Among Some Resistant Isolates

The expression of *tet38* in the presence of increasing amounts of fosfomycin with 0, 1/8 MIC, 1/4 MIC, and 1/2 MIC concentrations was determined by qRT-PCR. Notably, the expression of the *tet38* gene in JP3187, JP3212, JP3244, JP3505 JP3535, JP3539, P3589, JP3592, and ATCC 29213 was upregulated with the increase in fosfomycin concentration as compared with the 0 MIC strains (**Figure 2** and **Table 4**). Also, 4.63-fold and 6.42-fold increases were noted in the expression of *tet38* in JP3505 cells treated with 1/8 MIC (64 mg/L) and 1/4 MIC (128 mg/L) fosfomycin, respectively, as compared with that in cells that were not treated with fosfomycin (**Table 5**). A further 8.46-fold increase was observed in those treated with 1/2 MIC (256 mg/L) fosfomycin.

TABLE 4 | Relative expression of target enzyme gene *murA* and efflux pump gene *tet38* in fosfomycin-susceptible and fosfomycin-resistant *S. aureus*.

Strains	Relative expression level of *murA*[a] (mean ± SD)	Relative expression level of *tet38*[a] (mean ± SD)
S1	0.77 ± 0.15	0.77 ± 0.13
S2	1.45 ± 0.10	1.48 ± 1.02
S3	0.40 ± 0.05	0.71 ± 0.21
S4	0.48 ± 0.01	1.55 ± 0.33
S5	0.48 ± 0.06	0.98 ± 0.35
JP3187	0.75 ± 0.09	1.71 ± 0.93
JP3189	0.35 ± 0.01	0.71 ± 0.25
JP3212	0.47 ± 0.01	**21.6 ± 5.75**
JP3235	1.47 ± 0.14	0.92 ± 0.34
JP3244	0.21 ± 0.04	1.24 ± 0.15
JP3505	0.23 ± 0.04	**2.65 ± 1.04**
JP3535	0.34 ± 0.03	**2.74 ± 0.37**
JP3539	0.39 ± 0.05	1.71 ± 0.48
JP3589	0.42 ± 0.08	0.54 ± 0.23
JP3592	0.40 ± 0.07	**143.36 ± 2.05**
JP3600	1.52 ± 0.23	**24.59 ± 0.17**

S1–S5 represent the 5 fosfomycin-susceptible S. aureus strains. ATCC 29213 served as the control strain. [a] The relative gene expression with more than 2-fold change compared with ATCC 29213 after fosfomycin induction is shown in bold.

Molecular Typing

The 11 fosfomycin-resistant *S. aureus* specimens were categorized into 9 STs (**Table 2**): ST1 (*n* = 1), ST5 (*n* = 3), ST59 (*n* = 1), ST7 (*n* = 1), ST239 (*n* = 1), ST965 (*n* = 1), ST4539 (*n* = 1), ST4739 (*n* = 1), and a new ST that was found in the current study (ST 5708) (*n* = 1).

Growth Rate

In order to gain quantitative insight into the fitness cost imposed by *tet38*-overexpressed isolates, the growth curves of

8 *tet38*-overexpressed *S. aureus* were recorded. We identified a fitness cost after fosfomycin induction. The growth of 8 *tet38*-overexpression strains was inhibited in LB at a subinhibitory concentration of fosfomycin (**Figure 3**).

DISCUSSION

Due to the unique mechanisms of action, fosfomycin exhibits significant antimicrobial activity against a broad spectrum of pathogens, including *S. aureus* (Goto, 1977). A review described that the susceptibility of *S. aureus* to fosfomycin ranged from 33.2% to 100% in the nine available studies [odds ratio (OD) = 91.7%, 95% confidence interval (CI): 88.7–94.9%] (Vardakas et al., 2016). In the current study, the susceptibility rate of fosfomycin in *S. aureus* was 94.5% (189/200). However, the prevalence of fosfomycin resistance in clinical isolates of *S. aureus* has been reported with increasing frequency in many areas (Del Rio et al., 2014; Mihailescu et al., 2014; Shi et al., 2014).

The resistance mechanism of fosfomycin in Gram-negative bacteria has been widely reported; also, in a previous study, we reported the resistance of fosfomycin in ESBL-producing *Escherichia coli* (Bi et al., 2017). Fosfomycin enters the cell via two transporters, GlpT and UhpT, and mutations or insertions in *glpT* and/or *uhpT* genes result in the loss of function (Takahata et al., 2010). According to the study by Castaneda-Garcia et al. (2009), *glpT* inactivation played an essential role in the resistance to fosfomycin in *Pseudomonas aeruginosa* (Castaneda-Garcia et al., 2009). The *murA* gene is also closely related to fosfomycin resistance (Takahata et al., 2010; Couce et al., 2012). In addition, fosfomycin activity can be inhibited via the catalytic activity of FosA, FosB, and FosC, respectively (Garcia et al., 1995; Lee et al., 2012).

Among Gram-positive bacteria, the resistance mechanism of fosfomycin is rarely reported. In the current study, none of

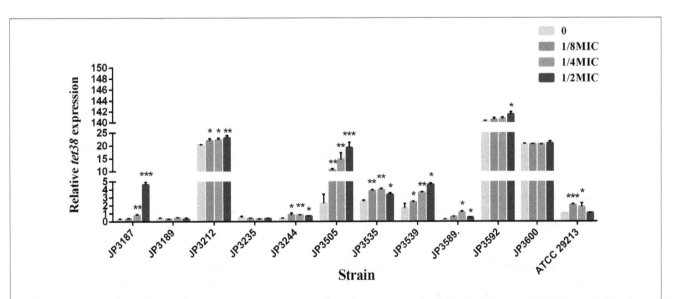

FIGURE 2 | The relative expression of efflux pump gene *tet38* in fosfomycin-resistant *S. aureus* exposed to 0, 1/8 MIC, 1/4 MIC, and 1/2 MIC concentrations. Bars indicate the mean values, and asterisks denote the significant difference of expression ($P < 0.05$).

TABLE 5 | Relative expression of efflux pump gene *tet38* in fosfomycin-resistant *S. aureus* exposed to different concentrations of fosfomycin.

Strains	The relative expression level of *tet38*[a] (mean ± SD)			
	0 MIC	1/8 MIC	1/4 MIC	1/2 MIC
JP3187	0.25 ± 0.09	0.32 ± 0.08	**0.77 ± 0.10**	**4.64 ± 0.25**
JP3189	0.38 ± 0.08	0.32 ± 0.01	0.43 ± 0.07	0.32 ± 0.13
JP3212	20.32 ± 0.10	21.89 ± 0.69	22.22 ± 0.56	23.02 ± 0.8
JP3235	0.53 ± 0.12	0.36 ± 0.08	0.33 ± 0.03	0.37 ± 0.06
JP3244	0.35 ± 0.06	**0.81 ± 0.20**	**0.83 ± 0.01**	0.68 ± 0.03
JP3505	2.27 ± 0.91	**10.51 ± 0.38**	**14.57 ± 2.12**	**19.21 ± 1.65**
JP3535	2.50 ± 0.12	3.82 ± 0.12	3.95 ± 0.14	3.34 ± 0.17
JP3539	1.67 ± 0.45	2.40 ± 0.08	**3.60 ± 0.08**	**4.60 ± 0.14**
JP3589	0.27 ± 0.02	**0.57 ± 0.06**	1.13 I'± 0.14	0.51 ± 0.01
JP3592	140.27 ± 0.05	140.48 ± 0.30	140.65 ± 0.23	141.47 ± 0.36
JP3600	20.58 ± 0.20	20.62 ± 0.04	20.47 ± 0.08	20.93 ± 0.72

[a]*The relative gene expression with more than 2-fold change compared with 0 MIC after fosfomycin induction is shown in bold.*

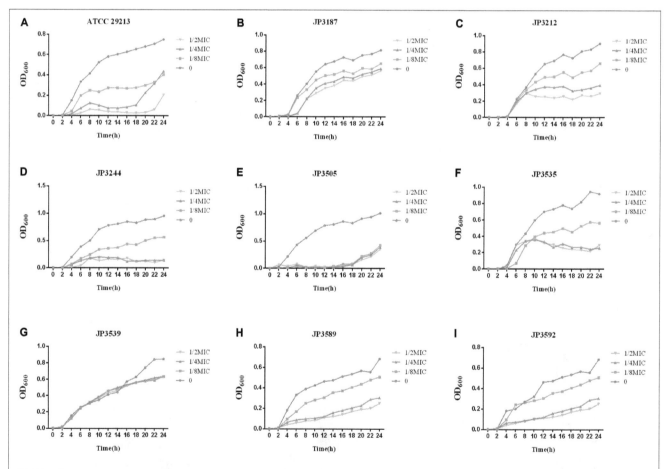

FIGURE 3 | Growth curves at different fosfomycin concentrations in *tet38*-overexpression *S. aureus*. The values shown are the average of three independent experiments. Different colors of lines represent different concentrations of fosfomycin. **(A)** Growth of control strain ATCC 29213. **(B–I)** Growth of 8 *tet38*-overexpression isolates.

the resistant strains carried the *fosA*, *fosB*, *fosC*, *fosD*, or *fosX* gene, indicating that these genes might not be the primary factors mediating the resistance of *S. aureus* against fosfomycin. Other studies have shown that the prevalence of fosfomycin resistance genes (*fosA*, *fosB*, and *fosC*) was not the predominant factor contributing to resistance in *S. aureus* (Xu et al., 2017). In addition, a total of 12 mutations were found in 11 strains of fosfomycin-resistant *S. aureus* by sequencing analysis. Of these, 3 were detected in *uhpT*, and TypeA$_{uhpT}$ was carried only by fosfomycin-resistant strain JP3212, while TypeI$_{uhpT}$ and TypeII$_{uhpT}$ were found in both fosfomycin-resistant and fosfomycin-sensitive strains, which likely did not contribute to fosfomycin resistance. Within the *glpT* gene of 11 drug-resistant strains, 2 mutations TypeA–B$_{glpT}$ were observed only in the drug-resistant strains. On the other hand, mutation TypeI$_{glpT}$ was widely detected in both drug-resistant and susceptible strains. Intriguingly, TypeB$_{glpT}$, which generated a stop codon (TA$_{1064}$G) at position 335 (**Figure 1**), was harbored in JP3535. Also, we found a mutation (TypeII$_{glpT}$) merely in the fosfomycin-sensitive strains. Of the five *murA* gene mutations found in the drug-resistant strains, TypeI$_{murA}$ and TypeII$_{murA}$ could also be found in susceptible strains, and the remaining three mutations (TypeA–C$_{murA}$) were found only in drug-resistant strains (TypeA$_{murA}$: JP3505; TypeB$_{murA}$: JP3589; TypeC$_{murA}$: JP3189, JP3235, JP3244; JP3592). In addition, TypeI$_{murA}$ was also found in fosfomycin-resistant strains (10/11). Among the above mutations, four mutation sites, TypeA$_{glpT}$, TypeB$_{glpT}$, TypeC$_{murA}$, and TypeII$_{murA}$, were consistent with those reported (Fu et al., 2015). We also found that the frequency of *murA* mutation in *S. aureus* was high, which might play a major role in mediating fosfomycin resistance, which needs an in-depth investigation.

Although several studies have mentioned that the overexpression of the *murA* gene can greatly increase the MICs of fosfomycin, the difference in *murA* expression between fosfomycin-sensitive and fosfomycin-resistant *S. aureus* has not been reported (Garcia et al., 1995; Olesen et al., 2014). In the current study, the results of qRT-PCR revealed a significant difference between the fosfomycin-resistant and fosfomycin-susceptible *S. aureus* with respect to the expression of *murA* as compared with that of *S. aureus* ATCC 29213. However, statistical differences could not be detected between two types of strains (**Table 4**), indicating that the overexpression of target gene *murA* has no role in conferring fosfomycin resistance in the strains identified in this study. Interestingly, some resistant strains showed a downward trend in the expression of *murA*, suggesting that the role of the *murA* gene in fosfomycin needs to be studied further.

Recent studies have shown that the *tet38* gene exerts a specific effect on fosfomycin resistance. According to the study by Truong-Bolduc, the overexpression of *tet38* resulted in a fourfold increase in the MIC of fosfomycin compared with that of the parent strain (Truong-Bolduc et al., 2018). The results of the current study showed that the expression of the *tet38* efflux pump gene in fosfomycin-resistant strains JP3212, JP3535, JP3592, and JP3600 was significantly higher than that in the control strain ATCC29213 and the susceptible strains ($P = 0.007$, $P = 0.002$, $P < 0.001$, $P < 0.001$, respectively). Furthermore, under the treatment of 0, 1/8 MIC, 1/4 MIC, and 1/2 MIC with fosfomycin, we found that the expression of efflux pump gene *tet38* was upregulated in most resistant isolates, even in the reference strain ATCC 29213. Although nonsense mutation was detected in *uhpT*, *glpT*, and *murA* genes, the level of *tet38* in JP3600 was high even without the drug, which might explain the resistance to fosfomycin. This phenomenon suggests that the

tet38 efflux pump plays a critical role in mediating fosfomycin resistance. Reportedly, abscess and other factors can promote the expression of *tet38* (Chen and Hooper, 2018), and the current study has shown that the stimulation of the drug also enhances the expression of the efflux pump, albeit the specific mechanism remains to be studied further. Moreover, the overexpression of *tet38* can also lead to changes in the cost of bacterial fitness. Some studies have demonstrated that the global regulator MgrA functions as a direct regulator of *tetR21*, which is a TetR-like regulator of the *tet38* efflux pump gene. TetR21 acts as a repressor of tet38 expression and may also regulate the expression of other bacterial resistance determinants (Truong-Bolduc et al., 2005, 2015). We speculated that the high expression of the *tet38* gene in *S. aureus* might be related to the regulation of TetR-like regulator TetR21 and the global regulator MgrA. We will also continue to focus on these phenomena in other bacteria in future studies.

MLST analyses designated three fosfomycin-resistant *S. aureus* isolated to ST5. Combined with drug sensitivity, we found that the ST5 resistant strains were resistant to at least five antibiotics. Among 11 fosfomycin-resistant strains, 72.7% were MDR strains, and further follow-up treatment was essential. Wu et al. (2018) reported that ST5 and ST239 strains were usually resistant to fosfomycin and constituted the predominant HA-MRSA clones in China. The new sequence type found in the resistant strain has been submitted to the repository (see text footnote 2).

CONCLUSION

A total of 11 fosfomycin-resistant strains were screened out from 200 *S. aureus* isolates, and the mechanism was explored. Our findings indicated that *fosA*, *fosB*, *fosC*, *fosD*, and *fosX* genes might not be the major resistant mechanism of *S. aureus* to fosfomycin. The mutations within the *glpT*, *uhpT*, and *murA* genes might play a critical role in conferring fosfomycin resistance. However, the role of overexpression of *murA* in fosfomycin resistance needs to be discussed further in *S. aureus*. Also, the phenomenon of overexpression in the *tet38* gene under a subinhibitory concentration of fosfomycin needs to be investigated further.

AUTHOR CONTRIBUTIONS

WX conducted the experiments, analyzed the data, and wrote the manuscript. TC participated in experiments and writing. HW and WZ provided fosfomycin-resistant strains and participated in the analysis of results. KY and QW participated in the analysis of the results. TZ helped to design the study. YX and XZ designed the study and corrected the manuscript. All authors read and approved the manuscript.

FUNDING

This study was supported by a research grant from the National Natural Science Foundation of China (no. 81171614).

REFERENCES

Bi, W., Li, B., Song, J., Hong, Y., Zhang, X., Liu, H., et al. (2017). Antimicrobial susceptibility and mechanisms of fosfomycin resistance in extended-spectrum beta-lactamase-producing *Escherichia coli* strains from urinary tract infections in Wenzhou. China. *Int. J. Antimicrob. Agents* 50, 29–34. doi: 10.1016/j.ijantimicag.2017.02.010

Castaneda-Garcia, A., Rodriguez-Rojas, A., Guelfo, J. R., and Blazquez, J. (2009). The glycerol-3-phosphate permease GlpT is the only fosfomycin transporter in *Pseudomonas aeruginosa*. *J. Bacteriol.* 191, 6968–6974. doi: 10.1128/jb.00748-09

Chen, C., and Hooper, D. C. (2018). Effect of *Staphylococcus aureus* Tet38 native efflux pump on in vivo response to tetracycline in a murine subcutaneous abscess model. *J. Antimicrob. Chemother.* 73, 720–723. doi: 10.1093/jac/dkx432

Chen, C., Xu, X., Qu, T., Yu, Y., Ying, C., Liu, Q., et al. (2014). Prevalence of the fosfomycin-resistance determinant, fosB3, in Enterococcus faecium clinical isolates from China. *J. Med. Microbiol.* 63, 1484–1489. doi: 10.1099/jmm.0.077701-0

Clinical and Laboratory Standards Institute [CLSI] (2018). *Performance Standards Forantimicro-Bial Susceptibility Testing: Twenty Eighth Informational Supplement M100-S28.* Wayne, PA: CLSI.

Couce, A., Briales, A., Rodriguez-Rojas, A., Costas, C., Pascual, A., and Blazquez, J. (2012). Genomewide overexpression screen for fosfomycin resistance in *Escherichia coli*: MurA confers clinical resistance at low fitness cost. *Antimicrob. Agents Chemother.* 56, 2767–2769. doi: 10.1128/aac.06122-11

Del Rio, A., Gasch, O., Moreno, A., Pena, C., Cuquet, J., Soy, D., et al. (2014). Efficacy and safety of fosfomycin plus imipenem as rescue therapy for complicated bacteremia and endocarditis due to methicillin-resistant *Staphylococcus aureus*: a multicenter clinical trial. *Clin. Infect. Dis.* 59, 1105–1112. doi: 10.1093/cid/ciu580

Enright, M. C., and Spratt, B. G. (1999). Multilocus sequence typing. *Trends Microbiol.* 7, 482–487.

Etienne, J., Gerbaud, G., Fleurette, J., and Courvalin, P. (1991). Characterization of staphylococcal plasmids hybridizing with the fosfomycin resistance gene fosB. *FEMS Microbiol. Lett.* 68, 119–122. doi: 10.1111/j.1574-6968.1991.tb04580.x

Fu, Z., Ma, Y., Chen, C., Guo, Y., Hu, F., Liu, Y., et al. (2015). Prevalence of Fosfomycin Resistance and Mutations in murA, glpT, and uhpT in Methicillin-Resistant *Staphylococcus aureus* strains isolated from blood and cerebrospinal fluid samples. *Front. Microbiol.* 6:1544. doi: 10.3389/fmicb.2015.01544

G, C. B., Sahukhal, G. S., and Elasri, M. O. (2019). Role of the msaABCR Operon in Cell Wall Biosynthesis, Autolysis, Integrity, and Antibiotic Resistance in *Staphylococcus aureus*. *Antimicrob. Agents Chemother.* 63:e00680-19.

Garcia, P., Arca, P., and Evaristo Suarez, J. (1995). Product of fosC, a gene from *Pseudomonas syringae*, mediates fosfomycin resistance by using ATP as cosubstrate. *Antimicrob. Agents Chemother.* 39, 1569–1573. doi: 10.1128/aac.39.7.1569

Gatadi, S., Madhavi, Y. V., Chopra, S., and Nanduri, S. (2019). Promising antibacterial agents against multidrug resistant *Staphylococcus aureus*. *Bioorg. Chem.* 92:103252. doi: 10.1016/j.bioorg.2019.103252

Goto, S. (1977). Fosfomycin, antimicrobial activity in vitro and in vivo. *Chemotherapy* 23(Suppl. 1), 63–74. doi: 10.1159/000222028

Lee, S. Y., Park, Y. J., Yu, J. K., Jung, S., Kim, Y., Jeong, S. H., et al. (2012). Prevalence of acquired fosfomycin resistance among extended-spectrum beta-lactamase-producing *Escherichia coli* and *Klebsiella pneumoniae* clinical isolates in Korea and IS26-composite transposon surrounding fosA3. *J. Antimicrob. Chemother.* 67, 2843–2847. doi: 10.1093/jac/dks319

Liu, B. H., Lei, C. W., Zhang, A. Y., Pan, Y., Kong, L. H., Xiang, R., et al. (2017). Colocation of the Multiresistance Gene cfr and the Fosfomycin Resistance Gene fosD on a Novel Plasmid in *Staphylococcus arlettae* from a Chicken Farm. *Antimicrob. Agents Chemother.* 61:e01388-17.

Mehraj, J., Witte, W., Akmatov, M. K., Layer, F., Werner, G., and Krause, G. (2016). Epidemiology of *Staphylococcus aureus* nasal carriage patterns in the community. *Curr. Top. Microbiol. Immunol.* 398, 55–87.

Michalopoulos, A. S., Livaditis, I. G., and Gougoutas, V. (2011). The revival of fosfomycin. *Int. J. Infect. Dis.* 15, e732–e739. doi: 10.1016/j.ijid.2011.07.007

Mihailescu, R., Furustrand Tafin, U., Corvec, S., Oliva, A., Betrisey, B., Borens, O., et al. (2014). High activity of Fosfomycin and Rifampin against methicillin-resistant *Staphylococcus aureus* biofilm in vitro and in an experimental foreign-body infection model. *Antimicrob. Agents Chemother.* 58, 2547–2553. doi: 10.1128/aac.02420-12

Nakaminami, H., Noguchi, N., Nishijima, S., Kurokawa, I., and Sasatsu, M. (2008). Characterization of the pTZ2162 encoding multidrug efflux gene qacB from *Staphylococcus aureus*. *Plasmid* 60, 108–117. doi: 10.1016/j.plasmid.2008.04.003

Olesen, S. H., Ingles, D. J., Yang, Y., and Schonbrunn, E. (2014). Differential antibacterial properties of the MurA inhibitors terreic acid and fosfomycin. *J. Basic Microbiol.* 54, 322–326. doi: 10.1002/jobm.201200617

Shi, J., Mao, N. F., Wang, L., Zhang, H. B., Chen, Q., Liu, H., et al. (2014). Efficacy of combined vancomycin and fosfomycin against methicillin-resistant *Staphylococcus aureus* in biofilms in vivo. *PLoS One* 9:e113133. doi: 10.1371/journal.pone.0113133

Shorr, A. F., Pogue, J. M., and Mohr, J. F. (2017). Intravenous fosfomycin for the treatment of hospitalized patients with serious infections. *Expert Rev. Anti Infect. Ther.* 15, 935–945. doi: 10.1080/14787210.2017.1379897

Silver, L. L. (2017). Fosfomycin: mechanism and resistance. *Cold Spring Harb. Perspect. Med.* 7:a025262. doi: 10.1101/cshperspect.a025262

Takahata, S., Ida, T., Hiraishi, T., Sakakibara, S., Maebashi, K., Terada, S., et al. (2010). Molecular mechanisms of fosfomycin resistance in clinical isolates of *Escherichia coli*. *Int. J. Antimicrob. Agents* 35, 333–337. doi: 10.1016/j.ijantimicag.2009.11.011

Truong-Bolduc, Q. C., Bolduc, G. R., Medeiros, H., Vyas, J. M., Wang, Y., and Hooper, D. C. (2015). Role of the Tet38 Efflux Pump in *Staphylococcus aureus* internalization and survival in epithelial cells. *Infect. Immun.* 83, 4362–4372. doi: 10.1128/iai.00723-15

Truong-Bolduc, Q. C., Dunman, P. M., Strahilevitz, J., Projan, S. J., and Hooper, D. C. (2005). MgrA is a multiple regulator of two new efflux pumps in *Staphylococcus aureus*. *J. Bacteriol.* 187, 2395–2405. doi: 10.1128/jb.187.7.2395-2405.2005

Truong-Bolduc, Q. C., Wang, Y., and Hooper, D. C. (2018). Tet38 efflux pump contributes to fosfomycin resistance in *Staphylococcus aureus*. *Antimicrob. Agents Chemother.* 62:e00927-18.

Ushanov, L., Lasareishvili, B., Janashia, I., and Zautner, A. E. (2020). Application of *Campylobacter jejuni* phages: challenges and perspectives. *Animals* 10:279. doi: 10.3390/ani10020279

Vardakas, K. Z., Legakis, N. J., Triarides, N., and Falagas, M. E. (2016). Susceptibility of contemporary isolates to fosfomycin: a systematic review of the literature. *Int. J. Antimicrob. Agents* 47, 269–285. doi: 10.1016/j.ijantimicag.2016.02.001

Wang, Y., Lin, J., Zhang, T., He, S., Li, Y., Zhang, W., et al. (2020). Environmental contamination prevalence, antimicrobial resistance and molecular characteristics of methicillin-resistant *Staphylococcus aureus* and *Staphylococcus epidermidis* isolated from secondary schools in Guangzhou, China. *Int. J. Environ. Res. Public Health* 17:623. doi: 10.3390/ijerph17020623

Wijesinghe, G., Dilhari, A., Gayani, B., Kottegoda, N., Samaranayake, L., and Weerasekera, M. (2019). Influence of laboratory culture media on in vitro growth, adhesion, and biofilm formation of *Pseudomonas aeruginosa* and *Staphylococcus aureus*. *Med. Princ. Pract.* 28, 28–35. doi: 10.1159/000494757

Molecular Mechanisms and Epidemiology of Fosfomycin Resistance in Staphylococcus aureus Isolated...

163

Wu, D., Chen, Y., Sun, L., Qu, T., Wang, H., and Yu, Y. (2018). Prevalence of Fosfomycin Resistance in Methicillin-Resistant *Staphylococcus aureus* isolated from patients in a University Hospital in China from 2013 to 2015. *Jpn. J. Infect. Dis.* 71, 312–314. doi: 10.7883/yoken.jjid.2018.013

Xu, S., Fu, Z., Zhou, Y., Liu, Y., Xu, X., and Wang, M. (2017). Mutations of the Transporter Proteins GlpT and UhpT confer fosfomycin resistance in *Staphylococcus aureus. Front. Microbiol.* 8:914. doi: 10.3389/fmicb.2017.00914

Zhang, X., Bi, W., Chen, L., Zhang, Y., Fang, R., Cao, J., et al. (2020). Molecular mechanisms and epidemiology of fosfomycin resistance in enterococci isolated from patients at a teaching hospital in China, 2013-2016. *J. Glob. Antimicrob. Resist.* 20, 191–196. doi: 10.1016/j.jgar.2019.08.006

13

Over-Expression of IS*Aba1*-Linked Intrinsic and Exogenously Acquired OXA Type Carbapenem-Hydrolyzing-Class D-ß-Lactamase-Encoding Genes is Key Mechanism Underlying Carbapenem Resistance in *Acinetobacter baumannii*

Marcus Ho-yin Wong[1†], Bill Kwan-wai Chan[1†], Edward Wai-chi Chan[1] and Sheng Chen[1,2]*

[1] State Key Laboratory of Chemical Biology and Drug Discovery, The Hong Kong Polytechnic University, Kowloon, Hong Kong, [2] Department of Infectious Diseases and Public Health, Jockey Club College of Veterinary Medicine and Life Sciences, City University of Hong Kong, Kowloon, Hong Kong

*Correspondence:
Sheng Chen
shechen@cityu.edu.hk

†These authors have contributed equally to this work

Acinetobacter baumannii is an important clinical pathogen which often causes fatal infections among seriously ill patients. Treatment options for managing infections caused by this organism have become limited as a result of emergence of carbapenem resistant strains. In the current study, whole genome sequencing, gene expression studies and enzyme kinetics analyses were performed to investigate the underlying carbapenem resistance mechanisms in fourteen clinical *A. baumannii* strains isolated from two hospitals, one each in Hong Kong and Henan Province, People's Republic of China. A large majority of the *A. baumannii* strains (11/14) were found to belong to the International Clone II (IC-II), among which six were ST208. Twelve of these strains were carbapenem resistant and found to either harbor bla_{OXA-23}/bla_{OXA-72}, or exhibit over-expression of the bla_{OXA-51} gene upon IS*Aba1* insertion. Enzymatic assay confirmed that the OXA variants, including those of bla_{OXA-51}, exhibited strong carbapenem-degrading activities. In terms of other intrinsic mechanisms, a weak correlation was observed between reduced production of outer membrane porin CarO/expression resistance-nodulation-division (RND) efflux AdeB and phenotypic resistance. This finding implied that over-production of carbapenem-hydrolyzing-class D-ß-lactamases (CHDLs), including the intrinsic bla_{OXA-51} gene and the acquired bla_{OXA-23} and bla_{OXA-24} elements, is the key mechanism of carbapenem resistance in *A. baumannii*. This view is confirmed by testing the effect of NaCl, a known bla_{OXA} inhibitor, which was found to cause reduction in carbapenem MIC by twofolds to eightfolds, suggesting that inhibiting OXA type carbapenemases represents the most effective strategy to control phenotypic carbapenem resistance in *A. baumannii*.

Keywords: *Acinetobacter baumannii*, carbapenem resistance, OXA-23, OXA-51, mechanisms

INTRODUCTION

Acinetobacter baumannii is an important Gram-negative pathogen that often causes serious hospital infections, especially among immunocompromised patients in intensive care units (ICUs) (Bergogne-Berezin and Towner, 1996). The increasing mortality due to *A. baumannii* infections is of major concern as this pathogen exhibits the potential to evolve into carbapenem resistant variants through acquiring antibiotic resistance-encoding mobile genetic elements, which is often exacerbated by the intrinsic low membrane permeability of this organism. These features render *A. baumannii* one of the bacterial pathogens that exhibits the highest resistance rate in clinical settings (Peleg et al., 2008). In 2013, the United States Center for Disease Control and Prevention estimated that as many as 11,500 *A. baumannii* infections occurred annually, among which 63% were multidrug resistant, resulting in 500 deaths (Queenan et al., 2012). Likewise, *A. baumannii* is responsible for more than 1/5 of all clinical Gram-negative bacterial infections in Hong Kong and other Asia-Pacific regions, with a high portion being multidrug resistant (Liu et al., 2012). Recently, the World Health Organization has listed carbapenem-resistant *A. baumannii* to be "Priority 1: Critical" in its "Global Priority List of Antibiotic-Resistant Bacteria to Guide Research, Discovery and Development of New Antibiotics," further highlighting the worsen situation caused by this pathogen (World Health Organisation, 2017).

Carbapenem resistance in *A. baumannii* has been attributed to intrinsic cellular mechanisms, including loss of outer membrane porins (OMP) and over-expression of efflux pumps, which could result in alteration of cytoplasmic antimicrobial drug concentration and hence its bactericidal effect (Magnet et al., 2001; Siroy et al., 2005). Several OMPs, including CarO, HMP-AB and OmpW, were found to be involved in transportation of β-lactams across cytoplasmic membrane of this bacterial pathogen (Gribun et al., 2003; Siroy et al., 2006). While OMPs are responsible for the uptake of antibiotics, the multi-drug efflux systems are believed to be involved in removal of drugs by pumping them out of the cell. In particular, the resistance-nodulation-division (RND) type efflux pumps, have long been hypothesized to play a role in rendering resistance toward various antibiotics. In *A. baumannii*, the most extensively studied RND efflux system is the *adeABC* gene product, which exhibits substrate specificity toward various β-lactams, including fluoroquinolones, aminoglycosides, tetracyclines and chloramphenicol (Higgins et al., 2004). Nevertheless, evidence confirming a direct linkage between carbapenem susceptibility and the presence/absence of these porin proteins and efflux systems in *A. baumannii* is currently not available.

Enzymatic mechanisms have been regarded as the key factors that mediate development of carbapenem resistance in Gram negative bacteria, including *A. baumannii*. Instead of bla_{IMP}, bla_{VIM} and bla_{NDM} which are commonly identified in other bacterial pathogens, the carbapenem-hydrolyzing-class-D β-lactamases (CHDLs) are regarded as key determinants underlying the emergence of carbapenem-resistant *A. baumannii* (Poirel and Nordmann, 2006). CHDLs denote the OXA-type β-lactamases which exhibit carbapenem hydrolyzing activity.

There are various types of bla_{OXA} genes which are known to be harbored by *A. baumannii*, including bla_{OXA-51}, bla_{OXA-23}, $bla_{OXA-24/40}$, bla_{OXA-58}, $bla_{OXA-143}$, and $bla_{OXA-235}$ (Higgins et al., 2013; Evans and Amyes, 2014). A considerable number of studies have been conducted on enzymes encoded by these resistance genes due to their uniqueness in *A. baumannii*, particularly the bla_{OXA-51}-like β-lactamases, the genetic determinant of which is inherent in *A. baumannii* chromosome and can be readily overexpressed as a result of promoter activation by insertion sequences such as IS*Aba1* (Turton et al., 2006). Apart from this chromosomal resistance gene, plasmid-borne bla_{OXA-23}-like, $bla_{OXA-24/40}$-like, and bla_{OXA-58}-like elements are also frequently identified in resistant isolates. Among them, bla_{OXA-23} is the most prevalent CHDL-encoding element in carbapenem-resistant *A. baumannii* worldwide (Mugnier et al., 2010). A previous study in China reported that 96.5% of carbapenem-resistant *A. baumannii* isolates carried bla_{OXA-23}-like elements, and that over 96% of those isolates belonged to the Clonal Complex CC92 (Ji et al., 2014). In Hong Kong, the majority of carbapenem-resistant *A. baumannii* were bla_{OXA-23}-like carrier that belonged to sequence type ST26 (Ho et al., 2010). Similarly, dissemination of bla_{OXA-23}-bearing *A. baumannii* was also observed in other Asian countries, including Taiwan, Japan, and Korea (Peleg et al., 2008).

A comprehensive study was performed in 2013 to investigate the interplay between intrinsic and extrinsic mechanisms in mediating development of antimicrobial resistance in *A. baumannii*, including efflux systems, membrane porins, and production of CHDL β-lactamases (Rumbo et al., 2013). The study concluded that the bla_{OXA-24} and bla_{OXA-58} are the major determinants of carbapenem resistance in this organism, and that bla_{OXA-51} and porin proteins were not involved in antimicrobial resistance of bla_{OXA-24} and bla_{OXA-58}-carrying isolates (Rumbo et al., 2013). Nevertheless, the exact role of intrinsic mechanisms in mediating carbapenem resistant phenotypes in *A. baumannii* strains carrying bla_{OXA-23} and bla_{OXA-51} remained unclear. In this work, we showed that intrinsic resistance mechanisms including RND-mediated efflux and reduced expression of porin proteins did not play a major role in mediating onset of carbapenem resistance in *A. baumannii*. Instead, the phenotype was mainly conferred by CHDL encoded by the bla_{OXA-23}, bla_{OXA-72}, and bla_{OXA-51}-like genes. In addition, we identified several variants of bla_{OXA-51}, which exhibited carbapenem-hydrolyzing activities that resemble those encoded by bla_{OXA-23} in terms of substrate profile, as over-expression of these bla_{OXA-51} variants in *A. baumannii* upon insertional activation by IS*Aba1* conferred the host strain a carbapenem resistant phenotype identical to bla_{OXA-23}-carrying strains.

MATERIALS AND METHODS

Bacterial Isolates

A total of 14 representative *Acinetobacter baumannii* clinical strains were first included in the genome sequencing, gene expression study, and western blot analysis as described below. The strains were isolated from patients of two hospitals, one each in Hong Kong and Henan Province, People's Republic of China, during the period between 2000 and 2013. These strains exhibited various carbapenem resistance phenotypes and genotypes. The genetic identity of these isolates was confirmed by the Vitek II bacterial identification system prior to further analysis. The ethic approval for this study was covered by human subject ethic approval, 2018-039, approved by the Second Affiliated Hospital of Zhejiang University, Zhejiang, China. An addition 453 clinical carbapenem-resistant *A. baumannii* strains isolated from four different regions of China, were included in the screening of bla_{OXA} genes in the latter part of the study. The experimental flow is illustrated by **Supplementary Figure S1**.

Antimicrobial Susceptibility Test

Minimal inhibitory concentration (MIC) of carbapenems was tested for the 14 *Acinetobacter baumannii* strains by using the microdilution method and interpreted according to CLSI guidelines (Clinical and Laboratory Standards Institute, 2016). Briefly, bacterial strains were grown on MH agar. Bacterial cell suspensions at a concentration equivalent to a 0.5 McFarland Standard were prepared and inoculated into microplate wells containing different concentrations of carbapenem. The final volume in each well was 150 µL. The effect of the efflux pump inhibitor Phenylalanine-arginine β-naphthylamide (PAβN) and CHDL inhibitor Sodium chloride on the susceptibility of the test strains to carbapenem was determined by adding the compounds to specific wells of the microtiter plate to produce a concentration of 30 µg/ml and 200 mM, respectively. The MIC test was repeated twice to ensure the accuracy of the result.

Whole Genome Sequencing and ST Typing of *Acinetobacter baumannii*

Whole genomic DNA was extracted from the strains using the Invitrogen™ PureLink™ Genomic DNA Mini kit, followed by sequencing with an Illumina® NextSeq 550 system. Raw reads generated in this study and the Illumina reads of 11 strains obtained from the NCBI database were trimmed or filtered to remove low-quality sequences and adaptors. Genome data were annotated with the RAST tool (Overbeek et al., 2014) and Prokka (Seemann, 2014). Scaffolds obtained were analyzed by Geneious 9.7. *A. baumannii* type strain ATCC19606 was used as reference throughout the analysis. ST profiles were determined according to the *A. baumannii* MLST (Oxford) database using sequences extracted from whole genome sequencing. Discrimination of International Clone II was based on analysis of the bla_{OXA-51} gene as described previously (Matsui et al., 2013).

qRT-PCR Analysis on Gene Expression

Overnight culture of *A. baumannii* isolate was inoculated into fresh LB broth until OD 0.6 was reached. Total RNA was extracted using the QIAGEN RNeasy® Mini Kit. The extracted RNA was further treated with the Invitrogen Turbo DNA-free™ Kit to remove any DNA contaminants. 1 µg of purified mRNA samples were reverse-transcribed to cDNA by using the Invitrogen™ SuperScript™ III First-Strand Synthesis SuperMix kit for qRT-PCR. Real-time PCR was performed on a Roche

LightCycler® 480 System and *Power*SYBR™ Green PCR Master Mix was used as the reaction medium. The parameters of PCR were as followed: the reaction mixture was first incubated at 95°C for 10 min for complete denaturation of template and activation of DNA polymerase; followed by 40 cycles of denaturation at 95°C for 10 s, annealing and polymerization at 60°C for 1 min. The melting temperature of PCR product was measured after completion of PCR to ensure the absent of non-specific PCR product. Expression level of endogenous genes was normalized with *gyrB* and *A. baumannii* ATCC19606 was used as control for comparison. The gene expression study was performed in triplicate. Primers used in this study are listed in **Supplementary Table S1**.

Western Blot of bla_{OXA-51}-Like Proteins

Cell lysates were solubilized by boiling with SDS running buffer for 10 min and subsequently separated by SDS-PAGE with 12% separating gel. Proteins were transferred to a PVDF membrane followed by blocking by skimmed milk for 1 h and incubated with mouse anti-OXA-51 antibody at 4°C overnight. The goat anti-mouse antibody was used as the secondary antibody. The signal was generated by HRP substrate and detected by chemiluminator. The broad range anti-GADPH (ABCAM) was used as loading control.

Further Screening of Carbapenem-Resistant *Acinetobacter baumannii* Clinical Isolates

An addition 453 clinical carbapenem-resistant *A. baumannii* strains, isolated from four different regions of China, were further screened for the presence of bla_{OXA-23}, presence of IS*Aba1* in the promoter region of bla_{OXA-23}, bla_{OXA-51} and presence of IS*Aba1* in the promoter region of bla_{OXA-51}. The primers sequences are shown in **Supplementary Table S1**. To screen for the presence of IS*Aba1* in the promoter region of bla_{OXA-23} or bla_{OXA-51}, PCR assay was performed using primer IS*Aba1*-F was used together with reverse primer of bla_{OXA-23} or bla_{OXA-51}. Strains that did not contain bla_{OXA-23} with insertion of IS*Aba1* in the promoter region were selected for Western-blot analysis as mentioned above to check for the over-expression of OXA-51 in these strains.

RESULTS AND DISCUSSION

Antimicrobial Susceptibility and Sequence Analysis of *Acinetobacter baumannii* Strains

Fourteen clinical *A. baumannii* strains were first tested for their susceptibility toward carbapenems. Resistance toward imipenem and meropenem was observable in 12 of the 14 strains, with MIC ranging from 8 to ≥64 µg/ml (**Table 1**). The fourteen strains were then subjected to whole-genome sequencing. Based on the sequences obtained, about half of the strains were found to belong to ST208 (6 out of 14), whereas three strains (AB2, AB5, and MH5) belonged to ST940. For the remaining five strains they belonged to different ST types. Only the three ST940 strains

TABLE 1 | Genetic and phenotypic characteristics of 14 *Acinetobacter baumannii* clinical strains tested in this study.

| Strain | Year/Origin | ST type (Oxford) | International clone | Presence of resistance determinants | | | | | | | MIC (µg/ml) | | | | |
				carO	adeB	adeRS	bla$_{OXA-51}$ variants	ISAba1-bla$_{OXA-51}$	bla$_{OXA-23/24/40}$	ISAba1-bla$_{OXA23}$	IMP[@]	IMP/PAβN	MER[@]	MER/PAβN	COL
AB1	2004, HK	208	IC II	+	+	–	OXA-83	+	–	–	16 (4)	16	32 (8)	32	1
AB2	2008, HK	940	Non-IC II	+	+	+	OXA-99	–	OXA-23	+	16 (8)	16	32 (16)	16	2
AB3	2011, HK	208	IC II	+	–	–	OXA-66	+	OXA-23#	+	32 (8)	32	≥64 (32)	32	2
AB4	2011, HK	253	IC II	+	+	+	OXA-66	–	OXA-23	+	≥64 (8)	≥64	≥64 (32)	≥64	2
AB5	2004, HK	940	Non-IC II	+	+	+	OXA-99	–	OXA-23	+	16 (4)	16	8 (8)	8	1
AB7	2011, HK	208	IC II	+	+	+	OXA-82	+	–	–	8 (4)	8	16 (16)	16	8
AB8	2003, HK	208	IC II	+	+	+	OXA-82	+	–	–	8 (8)	8	32 (16)	16	2
AB10	2000, HK	208	IC II	+	+	+	OXA-66	–	–	–	1 (0.25)	0.5	0.25 (0.25)	0.5	2
MH1	2000, HK	684	IC II	+	+	+	OXA-66	–	–	–	0.5 (0.5)	1	0.25 (0.125)	0.5	0.5
MH2	2010, HK	218	IC II	+	+	+	OXA-66	–	OXA-72	–	≥64 (64)	≥64	≥64 (≥64)	64	1
MH3	2011, HK	208	IC II	+	+	+	OXA-79	+	–	–	8 (4)	8	32 (8)	16	2
MH5	2006, HK	940	Non-IC II	+	–	–	OXA-99	–	OXA-23	+	32 (16)	16	32 (8)	4	1
MH6	2013, HN	195	IC II	+	+	+	OXA-66	–	OXA-23	+	32 (16)	16	32 (8)	8	2
MH7	2013, HN	369	IC II	+	+	+	OXA-66	–	OXA-23#	+	≥64 (32)	≥64	≥64 (16)	32	2

Presence of endogenous genes and other resistance determinants were investigated by analysis of whole genome sequences. [@]MIC performed in the presence of NaCl. #Chromosome-based. HK, Hong Kong; HN, Henan province, China. IMP, imipenem; MER, meropenem; COL, colistin; PAβN, Phenylalanine-arginine β-naphthylamide.

were found to belong to International Clone II (IC II) based on analysis on the intrinsic bla_{OXA-51} gene harbored by these strains (**Table 1** and **Supplementary Figure S6**). The findings corroborated with those in previous studies which reported the dissemination of *A. baumannii* Clonal Complex 92 strains within the Asia Pacific region, including Taiwan, South Korea and China (Kim et al., 2013). It has previously been demonstrated that the high genome plasticity of *A. baumannii* may result in sporadic loss of endogenous genes, altering the physiological status and hence antibiotic susceptibilies of the organism (Roca et al., 2012). In view of the possibility that resistance formation is due to loss of specific physiological functions, the relationship between presence of various intrinsic determinants of carbapenem sensitivity was determined; the determinants tested included the outer membrane porin-encoding genes *carO* and *ompA*, as well as the efflux gene *adeABC* and its regulator *adeRS*. It was found that all the test strains carried the intact *carO* and *ompA* genes without insertion of IS elements; this finding was consistent with that of a previous report (Rumbo et al., 2013). However, three strains (AB1, AB3, and MH5) were found to lack *adeRS*, with the latter two also lacking *adeB*. The intrinsic bla_{OXA-51} gene was detectable in all test strains, among them, the three ST940 strains were found to carry the variant gene bla_{OXA-99}, whereas the bla_{OXA-66}, bla_{OXA-79}, bla_{OXA-82} and bla_{OXA-83} variants were identified in the other strains. Interestingly, the ISAba1 element was found to be inserted into the promoter region of bla_{OXA-51} in five strains, all of which belonged to IC-II. Apart from carriage of various intrinsic CHDL genes, half of the strains were found to have acquired the bla_{OXA-23} gene, two of which were located in the chromosome. One strain was also found to harbor the bla_{OXA-72} element (a variant of bla_{OXA-24}) (**Table 1**). It has been described that

alteration of amino acids of the *adeRS* gene product could result in change of expression level of *adeB* (Wen et al., 2017). Sequences of *carO*, *adeB* and *adeRS* were then analyzed and aligned in attempt to establish their relationship with carbapenem susceptibility. However, it was shown that the genetic differences detectable in these genes were linked closely to their genetic types (IC-II and non IC-II) rather than carbapenem sensitivity (**Supplementary Figures S2–S5**). Other known carbapenemase genes such as bla_{NDM-1} were not detectable in the test strains. The combinational analysis of carbapenem resistance genotypes and their genetic characteristics showed that strains exhibiting carbapenem resistance were either carrying an additional CHDL gene (bla_{OXA-23} and bla_{OXA-24}) or having an ISAba1 linked upstream region in their bla_{OXA-51} element. Consistently, two carbapenem-susceptible isolates carried neither bla_{OXA-23} or bla_{OXA-24} nor insertion of ISAba1 in the intrinsic bla_{OXA-51} (**Tables 1, 2**).

Efflux Pumps Did Not Mediate Carbapenem Resistance in *Acinetobacter baumannii*

The effect of RND-efflux systems on carbapenem susceptibility in *A. baumannii* clinical strains was evaluated by supplementing Phenylalanine-arginine β-naphthylamide (PAβN) at a concentration of 30 μg/ml in determination of MIC toward carbapenem. As shown in **Table 1**, we found that addition of PAβN exhibited minimal effect on altering carbapenem MIC except for two strains (**Table 1**). This finding demonstrated that RND efflux pumps only play a minimal role in mediating carbapenem resistance in *A. baumannii* strains of hospital origins and that the resistance phenotype is mainly conferred by the bla_{OXA} enzymes.

TABLE 2 | Expression level of genes related to carbapenem resistance in *A. baumannii* strains.

Strain	Relative expression level of different genes by qPCR				
	carO	*adeB*	*adeR*	bla_{OXA-51}	bla_{OXA-23}
ATCC19606	1	1	1	1	n.a
AB1	1.53 ± 0.10	0.07 ± 0.01	n.a	25.75 ± 2.85	n.a
AB2	0.79 ± 0.09	0 ± 0.00	0.91 ± 0.01	1.53 ± 0.21	3.93 ± 0.31
AB3	1.1 ± 0.05	n.a	n.a	25.09 ± 3.06	3.14 ± 0.11
AB4	0.54 ± 0.06	0.04 ± 0.00	1.37 ± 0.02	0.98 ± 0.32	2.24 ± 0.06
AB5	0.53 ± 0.06	0 ± 0.01	0.92 ± 0.01	1.8 ± 0.10	3.82 ± 0.39
AB7	2.86 ± 0.12	0.31 ± 0.01	2.74 ± 0.21	58.26 ± 4.87	n.a
AB8	2.29 ± 0.11	0.25 ± 0.02	2.16 ± 0.16	53.27 ± 4.03	n.a
AB10	0.74 ± 0.01	0.2 ± 0.02	3.63 ± 0.28	2.81 ± 0.26	n.a
MH1	0.27 ± 0.01	0.12 ± 0.01	1.04 ± 0.08	2.46 ± 0.57	n.a
MH2	1.39 ± 0.15	0.2 ± 0.02	2.84 ± 0.30	1.39 ± 0.13	n.a
MH3	2.33 ± 0.15	0.17 ± 0.01	2.89 ± 0.19	64.96 ± 5.07	n.a
MH5	1.18 ± 0.28	n.a	n.a	7.16 ± 0.65	4.37 ± 0.36
MH6	1.13 ± 0.13	0.15 ± 0.01	3.44 ± 0.36	2.99 ± 0.45	7.64 ± 0.72
MH7	1.43 ± 0.13	0.13 ± 0.01	3.27 ± 0.50	2.25 ± 0.22	5.10 ± 0.16

Expression levels were normalized with ATCC19606 for carO, adeB, adeR and bla$_{OXA-51}$. Strains lacking the corresponding genes were depicted by "n.a." Expression of adeB was not detected in AB2 and AB5.

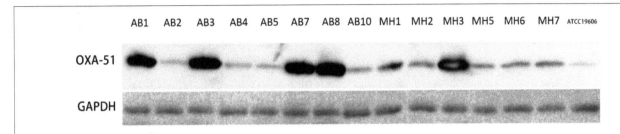

FIGURE 1 | Western blot analysis of *Acinetobacter baumannii* strains using OXA-51 specific antibody. The broad-range anti-GAPDH was used as loading control.

TABLE 3 | Surveillance of mechanisms of carbapenem resistance in clinical carbapenem-resistant *A. baumannii* isolates from different regions of China.

Characteristics of *A. baumannii* isolates from different sources		Guangdong, China	Zhejiang, China	Henan, China	Hong Kong, China	Total
Total No of strains of each source		163	173	72	45	453
Average MICs	MER	24.4	18.4	24.8	20.6	21.8
	IMP	26.8	16.2	24.6	22.4	22.0
	ERA	86.4	64.2	78.8	66.4	74.7
No of positive strains	bla_{OXA-51}	163	173	72	45	453
	ISAba1- bla_{OXA-51}	18	19	4	8	49
	bla_{OXA-23}	145	154	68	37	404
	ISAba1- bla_{OXA-23}	145	154	68	37	404
	Overexpression of OXA-51 (WB)[#]	18	19	4	8	49

MER, meropenem; IMP, imipenem; ERA, ertapenem. [#]OXA-51 expression level was determined by Western-blot using OXA-51 specific antibody developed in our lab.

To further investigate the role of various host determinants in mediating changes in carbapenem susceptibility, the expression level of various putative resistance genes, including the RND efflux pump gene *adeB*, its regulator *adeR*, the outer membrane porin gene *carO*, as well as the bla_{OXA-23} and bla_{OXA-51}-like β-lactamase-encoding elements, were further analyzed by RT-qPCR. The expression level of each gene was normalized by the gene encoding the gyrase protein subunit B (*gyrB*) of the *A. baumannii* type strain ATCC19606. The results are shown in **Table 2** and **Supplementary Figures S7–S11**. For *carO*, varied expression level was observed among the test strains, with most isolates exhibiting a level similar to or lower than that of ATCC19606. For the two susceptible strains, AB10 and MH1, *carO* expression was lower than that of ATCC19606 and most of the other carbapenem-resistant counterparts. The result is in line with a previous study, in which a decreased expression of *carO* has been described in carbapenem susceptible isolates recovered from Brazil (Fonseca et al., 2013). It should be noted that although strains AB7, AB8, and MH3 exhibited elevated *carO* expression by an amplitude >twofolds, their contribution to carbapenem resistance was hard to be addressed due to the presence of other major resistance mechanism, presence of OXA types of carbapenemases (**Tables 1, 2**).

An unexpected phenomenon regarding the *adeB* expression level of the test strains was observed. It was proposed that elevated expression of *adeABC* might contribute to reduced carbapenem susceptibility, possibly due to enhanced extrusion of intracellular antibiotics through efflux activity (Kim et al., 2013). Nevertheless, except for the two test strains AB3 and

MH5, which lacked *adeB*, all other test strains exhibited a very low transcript level of this efflux gene, with a range of 0.07 to 0.31 compared to ATCC19606. Transcript of *adeB* was not detected in strains AB2 and AB5. Of note, *adeB* expression in the two carbapenem sensitive strains AB10 and MH1 was similar to most of their resistant counterparts. In order to evaluate whether decreased *adeABC* expression was due to effect of transcription regulation, expression level of *adeR* was also examined in an attempt to determine the degree of correlation between the two. Contrary to the data on *adeB*, similar or higher transcription level of *adeR* was observed among the majority of the test isolates, ranging from 0.91 to 3.63 folds when compared to ATCC19606 (**Table 2**). Correlation between expression of *adeB* and *adeR*, as well as *adeR* and carbapenem susceptibility, therefore could not be established. Taken together, the results suggest that the *adeABC* gene plays a negligible role in mediating changes in carbapenem susceptibility, particularly in strains which harbor additional CHDL genes such as bla_{OXA-23} and bla_{OXA-24}. Indeed, the results of genotypic analysis corroborated with those of the expression study in that a lack of *adeABC* efflux system was observed in several resistant strains.

Overexpression of OXA-23 and Intrinsic OXA-51 Through ISAba1 Insertion Was the Major Mechanisms of Carbapenem Resistance

Antimicrobial susceptibility test revealed that all bla_{OXA-23} carriers were resistant to imipenem and meropenem but exhibited varied MIC values, presumably due to the fact that these strains carried various variants of bla_{OXA-23} and bla_{OXA-51}. Expression level of bla_{OXA-51} and bla_{OXA-23} was examined in an attempt to determine the degree of contribution of carbapenemases encoded by these genes to reduction in carbapenem susceptibility of the *A. baumannii* strains tested in this study. All bla_{OXA-23} genes were found to carry insertion in the promoter region by ISAba1. Consistently, expression level of the bla_{OXA-23} gene was found to be up-regulated 2.24 to 7.64 folds among the strains. Discrepancies between the effects of plasmid-borne and chromosome-based elements were not observed (**Tables 1, 2**). Among the 6 bla_{OXA-23} carriers which lacked an over-expressed bla_{OXA-51}, MIC values of imipenem and meropenem ranged from 16 to ≥ 64 µg/ml and 8 to ≥ 64 µg/ml, respectively. In particular, the higher transcript level of bla_{OXA-23} did not necessarily confer higher resistance level toward carbapenems. Since identical bla_{OXA-23} was harbored by all the strains, the possibility of varied activity toward carbapenem in individual variants can be ruled out. The lack of association between bla_{OXA-23} expression and susceptibility might then be attributed to physiological status of individual *A. baumannii* strains. Result of bla_{OXA-51} expression revealed consistency between ISAba1 insertion and transcript level of this endogenous carbapenemase. For the five test strains which carried the IS element, bla_{OXA-51} expression ranged from 25.09 to 64.96 folds compared to ATCC19606. To ensure that the overexpression of bla_{OXA-51} was consistent with their protein production, we took advantage of the monoclonal antibody specific to OXA-51 variants that produced by our lab to examine the production level of these OXA-51 variants by western blotting (**Figure 1**). It was shown that protein production correlated well with the qRT-PCR data, and that the five strains apparently over-produced the OXA-51 enzymes. The result confirmed that the ISAba1 insertion sequence is a key factor that promotes bla_{OXA-51} expression. To summarize, although the physiological status of individual strain may affect carbapenem susceptibility to some extent, resistance was observed only among *A. baumannii* strains which carried either ISAba1-bla_{OXA-51} or additional CHDL-encoding genes such as bla_{OXA23} and bla_{OXA-72}.

To confirm that overexpression of OXA-23 and intrinsic OXA-51 is the major mechanisms of carbapenem resistance in clinical *A. baumannii*, a total of 453 carbapenem-resistant clinical *A. baumannii* isolated from four different regions of China were screened for the presence of these two mechanisms (**Table 3**). Our results showed that 404/453 strains carried over-expressed OXA-23 with ISAba1 in the promoter region of bla_{OXA-23}, while the rest of 49 strains that did not carry bla_{OXA-23} exhibited an insertion of ISAba1 in the promoter region of bla_{OXA-51} and over-expression of OXA-51, which was confirmed by Western-blot using specific antibody to OXA-51 (**Table 3**). These data suggested that mechanisms of carbapenem resistance in clinical *A. baumannii* were mediated by either over-production of OXA-23 or OXA-51 through insertion of ISAba1 in their promoter region.

Correlation analysis of the enzymatic activity of OXA types carbapnemase and meropenem MIC of strains producing these enzymes indicated that: (1) *A. baumannii* strains that over-expressed OXA-23/OXA-24 regardless of the status of over-expression of OXA-51 variants generally displayed higher MIC of meropenem (≥ 16 µg/ml); (2) *A. baumannii* strains that over-expressed OXA-51 variants only displayed relatively low MIC of meropenem, with OXA-83 (32 µg/ml) being higher than OXA-79/OXA-83 (8 µg/ml); and (3) Western-blot experiments indicated that OXA-51 variants exhibited base line expression without the insertion of ISAba1, which is probably true for extrinsic OXAs. OXA variants with lower activity like OXA51 variants are needed to be overexpressed to counter carbapeneme resistance phenotype, while variants with high catalytic activity such as OXA-72 may not need to be overexpressed, its basic line expression might be enough to mediate high carbapenem resistance in *A. baumannii* in the case of MH2 in this study.

CONCLUSION

Acinetobacter baumannii is an important pathogen that may cause fatal infections in nosocomial settings. It was thought that the interplay of multiple resistance mechanisms, including over-expression of endogenous efflux systems, suppression of expression f porin proteins, reduced membrane permeability and carriage of CHDL-encoding elements could lead to carbapenem resistance in this bacterial pathogen. In the current study, through systematic characterization of a set of clinical *A. baumannii* strains with different OXA-23 and MIC profiles, we demonstrated that the RND efflux system and membrane porin proteins were not the key factors that conferred carbapenem resistance in the *A. baumannii* strains tested. Instead the OXA-23 and OXA-24 enzymes (OXA- 72 variant) were found to be the key elements underlying carbapenem resistance in *A. baumannii* strains as a result of insertion of the ISAba1 element, which provides a promoter for over-expression of the bla_{OXA-23} and bla_{OXA-23} genes (Nigro and Hall, 2016). In *A. baumannii* strains lacking these genes, carbapenem resistance was mainly due to the over-expression of bla_{OXA-51} variants, again through insertion of the promoter-bearing ISAba1 elements. Findings in this study emphasized the role of bla_{OXA} type enzymes in mediating carbapenem resistance in this major clinical pathogen. These data provided essential information for the design of new strategies to treat clinical infections caused by carbapenem-resistant *A. baumannii* strains.

AUTHOR CONTRIBUTIONS

MW and BC designed and performed the research, and drafted the manuscript. EC edited the manuscript. SC supervised the study and edited the manuscript.

FUNDING

This work was supported by the Health and Medical Research Fund of the Food and Health Bureau, Hong Kong (15141322) to SC.

REFERENCES

Bergogne-Berezin, E., and Towner, K. J. (1996). Acinetobacter spp. as nosocomial pathogens: microbiological, clinical, and epidemiological features. *Clin. Microbiol. Rev.* 9, 148–165. doi: 10.1128/cmr.9.2.148

Clinical and Laboratory Standards Institute (2016). *Performance Standards for Antimicrobial Susceptibility Testing: Twenty-sixth Informational Supplement M100-S26.* Wayne, PA: CLSI.

Evans, B. A., and Amyes, S. G. (2014). OXA β-lactamases. *Clin. Microbiol. Rev.* 27, 241–263. doi: 10.1128/CMR.00117-113

Fonseca, E. L., Scheidegger, E., Freitas, F. S., Cipriano, R., and Vicente, A. C. (2013). Carbapenem-resistant *Acinetobacter baumannii* from Brazil: role of carO alleles expression and blaOXA-23 gene. *BMC Microbiol.* 13:245. doi: 10.1186/1471-2180-13-245

Gribun, A., Nitzan, Y., Pechatnikov, I., Hershkovits, G., and Katcoff, D. J. (2003). Molecular and structural characterization of the HMP-AB gene encoding a pore-forming protein from a clinical isolate of *Acinetobacter baumannii. Curr. Microbiol.* 47, 434–443.

Higgins, P. G., Pérez-Llarena, F. J., Zander, E., Fernández, A., Bou, G., and Seifert, H. (2013). OXA-235, a novel class D β-lactamase involved in resistance to carbapenems in *Acinetobacter baumannii. Antimicrob. Agents Chemother.* 57, 2121–2126. doi: 10.1128/AAC.02413-2412

Higgins, P. G., Wisplinghoff, H., Stefanik, D., and Seifert, H. (2004). Selection of topoisomerase mutations and overexpression of adeB mRNA transcripts during an outbreak of *Acinetobacter baumannii. J. Antimicrob. Chemother.* 54, 821–823. doi: 10.1093/jac/dkh427

Ho, P. L., Ho, A. Y., Chow, K. H., Lai, E. L., Ching, P., and Seto, W. H. (2010). Epidemiology and clonality of multidrug-resistant *Acinetobacter baumannii* from a healthcare region in Hong Kong. *J. Hosp. Infect.* 74, 358–364. doi: 10.1016/j.jhin.2009.10.015

Ji, S., Chen, Y., Ruan, Z., Fu, Y., Ji, J., Fu, Y., et al. (2014). Prevalence of carbapenem-hydrolyzing class D β-lactamase genes in *Acinetobacter* spp. isolates in China. *Eur. J. Microbiol. Infect. Dis.* 33, 989–997. doi: 10.1007/s10096-013-2037-z

Kim, D. H., Choi, J.-Y. Y., Kim, H. W., Kim, S. H., Chung, D. R., Peck, K. R., et al. (2013). Spread of carbapenem-resistant *Acinetobacter baumannii* global clone 2 in Asia and AbaR-type resistance islands. *Antimicrob. Agents Chemother.* 57, 5239–5246. doi: 10.1128/AAC.00633-613

Liu, Y.-M. M., Chen, Y.-S. S., Toh, H.-S. S., Huang, C.-C. C., Lee, Y.-L. L., Ho, C.-M. M., et al. (2012). In vitro susceptibilities of non-*Enterobacteriaceae* isolates from patients with intra-abdominal infections in the Asia-Pacific region from 2003 to 2010: results from the study for monitoring antimicrobial resistance trends (SMART). *Int. J. Antimicrob. Agents* 40(Suppl.), S11–S17. doi: 10.1016/S0924-8579(12)70004-3

Magnet, S., Courvalin, P., and Lambert, T. (2001). Resistance-nodulation-cell division-type efflux pump involved in aminoglycoside resistance in *Acinetobacter baumannii* strain BM4454. *Antimicrob. Agents Chemother.* 45, 3375–3380. doi: 10.1128/AAC.45.12.3375-3380.2001

Matsui, M., Suzuki, S., Suzuki, M., Arakawa, Y., and Shibayama, K. (2013). Rapid discrimination of *Acinetobacter baumannii* international clone II lineage by pyrosequencing SNP analyses of bla(OXA-51-like) genes. *J. Microbiol. Methods* 94, 121–124. doi: 10.1016/j.mimet.2013.05.014

Mugnier, P. D., Poirel, L., Naas, T., and Nordmann, P. (2010). Worldwide dissemination of the blaOXA-23 carbapenemase gene of *Acinetobacter baumannii. Emerg. Infect. Dis.* 16, 35–40. doi: 10.3201/eid1601.090852

Nigro, S. J., and Hall, R. M. (2016). Structure and context of acinetobacter transposons carrying the oxa23 carbapenemase gene. *J. Antimicrob. Chemother.* 71, 1135–1147. doi: 10.1093/jac/dkv440

Overbeek, R., Olson, R., Pusch, G. D., Olsen, G. J., Davis, J. J., Disz, T., et al. (2014). The SEED and the rapid annotation of microbial genomes using subsystems technology (RAST). *Nucleic Acids Res.* 42, D206–D214. doi: 10.1093/nar/gkt1226

Peleg, A. Y., Seifert, H., and Paterson, D. L. (2008). *Acinetobacter baumannii*: emergence of a successful pathogen. *Clin. Microbio. Rev.* 21, 538–582. doi: 10.1128/CMR.00058-57

Poirel, L., and Nordmann, P. (2006). Carbapenem resistance in *Acinetobacter baumannii*: mechanisms and epidemiology. *Clin. Microbiol. Infect.* 12, 826–836. doi: 10.1111/j.1469-0691.2006.01456.x

Queenan, A. M., Pillar, C. M., Deane, J., Sahm, D. F., Lynch, A. S., Flamm, R. K., et al. (2012). Multidrug resistance among acinetobacter spp. in the USA and activity profile of key agents: results from CAPITAL surveillance 2010. *Diagn. Microbiol. Infect. Dis.* 73, 267–270. doi: 10.1016/j.diagmicrobio.2012.04.002

Roca, I., Espinal, P., Vila-Farres, X., and Vila, J. (2012). The *Acinetobacter baumannii* oxymoron: commensal hospital dweller turned pan-drug-resistant menace. *Front. Microbiol.* 3:148. doi: 10.3389/fmicb.2012.00148

Rumbo, C., Gato, E., López, M., Ruiz de Alegría, C., Fernández-Cuenca, F., Martínez-Martínez, L., et al. (2013). Contribution of efflux pumps, porins, and β-lactamases to multidrug resistance in clinical isolates of *Acinetobacter baumannii. Antimicrob. Agents Chemother.* 57, 5247–5257. doi: 10.1128/AAC.00730-713

Seemann, T. (2014). Prokka: rapid prokaryotic genome annotation. *Bioinformatics* 30, 2068–2069. doi: 10.1093/bioinformatics/btu153

Siroy, A., Cosette, P., Seyer, D., Lemaitre-Guillier, C., Vallenet, D., Van Dorsselaer, A., et al. (2006). Global comparison of the membrane subproteomes between a multidrug-resistant *Acinetobacter baumannii* strain and a reference strain. *J. Proteome Res.* 5, 3385–3398. doi: 10.1021/pr060372s

Siroy, A., Molle, V., Lemaître-Guillier, C., Vallenet, D., Pestel-Caron, M., Cozzone, A. J., et al. (2005). Channel formation by CarO, the carbapenem resistance-associated outer membrane protein of *Acinetobacter baumannii. Antimicrob. Agents Chemother.* 49, 4876–4883. doi: 10.1128/AAC.49.12.4876-4883.2005

Turton, J. F., Ward, M. E., Woodford, N., Kaufmann, M. E., Pike, R., Livermore, D. M., et al. (2006). The role of ISAba1 in expression of OXA carbapenemase genes in *Acinetobacter baumannii. FEMS Microbiol. Lett.* 258, 72–77. doi: 10.1111/j.1574-6968.2006.00195.x

Wen, Y., Ouyang, Z., Yu, Y., Zhou, X., Pei, Y., Devreese, B., et al. (2017). Mechanistic insight into how multidrug resistant *Acinetobacter baumannii* response regulator AdeR recognizes an intercistronic region. *Nucleic Acids Res.* 45, 9773–9787. doi: 10.1093/nar/gkx624

World Health Organisation (2017). *Global Priority List of Antibiotic-resistant Bacteria to Guide Research, Discovery, and Development of New Antibiotics.* Geneva: WHO Press.

14

Amoxicillin Increased Functional Pathway Genes and Beta-Lactam Resistance Genes by Pathogens Bloomed in Intestinal Microbiota Using a Simulator of the Human Intestinal Microbial Ecosystem

Lei Liu[1†], Qing Wang[1,2†], Huai Lin[1], Ranjit Das[1], Siyi Wang[1], Hongmei Qi[1], Jing Yang[1], Yingang Xue[3], Daqing Mao[4] and Yi Luo[1*]*

[1] College of Environmental Science and Engineering, Ministry of Education Key Laboratory of Pollution Processes and Environmental Criteria, Nankai University, Tianjin, China, [2] Hebei Key Laboratory of Air Pollution Cause and Impact (preparatory), College of Energy and Environmental Engineering, Hebei University of Engineering, Handan, China, [3] Key Laboratory of Environmental Protection of Water Environment Biological Monitoring of Jiangsu Province, Changzhou Environmental Monitoring Center, Changzhou, China, [4] School of Medicine, Nankai University, Tianjin, China

Correspondence:
Daqing Mao
maodq@nankai.edu.cn
Yi Luo
luoy@nankai.edu.cn

Antibiotics are frequently used to treat bacterial infections; however, they affect not only the target pathogen but also commensal gut bacteria. They may cause the dysbiosis of human intestinal microbiota and consequent metabolic alterations, as well as the spreading of antibiotic resistant bacteria and antibiotic resistance genes (ARGs). In vitro experiments by simulator of the human intestinal microbial ecosystem (SHIME) can clarify the direct effects of antibiotics on different regions of the human intestinal microbiota, allowing complex human microbiota to be stably maintained in the absence of host cells. However, there are very few articles added the antibiotics into this in vitro model to observe the effects of antibiotics on the human intestinal microbiota. To date, no studies have focused on the correlations between the bloomed pathogens caused by amoxicillin (AMX) exposure and increased functional pathway genes as well as ARGs. This study investigated the influence of 600 mg day^{-1} AMX on human intestinal microbiota using SHIME. The impact of AMX on the composition and function of the human intestinal microbiota was revealed by 16S rRNA gene sequencing and high-throughput quantitative PCR. The results suggested that: (i) AMX treatment has tremendous influence on the overall taxonomic composition of the gut microbiota by increasing the relative abundance of *Klebsiella* [linear discriminant analysis (LDA) score = 5.26] and *Bacteroides uniformis* (LDA score = 4.75), as well as taxonomic diversity (Simpson, $P = 0.067$, T-test; Shannon, $P = 0.061$, T-test), and decreasing the members of *Parabacteroides* (LDA score = 4.18), *Bifidobacterium* (LDA score = 4.06), and *Phascolarctobacterium* (LDA score = 3.95); (ii) AMX exposure significantly enhanced the functional pathway genes and beta-lactam resistance genes, and the bloomed pathogens were strongly correlated with the metabolic and immune system diseases gene numbers ($R = 0.98$, $P < 0.001$) or *bl2_len* and *bl2be_shv2* abundance ($R = 0.94$, $P < 0.001$); (iii) the changes caused by AMX were "SHIME-compartment" different with more significant alteration in ascending colon, and the effects were permanent, which could not be restored after 2-week AMX discontinuance. Overall results demonstrated negative side-effects of AMX, which should be considered for AMX prescription.

Keywords: amoxicillin, antibiotic resistance genes (ARGs), functional pathway genes, human intestinal microbiota, simulator of the human intestinal microbial ecosystem (SHIME)

INTRODUCTION

Human intestinal microbiota co-exists in symbiosis with human beings and comprises with about 150 times more genes than the human genome, which makes intestinal microbiota become "another" genome of human beings (Qin et al., 2010). Moreover, human intestinal microbiota has been demonstrated to provide numerous important functions for the human health, including fermentation of indigestible dietary polysaccharides, synthesis of essential amino acids, and vitamins, modulation of the immune function and protection from the pathogens, as well as metabolism of the xenobiotic drugs (Chow et al., 2010; Yatsunenko et al., 2012; Cabreiro et al., 2013). Both human and veterinary antibiotics were detected in the collective gut of the Chinese population through our previous research (Wang et al., 2020). The antibiotics in our gut would kill or prevent the growth of commensal beneficial bacteria, which would cause the dysbiosis of intestinal microbiota, resulting multiple human diseases (Blaser, 2016; Ianiro et al., 2016; Flandroy et al., 2018; Kho and Lal, 2018). Antibiotics may also promote the spreading of antibiotic resistant bacteria (ARB) and antibiotic resistance genes (ARGs) in the human gut (Stecher et al., 2013; Barraud et al., 2018). One of the most commonly prescribed antibiotic in clinical and residential applications is amoxicillin (AMX), an inexpensive oral penicillin-type, beta-lactam antibiotic that kills a broad spectrum of bacteria by interfering with the synthesis of bacterial cell wall peptidoglycan layer (Zapata and Quagliarello, 2015; Zhang et al., 2015). The influence of AMX on human intestinal microbiota by *in vivo* research has been well studied and recorded, including human (Ladirat et al., 2014a; Pallav et al., 2014; Vrieze et al., 2014; Zaura et al., 2015; Oh et al., 2016) and human microbiota associated-animal models (Barc et al., 2008; Collignon et al., 2008; Collignon et al., 2010). Oh et al. (2016) noticed that AMX increased the abundance of *Klebsiella* in human intestinal microbiota. As a typical Gram-negative bacterial pathogen, *K. pneumoniae* is ubiquitous in the environment and symbioses in the human gut (Rock et al., 2014). However, the bloom of *K. pneumoniae* in human gut is often related to unhealthy status (Pena et al., 1997; Wiener-Well et al., 2010; Gorrie et al., 2017). Furthermore, no studies have suggested the bloom of *K. pneumoniae* caused by AMX exposure contributed to the increase of functional pathway genes and beta-lactam resistance genes.

Previous reports have revealed that changes of intestinal microbiota by AMX exposure are region-dependent and more significant effects were observed in the proximal colon than in the

distal colon (Ladirat et al., 2014b; Marzorati et al., 2017). *In vivo* experiments detected the fecal samples that generally stand for the distal intestinal microbiota, which could not reveal the impacts of antibiotics on different gut regions. Moreover, *in vitro* experiment using simulator of the human intestinal microbial ecosystem (SHIME) can elucidate the direct effects of medicines on different regions of the human intestinal microbiota, which allows the complex human microbiota to be stably maintained in the absence of host cells (Van de Wiele et al., 2015). The SHIME model is known to be a useful tool for the *in vitro* study, which has already been used to identify the influence of bacteria and compounds on the colon microbiota, including probiotics such as *Clostridium cluster* XIVa and *Bifidobacterium longum* (Van den Abbeele et al., 2013; Truchado et al., 2015), prebiotics and prebiotics like compounds such as inulin, polyphenols and orange juice (Kemperman et al., 2013; Duque et al., 2016; Selak et al., 2016), and other toxic compounds such as Chlorpyrifos and Arsenic (Reygner et al., 2016; Yu et al., 2016). However, to the best of our knowledge, there are very few research that applied antibiotics into the SHIME model (Van den Abbeele et al., 2012; Bussche et al., 2015; Marzorati et al., 2017; Ichim et al., 2018; El Hage et al., 2019; Liu et al., 2020). These articles focused on the benefit of the mucosal environment, high-fiber diets, probiotic, and propionate-producing consortium in human intestinal microbiota. The effects of antibiotics, including AMX and other antibiotics mixture, vancomycin, and clindamycin, were limited on microbiota composition and metabolite. Also, there was little information available to demonstrate the link between the bloomed pathogens and functional pathway genes or ARGs. Hence, there is a need to study the influence of AMX on human intestinal microbiota in the SHIME model that integrates the entire gastrointestinal tract and maintains microbiome stability over an extended timeframe (Van de Wiele et al., 2015).

Since the reasonable dosage of AMX for the adult human study is about 750 to 1,500 mg day^{-1}, and only half volume of the adult gut can be simulated in the SHIME model, here the direct effects of 600 mg day^{-1} of AMX on the composition and function of the human fecal microbiota were followed by the previous studies (Pallav et al., 2014; Reijnders et al., 2016). Three reactors (representing the ascending, transverse, and descending colon, respectively) that inoculated with human intestinal microbiota were studied for the three groups: immediately before AMX administration during 0 to 21 days (a control group), AMX-exposure during 22 to 28 days (an AMX treated group), and after the AMX discontinuance during 29 to 42 days (a recovery group). The 16S rRNA gene sequencing and high-throughput quantitative PCR (HT-qPCR) results revealed that AMX exposure caused a tremendous impact on the overall taxonomic composition of the gut microbiota, and increased functional pathway genes as well as ARGs. The changes were "SHIME-compartment" different with more significant modulation in the ascending colon, which could not be restored after 2-week AMX discontinuance. Therefore, the results of our research demonstrated a severe impact and a negative side-effect of AMX related to health problems, which should be considered as a fundamental aspect of the cost-benefit equation for its prescription.

MATERIALS AND METHODS

The SHIME Model Experimental Setup and Sampling

The SHIME set up was formed by five double-jacketed reactors designated as the stomach, small intestine, ascending colon, transverse colon, and descending colon, respectively (**Supplementary Figure S1**). The last three reactors were inoculated with a mixture of fecal microbiota from a healthy adult volunteer, who did not suffer from gastrointestinal diseases or take antibiotics in the previous 6 months according to previous classic studies (Yu et al., 2016; Wang et al., 2018). And the differences between individuals may be alleviated by same culture condition (Van den Abbeele et al., 2013). The study was approved by the Biomedical Ethics Committees of Nankai University. The participant has given written informed consent to understand the study purpose, procedures, risks, benefits, and rights. The details of the SHIME system and the startup process are summarized in the **Supplementary Material**.

As shown in **Supplementary Figure S1**, during the first 2 weeks (0 to 14 days) of the experiment, control nutritional medium was added into the reactors to stabilize the microbial community. After this period, the SHIME was sequentially exposed to nutritious medium (15 to 21 days), and nutritious medium + 600 mg day^{-1} AMX (22 to 28 days), each time system was maintained for 1-week. Then a nutritious medium was added and observed for another 2-weeks (29 to 42 days). Samples were collected and analyzed at six time points of 14, 21, 24, 28, 35, and 42 days from the ascending colon, transverse colon and descending colon, respectively. Each of the 18 samples is a mixture of three samples collected at specific time intervals in a day (Liu et al., 2020), and AMX was added after samples (C-A2, C-T2, and C-D2) had been collected in 22 days and discontinued after samples (AMX-A2, AMX-T2, and AMX-D2) had been collected in 29 days. Therefore, these samples were divided into three groups: before AMX administration during 0 to 21 days (control group), AMX exposure during 22 to 28 days (AMX treatment group) and after the AMX discontinuance during 29 to 42 days (recovery group), which were according to previous classic studies (Yu et al., 2016; Wang et al., 2018). Specifically, during each sampling time, three sterilized centrifuge tubes (50 ml) were used to collect

the samples (10 ml) flow out from each colon vessel of the SHIME, respectively, and these samples were initially stored at −4°C (Van de Wiele et al., 2010; Yu et al., 2016). After all the samples were collected in each sampling day, three samples from the same vessel were mixed into one sterilized centrifuge tube (50 ml), which was operated in a super-clean bench. Then the samples were centrifuged at 10,400 g for 10 min, and the separated supernatants and pellets were stored at −80°C for further analyses.

16S rRNA Gene Sequencing and Analysis

Total DNA was extracted from the samples using the E.Z.N.A. stool DNA Kit (Omega, United States) according to the manufacturer's protocols. The V3–V4 region of the bacterial 16S rRNA gene was amplified by polymerase chain reaction (PCR) using primers 341F 5′-CCTAYGGGRBGCASCAG-3′ and 806R 5′-GGACTACNNGGGTATCTAAT-3′ (95°C for 2 min, followed by 27 cycles at 95°C for 30 s, 55°C for 30 s, and 72°C for 30 s, and a final extension at 72°C for 5 min). Amplicons were paired-end sequenced (PE250) on Illumina Hiseq2500 platform. In the end, a total of 651,502 tags were obtained. The raw reads were deposited into the NCBI Sequence Read Archive (SRA) database under the accession number of SRR9330193–SRR9330210. The details of bacterial DNA extraction and PCR amplification of the 16S rRNA gene are described in the **Supplementary Material**.

Raw Illumina fastq files were de-multiplexed, quality-filtered, and analyzed using Quantitative Insights Into Microbial Ecology (QIIME) (Caporaso et al., 2010). The 16S rRNA gene sequences were classified taxonomically using the Ribosomal Database Project (RDP), and classifier 2.0.1 (Wang et al., 2007). The AMX exposure on alpha diversity was further measured by the taxon richness (Chao1 index), evenness (Simpson index), and diversity index (Shannon index) using all recommended samples. Besides, beta diversity of microbiota communities at baseline and after antibiotics were portrayed by nonmetric multidimensional scaling (NMDS) and principal coordinate analysis (PCoA) of weighted and unweighted UniFrac distances. Linear discriminant analysis effect size (LEfSe) analysis was performed to determine the bacterial taxa that significantly differed between the control and AMX exposure group using Galaxy application tool (Segata et al., 2011). Functional predictions of microbial community were performed to visualize the distribution of functional pathway genes in the three parts of the colon with different treatments using Phylogenetic Investigation of Communities by Reconstruction of Unobserved States (PICRUSt) (Langille et al., 2013). The accuracy of PICRUSt for the detection of these more challenging functional groups was good (minimum accuracy = 0.82), suggesting that their inference of gene abundance across various types of functions was reliable, and PICRUSt predictions had high agreement with metagenome sample abundances across all body sites (Spearman r = 0.82, P < 0.001). PICRUSt has been successfully manipulated in many previous research for predicting microbial function of human intestinal microbiota (McHardy et al., 2013; Bunyavanich et al., 2016; Labus et al., 2017; Puri et al., 2018). The details of taxonomical classification, LEfSe analysis, and functional predictions are described in the **Supplementary Material**.

High-Throughput Quantitative PCR (HT-qPCR) and Analysis

High-throughput quantitative PCR reactions were performed to visualize the variation of ARGs during the treatment using Wafergen SmartChip Real-time PCR system, conducted by Anhui MicroAnaly Gene Technologies Co., Ltd. (Anhui, China). A total of 108 primer sets were used (Excel S1), including 102 primer sets to target the almost all major classes of ARGs found in the Chinese human gut microbiota (Hu et al., 2013), five mobile genetic elements (MGEs), and one 16S rRNA gene. The results were analyzed with SmartChip qPCR Software by excluding the wells with multiple melting peaks or amplification efficiency beyond the range (90–110%). Then data were screened with the conditions that a threshold cycle (CT) must be <31 and positive samples should have three replicates simultaneously. The details of HT-qPCR analysis are described in the **Supplementary Material**.

Data Analysis

All the results were expressed as mean values and standard deviations. The statistical analysis was performed with SPSS 17.0 software (SPSS Inc., Chicago, IL, United States). The T-test was conducted to compare the differences between the groups, and all the statistical tests were two-tailed. The statistical significance was set at three different levels ($*P < 0.05$, $**P < 0.01$, and $***P < 0.001$). Spearman test, Mantel test, and Procrustes test for correlation analysis between the microbiota and the functional pathway genes or ARGs were performed in R with the vegan package. Correlations between the pairs of variables were considered to be significant at $R > 0.6$, and P values were <0.05. The Gephi (V 0.9.1) software was used to visualize the bipartite network graphs using the Force Atlas algorithm.

RESULTS

AMX Exposure Increased Microbiota Diversity

The effects of 600 mg day^{-1} AMX treatment on the gut bacterial community were revealed by the 16S rRNA gene sequencing of fecal samples collected from three different vessels designated as ascending, transverse, and descending colon. The vessels were set up for three groups: before AMX administration during 0 to 21 days (control group), AMX exposure during 22 to 28 days (AMX treatment group) and after the AMX discontinuance during 29 to 42 days (recovery group). The alpha diversity of the fecal microbiota was assessed in each group. The taxon richness (Chao1 index), evenness (Simpson index), and diversity index (Shannon index) of the three groups are shown in **Figure 1**. As compared with the control group, a substantially rising in the evenness (Simpson, $P = 0.067$, T-test) and diversity (Shannon, $P = 0.061$, T-test) was observed in the AMX treatment groups; however, no change occurred in the microbiota richness (Chao1, $P = 0.564$, T-test). Moreover, data displayed that an increasing of microbiota evenness and diversity caused by the AMX treatments

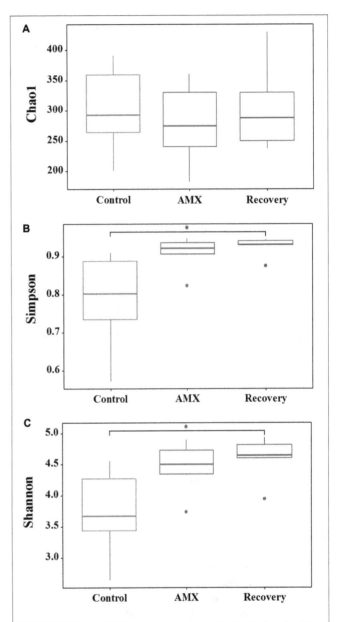

FIGURE 1 | Effects of AMX treatment on gut microbiota alpha diversity of the control (green), AMX (red), and recovery (blue) groups. The Chao1 index **(A)** was used to calculate the community richness, Simpson index **(B)** was used to calculate the community evenness, and Shannon index **(C)** was used to calculate the community diversity within each of the three groups (control, AMX, and recovery). Statistical significance between each of the three groups were analyzed using the T test at a significance level of 0.05.

was continued after two weeks of AMX discontinuance (Simpson, $P = 0.044$, T-test; Shannon, $P = 0.028$, T-test).

In addition, the beta diversity of the microbial communities and weighted UniFrac distance was also affected by AMX treatment. As shown in **Figure 2** and **Supplementary Figure S2**, the samples collected after the AMX treatment were differed from the control group, because the two groups clustered far away from each other in both UniFrac NMDS and PCoA analyses. The average weighted UniFrac distance between the AMX treatment

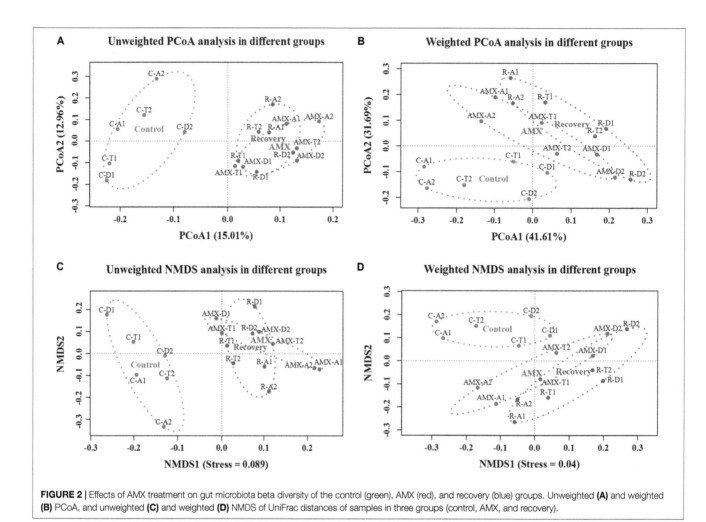

FIGURE 2 | Effects of AMX treatment on gut microbiota beta diversity of the control (green), AMX (red), and recovery (blue) groups. Unweighted **(A)** and weighted **(B)** PCoA, and unweighted **(C)** and weighted **(D)** NMDS of UniFrac distances of samples in three groups (control, AMX, and recovery).

group and control group (AMX vs control) was significantly higher ($P < 0.001$, T-test) than that within the control group (control vs control). Similarly, the beta diversity results showed that the gut microbial composition remained comparable after 2-week of AMX discontinuance because these samples were clustered together with the AMX treatment groups observed in both UniFrac NMDS and PCoA analyses. The average weighted UniFrac distance between the recovery group and the control group (recovery vs control) was also significantly higher ($P < 0.001$, T-test) than the control group (control vs control).

AMX Exposure Changed Microbiota Community Composition

The bacterial community compositions and their shifts at the phylum and genus levels after AMX exposure are shown in **Figure 3** and **Supplementary Figure S3**. Based on the 16S rRNA gene analysis, the taxonomic assignment was related to most four dominant phyla such as *Bacteroidetes, Firmicutes, Proteobacteria,* and *Synergistetes,* which accounted for 96.5 to 97.9% of the total community (**Figure 3A**). However, a noticeable increase in abundance of *Bacteroidetes* (from 16.3 to 19.9%) and *Synergistetes* (from 8.6 to 13.2%), and decrease of *Proteobacteria* (from 59.6 to 50.7%) were seen after AMX treatment. The shifted

phenomena (*Bacteroidete* from 13.3 to 23.2%; *Proteobacteria* from 68.8 to 57.8%) were more prominent in the ascending colon than the transverse and descending colons (**Supplementary Figure S3A**). A significant alteration in the communities was also observed at the phylum level (*Bacteroidetes* from 19.9 to 30.5%; *Proteobacteria* from 50.7 to 39.4%) after 2-week of AMX discontinued.

At the genus level, the *Bacteroides, Klebsiella, Megasphaera,* and *Pseudomonas* were predominant (**Figure 3B**). The antibiotic-treated subjects were shown to be substantially overgrown by *Bacteroides* (from 9.8 to 15.0%), *Klebsiella* (from 1.5 to 18.1%) and *Pyramidobacter* (from 0.8 to 10.0%), and declined in the percentage of *Cloacibacillus* (from 6.2 to 2.5%) and *Parabacteroides* (from 4.5 to 1.7%). Similarly, the changes of *Bacteroides* (from 8.4 to 20.5%) and *Klebsiella* (from 1.6 to 32.9%) were more evident in the ascending colon (**Supplementary Figure S3B**). As shown in **Figure 3B**, during the recovery period, it observed that the gut microbiota was not fully recuperated. Only, *Bacteroides* was inclined by abundance from 15.0 to 23.4%; however, all others were less retrieved (*Klebsiella* from 18.1% to 10.9%; *Pyramidobacte* from 10.0 to 8.5%; *Cloacibacillus* from 2.5 to 4.3%; *Parabacteroides* from 1.7 to 3.7%).

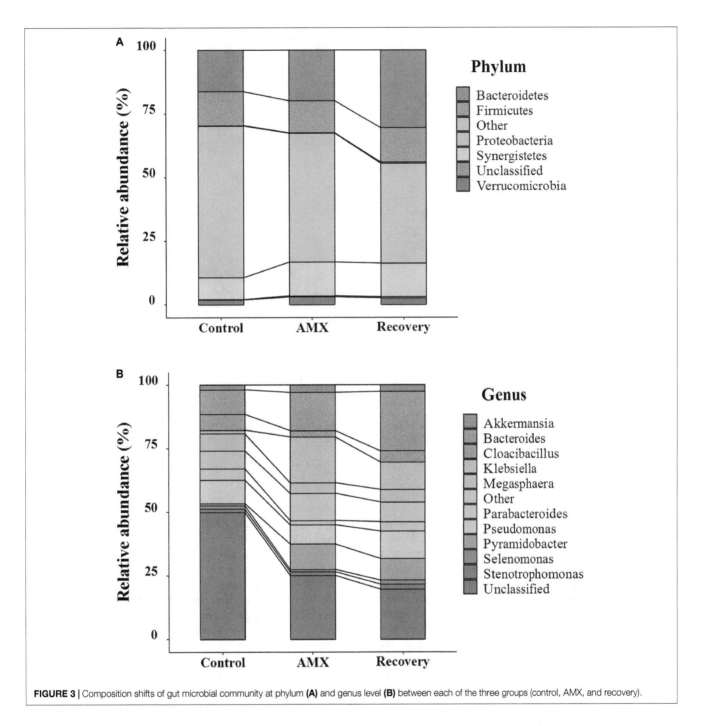

FIGURE 3 | Composition shifts of gut microbial community at phylum **(A)** and genus level **(B)** between each of the three groups (control, AMX, and recovery).

The LEfSe showed that the AMX exposure caused an obvious decrease in several taxa, including the members of *Parabacteroides* [linear discriminant analysis (LDA) score = 4.18], *Bifidobacterium* (LDA score = 4.06), and *Phascolarctobacterium* (LDA score = 3.95) (**Figure 4A**). The variation was accompanied by significant increases in the relative abundances of *Klebsiella* (LDA score = 5.26), and *Bacteroides uniformis* (LDA score = 4.75). However, after 2-week of AMX discontinuance, the decrease of *Bifidobacterium* (LDA score = 3.88), and increase of *Klebsiella* (LDA score = 4.67) and *Bacteroides uniformis*

(LDA score = 4.65) were still recognizable as compare with the control group (**Figure 4B**).

AMX Exposure Increased Functional Pathway Genes

The hierarchy cluster heatmap analysis using metagenomic 16S rRNA gene sequencing was predicted by PICRUSt. Results showed that functional pathway genes, which included cellular processes, environmental information processing, genetic information processing, human diseases, metabolism, and

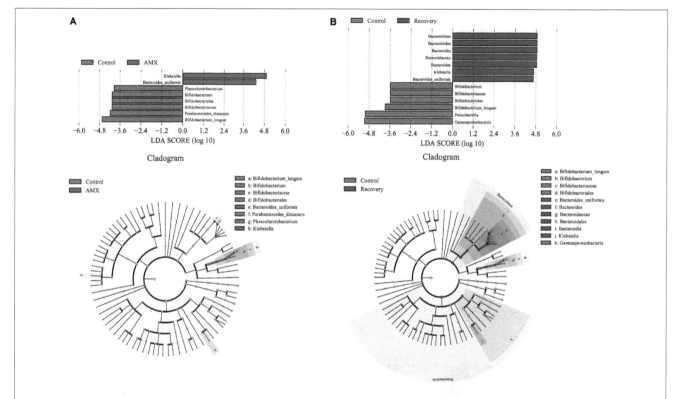

FIGURE 4 | LDA score and cladogram of LEfSe comparison analysis between the control and AMX groups **(A)**, and between the control and recovery groups **(B)**. The red, green, or blue shading depicts bacterial taxa that were significantly higher in either the control, AMX or recovery groups, as indicated. Selection of discriminative taxa between the control and AMX groups or between the control and recovery groups were based on an LDA score cutoff of 3.0, and differences in the relative abundances of taxa were statistically determined based on a Mann–Whitney test at a significance level of 0.05.

organismal systems were more abundant in the antibiotic exposure group than in the control group that represented by the ascending colon (**Figure 5**). For instance, as compared to the AMX-free sample C-A2, collected from the ascending colon before AMX administration, the gene numbers of human diseases related-pathways were 2.4–3.8 times enriched in the AMX exposed sample AMX-A2 that obtained after AMX treatment for 7 days. Similarly, the numbers of genes respect to functional pathways, for examples, membrane transport, transcription, xenobiotics biodegradation, metabolism, and excretory system were nearly 4.6–5.3 folds enriched in the AMX-A2 sample than C-A2. Moreover, these pathways were still maintained at a higher level (approximately 2.2–2.5 times enhanced than the control group) after the recovery phase.

To investigate whether the OTUs correlated with the functional pathway genes, the Mantel test and Procrustes analysis were used. The results showed that OTUs from the ascending, transverse, and descending colons were moderately correlated with the numbers of functional pathway genes (Mantel test, $R = 0.743$, $P < 0.001$). The Procrustes analysis indicated that OTUs obtained from the 16S rRNA gene data and the functional genes could be clustered according to the type of sample, which further exhibited a goodness-of-fit test ($R = 0.669$, $P < 0.001$, and 9,999 permutations) based on the Bray–Curtis dissimilarity metrics (**Supplementary Figure S4A**). As shown in **Figure 5**, the results demonstrated the co-occurrence

patterns of significantly shifted microbial taxa and functional pathway genes during AMX-treatment. It can be seen that the abundances of most imminent bacteria after AMX exposure such as *Bacteroides uniformis* and *Klebsiella* were positively associated with the gene numbers of functional pathways; however, the suppressed bacteria like *Phascolarctobacterium* and *Parabacteroides* were negatively associated (**Figure 5**). Specifically, the correlation coefficients of *Klebsiella* with the gene numbers of the digestive system, immune system, and metabolic diseases were about 0.98 ($P < 0.001$) and the correlation coefficients of *Phascolarctobacterium* abundance with gene numbers of signaling molecules and interaction, transport and catabolism, endocrine system, cell growth, and death were about −0.77 ($P < 0.01$).

AMX Exposure Increased the Abundance of Beta-Lactam and Tetracycline Resistance Genes

The relative abundances of ARGs such as beta-lactam and tetracycline resistance genes were substantially higher in the AMX exposure group as compared to the control group, while the multidrug-resistant ARGs and transposase were lower in the AMX exposure group (**Figure 6**). Notably, the relative log abundance of *bl2_len, bl2b_tem1,* and *bl2be_ctxm* (aminoglycoside) were about 1.6–2.4 log units higher after AMX

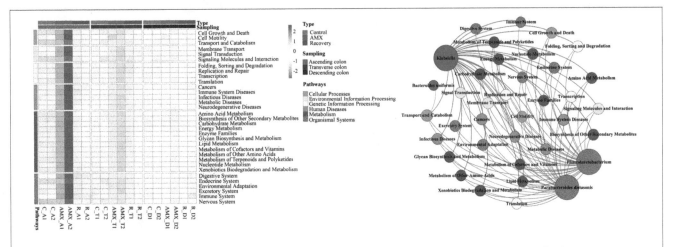

FIGURE 5 | Heatmap of human disease-related pathways in the three parts of colon within three groups and the network analysis revealing the co-occurrence patterns between microbial taxa abundance and functional pathway gene number. Heatmap colors reflect relative abundance from low (blue) to high (red). The nodes in network were colored according to types of functional pathway genes and microbial genera that increased (red) or decreased (green) after AMX exposure, and the edges were colored according to positive (red) or negative (blue) correlation. A connection represents strong and significant (P value < 0.05, R > 0.6) correlation. The size of each node is proportional to the number of connections, that is, degree.

treatment (AMX-A2) than in control (C-A2). Similarly, the *tetb*, *tetc*, and *tetr* (tetracycline) were about 1.4–2.5 log units higher than the control group. Besides, the reductions of relative log abundance in the ARGs such as *mdte* and *tolc* (multidrug) were about 1.2 log units after AMX treatment (AMX-A2) than control (C-A2), and *Tn22* (transposase) was 3.0 log units. Similarly, these ARGs were unable to return at the baseline level following the recovery procedure with about 0.6 to 3.2 log units change of relative abundance compared with the control group.

To investigate whether the OTUs correlated with the resistome composition, Mantel test and Procrustes analysis were also performed to correlate the OTUs with the resistome using ascending, transverse and descending colons' samples. Our results showed that OTUs were strongly correlated to the ARG profiles (Mantel test, $R = 0.895$, $P < 0.001$). The Procrustes analysis demonstrated that the bacterial OTUs and the ARGs in HT-qPCR data could be clustered by the type of sample and exhibited a goodness-of-fit-test ($R = 0.941$, $P < 0.001$, and 9,999 permutations) by Bray-Curtis dissimilarity metrics (**Supplementary Figure S4B**). The network analyses of co-occurrence patterns between the significantly changed microbial taxa after AMX treatment and ARG subtypes were shown in **Figure 6**. Interestingly, a very similar pattern of results was observed between the microbial taxa and functional pathway genes. The abundance of bacteria that significantly decreased after AMX treatment was positively associated with multidrug ARGs, while the abundance of increased bacteria was positively associated with beta-lactam resistance genes. For example, the moderate correlation coefficient of *Bifidobacterium longum* with *acra* abundance was 0.70 ($P < 0.05$), and for *Phascolarctobacterium* with *acrb* and *mdte* were 0.67 ($P < 0.05$). The strong correlations were found in the abundance of *Klebsiella* with the abundances of *bl2_len*, *bl2b_tem1*, and *bl2be_shv2* ($R = 0.9$, $P < 0.001$), and in *Bacteroides uniformis* with *bl2_len* and *bl2be_shv2* ($R = 0.8$, $P < 0.01$).

DISCUSSION

AMX Treatment Has a Tremendous Influence on the Overall Taxonomic Composition and Biodiversity

The SHIME model was stably operated in this study because the predominant phyla of *Bacteriodetes*, *Proteobacteria*, *Synergistetes*, and *Firmicutes* in the gut microbiome was previously demonstrated Yu et al. (2016). *Firmicutes* and *Bacteroidetes* are usually dominate in the microbiota of a healthy subject, however in the control microbiota of SHIME, *Proteobacteria* is majoritarian. For *in vivo* studies, highest percentage of *Proteobacteria* had also been observed in fecal samples from healthy human and animals (Gao et al., 2015; Li et al., 2015). Our previous *in vitro* study also discovered this phenomenon (Liu et al., 2020).

It has been reported that *in vivo* experiments of AMX caused by tiny effects on human gut microbiota composition (Vrieze et al., 2014; Reijnders et al., 2016). However, a definite shift in the phylum level in our research may attribute to the absence of disturbances from neurohumoral regulation, the individual differences, dietary habits, and physiological status using *in vitro* SHIME (Karl et al., 2018). The decrease of *Proteobacteria* shown in our study may also attribute to AMX is more effective for sensitive Gram-negative bacteria that belonging to *Proteobacteria* by interfering with the synthesis of bacterial cell wall peptidoglycan layer (Zapata and Quagliarello, 2015). And *Bacteroides uniformis* belonging to *Bacteroidetes* may be resistant to AMX to make them survive, because of the strong correlations were found in their abundance with *bl2_len* and *bl2be_shv2* ($R = 0.8$, $P < 0.01$). Some studies even showed the opposite phenomena like increasing of *Proteobacteria* and decreasing of *Bacteroidetes*, which might be caused by the combined effects with other antibiotics

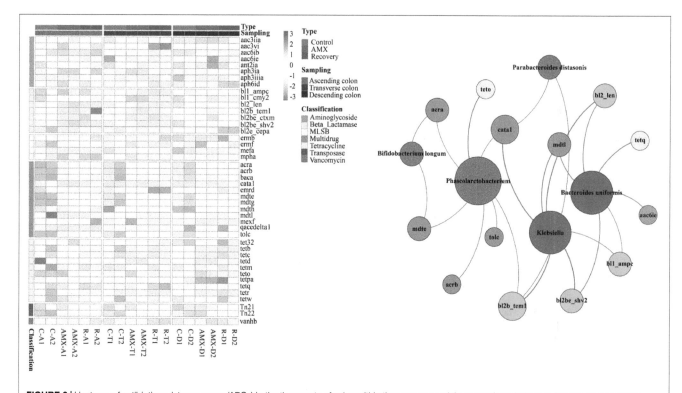

FIGURE 6 | Heatmap of antibiotic resistance genes (ARGs) in the three parts of colon within three groups and the network analysis revealing the co-occurrence patterns between abundance of microbial taxa and that of ARG subtypes. Heatmap colors reflect relative abundance from low (blue) to high (red). The nodes in network were colored according to ARG types and microbial genera that increased (red) or decreased (green) after AMX exposure, and the edges were colored according to positive (red) or negative (blue) correlation. A connection represents strong and significant (P value < 0.05, R > 0.6) correlation. The size of each node is proportional to the number of connections, that is, degree.

such as clarithromycin, fosfomycin, and metronidazole (Oh et al., 2016; Ishikawa et al., 2017). However, at the genus level, the blooming of intestinal microbiota such as *Bacteroides uniformis* and *Klebsiella* and decrease of *Bifidobacterium* occurred following AMX administration. These data were further supported by earlier reports (Ladirat et al., 2014a; Oh et al., 2016; Marzorati et al., 2017), while an increase of *Parabacteroides* was found in another study (Kabbani et al., 2017).

Amoxicillin treatment affected a vast number of sensitive intestinal bacterial species that directly engrossed their corresponding functions. As a result, the functionally redundant resistant intestinal bacterial species were initially present at low levels and became more abundant. Thus, to compensate this loss of function to maintain community function, and species with closer evolutionary relationship usually have more similar functions (Moya and Ferrer, 2016). For example, Van den Abbeele et al. (2012) have found that during antibiotic treatment, the abundance of antibiotic-resistant *Pediococcus acidilactici* was enlarged, while the amount of sensitive *Lactobacillus mucosae* was declined. Similarly, in this study, a reduction of sensitive *Parabacteroides* might be replaced by resistant *Bacteroides* species. Although the metabolic function of the intestinal microbiota could recover quickly, the unrestored composition of the intestinal microbiota was supported by increasing ARB,

which may pose a significant therapeutic challenge and that needs more attention.

As demonstrated by several studies that administration of antibiotics is significantly associated with decrease in microbial community diversity and richness, our results that AMX exposure increased the microbial diversity seems counterintuitive (Dethlefsen et al., 2008). The study by Vrieze et al. (2014) discovered a trend toward increased taxonomic diversity after AMX exposure, which was in accordance with our study. However, in some other studies no significant effect on microbiome diversity was found, which were opposed to our study (Pallav et al., 2014; Zaura et al., 2015; Reijnders et al., 2016). For this phenomenon, the possible reason was that AMX resistant intestinal bacterial species could bloom and compensate for or even surpassed the loss of AMX sensitive species. Intestinal microbiota with higher biodiversity was usually more resistant to the perturbation and colonization by pathogens, which might help in maintaining the intestinal homeostasis (Li et al., 2016). However, the improved biodiversity by AMX exposure that discovered in our study is mainly caused by increased abundance of AMX resistant intestinal bacterial species, which included opportunistic pathogen of the human intestine. This phenomenon may not be considered healthy for people because the increasing of opportunistic pathogens may be related to some human diseases that may cause the transmission and diffusion of ARGs.

Pathogen Contribute to the Increased Human Disease Pathway Genes and Beta-Lactam Resistance Genes

Some research articles have not mentioned the significant alteration of metabolic functions of the gut microbiota after AMX treatment (Vrieze et al., 2014; Reijnders et al., 2016), while the disruption of the metabolic activity of microbiota (increased in succinate and monosaccharide and oligosaccharide levels) in the fecal samples were found elsewhere (Ladirat et al., 2014a). Moreover, this study found that *Klebsiella* was positively associated with the gene numbers of functional pathways including cancer, metabolic and immune diseases, and other human diseases, which have not been reported yet in other research articles. *K. pneumoniae* is a typical Gram-negative bacterial pathogen, which frequently colonizes in the human gut and processes to infection diseases (Pena et al., 1997; Wiener-Well et al., 2010; Gorrie et al., 2017). The increase of the relative abundance of intestinal *Klebsiella* genus has been reported to associate with diverse human diseases such as pneumonia, inflammation, Crohn's disease, colitis, cystitis, liver abscess, and wound infections (Schneditz et al., 2014; Atarashi et al., 2017). All above findings suggested that *Klebsiella* might contribute to increase the pathway genes, including cancer, immune system diseases, infectious diseases, metabolic diseases, and neurodegenerative diseases.

It is also known from the literature that frequent use of antibiotics such as AMX may cause the transmission and proliferation of ARB and ARGs (Canton and Morosini, 2011; Zaura et al., 2015; Lenart-Boron et al., 2016). This study further demonstrated that the beta-lactamase resistance genes and the potential co-selected ARGs were increased after AMX exposure. The co-occurrence patterns between abundance of microbial taxa and that of ARG subtypes (**Figure 6**) showed that *Bacteroides uniformis* and *Klebsiella* might contributed to the increasing of ARGs including beta-lactam, tetracycline, and multidrug resistance. Therefore, treatment with AMX increases the number of resistance genes, even those not directly related to the antibiotic ingested. *Bacteroides uniformis* and *Klebsiella* are ubiquitous in the environment and are commensal in the human gut, notably the increased of their population, especially for *Klebsiella* is not usually considered as healthy. Moreover, resistance to beta-lactams via beta-lactamase production has mostly been described in *Klebsiella* spp. (Madhi et al., 2013; Marco et al., 2017). *Bifidobacterium* and *Parabacteroides* are most common or novel probiotics (Pinto-Sanchez et al., 2017; Wu et al., 2019), and the decreasing of these probiotics may cause dysbiosis of gut microbiota, which also leads to human health problem (Wischmeyer et al., 2016; George Kerry et al., 2018).

AMX Caused "SHIME-Compartment" Different and Permanent Alterations

In this study, *Klebsiella* and *Bacteroides uniformis* were found to be more significantly enriched in the ascending colon than other two colonic-regions, which was in keeping with the previous reports of the alteration in intestinal microbiota by exposure of antibiotics mixture and other toxic compounds like chlorpyrifos

and arsenic (Reygner et al., 2016; Yu et al., 2016; Marzorati et al., 2017). These studies revealed the "SHIME-compartment" specific effects that could be due to the inconsistent biodegradation of multiple compounds, gut microbiome community, and pH in different colon regions (Reygner et al., 2016; Yu et al., 2016; Marzorati et al., 2017). Moreover, a large number of functional pathways related genes was also shown to be increased in the ascending colon after AMX exposure, which further clarified that the primary effect observed at the level of the microbiota could also be identified at the genomic and metabolic levels (Garcia-Villalba et al., 2017; Wang et al., 2018). The intestinal microbiota is a key "organ" for the individual's health, and its response to AMX is started from the proximal colon and hence observed more obvious shifts there. This phenomenon suggested that more studies should focus on the proximal colon; however, it may be challenging to study by *in vivo* experiments that usually analysis the feces standing for the distal intestinal microbiota.

Furthermore, these AMX effects were still evident for at least 2 weeks after the AMX discontinuance, although the resilient tendency of microbial composition, functional pathway genes and ARGs were also observed. Pallav et al. (2014) revealed that AMX mediated opportunistic pathogen such as *Escherichia/Shigella* persisted up to 42 days after the interruption of antibiotic therapy. Similar phenomenon was also reported by Zwittink et al. (2018), whose work primarily discovered a 5 days treatment with combined of AMX and ceftazidime allowed *Enterococcus* to thrive and remain dominant up to 2 weeks, while the abundance of *Bifidobacterium* remained decreased till postnatal of 6 weeks after antibiotic treatment discontinuation. Therefore, our results demonstrated a serious negative side-effect of AMX, which could be persistent and different in the specific colon region and should be considered as an essential aspect of the risk assessment for AMX prescription.

PERSPECTIVES

Typical antibiotics have been detected in the collective gut of the Chinese population in our previous research, which provided a reference for this study of the effects of AMX on human gut microbiota (Wang et al., 2020). This study provides the originality of being able to control the effect of antibiotics in the different parts of the colon, evaluating in situ the alterations of the microbiota. Although SHIME has been successfully manipulated according to previous classic studies (Van den Abbeele et al., 2013; Yu et al., 2016; Wang et al., 2018), there were still three limitations of this study. First, AMX could not be absorbed by SHIME on the small intestine nor interact with the upper microbiota, which make the burden reaching the colon in the SHIME is much higher comparing to practical exposure to human colon. Considering that about 77 to 93% AMX is absorbed by the gastrointestinal tract and their interaction with the upper microbiota, the putative exposure dosage of AMX in colon is about 10% of the original oral dosage (Spyker et al., 1977; Arancibia et al., 1980; Huttner et al., 2019). This model is better to include the interaction with the human cell to get a closer result to *in vivo*, which is also a very good suggestion. Therefore, we would like to use 60 mg day^{-1} AMX (10% of this study) and include interaction with the human cell in our future work, with which the results would be close to *in vivo*. Second, this study lack of biological replicates and appropriate controls, which makes it difficult to interpret the results in relation to the microbial community variations and changes observed. Therefore, we would collect biological replicates and run a parallel experiment with blank medium at T0 and other timelines in our future study to negate any background noise and make the research scientifically reasonable. Another limitation is that the composition of the microbiota from the donor has not been analyzed before introducing it into the simulator. The composition of the initial microbiota from the donor may affect the stabilized microbiota in SHIME. Therefore, we would analyze the composition of the microbiota from the donor before introducing it into the simulator and compare the stabilized microbiota in SHIME that using multiple donors either by mixing their fecal samples or adding individually to explore the effects of initial microbiota composition in our future work, which would make this study more interesting. Although our work has these limitations, our findings would be valuable for directing future work. The findings in this study suggested several numbers of opportunities for additional study. One avenue is to expand the analysis to incorporate multi-omics approaches of the metagenome, metatranscriptome, and metabolome. Functional and metabolite analysis by multi-omics approaches would refine the results of predicting microbial function. Including interaction with the human cell in the fermentation vessels or manipulate *in vivo* study is also a good avenue to confirm the actual AMX's effects on cancers, metabolic and immune diseases, and other human diseases that found in our *in vitro* experiments. On the other hand, the studies of virome and fungome may exert the substantial influences on the intestinal microbiome. Thus, an expanded analysis of other microorganisms will also be necessary. It is of interest to investigate the impacts of different kinds of antibiotics and a mixture of them on the gut microbiota. Moreover, research on the restoration effects of some prebiotics, probiotics, and synbiotics during and after antibiotic therapy is promising, which may help to discover several clinical strategies and restore side effects caused by antibiotics. As the increasing of opportunistic pathogens, functional genes and ARGs by antibiotics exposure may pose a significant therapeutic challenge, it should be more critical to take some efficient measures to reduce or even eliminate the effects caused by antibiotic treatment.

CONCLUSION

Exposure to AMX had significantly altered the overall taxonomic composition of the gut microbiota with increasing taxonomic richness, functional pathway genes, and beta-lactam resistance genes. The changes were "SHIME-compartment" different and more substantial effect was observed in the ascending colon. The shifted human gut microbiota could not be restored after

2 weeks' of AMX discontinued. Importantly, most of the functional pathway genes and quantified beta-lactam resistance genes are positively associated with bacteria that increased after AMX exposure. Our results may open up new perspectives for the assessing of direct effects by antibiotics on the intestinal microbiota – a key "organ" in individual health. The results demonstrated the negative side-effects of AMX and should be considered for AMX prescription.

ETHICS STATEMENT

The study was approved by the Biomedical Ethics Committees of Nankai University. The participant has given written informed consent to confirm they understand the study purpose, procedures, risks, benefits, and rights.

AUTHOR CONTRIBUTIONS

LL carried out the laboratory work, analyzed the data, and wrote the manuscript. QW provided suggestions in the manuscript preparation and revised this manuscript. RD edited the language and improved the clarity of this manuscript. HL, SW, HQ, and JY carried out the laboratory work. YX provided funding support. DM and YL guided the laboratory work and revised this manuscript. All authors read and approved the final manuscript.

FUNDING

This study was sponsored by the Key projects of the National Natural Science Foundation of China (41831287), China National Funds for Distinguished Young Scientists (41525013), National Natural Science Foundation of China (31870351, 41703088, 31670509, and 21607016), Key projects of Research and Development of Hebei Province (19273707D), and Key projects of Tianjin Natural Science Foundation (19JCZDJC40800).

ACKNOWLEDGMENTS

The authors express the sincerest thanks to Professor Bing Wu at Nanjing University for the guidance of constructing SHIME model, and Guangzhou Gene Denovo Co., Ltd. and Anhui MicroAnaly Gene Technologies Co., Ltd. for genome sequencing and analysis.

REFERENCES

Arancibia, A., Guttmann, J., Gonzalez, G., and Gonzalez, C. (1980). Absorption and disposition kinetics of amoxicillin in normal human subjects. *Antimicrob. Agents Chemother.* 17, 199–202. doi: 10.1128/aac.17.2.199

Atarashi, K., Suda, W., Luo, C., Kawaguchi, T., Motoo, I., Narushima, S., et al. (2017). Ectopic colonization of oral bacteria in the intestine drives TH1 cell induction and inflammation. *Science* 358, 359–365. doi: 10.1126/science. aan4526

Barc, M. C., Charrin-Sarnel, C., Rochet, V., Bourlioux, F., Sandre, C., Boureau, H., et al. (2008). Molecular analysis of the digestive microbiota in a gnotobiotic mouse model during antibiotic treatment: influence of *Saccharomyces boulardii*. *Anaerobe* 14, 229–233. doi: 10.1016/j.anaerobe.2008.04.003

Barraud, O., Peyre, M., Couve-Deacon, E., Chainier, D., Bahans, C., Guigonis, V., et al. (2018). Antibiotic resistance acquisition in the first week of life. *Front. Microbiol.* 9:1467. doi: 10.3389/fmicb.2018.01467

Blaser, M. J. (2016). Antibiotic use and its consequences for the normal microbiome. *Science* 352, 544–545. doi: 10.1126/science.aad9358

Bunyavanich, S., Shen, N., Grishin, A., Wood, R., Burks, W., Dawson, P., et al. (2016). Early-life gut microbiome composition and milk allergy resolution. *J. Allergy Clin. Immunol.* 138, 1122–1130. doi: 10.1016/j.jaci.2016.03.041

Bussche, J. V., Marzorati, M., Laukens, D., and Vanhaecke, L. (2015). Validated high resolution mass spectrometry-based approach for metabolomic fingerprinting of the human gut phenotype. *Anal. Chem.* 87, 10927–10934. doi: 10.1021/acs. analchem.5b02688

Cabreiro, F., Au, C., Leung, K. Y., Vergara-Irigaray, N., Cocheme, H. M., Noori, T., et al. (2013). Metformin retards aging in *C. elegans* by altering microbial folate and methionine metabolism. *Cell* 153, 228–239. doi: 10.1016/j.cell.2013.02.035

Canton, R., and Morosini, M. I. (2011). Emergence and spread of antibiotic resistance following exposure to antibiotics. *FEMS Microbiol. Rev.* 35, 977–991. doi: 10.1111/j.1574-6976.2011.00295.x

Caporaso, J. G., Kuczynski, J., Stombaugh, J., Bittinger, K., Bushman, F. D., Costello, E. K., et al. (2010). QIIME allows analysis of high-throughput community sequencing data. *Nat. Methods* 7, 335–336. doi: 10.1038/nmeth. f.303

Chow, J., Lee, S. M., Shen, Y., Khosravi, A., and Mazmanian, S. K. (2010). Host-bacterial symbiosis in health and disease. *Adv. Immunol.* 107, 243–274. doi: 10.1016/S0065-2776(10)07001-X

Collignon, A., Bouttier, S., Lambert, S., Hoys, S., and Barc, M.-C. (2008). Gnotobiotic mouse model to study the effect of antibiotics on human faecal microbiota. *Microb. Ecol. Health Dis.* 20, 204–206. doi: 10.1080/08910600802408137

Collignon, A., Sandre, C., and Barc, M. C. (2010). *Saccharomyces boulardii* modulates dendritic cell properties and intestinal microbiota disruption after antibiotic treatment. *Gastroenterol. Clin. Biol.* 34, S71–S78. doi: 10.1016/S0399-8320(10)70024-5

Dethlefsen, L., Huse, S., Sogin, M. L., and Relman, D. A. (2008). The pervasive effects of an antibiotic on the human gut microbiota, as revealed by deep 16S rRNA sequencing. *PLoS Biol.* 6:e280. doi: 10.1371/journal.pbio.0060280

Duque, A. L. R. F., Monteiro, M., Adorno, M. A. T., Sakamoto, I. K., and Sivieri, K. (2016). An exploratory study on the influence of orange juice on gut microbiota using a dynamic colonic model. *Food Res. Int.* 84, 160–169. doi: 10.1016/j. foodres.2016.03.028

El Hage, R., Hernandez-Sanabria, E., Calatayud Arroyo, M., Props, R., and Van de Wiele, T. (2019). Propionate-producing consortium restores antibiotic-induced dysbiosis in a dynamic *in vitro* model of the human intestinal microbial ecosystem. *Front. Microbiol.* 10:1206. doi: 10.3389/fmicb.2019.01206

Flandroy, L., Poutahidis, T., Berg, G., Clarke, G., Dao, M. C., Decaestecker, E., et al. (2018). The impact of human activities and lifestyles on the interlinked microbiota and health of humans and of ecosystems. *Sci. Total Environ.* 627, 1018–1038. doi: 10.1016/j.scitotenv.2018.01.288

Gao, Z., Guo, B., Gao, R., Zhu, Q., and Qin, H. (2015). Microbiota disbiosis is associated with colorectal cancer. *Front. Microbiol.* 6:20. doi: 10.3389/fmicb. 2015.00020

Garcia-Villalba, R., Vissenaekens, H., Pitart, J., Romo-Vaquero, M., Espin, J. C., Grootaert, C., et al. (2017). Gastrointestinal simulation model TWIN-SHIME shows differences between human urolithin-metabotypes in gut microbiota composition, pomegranate polyphenol metabolism, and transport along the

intestinal tract. *J. Agric. Food Chem.* 65, 5480–5493. doi: 10.1021/acs.jafc. 7b02049

George Kerry, R., Patra, J. K., Gouda, S., Park, Y., Shin, H. S., and Das, G. (2018). Benefaction of probiotics for human health: a review. *J. Food Drug Anal.* 26, 927–939. doi: 10.1016/j.jfda.2018.01.002

Gorrie, C., Mirceta, M., Wick, R., Edwards, D., Thomson, N., Strugnell, R., et al. (2017). Gastrointestinal carriage is a major reservoir of *Klebsiella pneumoniae* infection in intensive care patients. *Clin. Infect. Dis.* 65, 208–215. doi: 10.1093/cid/cix270

Hu, Y., Yang, X., Qin, J., Lu, N., Cheng, G., Wu, N., et al. (2013). Metagenome-wide analysis of antibiotic resistance genes in a large cohort of human gut microbiota. *Nat. Commun.* 4, 2151–2249. doi: 10.1038/ncomms3151

Huttner, A., Bielicki, J., Clements, M. N., Frimodt-Møller, N., Muller, A. E., Paccaud, J. P., et al. (2019). Oral amoxicillin and amoxicillin–clavulanic acid: properties, indications and usage. *Clin. Microbiol. Infect.* doi: 10.1016/j.cmi. 2019.11.028 [Epub ahead of print].

Ianiro, G., Tilg, H., and Gasbarrini, A. (2016). Antibiotics as deep modulators of gut microbiota: between good and evil. *Gut* 65, 1906–1915. doi: 10.1136/gutjnl-2016-312297

Ichim, T. E., Kesari, S., and Shafer, K. (2018). Protection from chemotherapy- and antibiotic-mediated dysbiosis of the gut microbiota by a probiotic with digestive enzymes supplement. *Oncotarget* 9, 30919–30935. doi: 10.18632/oncotarget. 25778

Ishikawa, D., Sasaki, T., Osada, T., Kuwahara-Arai, K., Haga, K., Shibuya, T., et al. (2017). Changes in intestinal microbiota following combination therapy with fecal microbial transplantation and antibiotics for ulcerative colitis. *Inflamm. Bowel Dis.* 23, 116–125. doi: 10.1097/Mib.0000000000000975

Kabbani, T. A., Pallav, K., Dowd, S. E., Villafuerte-Galvez, J., Vanga, R. R., Castillo, N. E., et al. (2017). Prospective randomized controlled study on the effects of *Saccharomyces boulardii* CNCM I-745 and amoxicillin-clavulanate or the combination on the gut microbiota of healthy volunteers. *Gut Microbes* 8, 17–32. doi: 10.1080/19490976.2016.1267890

Karl, J. P., Hatch, A. M., Arcidiacono, S. M., Pearce, S. C., Pantoja-Feliciano, I. G., Doherty, L. A., et al. (2018). Effects of psychological, environmental and physical stressors on the gut microbiota. *Front. Microbiol.* 9:2013. doi: 10.3389/fmicb.2018.02013

Kemperman, R. A., Gross, G., Mondot, S., Possemiers, S., Marzorati, M., Van de Wiele, T., et al. (2013). Impact of polyphenols from black tea and red wine/grape juice on a gut model microbiome. *Food Res. Int.* 53, 659–669. doi: 10.1016/j. foodres.2013.01.034

Kho, Z. Y., and Lal, S. K. (2018). The human gut microbiome - a potential controller of wellness and disease. *Front. Microbiol.* 9:1835. doi: 10.3389/fmicb. 2018.01835

Labus, J. S., Hollister, E. B., Jacobs, J., Kirbach, K., Oezguen, N., Gupta, A., et al. (2017). Differences in gut microbial composition correlate with regional brain volumes in irritable bowel syndrome. *Microbiome* 5:49. doi: 10.1186/s40168-017-0260-z

Ladirat, S. E., Schoterman, M. H. C., Rahaoui, H., Mars, M., Schuren, F. H. J., Gruppen, H., et al. (2014a). Exploring the effects of galacto-oligosaccharides on the gut microbiota of healthy adults receiving amoxicillin treatment. *Br. J. Nutr.* 112, 536–546. doi: 10.1017/S0007114514001135

Ladirat, S. E., Schuren, F. H. J., Schoterman, M. H. C., Nauta, A., Gruppen, H., and Schols, H. A. (2014b). Impact of galacto-oligosaccharides on the gut microbiota composition and metabolic activity upon antibiotic treatment during *in vitro* fermentation. *FEMS Microbiol. Ecol.* 87, 41–51. doi: 10.1111/1574-6941. 12187

Langille, M. G., Zaneveld, J., Caporaso, J. G., McDonald, D., Knights, D., Reyes, J. A., et al. (2013). Predictive functional profiling of microbial communities using 16S rRNA marker gene sequences. *Nat. Biotechnol.* 31, 814–821. doi: 10.1038/nbt.2676

Lenart-Boron, A., Wolny-Koladka, K., Stec, J., and Kasprowic, A. (2016). Phenotypic and molecular antibiotic resistance determination of airborne coagulase negative *Staphylococcus* spp. strains from healthcare facilities in Southern Poland. *Microb. Drug Resist.* 22, 515–522. doi: 10.1089/mdr.2015. 0271

Li, D. T., Wang, P., Wang, P. P., Hu, X. S., and Chen, F. (2016). The gut microbiota: a treasure for human health. *Biotechnol. Adv.* 34, 1210–1224. doi: 10.1016/j. biotechadv.2016.08.003

Li, S., Zhang, C., Gu, Y., Chen, L., Ou, S., Wang, Y., et al. (2015). Lean rats gained more body weight than obese ones from a high-fibre diet. *Br. J. Nutr.* 114, 1188–1194. doi: 10.1017/S0007114515002858

Liu, L., Wang, Q., Wu, X., Qi, H., Das, R., Lin, H., et al. (2020). Vancomycin exposure caused opportunistic pathogens bloom in intestinal microbiome by simulator of the human intestinal microbial ecosystem (SHIME). *Environ. Pollut.* doi: 10.1016/j.envpol.2020.114399 [Epub ahead of print].

Madhi, F., Biscardi, S., Bingen, E., Jaby, O., Epaud, R., and Cohen, R. (2013). Combined relay therapy with oral cefixime and clavulanate for febrile urinary tract infection caused by extended-spectrum beta-lactamase-producing *Escherichia coli*. *Pediatr. Infect. Dis. J.* 32, 96–97. doi: 10.1097/INF. 0b013e318271f369

Marco, R. H., Olmos, E. G., Breton-Martinez, J. R., Perez, L. G., Sanchez, B. C., Fujkova, J., et al. (2017). Community-acquired febrile urinary tract infection caused by extended-spectrum beta-lactamase-producing bacteria in hospitalised infants. *Enferm. Infecc. Microbiol. Clin.* 35, 287–292. doi: 10.1016/j.eimc.2016.01.012

Marzorati, M., Vilchez-Vargas, R., Bussche, J. V., Truchado, P., Jauregui, R., El Hage, R. A., et al. (2017). High-fiber and high-protein diets shape different gut microbial communities, which ecologically behave similarly under stress conditions, as shown in a gastrointestinal simulator. *Mol. Nutr. Food Res.* 61, 1600150. doi: 10.1002/mnfr.201600150

McHardy, I. H., Goudarzi, M., Tong, M., Ruegger, P. M., Schwager, E., Weger, J. R., et al. (2013). Integrative analysis of the microbiome and metabolome of the human intestinal mucosal surface reveals exquisite inter-relationships. *Microbiome* 1:17. doi: 10.1186/2049-2618-1-17

Moya, A., and Ferrer, M. (2016). Functional redundancy-induced stability of gut microbiota subjected to disturbance. *Trends Microbiol.* 24, 402–413. doi: 10.1016/j.tim.2016.02.002

Oh, B., Kim, B. S., Kim, J. W., Kim, J. S., Koh, S. J., Kim, B. G., et al. (2016). The effect of probiotics on gut microbiota during the *Helicobacter pylori* eradication: randomized controlled trial. *Helicobacter* 21, 165–174. doi: 10.1111/hel.12270

Pallav, K., Dowd, S. E., Villafuerte, J., Yang, X., Kabbani, T., Hansen, J., et al. (2014). Effects of polysaccharopeptide from *Trametes versicolor* and amoxicillin on the gut microbiome of healthy volunteers: a randomized clinical trial. *Gut Microbes* 5, 458–467. doi: 10.4161/gmic.29558

Pena, C., Pujol, M., Ricart, A., Ardanuy, C., Ayats, J., Linares, J., et al. (1997). Risk factors for faecal carriage of *Klebsiella pneumoniae* producing extended spectrum beta-lactamase (ESBL-KP) in the intensive care unit. *J. Hosp. Infect.* 35, 9–16. doi: 10.1016/s0195-6701(97)90163-8

Pinto-Sanchez, M. I., Hall, G. B., Ghajar, K., Nardelli, A., Bolino, C., Lau, J. T., et al. (2017). Probiotic *Bifidobacterium longum* NCC3001 reduces depression scores and alters brain activity: a pilot study in patients with irritable bowel syndrome. *Gastroenterology* 153, 448–459. doi: 10.1053/j.gastro.2017.05.003

Puri, P., Liangpunsakul, S., Christensen, J. E., Shah, V. H., Kamath, P. S., Gores, G. J., et al. (2018). The circulating microbiome signature and inferred functional metagenomics in alcoholic hepatitis. *Hepatology* 67, 1284–1302. doi: 10.1002/hep.29623

Qin, J. J., Li, R. Q., Raes, J., Arumugam, M., Burgdorf, K. S., Manichanh, C., et al. (2010). A human gut microbial gene catalogue established by metagenomic sequencing. *Nature* 464, 59–65. doi: 10.1038/nature08821

Reijnders, D., Goossens, G. H., Hermes, G. D., Neis, E. P., van der Beek, C. M., Most, J., et al. (2016). Effects of gut microbiota manipulation by antibiotics on host metabolism in obese humans: a randomized double-blind placebo-controlled trial. *Cell Metab.* 24, 63–74. doi: 10.1016/j.cmet.2016.06.016

Reygner, J., Joly Condette, C., Bruneau, A., Delanaud, S., Rhazi, L., Depeint, F., et al. (2016). Changes in composition and function of human intestinal microbiota exposed to chlorpyrifos in oil as assessed by the SHIME® model. *Int. J. Environ. Res. Public Health* 13:1088. doi: 10.3390/ijerph13111088

Rock, C., Thom, K. A., Masnick, M., Johnson, J. K., Harris, A. D., and Morgan, D. J. (2014). Frequency of *Klebsiella pneumoniae* carbapenemase (KPC)-producing and non-KPC-producing Klebsiella species contamination of healthcare workers and the environment. *Infect. Control Hosp. Epidemiol.* 35, 426–429. doi: 10.1086/675598

Schneditz, G., Rentner, J., Roier, S., Pletz, J., Herzog, K. A., Bucker, R., et al. (2014). Enterotoxicity of a nonribosomal peptide causes antibiotic-associated colitis. *Proc. Natl. Acad. Sci. U.S.A.* 111, 13181–13186. doi: 10.1073/pnas.140327 4111

Segata, N., Izard, J., Waldron, L., Gevers, D., Miropolsky, L., Garrett, W. S., et al. (2011). Metagenomic biomarker discovery and explanation. *Genome Biol.* 12:R60. doi: 10.1186/gb-2011-12-6-r60

Selak, M., Riviere, A., Moens, F., Van den Abbeele, P., Geirnaert, A., Rogelj, I., et al. (2016). Inulin-type fructan fermentation by bifidobacteria depends on the strain rather than the species and region in the human intestine. *Appl. Microbiol. Biotechnol.* 100, 4097–4107. doi: 10.1007/s00253-016-7351-9

Spyker, D. A., Rugloski, R. J., Vann, R. L., and O'Brien, W. M. (1977). Pharmacokinetics of amoxicillin: dose dependence after intravenous, oral, and intramuscular administration. *Antimicrob. Agents Chemother.* 11, 132–141. doi: 10.1128/aac.11.1.132

Stecher, B., Maier, L., and Hardt, W. D. (2013). 'Blooming' in the gut: how dysbiosis might contribute to pathogen evolution. *Nat. Rev. Microbiol.* 11, 277–284. doi: 10.1038/nrmicro2989

Truchado, P., Van den Abbeele, P., Riviere, A., Possemiers, S., De Vuyst, L., and Van de Wiele, T. (2015). *Bifidobacterium longum* D2 enhances microbial degradation of long-chain arabinoxylans in an *in vitro* model of the proximal colon. *Beneficial Microbes* 6, 849–860. doi: 10.3920/Bm2015.0023

Van de Wiele, T., Gallawa, C. M., Kubachka, K. M., Creed, J. T., Basta, N., Dayton, E. A., et al. (2010). Arsenic metabolism by human gut microbiota upon *in vitro* digestion of contaminated soils. *Environ. Health Perspect.* 118, 1004–1009. doi: 10.1289/ehp.0901794

Van de Wiele, T., Van den Abbeele, P., Ossieur, W., Possemiers, S., and Marzorati, M. (2015). "The simulator of the human intestinal microbial ecosystem (SHIME®)," in *The Impact of Food Bioactives on Health: In Vitro and Ex Vivo Models*, eds K. Verhoeckx, P. Cotter, I. López-Expósito, C. Kleiveland, T. Lea, A. Mackie, et al. (Cham: Springer International Publishing), 305–317. doi: 10.1007/978-3-319-16104-4_27

Van den Abbeele, P., Belzer, C., Goossens, M., Kleerebezem, M., De Vos, W. M., Thas, O., et al. (2013). Butyrate-producing *Clostridium cluster* XIVa species specifically colonize mucins in an *in vitro* gut model. *ISME J.* 7, 949–961. doi: 10.1038/ismej.2012.158

Van den Abbeele, P., Roos, S., Eeckhaut, V., MacKenzie, D. A., Derde, M., Verstraete, W., et al. (2012). Incorporating a mucosal environment in a dynamic gut model results in a more representative colonization by *Lactobacilli*. *Microb. Biotechnol.* 5, 106–115. doi: 10.1111/j.1751-7915.2011.00308.x

Vrieze, A., Out, C., Fuentes, S., Jonker, L., Reuling, I., Kootte, R. S., et al. (2014). Impact of oral vancomycin on gut microbiota, bile acid metabolism, and insulin sensitivity. *J. Hepatol.* 60, 824–831. doi: 10.1016/j.jhep.2013.11.034

Wang, Q., Duan, Y. J., Wang, S. P., Wang, L. T., Hou, Z. L., Cui, Y. X., et al. (2020). Occurrence and distribution of clinical and veterinary antibiotics in the faeces of a Chinese population. *J. Hazard. Mater.* 383, 121129. doi: 10.1016/j.jhazmat. 2019.121129

Wang, Q., Garrity, G. M., Tiedje, J. M., and Cole, J. R. (2007). Naive Bayesian classifier for rapid assignment of rRNA sequences into the new bacterial taxonomy. *Appl. Environ. Microbiol.* 73, 5261–5267. doi: 10.1128/Aem.00062-07

Wang, Y., Rui, M., Nie, Y., and Lu, G. (2018). Influence of gastrointestinal tract on metabolism of bisphenol A as determined by *in vitro* simulated system. *J. Hazard. Mater.* 355, 111–118. doi: 10.1016/j.jhazmat.2018.05.011

Wiener-Well, Y., Rudensky, B., Yinnon, A. M., Kopuit, P., Schlesinger, Y., Broide, E., et al. (2010). Carriage rate of carbapenem-resistant *Klebsiella pneumoniae* in hospitalised patients during a national outbreak. *J. Hosp. Infect.* 74, 344–349. doi: 10.1016/j.jhin.2009.07.022

Wischmeyer, P. E., McDonald, D., and Knight, R. (2016). Role of the microbiome, probiotics, and 'dysbiosis therapy' in critical illness. *Curr. Opin. Crit. Care* 22, 347–353. doi: 10.1097/MCC.0000000000000321

Wu, T. R., Lin, C. S., Chang, C. J., Lin, T. L., Martel, J., Ko, Y. F., et al. (2019). Gut commensal *Parabacteroides goldsteinii* plays a predominant role in the anti-obesity effects of polysaccharides isolated from *Hirsutella sinensis*. *Gut* 68, 248–262. doi: 10.1136/gutjnl-2017-315458

Yatsunenko, T., Rey, F. E., Manary, M. J., Trehan, I., Dominguez-Bello, M. G., Contreras, M., et al. (2012). Human gut microbiome viewed across age and geography. *Nature* 486, 222–227. doi: 10.1038/nature11053

Yu, H., Wu, B., Zhang, X., Liu, S., Yu, J., Cheng, S., et al. (2016). Arsenic metabolism and toxicity influenced by ferric iron in simulated gastrointestinal tract and the roles of gut microbiota. *Environ. Sci. Technol.* 50, 7189–7197. doi: 10.1021/acs. est.6b01533

Zapata, H. J., and Quagliarello, V. J. (2015). The microbiota and microbiome in aging: potential implications in health and age-related diseases. *J. Am. Geriatr. Soc.* 63, 776–781. doi: 10.1111/jgs.13310

Zaura, E., Brandt, B. W., Teixeira de Mattos, M. J., Buijs, M. J., Caspers, M. P., Rashid, M. U., et al. (2015). Same exposure but two radically different responses to antibiotics: resilience of the salivary microbiome versus long-term microbial shifts in feces. *mBio* 6:e01693-15. doi: 10.1128/mBio.01693-15

Zhang, Q., Ying, G., Pan, C., Liu, Y., and Zhao, J. (2015). Comprehensive evaluation of antibiotics emission and fate in the river basins of China: source analysis, multimedia modeling, and linkage to bacterial resistance. *Environ. Sci. Technol.* 49, 6772–6782. doi: 10.1021/acs.est.5b00729

Zwittink, R. D., Renes, I. B., van Lingen, R. A., van Zoeren-Grobben, D., Konstanti, P., Norbruis, O. F., et al. (2018). Association between duration of intravenous antibiotic administration and early-life microbiota development in late-preterm infants. *Eur. J. Clin. Microbiol. Infect. Dis.* 37, 475–483. doi: 10.1007/s10096-018-3193-y

15

Prevalence, Genetic Diversity, and Temporary Shifts of Inducible Clindamycin Resistance *Staphylococcus aureus* Clones in Tehran, Iran: A Molecular–Epidemiological Analysis from 2013 to 2018

Mehdi Goudarzi[1]*, Nobumichi Kobayashi[2], Masoud Dadashi[3], Roman Pantůček[4], Mohammad Javad Nasiri[1], Maryam Fazeli[5], Ramin Pouriran[6], Hossein Goudarzi[1], Mirmohammad Miri[7], Anahita Amirpour[8] and Sima Sadat Seyedjavadi[9]

[1] Department of Microbiology, School of Medicine, Shahid Beheshti University of Medical Sciences, Tehran, Iran, [2] Department of Hygiene, School of Medicine, Sapporo Medical University, Sapporo, Japan, [3] Department of Microbiology, School of Medicine, Alborz University of Medical Sciences, Karaj, Iran, [4] Department of Experimental Biology, Faculty of Science, Masaryk University, Brno, Czechia, [5] Department of Virology, Pasteur Institute of Iran, Tehran, Iran, [6] School of Medicine, Shahid Beheshti University of Medical Sciences, Tehran, Iran, [7] Department of Critical Care and Anesthesiology, Imam Hossein Hospital, Shahid Beheshti University of Medical Sciences, Tehran, Iran, [8] Department of Internal Medicine, Shahid Beheshti University of Medical Sciences, Tehran, Iran, [9] Department of Mycology, Pasteur Institute of Iran, Tehran, Iran

*Correspondence:
Mehdi Goudarzi
gudarzim@yahoo.com;
m.goudarzi@sbmu.ac.ir

The prevalence of *Staphylococcus aureus* as an aggressive pathogen resistant to multiple antibiotics causing nosocomial and community-acquired infections is increasing with limited therapeutic options. Macrolide-lincosamide streptogramin B (MLSB) family of antibiotics represents an important alternative therapy for staphylococcal infections. This study was conducted over a period of five years from August 2013 to July 2018 to investigate the prevalence and molecular epidemiology in Iran of inducible resistance in *S. aureus*. In the current study, 126 inducible methicillin-resistant *S. aureus* (MRSA) (*n* = 106) and methicillin-sensitive *S. aureus* (MSSA) (*n* = 20) isolates were characterized by *in vitro* susceptibility analysis, resistance and virulence encoding gene distribution, phenotypic and genotypic analysis of biofilm formation, prophage typing, *S. aureus* protein A locus (*spa*) typing, staphylocoagulase (SC) typing, staphylococcal cassette chromosome *mec* (SCC*mec*) typing, and multilocus sequence typing. Of the 126 isolates, 76 (60.3%) were classified as hospital onset, and 50 (39.7%) were classified as community onset (CO). Biofilm formation was observed in 97 strains (77%). A total of 14 sequence types (STs), 26 *spa* types, 7 coagulase types, 9 prophage types, 3 *agr* types (no *agr* IV), and 9 clonal complexes (CCs) were identified in this study. The prevalence of the inducible MLSB (iMLSB) *S. aureus* increased from 7.5% (25/335) to 21.7% (38/175) during the study period. The iMLSB MRSA isolates were distributed in nine CCs, whereas the MSSA isolates were less diverse, which mainly belonged to CC22 (7.95%) and CC30 (7.95%). High-level mupirocin-resistant strains belonged to ST85-SCC*mec* IV/t008 (*n* = 4), ST5-SCC*mec* IV/t002 (*n* = 4), ST239-SCC*mec* III/t631 (*n* = 2), and ST8-SCC*mec* IV/t064 (*n* = 2) clones, whereas low-level mupirocin-resistant strains belonged to ST15-SCCmec IV/t084 ($n = 5$), ST239-SCCmec III/t860 ($n = 3$), and ST22-SCCmec IV/t790 ($n = 3$) clones. All the fusidic acid–resistant iMLSB isolates were MRSA and belonged to ST15-SCCmec IV/t084 ($n = 2$), ST239-SCCmec III/t030 ($n = 2$), ST1-SCCmec V/t6811 ($n = 1$), ST80-SCCmec IV/t044 ($n = 1$), and ST59-SCCmec IV/t437 ($n = 1$). The CC22 that was predominant in 2013–2014 (36% of the isolates) had almost disappeared in 2017–2018, being replaced by the CC8, which represented 39.5% of the 2017–2018 isolates. This is the first description of temporal shifts of iMLSB *S. aureus* isolates in Iran that identifies predominant clones and treatment options for iMLSB *S. aureus*–related infections.

Keywords: methicillin-resistant *S. aureus*, methicillin-susceptible *S. aureus*, inducible resistance, staphylocoagulase, SCCmec, *agr* allotype, MLST

INTRODUCTION

Staphylococcus aureus is one of the most common aggressive pathogen that causes many diseases in humans and animals such as skin and soft tissue infections, osteomyelitis, bacteremia, and endocarditis (Gordon and Lowy, 2008). The expression of virulence factors promoting adhesion needs nutrients, and evasion of host immunologic responses including cell surface components (collagen-binding protein, clumping factor, fibronectin-binding protein, and elastin-binding protein), secreted factors (staphylokinase toxic shock syndrome toxin-1), hemolysin, exfoliative toxins (ETA and ETB), staphylococcal enterotoxins (SEs), and lipase and Panton–Valentine leukocidin (PVL), besides the presence of antibiotic resistance genes, turns *S. aureus* into a very pathogenic microorganism (Gordon and Lowy, 2008; Gould et al., 2012).

In addition to the aforementioned, the biofilm-forming of *S. aureus* strains can play a key role in pathogenesis and resistance to antimicrobials (Luther et al., 2018). The rate of infections due to *S. aureus*, especially the antibiotic-resistant strains, has dramatically increased recently, which is becoming a serious problem all over the world (Gould et al., 2012). Emerging simultaneous resistance to multiple antibacterial agents underscores the necessity for therapeutic alternatives for the treatment of bacterium-related infections (Pantosti et al., 2007; Dadashi et al., 2018). Although the use of effective antibiotics such as vancomycin, linezolid, and quinupristin-dalfopristin is considered appropriate for therapy, widespread utilization of these antibiotics has made the current usage of these therapeutic options often unsuccessful (Pantosti et al., 2007; Gould et al., 2012; Wang et al., 2012; Dadashi et al., 2018). In recent years, the use of macrolide–lincosamide–streptogramin group B (MLSB) antibiotics has been favored, which is regarded as an alternative approach to treating such infections (Patel et al., 2006). Clindamycin, a member of MLSB family, serves as one such effective therapeutic alternative for treating *S. aureus* infections, because of its proven efficacy, safety, convenience of administration (parenteral and oral), and excellent pharmacokinetic properties. However, one important issue in clindamycin administration is the potential emergence of inducible clindamycin resistance, which may increase the risk of clinical failure (Chavez-Bueno et al., 2005; Adhikari et al., 2017).

Recent published data indicate that there has been a concurrent worldwide increase in the prevalence of inducible clindamycin resistance in different areas (Abimanyu et al., 2012; Wang et al., 2012). Evidence of epidemiological researches has revealed that iMLSB *S. aureus* strains are mostly genetically distinct from each other. One of the most prevalent iMLSB *S. aureus* strains in the United States belongs to sequence type 8 (ST8) strains, whereas in European countries, the majority of iMLSB *S. aureus* strains circulating was affiliated with the clonal complexes CC5 and CC8 (Ilczyszyn et al., 2016). Many studies across the world have focused on molecular epidemiology and analysis of iMLSB *S. aureus* strains isolated from the clinic (Lewis and Jorgensen, 2005; Patel et al., 2006; Adhikari et al., 2017). In our country, data on the prevalence or genetic diversity of inducible clindamycin resistance among *S. aureus* are very unknown, and there have been no published data on the molecular epidemiological characterization of the inducible clindamycin-resistant *S. aureus* strains in Iran. Here we provide molecular characterization of iMLSB *S. aureus* strains. With this aim, phenotypic and genotypic resistance patterns, presence of different classes of prophages, biofilm-forming ability, presence of the *icaABCD*, adhesion genes, and virulence factors were assessed. Then, multilocus sequence typing (MLST), staphylococcal cassette chromosome *mec* (SCCmec), *agr*, *coa*, and *spa* typing methods were used to characterize the genotype of the iMLSB *S. aureus* strains. To the best of our knowledge, this is the first report on the molecular characterization of the inducible clindamycin-resistant *S. aureus* strains from Iran.

MATERIALS AND METHODS

Study Population, Bacterial Isolation, and Inducible Clindamycin Resistance Screening

A total of 1,161 non-duplicated clinical *S. aureus* isolates were obtained from different clinical specimens including wound, blood, pus, urine, sputum, conjunctivitis, and body fluids from both genders and all age groups of patients, over a period of 5 years from August 2013 to July 2018. This cross-sectional study was conducted in four hospitals affiliated to Shahid Beheshti

University of Medical Sciences (Loghman, Shohada, Taleghani, Emam Hossein). The processing of all samples was done in 2 h. Among these isolates, 126 *S. aureus* isolates were identified with iMLSB phenotype based on the routine biochemical techniques such as Gram staining; colony morphology comprising shape, size, color, and hemolysis patterns; catalase test; tube coagulase test; growth on mannitol salt agar; and DNase. Polymerase chain reaction (PCR) assay targeting the *S. aureus*-specific *nuc* gene was applied to verify the isolates (Goudarzi et al., 2016b). *Staphylococcus aureus* strains were studied to identify inducible resistance phenotypes according to the Clinical and Laboratory Standard Institute (CLSI) D-zone test. The D-zone test was performed by placing 15 µg erythromycin and 2 µg clindamycin disks at a spaced 15 to 26 mm apart from center to center on the Mueller–Hinton agar (Merck, Darmstadt, Germany) plate inoculated with a 0.5 McFarland-equivalent bacterial suspension. The results also were read at 16 to 18 h incubation at 37°C and ambient air, using transmitted and reflected light; inducible clindamycin resistance was verified if the clindamycin zone of inhibition adjacent to the erythromycin disk (D-shape) was flattened. A confirmatory microdilution broth test was done on all isolates for further confirmation. Briefly, any growth in the same well that contained 4 µg/mL erythromycin and 0.5 µg/mL clindamycin was set as a positive test and vice versa. *Staphylococcus aureus* ATCC 25923 was used to perform routine quality control of antibiotic disks. Confirmed isolates were kept into tryptic soy broth (TSB; Merck) with 20% glycerol at −70°C for molecular testing.

Hospital-onset (HO) *S. aureus* was set if the positive culture of *S. aureus* was obtained on or after 96 h of admission to a hospital. Community-onset (CO) *S. aureus* was set if the culture was obtained prior to 4 days of hospitalization with one or more of the following criteria: (1) a history of hospitalization, surgery, dialysis, or residence in a long-term care facility in 12 months prior to culture date or (2) the presence of a central vascular catheter within 2 days before *S. aureus* culture. Invasive *S. aureus* infection was defined according to the Centers for Disease Control and Prevention defining isolation of *S. aureus* from typically sterile body sites such as the blood, bone, fluids (pericardial, joint/synovial, peritoneal, cerebrospinal, and pleural), internal body sites (brain, lymph node, pancreas, ovary, liver, spleen, heart, and kidney), or other normally sterile sites (Goudarzi et al., 2016a). The Ethics Committee of the Shahid Beheshti University of Medical Sciences in Tehran, Iran, certified the protocol of this project (IR.SBMU. MSP.REC.1396.412).

Determining Resistance Pattern

Phenotypic methicillin resistance screening was performed by placing the cefoxitin disk (30 µg) on Mueller–Hinton agar (Merck), previously inoculated with a 0.5 McFarland-equivalent bacterial suspension. *In vitro* susceptibility of the isolates to kanamycin, ciprofloxacin, penicillin, quinupristin–dalfopristin, rifampin, tetracycline, linezolid, teicoplanin, amikacin, tobramycin, gentamicin, and trimethoprim–sulfamethoxazole (Mast; Merseyside, United Kingdom) was done according to the modified Kirby–Bauer disk diffusion method on Mueller–Hinton agar plates, as per CLSI recommendation. The European

Committee for Antimicrobial Susceptibility Testing (EUCAST) breakpoint was used for interpreting the results of fusidic acid and ceftriaxone disks. As specified by the CLSI guidelines, the broth microdilution method was applied for determining the minimum inhibitory concentration (MIC) of vancomycin and mupirocin. Minimum inhibitory concentration values of 8 to 256 and ≥512 µg/mL were established to show low-level and high-level mupirocin resistance (LLMUPR, HLMUPR) of the strains, in the respective order. As specified by the CLSI guidelines, MIC breakpoints for vancomycin were set as follows: susceptible, ≤2 µg/mL; intermediate, 4–8 µg/mL; and resistant, ≥16 µg/mL. Fusidic acid MICs were specified by the broth microdilution method and interpreted based on EUCAST guidelines. Minimum inhibitory concentration breakpoints were set as follows: susceptible, ≤1 µg/mL; and resistant, >1 µg/mL. The *S. aureus* ATCC 25923 and ATCC 29213 strains were put to test as control strains. Sigma Chemical Co. (St. Louis, MO, United States) provided the study with the powders of antibiotics.

DNA Extraction

To extract DNA, overnight cultures of *S. aureus* strains on 5% sheep blood agar (Merck) were used by applying the InstaGene Matrix kit (Bio-Rad, Hercules, CA, United States) following the manufacturer's instructions and adding lysostaphin (Sigma-Aldrich; St. Louis, United States) for bacterial lysis. Gel electrophoresis and NanoDrop 2000 spectrophotometer (Thermo, Wilmington, Delaware, United States) were applied, respectively, to test the quality and quantity of isolated *S. aureus* DNA (Goudarzi et al., 2016a,b). Seemingly, if the purity were appropriated, it would be applied as the template for PCR. Two hundred microliters of elution buffer [10 mM Tris–Cl, 0.5 mM EDTA (pH 9.0)] was applied to elute the extracted DNA, which was then kept at −20°C until use.

Detecting Antimicrobial Resistance Determinants and Virulence Factors

Polymerase chain reaction method was used for genotypic amplification of the *mecA* gene (Goudarzi et al., 2016a,b). Isolates exhibiting phenotypic resistance to particular antimicrobial agents were put to test for the presence of resistance genes [*mecA*, *vanA*, *vanB*, *mupB*, *mupA*, *fusA*, *fusB*, *fusC*, *erm*(A), *erm*(B), *erm*(C), *tet*(M), *ant* (4′)-*Ia*, *aac* (6′)-*Ie/aph* (2″), *aph* (3′)-*IIIa*] (Castanheira et al., 2010a; Nezhad et al., 2017). Virulence factors involved SE genes (*sea*, *seb*, *etb*, *sec*, *sed*, *see*, *seg*, *seh*, *sei*, and *sej*) (Monday and Bohach, 1999), exfoliative toxin genes (*eta* and *etb*), Panton–Valentine leukotoxin genes lukS-PV and lukF-PV (*pvl*), and toxic shock syndrome toxin genes (*tst*) (Goudarzi et al., 2016a; Nezhad et al., 2017).

Phenotypic Analysis of Biofilm Formation

Slime production assay or Congo red agar (CRA) method and microtiter plate (MtP) assay were recruited as *in vitro* methods for the detection of phenotypic biofilm formation. In CRA method, briefly, after preparation of CRA by adding 0.8 g of CR (Sigma-Aldrich; St. Louis, United States) to 1 L of brain heart infusion agar (Merck) and autoclaving it, filters used for add saccharose (36 g) (Sigma-Aldrich; St. Louis, United States) to CRA. Bacteria were inoculated on CRA and incubated at 37°C for 24 h and then overnight at room temperature. Biofilm formation was categorized in four levels based on colony color that strains appeared: (i) strong biofilm producer strains (very black colonies), (ii) moderate biofilm producer strains (black colonies), (iii) weak biofilm producer strains (gray colonies), and (iv) biofilm non-producer strains (red colonies) (Arciola et al., 2002; Yousefi et al., 2016).

The MtP assay as a quantitative method for biofilm detection was carried out as described previously. Concisely, an overnight culture of bacterial isolates in TSB (Merck) containing 1% glucose was diluted to 1:100 with fresh medium. Sterile MtP with flat-bottomed 96-well polystyrene was filled with 200 μL of the diluted culture and incubated at 37°C for 24 h. After incubation, wells were washed three times with 200 μL of phosphate-buffered saline (pH 7.2) to remove planktonic bacteria. Afterward, wells were fixed by 99% methanol, dried at room temperature, and then stained with 0.1% safranin. Safranin dye bound to the adherent cells was dissolved with 1 mL of 95% ethanol per well. As a negative control, 200 μL of TSB–1% glucose was used. The optical density (OD) of each well was measured using an enzyme-linked immunosorbent assay reader at a wavelength of 490 nm. Optical density cutoff defined as average OD of negative control + 3 × standard deviation of the negative control. Biofilm formation of strains was analyzed according to the absorbance of the safranin-stained attached cells and interpreted as per the criteria described by Stepanović et al. (2007). Accordingly, the degree of biofilm production was categorized into strong, moderate, weak, or without biofilm. For quality control, *Staphylococcus epidermidis* ATCC 35984 strain was used in each run.

Genetic Analysis of Biofilm Formation

Polymerase chain reaction assays for the detection of *icaABCD*, *cna*, *ebp*, *fnbB*, *fnbA*, *clfB*, *clfA*, and *bap* genes were performed as described previously (Nemati et al., 2009; Yousefi et al., 2016). Detection of arginine catabolic mobile elements for definitive confirmation of USA300 was performed as previously described by Diep et al. (2008).

Prophage Typing

iMLSB-positive *S. aureus* were characterized by prophage typing by using multiplex-PCR assay and oligonucleotide primers SGA, SGB, SGF (SGFa and SGFb), SGD, and SGL prophages as explained previously by Pantůček et al. (2004) and Rahimi et al. (2012).

Staphylococcus aureus Protein A Locus (*spa*) Typing

Staphylococcus aureus isolates underwent *spa* typing as recommended by Harmsen et al. (2003); all PCR products were Sanger sequenced in both directions. The sequences obtained were edited using the Chromas software (version 1.45;

Technelysium, Tewantin, Australia). Ridom SpaServer database[1] was applied in order to assign the *spa* type.

Staphylocoagulase Typing

Four sets of multiplex PCR reactions were used for assigning staphylocoagulase (SC) types (I–X) according to the procedure of Hirose et al. (2010). Set A contained primers for identifying SC types I, II, III, IVa, IVb, Va, and VI, whereas set B contained primers for identifying SC types VII, VIII, and X. Set 3 was used for identifying SC types IX and Vb. SC types IVa and IVb were distinguished using a set of four primers.

SCC*mec* Typing

The multiplex PCR amplification was done with specific primers for SCC*mec* typing, as recommended by Boye et al. (2007). The prototype strains applied as control strains for typing were *S. aureus* ATCC 10442 (type I), *S. aureus* N315 (type II), *S. aureus* 85/2082 (type III), *S. aureus* MW2 (type IV), *S. aureus* WIS 173 (type V), and *S. aureus* HDE288 (type VI).

agr Typing

Multiplex PCR was performed for *agr*-type detection using primer set comprising a common forward primer (pan-agr) and reverse primers (*agr*1, *agr*2, *agr*3, and *agr*4) specific to each *agr* group (Gilot et al., 2002).

Multilocus Sequence Typing

All the 126 *S. aureus* isolates with iMLSB phenotype were further characterized by MLST as described by Enright et al. (2000) by sequencing an internal fragment of seven unlinked housekeeping genes to identify the following allelic profiles: phosphate acetyltransferase (*pta*), carbamate kinase (*arcC*), triosephosphate isomerase (*tpi*), shikimate dehydrogenase (*aroE*), guanylate kinase (*gmk*), acetyl-coenzyme A acetyltransferase (*yqiL*), and glycerol kinase (*glp*). The purification of PCR products was done by performing the Qiagen PCR purification kit. In addition, the two strands were sequenced on the ABI Prism 377 automated sequencer (Applied Biosystems, Perkin-Elmer Co., Foster City, CA, United States). Finally, STs were submitted to the online MLST website through the submission of DNA sequences[2].

Ethics Statement

The current study protocol was approved by the Ethics Committee of the Shahid Beheshti University of Medical Sciences in Tehran, Iran (IR.SBMU.MSP.REC.1396.700). Written informed consent was obtained from participants.

RESULTS

Isolation and Identification of *S. aureus*

A total of 126 *S. aureus* isolates with inducible resistance phenotype were identified, including 106 methicillin-resistant

[1] http://www.spaserver.ridom.de
[2] https://pubmlst.org/

S. aureus (MRSA) and 20 methicillin-sensitive *S. aureus* (MSSA) isolates representing 84.1 and 15.9% of isolates, respectively. Precisely, of 126 iMLSB *S. aureus* isolates, 41 were collected from female patients (32.6%), and the rest were collected from male patients (85, 67.4%). In the present study, 43 strains (34.1%) were isolated from wound, 32 (25.4%) from blood, 15 (11.9%) from body fluids, 14 (11.1%) from pus, 12 (9.5%) from urine, 7 (5.6%) from sputum, and 3 (2.4%) from conjunctiva. Of the 126 isolates, 76 (60.3%) were classified as HO, and 50 (39.7%) were classified as CO. According to the case notes, the rates of invasive and non-invasive *S. aureus* with iMLSB phenotype were found to be 37.3 and 62.7%, respectively. The patients' average age was 38 years. The patients were distributed in four age groups: 21 patients ≤20 years (16.7%), 60 patients between 21 and 45 years (47.6%), 30 patients between 46 and 65 years (23.8%), and 15 patients ≥65 years (11.9%). Regarding the occurrence of inducible resistance in *S. aureus* strains, data exhibited that most cases belonged to the age groups of 21 to 45 years between 2013 and 2017, whereas in 2018, more than half of the cases were found to be in the age group between 46 and 65 years. Patients with invasive infections and HO were older. Of 21 patients aged ≤20 years, 12 (57.1%) of 60 patients were between 21 and 45 years, 28 (46.7%) of 30 patients were between 46 and 65 years, and 9 (30%) had CO infections. However, among 15 patients aged ≥65 years, only 1 (6.7%) had CO infections. There were also trends toward an increasing incidence of HO infections in elderly patients.

Antimicrobial Susceptibility

The highest and lowest rates of resistance in 126 *S. aureus* isolates tested were related to penicillin (91.3%) and fusidic acid (5.6%), respectively. The entire strains were susceptible to teicoplanin, linezolid, and vancomycin. Resistance to tested antibiotics was higher in MRSA than in MSSA. The rate of resistance to the tested antibiotics, with the exception of ciprofloxacin, was higher among HO *S. aureus* strains across CO *S. aureus* strains. The frequency of resistance rate among MRSA and MSSA strains to antimicrobial agents is presented in **Table 1**.

The entire *S. aureus* isolates were susceptible to vancomycin such that 15 isolates (11.9%) had MIC ≥ 0.5 μg/mL, 38 (30.2%) had MIC ≥ 1 μg/mL, and 73 (57.9%) exhibited MIC ≥ 2 μg/mL. The data of the microbroth dilution method illustrated that 23 isolates (18.3%) were mupirocin-resistant; of these, 11 (8.7%) and 12 (9.6%) were LLMUPR and HLMUPR, respectively. Of the 126 isolates of *S. aureus* with iMLSB phenotype, seven (5.6%) were fusidic acid-resistant. In total, 80.2% of isolates (101/126) were multidrug resistance (MDR), and the MDR rate for MRSA isolates (85.8%) was significantly higher than that for MSSA (50%). Information about simultaneous resistance patterns and distribution of clinical samples is presented in **Table 2**.

agr and SCC*mec* Typing

By using *agr* typing method, all 126 *S. aureus* isolates with iMLSB phenotype could be typed *agr* I–III. Of these isolates tested, 77 (10 MSSA and 67 MRSA) were *agr* I, 20 (MRSA) were *agr* II, and 29 (10 MSSA and 19 MRSA) were *agr* III. Staphylococcal cassette chromosome *mec* typing for MRSA isolates indicated that type IV was the predominant SCC*mec* type (57.6%, 61/106), followed by SCC*mec* III (33%, 35/106), SCC*mec* V (7.5%, 8/106), and SCC*mec* II (1.9%, 2/106). In addition, no MRSA isolates harbored SCC*mec* type I.

Determination of Adhesion and Biofilm Production Ability

Biofilm formation was observed in 97 strains (77%) using the CRA and MtP methods, whereas 29 strains (23%) were confirmed as non–biofilm producer strains. Of the total MRSA isolates, MtP detected 18 (17%) as weak, 23 (21.7%) as moderate, and 42 (39.6%) as strong biofilm producers. By CRA, 20 isolates (18.9%) were able to produce biofilm weakly, and 26 (24.5%) and 37 (34.9%) isolates presented moderate and potent biofilm formation, respectively. In MSSA isolates, MtP indicated weak biofilm production in five isolates (25), moderate biofilm production in three (15%), and strong biofilm production in six isolates (30%), whereas CRA detected four isolates (20%) as weak, five (25%) as moderate, and five (25%) as strong biofilm producers. The analysis of *icaA-D* genes among tested *S. aureus* strains showed that the most frequently detected gene was *icaD* (*n* = 92, 73%), followed by *icaA* (*n* = 90, 71.4%), *icaB* (*n* = 76, 60.3%), and *icaC* (*n* = 67, 53.2%). Overall, six different biofilm patterns were identified. **Figure 1** presents the distribution of *icaABCD* among tested strains. Regarding the presence of adhesion genes, the seven most frequent adhesion-related genes were *clfA* (93.7%, 118/126) followed by *clfB* (87.3%, 110/126), *fnbB* (61.9%, 78/126), *cna* (57.9%, 73/126), *fnbA* (54%, 68/126), *ebp* (50%, 63/126), and *bap* (3.2%, 8/126), respectively. The adhesion profiles are shown in **Figure 1**. None of the MSSA strains carried the *bap* gene. In MSSA strains, three different adhesion patterns including *clfA* + *clfB* + *fnbB* (50%, 10/20), *clfA* + *clfB* + *fnbB* + *fnbA* + *ebp* + *cna* (25%, 5/20), and *fnbB* + *fnbA* + *cna* (25%, 5/20) were observed. Apparently, higher diversity among the adhesion patterns from MRSA (six patterns) than those from MSSA (three patterns) was noticed.

Determination of Prophage Types and Toxin and Enterotoxin Encoding Genes

A total of 103 strains (81.7%) of the 126 inducible resistant *S. aureus* strains tested had one or more virulence genes. The most frequently attained virulence genes were *pvl* (23.8%, 30/126), followed by *sea* (19.8%, 25/126), *tst* (19%, 24/126), *sec* (11.1%, 14/126), *sed* (9.5%, 12/126), *seg* (4.8%, 6/126), *seb* (4%, 5/126), *see* (3.2%, 4/126), and *eta* (2.4%, 3/126), but *she*, *sei*, and *sej* encoding genes were detected in any of the total number of 126 isolates tested. In this analysis, six prophage types were grouped into seven separate prophage profiles. **Figure 1** provides a summary data of the number and frequency of prophage profiles among isolates tested.

The data for antibiotic resistance genes in *S. aureus* strains studied revealed that the most common gene was *mecA* in 106 strains (84.1%), followed by *erm*(A) in 43 strains (34.1%), *erm*(B) in 41 (32.5%), *erm*(C) in 361 (28.6%), *ant* (4′)-Ia in 35 (27.8%), *tet*(M) in 32 (25.4%), *aac* (6′)-Ie/*aph* (2″) in 29 (23%), *aph* (3′)-IIIa in 17 (13.5%), *mupA* in 12 (9.5%), *fusB* in 6 (4.8%) strains,

TABLE 1 | Antimicrobial resistance pattern of MRSA and MSSA isolates with iMLSB phenotype.

Antibiotic	106 MRSA isolates n (%)		20 MSSA isolates n (%)		Total n (%)
	Hospital onset	Community onset	Hospital onset	Community onset	
Penicillin	67(53.2)	39(31)	9(7.1)	–	115(91.3)
Gentamicin	76(60.3)	21(16.6)	5(4)	4(3.2)	106(84.1)
Tetracycline	45(35.7)	29(23)	9(7.1)	6(4.8)	89(70.6)
Kanamycin	34(27)	19(15.1)	8(6.3)	5(4)	66(52.4)
Ceftriaxone	41(32.5)	11(8.7)	7(5.6)	4(3.2)	63(50)
Amikacin	31(24.6)	17(13.5)	10(7.9)	1(0.8)	59(46.8)
Ciprofloxacin	23(18.2)	29(23)	5(4)	–	57(45.2)
Tobramycin	39(31)	5(4)	7(5.5)	–	51(40.5)
Rifampin	25(19.8)	9(7.1)	3(2.4)	2(1.6)	39(30.9)
Trimethoprim–sulfamethoxazole	17(13.5)	11(8.7)	5(4)	2(1.6)	35(27.8)
Quinupristin–dalfopristin	18(14.3)	9(7.1)	–	3(2.4)	30(23.8)
Mupirocin	13(10.3)	4(3.2)	5(4)	1(0.8)	23(18.3)
Fusidic acid	7(5.6)	–			7(5.6)

TABLE 2 | Resistant pattern and distribution of samples in 126 S. aureus strains isolated from clinical sources.

Simultaneous resistance to antibiotics	Resistance profile	Resistance pattern[a]	Type of samples[b] (n;%)	Number of isolates (%)
Nine	A	PG, GM, T, K, CIP, TN, SYN, RI, TS	W (6; 40), B (3; 20), BF (2; 13.3), U (4; 26.7),	15 (11.9)
Eight	B	PG, GM, T, K, CRO, AK, CIP, TN	W (9; 52.9), B (5; 29.4), P (3; 17.7)	17 (13.5)
	C	PG, GM, T, K, CRO, RI, TS, MUP	W (4; 33.3), B (3; 25), P (2; 16.7), BF (2; 16.7), S (1; 8.3)	12 (9.5)
	D	PG, GM, T, CRO, AK, RI, MUP, TS	W (3; 37.5), BF (1; 12.5), P (4; 50)	8 (6.3)
Seven	E	PG, GM, T, K, CRO, AK, CIP	W (4; 26.8), B (3; 20), BF (2; 13.3), U (2; 13.3), P (2; 13.3), S (2; 13.3)	15 (11.9)
	F	PG, GM, T, CRO, AK, TN, FC	B (5; 100)	5 (4)
Six	G	PG, GM, T, AK, CIP, SYN	W (5; 50), BF (3; 30), U (2; 20)	10 (7.9)
Five	H	PG, GM, T, K, TN	W (3; 42.9), B (3; 42.9), C (1; 14.2)	7 (5.6)
	I	PG, GM, CRO, TN, SYN	BF (2; 40), C (1; 20), P (1; 20), U (1; 20)	5 (4)
	J	PG, GM, TN, MUP, FC	W (2; 100)	2 (1.6)
Four	K	PG, GM, AK, RI	B (2; 50), BF (1; 25), P (1; 25)	4 (3.2)
	L	PG, GM, CRO, MUP	C (1; 100)	1 (0.8)
Two	M	PG, GM	S (4; 80), U (1; 20)	5 (4)
One	N	PG	W (5; 55.6), B (4; 44.4)	9 (7.1)
Without	O	–	W (2; 18.2), B (4; 36.3), U (2; 18.2), P (1; 9.1), BF (2; 18.2)	11 (8.7)

[a]PG, penicillin; CRO, ceftriaxone; GM, gentamicin; K, kanamycin; AK, amikacin; TN, tobramycin; T, Tetracycline; CIP, ciprofloxacin; TS, trimethoprim–sulfamethoxazole; RI, rifampicin; MUP, mupirocin; FC, fusidic acid; SYN, quinupristin–dalfopristin. [b]B, blood; W, wound; P, pus; BF, body fluid; U, urine; S, sputum; C, conjunctiva.

and fusC in 1 strain. vanB, mupB, and fusA genes were not detected in none of experimented isolates.

SC Typing

In the present study, all isolates could be typed by SC typing method. These isolates were distinguished into seven SC types (I–VI). The predominant SC type was III and included 56 isolates (44.4%), followed by II (28.6%, 36/126), IVa (9.5%, 12/126),

VI (7.9%, 10/126), I (4%, 5/126), V (4%, 5/126), and IVb (1.6%, 2/126). A total of seven SC types and two types (II and IVa) were detected in MSSA isolates.

MLST and spa Typing

All the isolates were typed by spa and MLST. A total of 26 spa types were attained in the entire 126 S. aureus. The isolates identified as invasive S. aureus were assigned to particular t790,

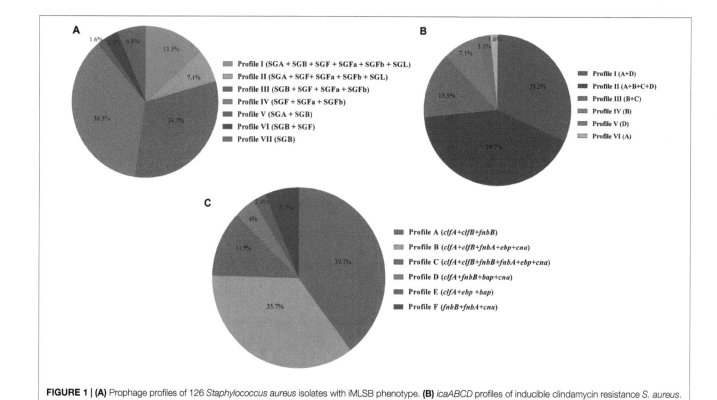

FIGURE 1 | (A) Prophage profiles of 126 *Staphylococcus aureus* isolates with iMLSB phenotype. (B) *icaABCD* profiles of inducible clindamycin resistance *S. aureus*.
(C) Adhesion profiles of *S. aureus* isolates investigated in this study.

t002, t008, t064, t030, t037, and t631 *spa* types. For CO, the isolates were assigned to *spa* types t005, t1869, t019, t021, t10795, t6811, t002, t045, t008, t065, t030, and t037. Among MSSA isolates, the most common *spa* types were t021, t005, t1869, and t318 representing 35 (7/20), 25 (5/20), 25 (5/20), and 15% (3/20), and among MRSA isolates, the top four *spa* types were t037, t437, t030, and t008 representing 10.4 (11/106), 9.4 (10/106), 8.5 (9/106), and 7.5% (8/106) of isolates. Multilocus sequence typing identified 14 ST types in both MRSA and MSSA isolates, namely, ST22 (14.3%, 18/126), ST30 (11.9%, 15/126), ST1 (1.6%, 2/126), ST772 (4.8%, 6/126), ST8 (10.3%, 13/126), ST239 (23%, 29/126), ST585 (1.6%, 2/126), ST5 (5.63%, 7/126), ST225 (1.6%, 2/126), ST80 (9.5%, 12/126), ST59 (4.8%, 6/126), ST338 (3.2%, 4/126), ST15 (4%, 5/126), and ST45 (4%, 5/126), which were further grouped into nine CCs including CC1, 5, 8, 15, 22, 30, 45, 59, and 80. Among MSSA, CC22 and CC30 were the dominant clones, each clone with 50% (10/20) of the isolates being assigned to these genotypes, and all were recovered from non-invasive *S. aureus* and both CO (55%, 11/20) and HO (45%, 9/20) cases. CC8 (41.5%, 44/106), CC80 (11.3%, 124/106), and CC5 (8.5%, 9/106) were the top three CCs in MRSA isolates. **Table 3** represents the analysis of *S. aureus* clones obtained from patients based on invasive and non-invasive infections.

Temporal Changes in Inducible Resistant *S. aureus* Genotypes

Table 4 gives information about the percentage of inducible resistant *S. aureus* strains assigned to each CC for each year

between 2013 and 2018. The prevalence of inducible resistance *S. aureus* isolates elevated in the experiment from 19.8% in 2013–2014 to 30.2% in 2017–2018. Apart from 2013 to 2014 in which CC22 genotype was the most prevalent CC among inducible resistance isolates (36%, 9/25), in the remaining years of study (2014–2018), the CC8 isolates were the most predominant genotype. The CC8, as a predominate genotype, was at its most prevalent in 2016–2017 (41.6%, 10/24). Its prevalence increased during the study period from 20% in 2013–2014 (5/25) to 39.5% (15/38) in 2017–2018. By contrast, the prevalence rate of CC22 decreased from 36% in 2013–2014 to 0% in 2017–2018. The CC30, the third predominated CC among our clinical isolates, had its most prevalence in 2017–2018 (18.4%, 7/38). The prevalence of this type varied dramatically each year during 2013–2018; despite a decrease to 8% (2/25) in 2013–2014, a slight increase in the prevalence of this type was noted during 2014–2015 (9.5%, 2/21) and 2015–2016 (16.7%, 3/18), followed by an overall decrease to 4.2% (1/24) in 2016–2017. The prevalence of this type increased to 18.4% (7/38) in 2017–2018.

The first CC45 isolates were found in 2015–2016. The prevalence of this genotype diminished during the study period from 22.2% (4/18) in 2015–2016 to 4.2% (1/24) in 2016–2017 apart from 2017–2018 when no CC45 was detected. The CC45 was the second predominant genotype in 2015–2016 (22.2%, 4/18). The CC15, absent during 2013–2016, was detected during 2016–2017 (8.3%, 2/24), but remained at relatively low prevalence (7.9%, 3/38) in 2017–2018.

TABLE 3 | Analysis of S. aureus clones obtained from patients based on invasive and non-invasive infections.

Clonal complex (CC)	Molecular types	Invasive S. aureus		Non-invasive S. aureus		Total, n (%)
		Community onset, n (%)	Hospital onset, n (%)	Community onset, n (%)	Hospital onset, n (%)	
CC22	ST22-SCCmec IV/t852	0(0)	0(0)	0(0)	2(100)	2(1.6)
	ST22-SCCmec IV/t790	0(0)	3(60)	0(0)	2(40)	5(4)
	ST22-SCCmec IV/t005	0(0)	0(0)	0(0)	1(100)	1(0.7)
	ST22/t005	0(0)	0(0)	2(40)	3(60)	5(4)
	ST22/t1869	0(0)	0(0)	4(80)	1(20)	5(4)
CC30	ST30-SCCmec IV/t605	0(0)	0(0)	0(0)	2(100)	2(1.6)
	ST30-SCCmec IV/t019	0(0)	0(0)	3(100)	0(0)	3(2.4)
	ST30/t318	0(0)	0(0)	0(0)	3(100)	3(2.4)
	ST30/t021	0(0)	0(0)	5(71.4)	2(28.6)	7(5.5)
CC1	ST772-SCCmec IV/t10795	0(0)	0(0)	3(60)	2(40)	5(4)
	ST772-SCCmec IV/t657	0(0)	0(0)	0(0)	1(100)	1(0.7)
	ST1-SCCmec IV/t6811	0(0)	0(0)	1(50)	1(50)	2(1.6)
CC5	ST5-SCCmec IV/t002	2(28.6)	3(42.8)	1(14.3)	1(14.3)	7(5.5)
	ST225-SCCmec II/t045	0(0)	0(0)	1(50)	1(50)	2(1.6)
CC8	ST8-SCCmec IV/t008	1(12.5)	3(37.5)	4(50)	0(0)	8(6.3)
	ST8-SCCmec IV/t064	2(40)	2(40)	1(20)	0	5(4)
	ST585-SCCmec III/t713	0(0)	0(0)	0(0)	2(100)	2(1.6)
	ST239-SCCmec III/t030	0	4(44.4)	1(11.2)	4(44.4)	9(7.1)
	ST239-SCCmec III/t037	7(63.6)	1(9.1)	0(0)	3(27.3)	11(8.7)
	ST239-SCCmec III/t631	0(0)	1(25)	0(0)	3(75)	4(3.2)
	ST239-SCCmec III/t860	0(0)	0(0)	0(0)	3(100)	3(2.4)
	ST239-SCCmec III/t388	0(0)	0(0)	0(0)	2(100)	2(1.6)
CC80	ST80-SCCmec IV/t044	0(0)	6(75)	0(0)	2(25)	8(6.3)
	ST80-SCCmec IV/t131	0(0)	0(0)	2(50)	2(50)	4(3.2)
CC59	ST59-SCCmec IV/t437	3(50)	2(33.3)	0(0)	1(16.7)	6(4.8)
	ST338-SCCmec III/t437	0(0)	0(0)	0(0)	4(100)	4(3.2)
CC15	ST15-SCCmec IV/t084	2(40)	1(20)	0(0)	2(40)	5(4)
CC45	ST45-SCCmec IV/t038	4(80)	0(0)	1(20)	0(0)	5(4)

TABLE 4 | Distribution of characterized S. aureus isolates with iMLSB phenotype by year.

S. aureus clones	2013–2014, n (%)	2014–2015, n (%)	2015–2016, n (%)	2016–2017, n (%)	2017–2018, n (%)	Total, n (%)
CC8	5(11.4)	8(18.2)	6(13.6)	10(22.7)	15(34.1)	44(34.9)
CC22	9(50)	5(27.8)	1(5.6)	3(16.6)	0(0)	18(14.3)
CC30	2(13.3)	2(13.3)	3(20)	1(6.7)	7(46.7)	15(11.9)
CC80	3(25)	0(0)	0(0)	4(33.3)	5(41.7)	12(9.5)
CC59	0(0)	1(10)	0(0)	2(20)	7(70)	10(7.9)
CC5	2(22.2)	3(33.4)	2(22.2)	1(11.1)	1(11.1)	9(7.1)
CC1	4(50)	2(25)	2(25)	0(0)	0(0)	8(6.4)
CC45	0(0)	0(0)	4(80)	1(20)	0(0)	5(4)
CC15	0(0)	0(0)	0(0)	2(40)	3(60)	5(4)
Total	25(19.8)	21(16.7)	18(14.3)	24(19)	38(30.2)	126(100)

The CC59 isolates were not detected between 2013–2014 and 2015–2016. The CC59 isolates were detected for the first time in 2014–2015 (4.8%, 1/21), and increased to 8.3% (2/24) in 2016–2017. This genotype was present at its greatest prevalence in 2017–2018, accounting for 18.4% (7/38) of inducible resistance strains. The prevalence of CC80 varied dramatically during the 5-year period, this genotype was not identified among any of the 2014–2015 and 2015–2016 tested strains. In 2013–2014, only 12% (3/25) of isolates exhibited this genotype. An increase in the prevalence of this genotype was noted between 2016 and 2017 to 16.7% (4/24), followed by a decline to 13.2% (5/38) in 2017–2018. The CC5 genotype was present in each year between 2013 and 2018. The highest prevalence of this genotype occurred in 2014–2015 (14.3%, 3/21), followed by 11.1% (2/18) between 2015 and

Antimicrobial Resistance: Public Health Challenges

2016. Overall, the prevalence of this genotype diminished during the study period from 8% (2/25) in 2013–2014 to 2.6% (1/38) in 2017–2018. The CC1 isolates were not identified between 2016 and 2018. It was the third predominant genotype in 2013–2014, accounting for 16% (4/25) of examined isolates, but it dropped to 9.5% (2/21) in 2014–2015 and then indicated an increase in 2015–2016 (11.1%, 2/18).

Observations on Inducible Clindamycin-Resistant *S. aureus* Clones

The molecular characteristics of the isolates related to each genotype of inducible resistance MRSA and MSSA are shown in **Table 5**. Meanwhile, the details of each clonal lineage are explained below.

CC1

In this study, most of the isolates identified as CC1/ST772-MRSA-V were represented by *spa* type t10795 (83.3%, 5/6). Among the CC1/ST772-MRSA-V isolates, resistance to aminoglycosides encoded by *aac (6′)-Ie/aph (2″)* and *aph (3′)-IIIa*, and tetracycline encoded by *tet(M)* was common. Three isolates (60%) were able to produce biofilm strongly. The finding indicated that *fnbB* gene was present in all of the CC1 isolates. *icaA* and *icaD* were the most prevalent biofilm-related genes. More than half of the isolates (60%) carried *pvl* genes. The one remaining CC1/ST772-MRSA-V isolate was assigned to *spa* type t657 and *coa* type IVa. This isolate exhibited resistance to multiple antibiotics and harbored resistance genes *mecA* and *erm*(C); meanwhile, enterotoxin genes *sea* + *seb* carried simultaneously. The CC1/ST1-MRSA-V isolates exhibited *spa* type, t6811. One isolate carried *fusc* and exhibited resistance to fusidic acid at MIC 32 µg/mL. MDR pattern was detected among these isolates. Both isolates were identified to be biofilm producers albeit weakly. Toxin gene differs from those detected in CC1/ST772-MRSA-V found among the CC1/ST1-MRSA-V isolates, namely, *sec*. All the isolates exhibited erythromycin resistance encoded by *erm*(C).

CC5

All CC5/ST5-MRSA-IV isolates were assigned to single *spa* type t002. This isolates carried the enterotoxin genes *sea* (42.9%, 3/7) and *sed* + *seg* (42.9%, 3/7) and the toxin *tst* (42.9%, 3/7). Among the CC5/ST5-MRSA-IV isolates, resistance to erythromycin encoded by *erm*(A), tetracycline encoded by *tet(M)*, and mupirocin encoded by *mupA* was common. Five of HLMUPR strains, which harbored the *mupA* gene, belonged to this CC (41.7%, 5/12). Nearly 60% of all isolates that occurred in these clones showed moderate biofilm formation. The remaining 40% were not able to produce biofilm. The top three adhesion-related genes among CC5 isolates were *clfA* (100%, 9/9), *clfB* (77.8%, 7/9), *ebp* (75%, 6/9), and *cna* (75%, 6/9). Of nine CC5 isolates, *icaA* and *icaD* were found in seven isolates, whereas *icaB* and *icaC* were detected in six isolates. The other CC5 genotypes identified (CC5/ST225-MRSA-II) were assigned to *spa* type t045, which exhibited resistance to multiple antibiotics including aminoglycosides resistance encoded by *ant (4′)-Ia (2)* and *aac (6′)-Ie/aph (2″)* genes. *tst* encoding gene

was detected in all isolates. All CC5/ST225-MRSA-II showed strong biofilm formation. The predominant prophage profile was SGF + SGFa + SGFb.

CC8

In this study, CC8 was represented by ST8-MRSA-IV (29.6%, 13/44), ST239-MRSA-III (65.9%, 29/44), and ST585-MRSA-III (4.5%, 4/44). *spa* types t008 (61.5%, 8/13) and t064 (38.5%, 5/13) predominated among the CC8/ST8-MRSA-IV isolates. Among 13 ST8-MRSA-IV strains, 8 isolates harbored the *arcA* and *opp3AB* genes and confirmed as USA300. The majority of CC/ST8-MRSA-IV (USA300), as a major global epidemic clone that has been noticed for its rapidity dissemination within the community and hospitals isolates, exhibited resistance to aminoglycosides encoded by *aph (3′)-IIIa* (61.5%, 8/13). Resistance to erythromycin encoded by *erm*(C) (38.5%, 5/13) and tetracycline encoded by *tet(M)* (38.5%, 5/13) was also detected in this genotype. Six strains belonging to CC/ST8-MRSA-IV clone demonstrated the HLMUPR phenotype and carried *mupA* gene. The findings showed that the majority of the isolates (77%, 10/13) was able to produce biofilm, although at different intensities. Nine isolates in this clone harbored the *pvl* genes (69.2%); the rest of four isolates carried the *sed* gene (30.8%).

The majority of CC8/ST239-MRSA-III isolates were assigned to *spa* type t037 (37.9%, 11/29), followed by t030 (31.1%, 9/29), t631 (13.8%, 4/29), t860 (10.3%, 3/29), and t388 (6.9%, 2/29). Resistance to multiple antibiotics simultaneously was identified in this genotype. Fusidic acid resistance encoded by *fusc* (6.9%, 2/29); tetracycline resistance encoded by *tet(K)* (41.4%, 12/29); aminoglycoside resistance encoded by *ant (4′)-Ia* (58.6%, 17/29), *aac (6′)-Ie/aph (2″)* (37.9%, 11/29), and *aph (3′)-IIIa* (6.9%, 2/29); and mupirocin resistance encoded by *mupA* (6.9%, 2/29) were also noted. Almost more than half of the isolates carried *sea* (55.2%, 16/29), 48.3% (14/29) carried *tst*, and 17.2% (5/29) carried *sec* only three isolates harboring *seg* gene. All three ST239-SCC*mec* III/t860 isolates carried *eta* and demonstrated the LLMUPR phenotype. The CC8/ST239-MRSA-III isolates displayed high levels of biofilm production (86.2%, 25/29). Regarding the biofilm-related genes, the *icaD* (70.5%, 31/44) was common, followed by *icaA* (68.2%, 30/44), *icaB* (68.2%, 30/44), and *icaC* (61.4%, 27/44). The top three adhesion-related genes among CC8 isolates were *clfA* (100%, 44/44), *clfB* (86.4%, 38/44), and *cna* (86.4%, 38/44).

Two remaining CC8/ST585-MRSA-III isolates were assigned to *spa* type t713 and carried multiple resistance genes, that is, *tet(M)*, *erm*(C), and enterotoxin genes *see*. Both of these strains indicated strong biofilm formation. The majority of the CC8 isolates was found to harbor SGF + SGFa + SGFb proghages.

CC15

The five CC15/ST15 MRSA-IV isolates identified revealed the same *spa*, *coa*, *agr*, and prophage profile. Fewer than half of the isolates were resistant to fusidic acid encoded by *fusB*. All CC15/ST15 MRSA-IV isolates carried *pvl* genes. More than half of the isolates were biofilm producers. All CC15 isolates were positive for *fnbB* gene, and 80% of the isolates were found to carry all of the biofilm-related genes (*icaA-D*). One isolate was found

TABLE 5 | Phenotypic and genotypic typing data for inducible resistance MRSA ($n = 106$) and MSSA ($n = 20$) isolates studied in Tehran, Iran, between 2013 and 2018.

CC	Genotype MRSA	Genotype MSSA	Antibiotic resistance spa	agr	coa	Phenotype profiles[a] (% indicated when not 100%)	Typing category results (n) Genotype (%)	Virulence genes (% indicated when not 100%)	Biofilm status[b] (% indicated when not 100%)	Prophage profile[c] (% indicated when not 100%)
22	ST22-MRSA-IV (8)		t852 (2), t790 (5)	I	III	A (14.2), B (42.9), D (42.9)	mecA (100), ant (4')-Ia (28.6), aac (6')-Ie/aph (2'') (42.9), erm(C) (57.1), erm(B) (42.9)	pvl (28.6), tst (42.9), sea (14.2)	W (57.1), S (42.9)	I (28.6), IV (71.4)
			t005 (1)	I	IVa	H	mecA, erm(A), erm(B)	pvl	S	I
		ST22-MSSA (10)	t005 (5), t1869 (5)	I	IVa	N (40), K (30), H (30)	erm(A) (50), aac (6')-Ie/aph (2'') (20), ant (4')-Ia (30), tet(M) (50), erm(B) (50)	sec (30)	N (50), W (30), S (20)	III (50), IV (50)
30	ST30-MRSA-IV (5)		t605 (2), t019 (3)	III	II	A (40), B (20), E (40)	mecA (100), erm(C) (60), aac (6')-Ie/aph (2'') (40), aph (3')-IIIa (20), tet(M) (20)	pvl (60), sea (40)	N (20), W (40), S (40)	I (60), V (40)
		ST30-MSSA (10)	t021 (7), t318 (3)	III	II	G (30), N (10), I (10), O (40), L (10)	erm(A) (10), erm(B) (20), erm(C) (50), ant (4')-Ia (30), aph (3')-IIIa (10), erm(B) (60)	sed (40), pvl (30)	N (10), W (20), M (30), S (40)	VI (10), VII (30), III (30), IV (30)
1	ST1-MRSA-IV (2)		t6811 (2)	III	IVb	E (50), F (50)	mecA (100), erm(A) (100), fusc (50)	sec	W	III
	ST772-MRSA-IV (6)		t10795 (5)	II	III	B (60), E (40)	mecA (100), aac (6')-Ie/aph (2'') (40), aph (3')-IIIa (60), tet(M) (60), erm(B) (100)	pvl (60), sea (40)	N (20), W (20), S (60)	I (40), IV (60)
			t657 (1)	II	IVa	I	mecA, erm(C)	sea + seb	S	VII
8	ST8-MRSA-IV (13)		t008 (8), t064 (5)	I	III	C (30.8), D (23.1), O (38.5), M (7.6)	mecA (100), mupA (46.1), aph (3')-IIIa (61.5), erm(C) (38.5), tet(M) (38.5), erm(B) (30.8)	pvl (69.2), sed (30.8)	N (23.1), W (38.4), M (23.1), S (15.4)	I (69.2), IV (30.8)
	ST239-MRSA-III (29)		t030 (9), t037 (11), t631 (4), t860 (3), t388 (2)	I	III	A (20.7), B (13.8), C (10.4), D (3.4), E (17.3), F (6.9), G (13.8), I (6.9), K (3.4), O (3.4)	mecA (100), mupA (6.9), fusB (6.9), erm(A) (51.7), erm(B) (17.3), erm(C) (44.8), ant (4')-Ia (58.6), aac (6')-Ie/aph (2'') (37.9), aph (3')-IIIa (6.9), tet(M) (41.3)	tst (48.3), sea (55.1), sec (17.3), seg (10.4), eta (10.4)	N (13.8), W (13.8), M (10.4), S (62)	III (41.4), IV (44.8), VII (13.8)
5	ST585-MRSA-III (2)		t713 (2)	I	III	I (50), E (50)	mecA (100), tet(M) (50), erm(C) (50)	see	S	IV
	ST5-MRSA-IV (7)		t002 (7)	II	II	C (42.9), D (14.2), H (42.9)	mecA (100), mupA (57.1), erm(A) (57.1), tet(M) (71.4)	tst (42.9), sea (42.9), sed + seg (42.9)	N (42.9), M (57.1)	IV
	ST225-MRSA-II (2)		t045 (2)	II	II	G	mecA (100), ant (4')-Ia (100), aac (6')-Ie/aph (2'') (100), erm(B) (50)	tst (100), sed (50)	S	VI
80	ST80-MRSA-IV (12)		t044 (8), t131 (4)	III	II	B (50), E (25), F (8.3), M (16.7)	mecA (100), fusB (8.3), ant (4')-Ia (41.7), aac (6')-Ie/aph (2'') (33.3), erm(A) (83.3)	pvl (33.3)	N (25), M (41.7), S (33.3)	III (58.4), VI (8.3), II (33.3)
59	ST59-MRSA-IV (6)		t437 (6)	I	VI	E (16.7), F (16.7), N (66.6)	mecA (100), fusB (16.7), erm(B) (33.3), erm(C) (66.7)	seb (66.7)	N (50), M (33.3), S (16.7)	III
	ST338-MRSA-III (4)		t437 (4)	I	VI	A (50), M (50)	mecA (100), ant (4')-Ia (75), aph (3')-IIIa (50), erm(B) (75)	see (50)	N (25), M (25), S (50)	III
15	ST15-MRSA-IV (5)		t084 (5)	II	I	C (40), J (40), O (20)	mecA (100), fusB (40), erm(B) (80)	pvl (100)	N (40), M (40), S (20)	II
45	ST45-MRSA-IV (5)		t038 (5)	I	V	A (80), G (20)	mecA (100), erm(A) (100), aac (6')-Ie/aph (2'') (60)	tst (40), sec (80)	N (40), M (60)	III (20), IV (80)

[a] Phenotypic profile are presented in **Table 2**. [b] W, weak producer; M, moderate producer; S, strong producer; N, non-producer. [c] Prophage profiles are presented in **Figure 1A**.

to carry none of the tested *ica* genes. All of the CC15 isolates possessed SGA + SGF + SGFa + SGFb + SGL prophage profile.

CC22

Three *spa* types t852, t790, and t005 and two spa types t005, t1869 predominated among the CC22/ST22-MRSA-IV isolates (44.4%, 8/18) and CC22/ST22-MSSA (55.6%, 10/18) isolates. Among the MRSA isolates, resistance to erythromycin encoded by *erm(C)* and aminoglycosides encoded by *aac (6′)-Ie/aph (2″)* were prevalent, whereas in MSSA isolates resistance to tetracycline encoded by *tet*(M) and that to aminoglycosides encoded by *ant (4′)-Ia (3)* were common. All the MRSA isolates were biofilm producers, whereas in MSSA isolates half of the isolates were able to produce biofilm. The results indicated that adhesion genes *clfA* and *clfB* were detected in all of the MRSA strains, and the most common *ica* genes were *icaA* and *icaB*. All the MSSA isolates carried *clfA*, *clfB*, and *fnbB* simultaneously, and *icaA* and *icaD* were the most prevalent biofilm-related genes. The isolates identified as CC22/ST22-MRSA-IV isolates showed a prevalence of 37.5% (3/8) for the *pvl* and *tst* genes. One isolate carried *sea* gene (12.5%, 1/8). The *sec* gene (30%, 3/10) was the only toxin gene detected among CC22/ST22-MSSA isolates. The carriage of *pvl* genes was more common among MRSA isolates than among MSSA isolates. The SGB + SGF + SGFa + SGFb prophage profile was detected in the majority of CC22 isolates.

CC30

CC/ST30 isolates were found in both MRSA and MSSA isolates. Among MSRA isolates, the most predominant *spa* types were t605 and t019, representing 40% (2/5) and 60% (3/5) of isolates. Multiple resistance genes including *erm(C)*, *aac (6′)-Ie/aph (2″)*, *aph (3′)-IIIa*, and *tet*(M) were identified among tested isolates. More than half of the CC/ST30-MRSA-IV isolates carried *pvl*, whereas isolates harboring *sea* were at a relatively low frequency. All CC/ST30-MRSA-IV isolates displayed agr type III and *coa* type II. Four isolates (80%) were able to produce biofilm, and the remaining 20% were non–biofilm producers. All the MRSA isolates carried biofilm (*icaA*, *icaB*, *icaC*, and *icaD*) and adhesion (*clfA*, *clfB*, and *fnbB*) related genes. In all the MSSA strains, *fnbA*, *cna*, and *icaA* genes were detected. Among MSSA isolates, *spa* types t021 and t318 represented 70% (7/10) and 30% (3/10) of isolates. Nearly 90% (9/10) of the CC/ST30-MSSA isolates could form biofilm at different intensities. Various prophage patterns with the majority of SGB (60%, 6/10) were identified among MSSA isolates. The majority of CC/ST30-MSSA isolates exhibited erythromycin resistance encoded by *erm*(B) (80%, 8/10), and *erm*(C) (50%, 5/10). The *pvl* and *sed* encoding genes were the only toxins produced by this genotype. The SGA + SGB + SGF + SGFa + SGFb + SGL was found as the most predominant prophage profile among CC/ST30-MRSA-IV isolates.

CC45

All ST45-MRSA-IV isolates were assigned a *spa* type t038, *agr* I, and *coa* V. The isolates that exhibited resistance to multiple antibiotics were confirmed among these isolates. More than half of them (60%) were biofilm producers. All of these isolates carried *icaB*, *clfA*, *clfB*, and *fnbB* encoding genes simultaneously. All ST45-MRSA-IV isolates possessed *erm*(A) gene. The carriage of *aac (6′)-Ie/aph (2″)* gene was found in 60% of isolates. The enterotoxin gene *sec* was present in 80% of isolates. Among prophage patterns, the SGF + SGFa + SGFb was common.

CC59

Two CC5 MRSA isolates were detected as one with ST59 and another one with ST338. All CC59 isolates indicated a single *spa* type, t437, *coa* type VI, and SGB-SGF-SGFa-SGFb phage pattern. All CC59/ST59 isolates were discriminated into SCC*mec* types IV. Two-thirds of ST59-MRSA-IV isolates carried *seb* gene; however, no other toxin genes were identified. Three isolates accounting for half (50%) of the entire ST59-MRSA-IV isolates were non–biofilm producers, and only one isolate showed strong biofilm formation. Results also demonstrated that the *icaA*, *icaD*, *clfA*, and *clfB* genes were detected in all of the CC59 isolates. Almost one-fifth of these isolates were resistant to fusidic acid encoded by *fusB* gene. Four and two ST59-MRSA-IV isolates carried *erm*(C) (66.7%) and *erm*(B) (33.3%), respectively. All CC59/ST338 isolates were assigned into an SCC*mec* type III. Half of CC59/ST338-MRSA-III isolates harbored *see* encoding gene. Other toxin-encoding genes were not noticed. The predominant isolates carried *erm*(B) (75%, 3/4), and aminoglycoside resistance encoded by *aph (3′)-IIIa* was also common among these isolates (50%, 2/4). All of the CC59 isolates possessed SGB + SGF + SGFa + SGFb prophage profile.

CC80

The CC80 isolates exhibited different *spa* types including t044 (66.7%, 8/12), t131 (33.3%, 4/12). All the ST80-MRSA-IV isolates assigned *agr* III and *coa* II. One-fourth of isolates were categorized as non–biofilm producers. The results exhibited that the *clfA* and *clfB* genes were explored in the entire CC80 isolates. The gene encoding for *icaD* (91.7%, 11/12) was the most prevalent biofilm-related gene among isolates.

The carriage of *pvl* genes was confirmed in one-third of tested isolates. Resistances to aminoglycosides encoded by *ant (4′)-Ia (41.7)* and *aac (6′)-Ie/aph (2″) (33.3)*, erythromycin encoded by *erm*(A), and fusidic acid encoded by *fusB* were common. The most prevalent prophage pattern was SGA + SGB + SGF + SGFa + SGFb + SGL.

DISCUSSION

This cross-sectional study provided several novel findings regarding the prevalence and genetic diversity of iMLSB-positive *S. aureus* strains isolated from clinical samples. It was observed that there was approximately a threefold increase in the prevalence of iMLSB *S. aureus* strains, from 7.5 to 21.7%, between 2013 and 2018. In contrast, Chavez-Bueno et al. (2005) suggested a significant decline in the trend for the prevalence of iMLSB phenotype from 93% in 1999 to 7% in 2002. Although our results markedly exhibited an increase in the prevalence of the inducible resistance among clinical *S. aureus* isolates in Iran, enhanced clinical and laboratory awareness of inducible resistance may also be responsible for this rise. Molecular epidemiology and prevalence of inducible resistance among *S. aureus* strains change geographically and dynamically (Monecke et al., 2011; Boswihi et al., 2016). In this experiment, the prevalence of iMLSB among *S. aureus* was found to be 10.9% with 84.1% MRSA and 15.9% MSSA isolates exhibiting iMLSB. This prevalence was lower than the rates reported from Nepal (21%) (Adhikari et al., 2017) and Jordan (76.7%) (Aqel et al., 2017), whereas it was higher than Brazil (7.9%) (Bottega et al., 2014). However, variable rates of iMLSB among *S. aureus* isolates have been reported in previously published data from Iran ranging from 4.1 to 20.7% (Memariani et al., 2009; Khashei et al., 2018). Regarding the increasing incidence of inducible resistance, our study suggests the necessity to revise the prescription of macrolides, which could cause a decline in resistance patterns. The investigated population and the prevalence of different clones in across various regions of the world could likely explain the striking differences in inducible clindamycin resistance.

In the present experiment, 18.3% of isolates tested were found to be resistant to mupirocin. This prevalence is higher than that reported rate in Jordan (5%) (Aqel et al., 2012) and other reports in France (2.2%) (Desroches et al., 2013) and Greece (1.6%) (Petinaki et al., 2004). A research performed by Abbasi-Montazeri et al. (2013) in Iran notified that 6% of *S. aureus* strains obtained from burn patients were detected as mupirocin-resistant. A high prevalence of resistance to mupirocin in this experiment indicates that there are unrestricted policies in the use of mupirocin for long periods and/or increasing trends of mupirocin prescription in our setup. Furthermore, we observed that 9.6 and 8.7% isolates had HLMUPR and LLMUPR phenotypes, respectively, which are higher than the rate stated in France (0.8%) (Desroches et al., 2013) and Korea (5%) (Yun et al., 2003). Different prevalence rates of HLMUPR *S. aureus* were reported from other researchers in Iran, 25% by Shahsavan et al. (2012) and 17% by Abbasi-Montazeri et al. (2013). We found that 9.5% of the examined isolates carried *mupA* gene, and all of them exhibited an HLMUPR phenotype. Researches from Spain (González-Domínguez et al., 2016) (27.2%) and Iran (Abbasi-Montazeri et al., 2013) (34%) revealed a higher rate of this gene among their *S. aureus* strains. Contrary to the study of Shahsavan et al. (2012), reporting *mupA* gene only in MRSA strains with cMLSB phenotype, the present data showed the existence of *mupA* gene in inducible resistance MRSA strains.

This study indicated that of 126 inducible clindamycin-resistant *S. aureus* isolates, 5.6% were fusidic acid–resistant, which was similar to those in Canada (7%) and Australia (7%); nonetheless, it was far lower than the values previously reported in Greece (62.4%) and Ireland (19.9%) (Castanheira et al., 2010a,b). In a multicenter experiment performed from 2007 to 2011 in three referral hospitals in Tehran, Iran, of 726 tested *S. aureus* isolates, 3% of isolates were found to be resistant to fusidic acid (Deotale et al., 2010). In our collections, we found that *fusB* and *fusC* were present in six strains and one strain, respectively. A previously studied experiment from China noted a higher rate of *fusB* gene (10.5%); on the other hand, *fusC* and *fusA* genes were not present in any of tested isolates (Yu et al., 2015). These data highlighted that *fusB* is the predominant determinant

responsible for resistance to fusidic acid among *S. aureus* in Iran. According to previously published data, different fusidic acid resistance rates were reported in both MRSA and MSSA strains. Notably, this study showed that fusidic acid resistance was only seen among MRSA isolates, which were in line with a report of China indicating that the prevalence of fusidic acid resistance among MRSA isolates was significantly higher than that among MSSA isolates (Yu et al., 2015).

According to the evidence, the ability to produce biofilm among *S. aureus* is diverse, with data ranging within 43 to 88% (Luther et al., 2018). Our results showed that, of the 126 isolates under investigation, 77% of strains could produce biofilm, whereas 23% were confirmed as non–biofilm producer strains. This finding is similar to those in Egypt (83.3%) (Gad et al., 2009), whereas based on a study of Iran biofilm production reported rate was 38.7% (a twofold decrease) (Mirzaee et al., 2014). In this study, the biofilm formability of MRSA isolates (78.3%) was higher than that of MSSA isolates (70%). Apparently, high capability of biofilm formation among MRSA strains was described by conducted studies from India (57.6%) (Mathur et al., 2006), China (66%) (Wang et al., 2010), and South Africa (37.8%) (Samie and Shivambu, 2011).

Data obtained from different studies suggest that the ability of biofilm formation in *S. aureus* strains is attributed to the expression of a wide range of virulence and adhesion factors of this bacterium (Nemati et al., 2009; Samie and Shivambu, 2011; Luther et al., 2018), but the correlation between the existence of specific virulence factor and biofilm production has been controversial. Researches has shown that *ica ABCD* and adhesion genes can affect the biofilm formation ability in *S. aureus*. In this study, the most frequent *ica* genes were *icaD* (73%), followed by *icaA* (71.4%), *icaB* (60.3%), and *icaC* (53.2%). According to an analysis by Mirzaee et al. (2014) on 31 clinical *S. aureus* isolates, *icaD*, *icaA*, and *icaC* genes with the exception of *icaB* were found in more than half of the isolates tested. In the study of Yousefi et al. (2016), of 39 isolates of *S. aureus* recovered from UTI patients, 69.2% were biofilm producers, and it was notable that all isolates carried *icaA*, *fnbA*, and *clfA* genes. In the current study, a high percentage of *icaABCD* genes made up 39.7% of the overall sample, which was close to a recent report in Iran (38.7%) (Mirzaee et al., 2014). The correlation between biofilm formation and the presence of adhesion genes is well established. In present survey, the most prevalent gene was *clfA* (93.7%), followed by *clfB* (87.3), *fnbB* (61.9%), *cna* (57.9%), *fnbA* (54%), *ebp* (50%), and *bap* (3.2%), respectively. The attained data are consistent with a previous finding from Iran, which has displayed the role of the *bap* gene in biofilm production rarely. Our findings indicated that isolates with more adhesion and *ica* encoding genes were strictly associated with biofilm formation. Overall, our data confirmed the high ability of biofilm formation among inducible resistance *S. aureus* strains, which helps *S. aureus* to persist in infections. This scenario draws attention from clinicians to use treatment protocols in patients potentially infected with these bacteria.

Based on the results of *coa* typing, the top three *coa* types were III (44.4%), II (28.6%), and IVa (9.5%). This result was in contrast with the previous report by Hirose et al. (2010) in Japan, which indicated that *coa* types II, VII, and I accounted for 91.9%, 3.9%, and 1.7% of isolates. We detected seven SC types (I–VI) among iMLSB *S. aureus* strains suggesting diverse genetic backgrounds of tested isolates in this region of Iran. In a research involving 157 *S. aureus* strains from clinical specimens, nine different patterns of *coa* gene were detected (Afrough et al., 2013). These findings were confirmed by results in Thailand (Janwithayanuchit et al., 2006) and Egypt (Omar et al., 2014) reported previously. Genetic variability in *coa* gene among studied isolates indicated that it could not be a predictor for specific iMLSB *S. aureus* strains.

In the present study, the findings revealed that seven different prophage profiles were identified in the isolates studied. A high diversity of prophage patterns among *S. aureus* isolates has been reported from the United States (Workman et al., 2006), Czech Republic (Pantůček et al., 2004) and Iran (Rahimi et al., 2012). Our data exhibited that SGFa-SGFb (36.5%) and SGB-SGFa-SGFb (31.7%) were the major prophage profiles, which was in accordance with the study of Rahimi et al. (2012). SGF-type prophages are associated with the immune evasion cluster typical for *S. aureus* isolated from humans (Kahánková et al., 2010). SGA has been reported to be common among *pvl*-positive MRSA-IV isolates. This finding was consistent with previous research, revealing that all the *pvl*-positive isolates harbored SGA prophage type (Rahimi et al., 2012). Notably, the PVL was the most frequently encoded toxin in the tested isolates (23.8%). Previously published data from England and the United States (Holmes et al., 2005) indicated that the prevalence of *pvl* encoding genes among *S. aureus* was low (1.6%). Nevertheless, previous reports all over the world had shown a high prevalence of *pvl* among *S. aureus* strains (Monecke et al., 2011; Boswihi et al., 2016; Goudarzi et al., 2016a). In Iran, the *pvl*-positive rate ranged from 7.4 to 55.6% in *S. aureus* isolates. In our research, a relatively low but increasing prevalence of *pvl*-positive *S. aureus* strains was noted. According to our report, a recent study from Ireland showed an ascending trend of *pvl* among MRSA strains (from 0.2 to 8.8%), whereas this trend was diminishing for MSSA strains (20–2.5%) (Shore et al., 2014). Although this difference can, to some extent, reflect the origin of isolates and the type of sample, this could also be because of different *pvl*-encoding phages among *S. aureus* strains.

Considering the genes encoding enterotoxins, the data analysis of the current study exhibited that 54.8% of isolates carried one or more SE genes, with the *sea* (19.8%) and *sec* (11.1%) genes being the most commonly found. The attained data are consistent with the reports previously obtained from Iran and Turkey estimating enterotoxigenic *S. aureus* strains in 45 and 62.6% of isolates tested, respectively (Imanifooladi et al., 2007; Aydin et al., 2011). Based on earlier studies, the *she*, *sei*, and *sej* encoding genes were rarely present in *S. aureus* isolated from clinical samples, and similarly, these genes were not detected in the present survey either.

The present study displayed diversity in the numbers and the molecular types of iMLSB *S. aureus* clones identified in our health care settings. According to the current results, CC8 was the most prevalent clone in both CO and HO *S. aureus* isolates. The prevalence of CC8 was increased from 2013–2014 (20%) to 2017–2018 (39.5%). These strains were found in association with *pvl*-encoding bacteriophage and HLMUPR,

which carried *mupA* gene, which is similar to those reported in Iran (Azimian et al., 2014), Kuwait (Boswihi et al., 2016), and Ireland (Shore et al., 2014). According to evidence, phenotypic and genotypic resistance pattern in the ST8-IV isolates was found to be varied. In accordance with our research, high resistance to aminoglycosides and low resistance to tetracycline in ST8-MRSA isolates were described previously by researchers (Shore et al., 2014; Boswihi et al., 2016). The enterotoxin gene *sed* was the solo toxin gene detected among the ST8-IV isolates. Variability in the enterotoxin genes within ST8-IV isolates was reported by several investigators (Shore et al., 2014; Boswihi et al., 2016). The detection of the ST8-IV isolates in our study is of concern and highlights transmissibility and rapidity of its spread as an international epidemic MRSA clone in Iran.

ST239-MRSA-III, one of the most successful and persistent clones, was the most predominant genotype in CC8. Multiresistant ST239 clone was previously reported in South American, European, and some Asian countries, including Kuwait and Saudi Arabia (Shore et al., 2014; Boswihi et al., 2016). In this study, ST239 had five important *spa* types (t030, t037, t631, t860, and 388). The data in this experiment indicated that half of ST239-SCC*mec* III/t631 strains exhibited HLMUPR phenotype and harbored *mupA* gene. These findings are in parallel with previous reports from Iran (Goudarzi et al., 2016a) and those reported in India and Kuwait (Abimanyu et al., 2012; Boswihi et al., 2016). All ST239-SCC*mec* III/t860 strains exhibited the LLMUPR phenotype, which was similar to findings in other countries including China and Kuwait (Boswihi et al., 2016; Liang et al., 2018). According to the molecular typing results, ST239-SCC*mec* III/030 with 20.5% and ST239-SCC*mec* III/037 with 25% were recognized as the most common multiresistant ST239- MRSA-III type. These results were consistent with previous research performed by Li et al. (2018), who demonstrated multiresistant ST239-SCC*mec* III/030 as the most predominant genotype in China from 2005 to 2013, which decreased significantly in 2016. During a 12-year period in Norway, Fossum and Bukholm (2006) indicated ST239 as the most prevalent MRSA clones, which became endemic in hospital environments in Norway. However, molecular characteristics, especially antibiotic resistance gene and virulence factors, of our ST239-MRSA-III strains were similar to those of ST239 strains reported in Kuwait, China, and Saudi Arabia (Lewis and Jorgensen, 2005; Boswihi et al., 2016). The emergence of ST239-MRSA-III may be due to the import of this clone from neighboring countries.

Increasing prevalence rate of CC8 and disappearance of CC22 between 2013 and 2018 highlighted replacement and the changing clonal structure of MRSA in this region of Iran. As summarized in **Table 5**, *pvl* encoding genes were detected in two isolates of ST22-SCC*mec* IV/t852 and one isolate of ST22-SCC*mec* IV/t005. These *pvl*-positive genotypes were mainly distributed at some geographic area including England, Australia, Ireland, Kuwait, Iran, Germany, Saudi Arabia, and Nepal (Monecke et al., 2011; Shore et al., 2014; Boswihi et al., 2016). Of note, the majority of the ST22-SCC*mec* IV/t790 isolates was related to the *tst* gene, demonstrated LLMUPR phenotype, and could exhibit multiresistance. A recent report in Ireland also displayed that most of *pvl*-positive ST22-MRSA-IV isolates were associated with resistance to gentamicin, trimethoprim, and ciprofloxacin and carried the *erm(C)*, *lnu(A)*, *aacA-aphD*, *aadD*, and *mupA* genes (Shore et al., 2014).

The ST22-MSSA isolates exhibited different antimicrobial resistance patterns including resistance to penicillin, gentamicin, tetracycline, kanamycin, rifampin, tobramycin, and amikacin. Our data are in concordance with a study conducted in Ireland, which reported the prevalence of low frequency of ST22-MSSA/t005 and ST22-MSSA/t1869 strains during the study period from 2002 to 2011. They indicated that ST22-MSSA was resistant to amikacin, ampicillin, fusidic acid, gentamycin, kanamycin, and tobramycin with multiple resistance genes *blaZ*, *aacA-aphD*, and *dfrS1* detected among these isolates (Shore et al., 2014).

Our data showed that 40% of the CC/ST30 isolates carried *pvl*, which belonged to MRSA and MSSA strains. PVL-positive CC30/ST30-IV strains have been described in Iran (Goudarzi et al., 2016a,b), Kuwait (Boswihi et al., 2016), and Ireland (Shore et al., 2014). Importantly, the prevalence of CC30/ST30 increased from 8% in 2013 to 18.4% in 2018 in our country. In this connection, Boswihi et al. exhibited ST30 as the second dominant MRSA genotypes in Kuwait hospitals, which decreased from 30% in 2001–2003 to 22% in 2006. They also showed a low prevalence of ST30-IV-MRSA among tested isolates (2.9%) (Boswihi et al., 2016). Surprisingly, all MRSA isolates carried biofilm and adhesion-related genes, and approximately 90% of the MSSA isolates were able to form biofilm at different intensities. In line with our study, Chamon et al. (2015) from Brazil showed biofilm production ability among ST30 strains. They also found *bbp* gene as a possible marker of this lineage. Congruent with the previous observations (Shore et al., 2014; Boswihi et al., 2016), all of our ST30 isolates belonged to *agr* type III, with different toxin and antimicrobial resistance patterns noted for this genotype.

As aforementioned, fewer than half of the CC/ST80-MRSA-IV isolates showed aminoglycoside resistance encoded by *ant (4')-Ia*, *aac (6')-Ie/aph (2'')*. Resistance to fusidic acid encoded by *fusB* was detected in one isolate. These results were different from a previous study conducted in Ireland, which exhibited all CC/ST80-MRSA-IV isolates were resistant to kanamycin and neomycin, encoded by *aph (3')-IIIa*. In addition, our data revealed that resistances to tetracycline, fusidic acid, and erythromycin encoded by *tet(K)*, *fusB*, and *erm(C)*, respectively, were frequent among tested isolates (Shore et al., 2014). The variations could be a result of differences in the genetic backgrounds of the *S. aureus* strains. The prevalence of CC/ST80-MRSA-IV increased from 12% in 2013 to 13.2% in 2018. This increasing rate of ST80-IV raises the concern that this strain is becoming endemic in our hospitals.

Based on the evidence, ST80-IV is acknowledged as a toxigenic virulent isolate. In the present study, *pvl*-positive CC/ST80-SCC*mec*/t044 isolates were confirmed by approximately half of the isolates. ST80-MRSA-MRSA isolates harboring the *pvl* genes

were previously reported from Kuwait, Malaysia, Singapore, and Ireland (Shore et al., 2014; Boswihi et al., 2016).

According to previously published data, CC/ST59 has limited geographical spread. In the present research CC/ST59 was present in 10 isolates, accounting for 7.9%. This clone was previously reported in Australia, Ireland, United Kingdom, Korea, Kuwait, and Taiwan (Monecke et al., 2011; Boswihi et al., 2016). In this study, the results revealed that our isolates carried resistance genes at a relatively low level, but *erm*(C) encoding resistance to erythromycin was noted in more than half of the isolates. Conversely, high frequencies of multiple resistance genes including *erm*(B), *aph (3')-IIIa*, and *tet*(K) were identified among tested isolates of a study performed in Ireland (Shore et al., 2014). Notably, resistance to fusidic acid encoded by *fusB* was also detected in one isolate, which was similar to the previous report from Ireland (Shore et al., 2014). According to this experiment, 66.7% of the isolates were positive for *seb* (60.4%) gene. This is inconsistent with the research conducted in Ireland showing that *seb* gene could be a possible marker of this lineage. The observed frequency of CC59/ST338-SCC*mec*III/t437 isolates was in accordance with previous reports, as this genotype is infrequently isolated (Li et al., 2013).

Another clone found among inducible resistance *S. aureus* strains was ST5-SCC*mec* IV/t002 (7.1%). Recent studies have shown the presence of CC/ST5- SCC*mec*IV/t002 clones in Asian and European countries, such as Iran, Japan, Korea, the United Arab Emirates, Kuwait, Ireland, and Australia (Monecke et al., 2011; Boswihi et al., 2016). The present data indicated that the prevalence of CC/ST5- SCC*mec*IV/t002 diminished during the study from 8% in 2013–2014 to 2.6% in 2017–2018. Conversely, a recent cross-sectional study performed in New Zealand on 3,323 patients from 2005 to 2011 documented seven most frequent MRSA clones. This study also indicated an ST5-SCC*mec*IV clone, which rapidly displaced ST30-SCC*mec*IV as the dominant CA-MRSA clone (Williamson et al., 2013). It was also observed that nearly half of ST5-SCC*mec*IV/t002 isolates were confirmed as HLMUPR strains. The finding of CC/ST5-SCC*mec*IV/t002 isolates in our screening indicated that resistance was observed for erythromycin encoded by *erm*(A), tetracycline encoded by *tet*(M), and mupirocin encoded by *mupA*. In an experiment conducted in 2010 in China, Song et al. (2013) revealed a different result. They showed a high prevalence of ST5-SCC*mec*IV/t002 among their clinical *S. aureus* isolates.

As shown in **Table 5**, the CC1 isolates belonged to two STs (ST772 and ST1). *spa* types t10795 and t657 pertained to ST772, whereas *spa* type t6811 was identified in ST1 isolates. ST772- SCC*mec*V, which is known as Bengal Bay clone, emerged in Bangladesh and was reported in New Zealand, Nepal, Italy, the United Arab Emirates, Malaysia, the United Kingdom, Ireland, Saudi Arabia, India, Australia, and Kuwait (Monecke et al., 2011; Shore et al., 2014; Boswihi et al., 2016). This clone was found in 6.4% of the examined isolates. All isolates were multiresistant and carried *aac (6')-Ie/aph (2'')*, *aph (3')-IIIa*, *tet*(M), and *erm(B)*. The attained data are in accordance to results of the study of Shore et al. (2014), which reported MDR pattern and carriage of *ant (4′)-Ia, aac (6′)-Ie/aph (2″)*, and *tet*(M) genes among CC1/ST772-SCC*mec*V isolates. The study demonstrated similarities in genetic characteristics including susceptibility to antibiotics and toxin-encoding genes of our ST772-SCC*mec*V isolates recently reported in Kuwait (Boswihi et al., 2016). Of two CC1/ST1-SCC*mec*V/t6811 isolates, one isolate carried *fusc* and exhibited resistance to fusidic acid at MIC 32 μg/mL. Boswihi et al. (2016) previously reported ST1-SCCmecV/t6811 carrying *fusC* gene from Kuwait.

In contrast to our study, which reported a low prevalence of ST15 (4%), a recent multicenter study performed in 25 European countries documented a relatively high prevalence of ST15 and reported it as the second most frequent clone across most of the European countries (Grundmann et al., 2014). In a study of 568 *S. aureus* isolates in 11 European countries, researchers reported a low level of this type among the tested isolates (Rolo et al., 2012). Our data demonstrated that all the ST15 isolates were *pvl*-positive and displayed the LLMUPR phenotype. The analysis of our previous study indicated that the most common mupirocin-resistant MRSA isolates belonged to ST15-SCC*mec* IV/t084 (Goudarzi et al., 2017), which is in line with the present data. Although ST15 is more frequently detected in MRSA, there are reports that indicate the high distribution of this type among MSSA strains (Monecke et al., 2011; Boswihi et al., 2016). It was notable that all ST15 isolates harbored SCC*mec* IV, *agr* type II, and *coa* type I and belonged to *spa* type t084. Different antimicrobial resistance patterns were noted among these isolates, which is in accordance with previous studies (Rolo et al., 2012; Grundmann et al., 2014; Goudarzi et al., 2017).

In contrast to a study conducted in Kuwait, which reported CC45 as one of the most epidemics MRSA isolates with different antimicrobial resistance patterns, in the current research, a low frequency of the CC45 (4%) was observed among examined isolates. In a study conducted in the South of Poland, 26.1% of *S. aureus* isolates were found to be related to CC45 (Ilczyszyn et al., 2016). This ST was at its most prevalent in 2015, when it accounted for 22.2% (4/18) of inducible resistance isolates, reduced to 4.2% (1/24) in 2016, and disappeared in 2017–2018.

The strengths of our research included examining the prevalence and temporal differences in iMLSB *S. aureus* strains. It was the first study on the molecular characterization of inducible clindamycin-resistant *S. aureus* strains from Iran. However, the present research had limitations. One limitation of our study was the modest sample size and the impossibility of using typing methods such as pulsed-field gel electrophoresis (PFGE). It was not possible either to correlate demographics data with circulating clones owing to a lack of data linking patient characteristics. Another important limitation of our study was *clfA*- and *clfB*-negative *S. aureus* strains, which were unusual and required further analysis using whole-genome sequencing and microarray system.

CONCLUSION

This was the first report of monitoring the prevalence and characterization of *S. aureus* isolates with the inducible resistance phenotype in Iran. Our investigation supports a detailed epidemiological survey on the prevalence and temporal differences in iMLSB *S. aureus* strains. It was ultimately attained that there is a considerable increasing trend for CC8 versus a decreasing trend for CC22. However, we revealed a shift in the clonal composition of MRSA isolates over time with the emphasis on a progressive replacement of CC22 clone by CC8 clones between 2013 and 2018. Indeed, our research indicated that iMLSB *S. aureus* isolates with similar genetic backgrounds exhibited specific virulence gene profiles, antimicrobial resistance patterns, and biofilm patterns. Increase in *S. aureus* with inducible resistance phenotype harboring SCC*mec*IV during the 5-year period makes sense that there is a shift in the iMLSB population from our community to hospital. Therefore, we conclude that there is a need for ongoing and nationwide surveillance studies to further evaluate of *S. aureus* with inducible resistance phenotype and to prevent these strains from becoming endemic in the Iranian hospitals.

ETHICS STATEMENT

The current study protocol was approved by the Ethics Committee of the Shahid Beheshti University of Medical Sciences in Tehran, Iran (IR.SBMU.MSP.REC.1396.700). Written informed consent was obtained from participants.

AUTHOR CONTRIBUTIONS

MG and HG conceived, designed, and supervised the study. MD, RaP, MN, MF, MM, SS, and AA performed the experiments. NK, RoP, and MG analyzed and interpreted the data. MG, HG, NK, SS, and RoP drafted and written the manuscript. All authors approved the final version of manuscript.

FUNDING

This study was supported financially by the grant (No. 12688) from Research Deputy of Shahid Beheshti University of Medical Sciences, Tehran, Iran.

ACKNOWLEDGMENTS

We are indebted to Dr. Edet E. Udo (Kuwait University) and Dr. Agnes Marie Sá Figueiredo (Universidade Federal do Rio de Janeiro) for providing reference strains of the *S. aureus*

REFERENCES

Abbasi-Montazeri, E., Khosravi, A. D., Feizabadi, M. M., Goodarzi, H., Khoramrooz, S. S., Mirzaii, M., et al. (2013). The prevalence of methicillin resistant Staphylococcus aureus (MRSA) isolates with high-level mupirocin resistance from patients and personnel in a burn center. Burns 39, 650–654. doi: 10.1016/j.burns.2013.02.005

Abimanyu, N., Murugesan, S., and Krishnan, P. (2012). Emergence of methicillin-resistant Staphylococcus aureus ST239 with high-level mupirocin and inducible clindamycin resistance in a tertiary care center in Chennai. South India. J. Clin. Microbiol. 50, 3412–3413. doi: 10.1128/JCM.01663-12

Adhikari, R., Shrestha, S., Barakoti, A., and Amatya, R. (2017). Inducible clindamycin and methicillin resistant Staphylococcus aureus in a tertiary care hospital. Kathmandu, Nepal. BMC. Infect. Dis. 17:483. doi: 10.1186/s12879-017-2584-5

Afrough, P., Pourmand, M. R., Sarajian, A. A., Saki, M., and Saremy, S. (2013). Molecular investigation of Staphylococcus aureus, coa and spa genes in Ahvaz hospitals, staff nose compared with patients clinical samples. Jundishapur. J. Microbiol. 6:e5377.

Aqel, A., Alzoubi, H., and Al-Zereini, W. (2017). Prevalence of inducible clindamycin resistance in methicillin-resistant Staphylococcus aureus: the first study in Jordan. J. Infect. Dev. Ctries. 11, 350–354. doi: 10.3855/jidc.8316

Aqel, A., Ibrahim, A., and Shehabi, A. (2012). Rare occurrence of mupirocin resistance among clinical Staphylococcus isolates in Jordan. Acta Microbiol. Immun. Hung 59, 239–247. doi: 10.1556/AMicr.59.2012.2.8

Arciola, C. R., Campoccia, D., Gamberini, S., Cervellati, M., Donati, E., and Montanaro, L. J. B. (2002). Detection of slime production by means of an optimised Congo red agar plate test based on a colourimetric scale in Staphylococcus epidermidis clinical isolates genotyped for ica locus. Biomaterials 23, 4233–4239. doi: 10.1016/S0142-9612(02)00171-0

Aydin, A., Sudagidan, M., and Muratoglu, K. (2011). Prevalence of staphylococcal enterotoxins, toxin genes and genetic-relatedness of foodborne Staphylococcus aureus strains isolated in the Marmara Region of Turkey. Int. J. Food. Microbiol. 148, 99–106. doi: 10.1016/j.ijfoodmicro.2011.05.007

Azimian, A., Havaei, S. A., Ghazvini, K., Khosrojerdi, M., Naderi, M., and Samiee, S. M. (2014). Isolation of PVL/ACME-positive, community acquired, methicillin-resistant Staphylococcus aureus (USA300) from Iran. J. Med. Microbiol. 2, 100–104.

Boswihi, S. S., Udo, E. E., and Al-Sweih, N. (2016). Shifts in the clonal distribution of methicillin-resistant Staphylococcus aureus in Kuwait hospitals: 1992-2010. PLoS One 11:e0162744. doi: 10.1371/journal.pone.0162744

Bottega, A., Rodrigues, M. D. A., Carvalho, F. A., Wagner, T. F., Leal, I. A. S., Santos, S. O. D., et al. (2014). Evaluation of constitutive and inducible resistance to clindamycin in clinical samples of Staphylococcus aureus from a tertiary hospital. Rev. Soc. Bras. Med. Trop. 47, 589–592. doi: 10.1590/0037-8682-0140-2014

Boye, K., Bartels, M. D., Andersen, I. S., Moeller, J. A., Westh, H. (2007). A new multiplex PCR for easy screening of methicillin-resistant Staphylococcus aureus SCCmec types I–V. J. Clin. Microbiol. 13, 725–727. doi: 10.1111/j.1469-0691.2007.01720.x

Castanheira, M., Watters, A. A., Bell, J. M., Turnidge, J. D., and Jones, R. N. (2010a). Fusidic acid resistance rates and prevalence of resistance mechanisms among Staphylococcus spp. isolated in North America and Australia, 2007-2008. Antimicrob. Agents. Chemother. 54, 3614–3617. doi: 10.1128/AAC.01390-09

Castanheira, M., Watters, A. A., Mendes, R. E., Farrell, D. J., and Jones, R. N. (2010b). Occurrence and molecular characterization of fusidic acid resistance mechanisms among Staphylococcus spp. from European countries (2008). J. Antimicrob. Chemother. 65, 1353–1358. doi: 10.1093/jac/dkq094

Chamon, R. C., Iorio, N. L. P., da Silva Ribeiro, S., Cavalcante, F. S., and dos Santos, K. R. N. (2015). Molecular characterization of Staphylococcus aureus isolates carrying the Panton-Valentine leukocidin genes from Rio de Janeiro hospitals. Diagn. Microbiol. Infect. Dis. 83, 331–334. doi: 10.1016/j.diagmicrobio.2015.09.004

Chavez-Bueno, S., Bozdogan, B., Katz, K., Bowlware, K. L., Cushion, N., Cavuoti, D., et al. (2005). Inducible clindamycin resistance and molecular epidemiologic trends of pediatric community-acquired methicillin-resistant Staphylococcus aureus in Dallas. Texas. Antimicrob. Agents. Chemother. 49, 2283–2288. doi: 10.1128/AAC.49.6.2283-2288.2005

Dadashi, M., Nasiri, M. J., Fallah, F., Owlia, P., Hajikhani, B., Emaneini, M., et al. (2018). Methicillin-resistant Staphylococcus aureus (MRSA) in Iran: a systematic review and meta-analysis. J. Glob. Antimicrob. Resist. 12, 96–103. doi: 10.1016/j.jgar.2017.09.006

Deotale, V., Mendiratta, D., Raut, U., and Narang, P. (2010). Inducible clindamycin resistance in Staphylococcus aureus isolated from clinical samples. Indian. J. Med. Microbiol. 28:124. doi: 10.4103/0255-0857.62488

Desroches, M., Potier, J., Laurent, F., Bourrel, A.-S., Doucet-Populaire, F., Decousser, J.-W., et al. (2013). Prevalence of mupirocin resistance among invasive coagulase-negative staphylococci and methicillin-resistant Staphylococcus aureus (MRSA) in France: emergence of a mupirocin-resistant MRSA clone harbouring mupA. J. Antimicrob. Chemother. 68, 1714–1717. doi: 10.1093/jac/dkt085

Diep, B. A., Stone, G. G., Basuino, L., Graber, C. J., Miller, A., des Etages, S. A., et al. (2008). The arginine catabolic mobile element and staphylococcal chromosomal cassette mec linkage: convergence of virulence and resistance in the USA300 clone of methicillin-resistant Staphylococcus aureus. J. Infect. Dis. 197, 1523–1530. doi: 10.1086/587907

Enright, M. C., Day, N. P., Davies, C. E., Peacock, S. J., and Spratt, B. G. (2000). Multilocus sequence typing for characterization of methicillin-resistant and methicillin-susceptible clones ofStaphylococcus aureus. J. Clin. Microbiol. 38, 1008–1015.

Fossum, A., and Bukholm, G. (2006). Increased incidence of methicillin-resistant Staphylococcus aureus ST80, novel ST125 and SCCmecIV in the south-eastern part of Norway during a 12-year period. J. Clin. Microbiol. 12, 627–633. doi: 10.1111/j.1469-0691.2006.01467.x

Gad, G. F. M., El-Feky, M. A., El-Rehewy, M. S., Hassan, M. A., Abolella, H., and El-Baky, R. M. A. (2009). Detection of icaA, icaD genes and biofilm production by Staphylococcus aureus and Staphylococcus epidermidis isolated from urinary tract catheterized patients. J. Infect. Dev. Countr. 3, 342–351. doi: 10.3855/jidc.241

Gilot, P., Lina, G., Cochard, T., and Poutrel, B. (2002). Analysis of the genetic variability of genes encoding the RNA III-activating components Agr and TRAP in a population of Staphylococcus aureus strains isolated from cows with mastitis. J. Clin. Microbiol. 40, 4060–4067. doi: 10.1128/jcm.40.11.4060-4067.2002

González-Domínguez, M., Seral, C., Potel, C., Sáenz, Y., Álvarez, M., Torres, C., et al. (2016). Genotypic and phenotypic characterization of methicillin-resistant Staphylococcus aureus (MRSA) clones with high-level mupirocin resistance. Diagn. Microbiol. Infect. Dis. 85, 213–217. doi: 10.1016/j.diagmicrobio.2016.02.021

Gordon, R. J., and Lowy, F. D. (2008). Pathogenesis of methicillin-resistant Staphylococcus aureus infection. Clin. Infect. Dis. 46(Suppl. 5), S350–S359. doi: 10.1086/533591

Goudarzi, M., Bahramian, M., Tabrizi, M. S., Udo, E. E., Figueiredo, A. M. S., Fazeli, M., et al. (2017). Genetic diversity of methicillin resistant Staphylococcus aureus strains isolated from burn patients in Iran: ST239-SCCmec III/t037 emerges as the major clone. Microb. Pathog. 105, 1–7. doi: 10.1016/j.micpath.2017.02.004

Goudarzi, M., Goudarzi, H., Figueiredo, A. M. S., Udo, E. E., Fazeli, M., Asadzadeh, M., et al. (2016a). Molecular characterization of methicillin resistant Staphylococcus aureus strains isolated from intensive care units in Iran: ST22-SCCmec IV/t790 emerges as the major clone. PLoS One 11:e0155529. doi: 10.1371/journal.pone.0155529

Goudarzi, M., Seyedjavadi, S. S., Azad, M., Goudarzi, H., and Azimi, H. (2016b). Distribution of spa types, integrons and associated gene cassettes in Staphylococcus aureus strains isolated from intensive care units of hospitals in Tehran, Iran. Arch. Clin. Infect. Dis. 11, 1–11.

Gould, I. M., David, M. Z., Esposito, S., Garau, J., Lina, G., Mazzei, T., et al. (2012). New insights into meticillin-resistant Staphylococcus aureus (MRSA) pathogenesis, treatment and resistance. Int. J. Antimicrob. Agents 39, 96–104. doi: 10.1016/j.ijantimicag.2011.09.028

Grundmann, H., Schouls, L. M., Aanensen, D. M., Pluister, G. N., Tami, A., Chlebowicz, M., et al. (2014). The dynamic changes of dominant clones of Staphylococcus aureus causing bloodstream infections in the European region: results of a second structured survey. Euro. Surveill. 19:20987. doi: 10.2807/1560-7917.es2014.19.49.20987

Harmsen, D., Claus, H., Witte, W., Rothgänger, J., Claus, H., Turnwald, D., et al. (2003). Typing of methicillin-resistant Staphylococcus aureus in a university hospital setting by using novel software for spa repeat determination and database management. *J. Clin. Microbiol.* 41, 5442–5448. doi: 10.1128/jcm.41. 12.5442-5448.2003

Hirose, M., Kobayashi, N., Ghosh, S., Paul, S. K., Shen, T., Urushibara, N., et al. (2010). Identification of Staphylocoagulase Genotypes I-X and Discrimination of Type IV and V Subtypes by Multiplex PCR Assay for Clinical Isolates of *Staphylococcus aureus. Jpn. J. Infect. Dis.* 63, 257–263.

Holmes, A., Ganner, M., McGuane, S., Pitt, T., Cookson, B., and Kearns, A. (2005). *Staphylococcus aureus* isolates carrying Panton-Valentine leucocidin genes in England and Wales: frequency, characterization, and association with clinical disease. *J. Clin. Microbiol.* 43, 2384–2390. doi: 10.1128/JCM.43.5.2384-2390. 2005

Ilczyszyn, W. M., Sabat, A. J., Akkerboom, V., Szkarlat, A., Klepacka, J., Sowa-Sierant, I., et al. (2016). Clonal structure and characterization of *Staphylococcus aureus* strains from invasive infections in paediatric patients from South Poland: association between age, spa types, clonal complexes, and genetic markers. *PLoS One* 11:e0151937. doi: 10.1371/journal.pone.015 1937

Imanifooladi, A., Sattari, M., Peerayeh, S. N., Hassan, Z., and Hossainidoust, S. (2007). Detection the *Staphylococcus aureus* producing enterotoxin isolated from skin infections in hospitalized patients. *Pak. J. Biol. Sci.* 10, 502–505.

Janwithayanuchit, I., Ngam-Ululert, S., Paungmoung, P., and Rangsipanuratn, W. (2006). Epidemiologic study of methicillin-resistant *Staphylococcus aureus* by coagulase gene polymorphism. *Scienceasia* 32, 127–132. doi: 10.2306/ scienceasia1513-1874.2006.32.127

Kahánková, J., Pantůček, R., Goerke, C., Růžičková, V., Holochová, P., and Doškař, J. (2010). Multilocus PCR typing strategy for differentiation of *Staphylococcus aureus* siphoviruses reflecting their modular genome structure. *Environ. Microbiol.* 12, 2527–2538. doi: 10.1111/j.1462-2920.2010. 02226.x

Khashei, R., Malekzadegan, Y., Sedigh Ebrahim-Saraie, H., and Razavi, Z. (2018). Phenotypic and genotypic characterization of macrolide, lincosamide and streptogramin B resistance among clinical isolates of staphylococci in southwest of Iran. *BMC. Res. Notes* 11:711. doi: 10.1186/s13104-018-3817-4

Lewis, J. S., and Jorgensen, J. H. (2005). Inducible clindamycin resistance in staphylococci: should clinicians and microbiologists be concerned? *Clin. Infect. Dis.* 40, 280–285. doi: 10.1086/426894

Li, J., Wang, L., Ip, M., Sun, M., Sun, J., Huang, G., et al. (2013). Molecular and clinical characteristics of clonal complex 59 methicillin-resistant *Staphylococcus aureus* infections in Mainland China. *PLoS One* 8:e70602. doi: 10.1371/journal. pone.0070602

Li, S., Sun, S., Yang, C., Chen, H., Yin, Y., Li, H., et al. (2018). The changing pattern of population structure of *Staphylococcus aureus* from bacteremia in China from 2013 to 2016: ST239-030-MRSA replaced by ST59-t437. *Front. Microbiol.* 9:332. doi: 10.3389/fmicb.2018.00332

Liang, B., Mai, J., Liu, Y., Huang, Y., Zhong, H., Xie, Y., et al. (2018). Prevalence and Characterization of *Staphylococcus aureus* isolated from women and Children in Guangzhou. *China. Front. Microbiol.* 9:2790. doi: 10.3389/fmicb.2018.02790

Luther, M. K., Parente, D. M., Caffrey, A. R., Daffinee, K. E., Lopes, V. V., Martin, E. T., et al. (2018). Clinical and genetic risk factors for biofilm-forming *Staphylococcus aureus. Antimicrob. Agents Chemother.* 62, e2252–e2217. doi: 10.1128/AAC.02252-17

Mathur, T., Singhal, S., Khan, S., Upadhyay, D., Fatma, T., and Rattan, A. (2006). Detection of biofilm formation among the clinical isolates of staphylococci: an evaluation of three different screening methods. *Indian J. Med. Microbiol.* 24:25. doi: 10.4103/0255-0857.19890

Memariani, M., Pourmand, M., Shirazi, M., Dallal, M., Abdossamadi, Z., and Mardani, N. (2009). The importance of inducible clindamycin resistance in enterotoxin positive *S. aureus* isolated from clinical samples. *Tehran. Univ. Med. J.* 67, 250–256.

Mirzaee, M., Najar-Peerayeh, S., Behmanesh, M., Forouzandeh-Moghadam, M., and Ghasemian, A.-M. (2014). Detection of intracellular adhesion (ica) gene and biofilm formation *Staphylococcus aureus* isolates from clinical blood cultures. *J. Med. Bacteriol.* 3, 1–7.

Monday, S. R., and Bohach, G. A. (1999). Use of multiplex PCR to detect classical and newly described pyrogenic toxin genes in staphylococcal isolates. *J. Clin. Microbiol.* 37, 3411–3414.

Monecke, S., Coombs, G., Shore, A. C., Coleman, D. C., Akpaka, P., Borg, M., et al. (2011). A field guide to pandemic, epidemic and sporadic clones of methicillin-resistant *Staphylococcus aureus. PLoS One* 6:e17936. doi: 10.1371/journal.pone. 0017936

Nemati, M., Hermans, K., Devriese, L. A., Maes, D., and Haesebrouck, F. (2009). Screening of genes encoding adhesion factors and biofilm formation in *Staphylococcus aureus* isolates from poultry. *Avian. Pathol.* 38, 513–517. doi: 10.1080/03079450903349212

Nezhad, R. R., Meybodi, S. M., Rezaee, R., Goudarzi, M., and Fazeli, M. (2017). Molecular characterization and resistance profile of methicillin resistant *Staphylococcus aureus* strains isolated from hospitalized patients in intensive care unit. *Tehran-Iran. Jundishapur. J. Microbiol.* 10:e41666. doi: 10.5812/jjm. 41666

Omar, N. Y., Ali, H. A. S., Harfoush, R. A. H., and El Khayat, E. H. (2014). Molecular typing of methicillin resistant *Staphylococcus aureus* clinical isolates on the basis of protein A and coagulase gene polymorphisms. *Int. J. Microbiol.* 2014:650328. doi: 10.1155/2014/650328

Pantosti, A., Sanchini, A., and Monaco, M. (2007). Mechanisms of antibiotic resistance in *Staphylococcus aureus. Future Microbiol.* 2, 323–334. doi: 10.2217/ 17460913.2.3.323

Pantůček, R., Doškař, J., Růžičková, V., Kašpárek, P., Oráčová, E., Kvardova, V., et al. (2004). Identification of bacteriophage types and their carriage in *Staphylococcus aureus. Arch. Virol.* 149, 1689–1703. doi: 10.1007/s00705-004-0335-6

Patel, M., Waites, K. B., Moser, S. A., Cloud, G. A., and Hoesley, C. J. (2006). Prevalence of inducible clindamycin resistance among community- and hospital-associated *Staphylococcus aureus* isolates. *J. Clin. Microbiol.* 44, 2481–2484. doi: 10.1128/JCM.02582-05

Petinaki, E., Spiliopoulou, I., Kontos, F., Maniati, M., Bersos, Z., Stakias, N., et al. (2004). Clonal dissemination of mupirocin-resistant staphylococci in Greek hospitals. *J. Antimicrob. Chemother.* 53, 105–108. doi: 10.1093/jac/dkh028

Rahimi, F., Bouzari, M., Katouli, M., and Pourshafie, M. R. (2012). Prophage and antibiotic resistance profiles of methicillin-resistant *Staphylococcus aureus* strains in Iran. *Arch. Virol.* 157, 1807–1811. doi: 10.1007/s00705-012-1361-4

Rolo, J., Miragaia, M., Turlej-Rogacka, A., Empel, J., Bouchami, O., Faria, N. A., et al. (2012). High genetic diversity among community-associated *Staphylococcus aureus* in Europe: results from a multicenter study. *PLoS One* 7:e34768. doi: 10.1371/journal.pone.0034768

Samie, A., and Shivambu, N. (2011). Biofilm production and antibiotic susceptibility profiles of *Staphylococcus aureus* isolated from HIV and AIDS patients in the Limpopo Province, South Africa. *Afr. J. Biotechnol.* 10, 14625–14636. doi: 10.5897/AJB11.1287

Shahsavan, S., Emaneini, M., Khoshgnab, B. N., Khoramian, B., Asadollahi, P., Aligholi, M., et al. (2012). A high prevalence of mupirocin and macrolide resistance determinant among *Staphylococcus aureus* strains isolated from burnt patients. *Burns* 38, 378–382. doi: 10.1016/j.burns.2011.09.004

Shore, A. C., Tecklenborg, S. C., Brennan, G. I., Ehricht, R., Monecke, S., and Coleman, D. C. (2014). Panton-Valentine leukocidin-positive *Staphylococcus aureus* in Ireland from 2002 to 2011: 21 clones, frequent importation of clones, temporal shifts of predominant methicillin-resistant *S. aureus* clones, and increasing multiresistance. *J. Clin. Microbiol.* 52, 859–870. doi: 10.1128/JCM. 02799-13

Song, Y., Du, X., Li, T., Zhu, Y., and Li, M. (2013). Phenotypic and molecular characterization of *Staphylococcus aureus* recovered from different clinical specimens of inpatients at a teaching hospital in Shanghai between 2005 and 2010. *J. Med. Microbiol.* 62, 274–282. doi: 10.1099/jmm.0.050971-0

Stepanović, S., Vuković, D., Hola, V., Bonaventura, G. D., Djukić, S., Ćirković, I., et al. (2007). Quantification of biofilm in microtiter plates: overview of testing conditions and practical recommendations for assessment of biofilm production by staphylococci. *APMIS* 115, 891–899. doi: 10.1111/j.1600-0463. 2007.apm_630.x

Wang, L., Liu, Y., Yang, Y., Huang, G., Wang, C., Deng, L., et al. (2012). Multidrug-resistant clones of community-associated meticillin-resistant *Staphylococcus aureus* isolated from Chinese children and the resistance genes to clindamycin and mupirocin. *J. Med. Microbiol.* 61, 1240–1247. doi: 10.1099/jmm.0.042663-0

Wang, L., Yu, F., Yang, L., Li, Q., Zeng, X. Z., and Xu, Y. (2010). Prevalence of virulence genes and biofilm formation among *Staphylococcus aureus* clinical isolates associated with lower respiratory infection. *Afr. J. Microbiol. Res.* 4, 2566–2569.

Williamson, D. A., Roberts, S. A., Ritchie, S. R., Coombs, G. W., Fraser, J. D., and Heffernan, H. (2013). Clinical and molecular epidemiology of methicillin-resistant *Staphylococcus aureus* in New Zealand: rapid emergence of sequence type 5 (ST5)-SCCmec-IV as the dominant community-associated MRSA clone. *PLoS One* 8:e62020. doi: 10.1371/journal.pone.0062020

Workman, M., Nigro, O. D., and Steward, G. F. (2006). Identification of prophage in Hawaiian coastal water isolate of *Staphylococcus Aureus*. *J. Young. Investig.* 15, 1–8.

Yousefi, M., Pourmand, M. R., Fallah, F., Hashemi, A., Mashhadi, R., and Nazari-Alam, A. (2016). Characterization of *Staphylococcus aureus* biofilm formation in urinary tract infection. *Iran J. Public Health* 45:485.

Yu, F., Liu, Y., Lu, C., Jinnan, L., Qi, X., Ding, Y., et al. (2015). Dissemination of fusidic acid resistance among *Staphylococcus aureus* clinical isolates. *BMC. Microbiol.* 15:210. doi: 10.1186/s12866-015-0552-z

Yun, H.-J., Lee, S. W., Yoon, G. M., Kim, S. Y., Choi, S., Lee, Y. S., et al. (2003). Prevalence and mechanisms of low-and high-level mupirocin resistance in staphylococci isolated from a Korean hospital. *J Antimicrob. Chemother.* 51, 619–623. doi: 10.1093/jac/dkg140

16

Characterization of Lytic Bacteriophages Infecting Multidrug-Resistant Shiga Toxigenic Atypical *Escherichia coli* O177 Strains Isolated from Cattle Feces

Peter Kotsoana Montso [1,2], Victor Mlambo [3] and Collins Njie Ateba [1,2]*

[1] Bacteriophage Therapy and Phage Bio-Control Laboratory, Department of Microbiology, Faculty of Natural and Agricultural Sciences, North-West University, Mmabatho, South Africa, [2] Food Security and Safety Niche Area, North-West University, Mmabatho, South Africa, [3] Faculty of Agriculture and Natural Sciences, School of Agricultural Sciences, University of Mpumalanga, Mbombela, South Africa

Correspondence:
Collins Njie Ateba
collins.ateba@nwu.ac.za

The increasing incidence of antibiotic resistance and emergence of virulent bacterial pathogens, coupled with a lack of new effective antibiotics, has reignited interest in the use of lytic bacteriophage therapy. The aim of this study was to characterize lytic *Escherichia coli* O177-specific bacteriophages isolated from cattle feces to determine their potential application as biocontrol agents. A total of 31 lytic *E. coli* O177-specific bacteriophages were isolated. A large proportion (71%) of these phage isolates produced large plaques while 29% produced small plaques on 0.3% soft agar. Based on different plaque morphologies and clarity and size of plaques, eight phages were selected for further analyses. Spot test and efficiency of plating (EOP) analyses were performed to determine the host range for selected phages. Phage morphotype and growth were analyzed using transmission electron microscopy and the one-step growth curve method. Phages were also assessed for thermal and pH stability. The spot test revealed that all selected phages were capable of infecting different environmental *E. coli* strains. However, none of the phages infected American Type Culture Collection (ATCC) and environmental *Salmonella* strains. Furthermore, EOP analysis (range: 0.1–1.0) showed that phages were capable of infecting a wide range of *E. coli* isolates. Selected phage isolates had a similar morphotype (an icosahedral head and a contractile tail) and were classified under the order Caudovirales, *Myoviridae* family. The icosahedral heads ranged from 81.2 to 110.77 nm, while the contractile tails ranged from 115.55 to 132.57 nm in size. The phages were found to be still active after 60 min of incubation at 37 and 40°C. Incremental levels of pH induced a quadratic response on stability of all phages. The pH optima for all eight phages ranged between 7.6 and 8.0, while at pH 3.0 all phages were inactive. Phage latent period ranged between 15 and 25 min while burst size ranged from 91 to 522 virion particles [plaque-forming unit (PFU)] per infected cell. These results demonstrate that lytic *E. coli* O177-specific bacteriophages isolated from cattle feces are highly stable and have the capacity to infect different *E. coli* strains, traits that make them potential biocontrol agents.

Keywords: atypical enterophagenic *E. coli* O177, bacteriophages, bacteriophage therapy, biocontrol, biological properties, multi-drug resistance, shiga-toxigenic *E. coli*

INTRODUCTION

Bacteriophages (phages) are self-replicating viruses, which are capable of infecting and lysing their specific host bacteria (1). They are ubiquitous organisms on Earth estimated to number at 10^{30}-10^{32} (2). Phages are relatively safe, nontoxic, and harmless to animals, plants, and humans (3, 4). They are found in various environments related to their host such as in food, soil, sewage water, feces, and farm environments (2). Several bacterial species such as *Campylobacter*, *Escherichia coli*, *Listeria*, *Salmonella*, *Pseudomonas*, and *Vibrio* species are used as hosts to isolate their specific bacteriophages (5–7). Because of their host specificity and nontoxicity, lytic phages are considered to be an alternative solution to combat antimicrobial-resistant pathogens. Outbreaks of listeriosis and widespread occurrence of multidrug resistance in *E. coli*, *Salmonella*, and *Staphylococcus* species have been reported in South Africa (8–11). However, there has been no attempt to use bacteriophages to control antibiotic-resistant pathogens, in either hospital settings or food industry.

Antibiotic resistance in foodborne pathogens, particularly *E. coli* species, remains a public health concern. Antibiotic-resistant pathogens do not only increase economic and social costs but are also responsible for severe infections in humans (12). In 2014, foodborne infections caused an estimated 600 million illnesses and 420,000 deaths across the globe (13). In addition, 978 listeriosis cases were reported in South Africa from 2017 to 2018, resulting in 183 deaths (11). The leading pathogenic bacteria of concern are *E. coli* O157, *Campylobacter*, *Listeria*, and *Salmonella* species (14). Moreover, recent reports revealed that non-O157 strains, particularly O26, O45, O103, O111, O121, and O145, exhibit multidrug resistance and are among the leading causes of foodborne infection (15).

In view of the above, several interventions, such as physical, chemical, and biological methods, have been devised and implemented at all levels of the food chain to combat foodborne infection and the spread of antibiotic-resistant pathogens (16). However, these conventional methods have significant drawbacks such as corrosion of food processing plants, environmental pollution, change of food matrices, development of antibiotic resistance, and toxic effects of chemical residues (17). In addition, application of chemical agents coupled with a lack of effective enforcement regulations in food may hamper international trade and thus affect the economy of the exporting country (16, 18). Therefore, lack of new antibiotics and inefficacy of conventional strategies to combat multidrug-resistant bacterial pathogens necessitate the search for alternative control strategies such as the use of bacteriophages. Given their biological properties as explained above, lytic phages can be applied at all levels of the food chain, including preharvest application. Preharvest intervention has the advantage of preventing the transmission of foodborne pathogens from food-producing animals to human.

Considering the virulence and antibiotic resistance profiles of the *E. coli* O177 strain, coupled with the lack of new antibiotics and limitations of conventional strategies to mitigate antibiotic resistance, there is a need to expand the search for novel bacteriophages for biocontrol application. Therefore, the current study was designed to isolate and characterize lytic

E. coli O177-specific bacteriophages as potential biocontrol agents. Stability and viability of the phages were determined under temperature and pH ranges that would be obtained in a live ruminant to assess their stability for preharvest use in these animals.

MATERIALS AND METHODS

Bacterial Strain

Multidrug-resistant and virulent atypical enteropathogenic *E. coli* O177 strain was used to isolate *E. coli* O177-specific bacteriophages. The atypical enteropathogenic *E. coli* O177 isolates were obtained from cattle feces and confirmed through PCR analysis. The isolates were further screened for the presence of virulence and antimicrobial gene determinants. Prior to phage isolation, 40 *E. coli* O177 isolates stored at −80°C were resuscitated on MacConkey agar and incubated at 37°C for 24 h. A single colony from each sample was transferred into 15-ml nutrient broth in 50-ml falcon tubes. The samples were incubated in a shaker (160 rpm) at 37°C for 3 h until the growth reached an optical density (OD) of 0.4–0.5 (600 nm).

Enrichment and Isolation Purification of *E. coli* O177-Specific Bacteriophages

Escherichia coli O177-specific bacteriophages were isolated from cattle feces using *E. coli* O177 environmental strain following the enrichment method (19, 20) with some modifications. Twenty fecal samples were collected from two commercial feedlots and two dairy farms. Samples were collected directly from the rectum using arm-length rectal gloves, placed in a cooler box containing ice packs, and transported to the laboratory. Five grams of each fecal sample was dissolved in 20 ml of lambda diluent and vortexed to obtain a homogeneous mixture. The mixture was centrifuged at 10,000 × *g* for 10 min using Hi Centrifuge SR (model: Z300, Germany) to sediment fecal matter and other impurities. An aliquot of 10 ml from the supernatant was extracted and filter-sterilized using a 0.22-μm pore-size syringe filter (GVS Filter Technology, USA) to obtain crude phage filtrates. For enrichment, 5 ml of each filtrate was added to 100 μl of exponential-phase (OD_{600} = 0.4–0.5) culture of each of the 40 *E. coli* O177 host strains in 10 ml of double-strength tryptic soya broth (TSB) supplemented with 2 mM of calcium chloride ($CaCl_2$). The samples were incubated in a shaking incubator (80 rpm) at 37°C for 24 h. After incubation, the samples were centrifuged at 10,000 × *g* for 10 min using Hi Centrifuge SR (Model: Z300, Germany) to remove bacterial cells and sample debris. The supernatant was filter-sterilized with a 0.22-μm pore-size Acrodisc syringe filter (GVS Filter Technology, USA) to obtain crude phage filtrates.

Subsequently, a spot test was performed to determine the presence of phages as previously described (19). Briefly, 100 μl of exponential-phase (OD_{600} = 0.4–0.5) culture of the bacterial host was mixed with 3 ml of soft agar (0.3% w/v agar) held at 50°C, then poured onto modified nutrient agar (MNA) plates so as to create a bacterial lawn, and allowed to solidify for 15 min. Ten microliters of each crude phage filtrate was spotted on bacterial lawn, and the plates were incubated at 37°C for 24 h. After incubation, the plates were observed for the presence of clear zones or plaques at inoculated points. Plaques were picked using a sterile pipette tip and suspended in 1 ml of lambda diluent [10 mM of Tris Cl (pH 7.5), 8 mM of $MgSO_4 \cdot 7H_2O$] in 2-μl Eppendorf tubes. The tubes were left at room temperature to allow phages to diffuse into the solution. The tubes were then centrifuged at 11,000 × g for 10 min, and the supernatant was filter-sterilized with a 0.22-μm pore-size Acrodisc syringe filter (GVS Filter Technology, Germany).

Bacteriophage Purification and Propagation

Bacteriophages were purified from single plaque isolates using the soft agar overlay method (21, 22). Plaque assay was performed, and the plates were incubated at 37°C for 24 h. After incubation, single plaques from each plate were picked based on their sizes and clarity using a sterile pipette tip and were resuspended in 1 ml of lambda diluent in 2-μl Eppendorf tubes. The tubes were left at 4°C for 24 h to allow phage to diffuse into the buffer. The tubes were then centrifuged at 10,000 × g for 10 min, and the supernatant was filter-sterilized using a 0.22-μm pore-size Acrodisc syringe filter (GVS Filter Technology, Germany). The purification process was repeated three consecutive times until homogeneous plaques were obtained for each phage isolate. Purified phages were propagated using E. coli O177 host bacteria. One hundred microliters of pure phage stocks was mixed with 100 μl of exponential-phase ($OD_{600} = 0.4$–0.5) culture of corresponding host(s) in a 50-ml falcon tube containing sterile 10-ml double-strength TSB supplemented with 2 mM of $CaCl_2$. The mixture was incubated in a shaking incubator (150 rpm) at 37°C for 24 h. After incubation, the samples were centrifuged at 8,000 × g for 10 min at 4°C, and the supernatant was filter-sterilized using a 0.22-μm pore-size Acrodisc syringe filter (GVS Filter Technology, Germany). Ten-fold serial dilutions were prepared, phage titers were determined using plaque assay, and the titers were expressed as PFU per milliliter. The stock phages were stored at 4°C for further analysis.

Characterization of Selected E. coli O177-Specific Bacteriophages

Host Range and Cross Infectivity of the Phage Isolates

The host range of eight selected phage isolates was evaluated against 50 bacterial hosts [13 E. coli O177, 12 E. coli O157, 12 E. coli O26, and 10 Salmonella species (environmental strains), 1 Pseudomonas aeruginosa (ATCC 27853), 1 Salmonella enterica (ATCC 12325), and 1 Salmonella typhimurium (ATCC 14028)], and all environmental species were isolated from cattle feces. Phage isolates were selected based on different plaque morphologies and clarity of the plaques and sizes. The spot test technique was performed to determine lytic spectrum activity of each phage isolates as previously described (21). The bacterial lawns of all the selected bacterial hosts were prepared on MNA plates. Ten microliters of phage stock (10^7–10^9 PFU/ml) was spotted on bacterial lawn and allowed to air-dry under laminar

airflow for 10 min. The plates were incubated at 37°C for 24 h. After incubation, the plates were observed for the presence of plaques at the point of application, and the phage lytic profiles were classified into three categories according to their clarity: clear, turbid, and no lysis (23). The test was performed in triplicates for each phage isolate.

Efficiency of Plating of Phages

Efficiency of plating (EOP) was performed to determine lytic efficiency of the phage in comparison with their suitable host bacteria as previously described (24), with modification. Fifteen bacterial strains (five E. coli O177, five E. coli O26, and five E. coli O157) were selected based on their sensitivity against the phages. Ten-fold serial dilutions of phages were prepared to obtain single plaques. An aliquot of 100 μl of each phage (1×10^4 PFU/ml) was mixed with 100 μl of exponential-phase ($OD_{600} = 0.4$–0.5) culture of each bacterium in 50-ml sterile falcon tubes and left for 10 min at room temperature to allow the phage to attach to the host. Then, 3 ml of soft agar (0.3% w/v) was added to the tube, and the mixture was poured onto MNA plates. Three independent assays were performed for each phage isolate. After solidifying, the plates were incubated at 37°C for 24 h. After incubation, the number of plaques per plate was counted. The EOP was calculated as the ratio between the average number of plaques on target host bacteria (PFUs) and average number of plaques of reference host bacteria (PFUs). The EOP was classified as high (EOP ≥ 0.5), moderate (EOP > 0.01 < 0.5), and low (EOP ≤ 0.1) based on the reproducible infection on the targeted bacteria (25). The following formula was used to calculate EOP values:

$$\text{Relative EOP} = \frac{\text{average number of plaques on targeted host bacteria (PFUs)}}{\text{average number of plaques on reference host bacteria (PFUs)}}$$

Transmission Electron Microscopy Analysis

Eight phage isolates were subjected to transmission electron microscopy (TEM), and phage morphotype was determined using negative staining techniques as previously described (26), with some modifications. Briefly, phages were propagated to obtain high titer (10^8–10^{11} PFU/ml). Ten milliliters of each phage (10^8–10^{11} PFU/ml) was concentrated in 50-ml falcon tubes by adding 10% (w/v) PEG, and the mixture was incubated at 4°C overnight to allow precipitation of the phage particles. After incubation, phage particles were sedimented by centrifugation at 11,000 × g for 10 min at 4°C. The supernatant was discarded, and the pellet was washed three times with 0.1 M ammonium acetate (pH 7.0). The pellet was resuspended in 200 μl of ammonium acetate. Ten microliters of concentrated phage solution was deposited on 200-mesh copper grids with carbon-coated formvar films. The phage particles were allowed to adsorb for 2 min, and excess liquid was drained off with a sterile filter paper. The grid was allowed to air-dry. A drop of 1% (w/v) ammonium molybdate (aqueous, pH 6.5) was added to negatively stain the phage particles and allowed to air-dry for 10–15 min. The grid containing the specimen (phage particles) was then loaded into a transmission electron microscope (model: FEI Tecnai; TEM, Czech Republic) and operated at 120 kV to scan and view phage images with a magnification range of 20,000–100,000. Micrographs were taken with a Gatan bottom-mounted camera using Digital Micrograph software at 80 kV and a magnification range of 20,000–250,000. The images were taken, and morphology characteristics were used to classify phage isolates as previously described (27).

Effect of Different Temperatures and pH on the Stability and Viability of Phages

Phage stability and viability were evaluated across different temperatures (37 and 40°C) over a 60-min period in a temperature-controlled incubator. The concentration of the host bacteria and phage titers was standardized before starting the experiment. One hundred microliters of exponential-phase culture [10^5 colony-forming unit (CFU)/ml] and 100 μl of phages (10^5 PFU/ml) was added to 10 ml of double-strength TSB supplemented with 2 mM of $CaCl_2$. The tubes were incubated in a preset shaking incubator at 37 and 40°C for 60 min, and samples were taken at 10, 30, and 60 min of incubation and assessed for viability and concentration using double-layer agar (22). Plaque assay was performed in triplicates for each sample, and the results were expressed as PFU per milliliter. For pH, phages were exposed to different pH levels (3.0, 4.5, 6.3, 7.0, 8.5, and 10.0) in a 48-h incubation period. Ten milliliters of sterile double-strength TSB (amended with 2 mM of $CaCl_2$) was distributed into 50-ml falcon tubes to prepare different pH solutions. The pH was adjusted using hydrochloric acid (HCL, 6M) or sodium hydroxide (NaOH, 6M). One hundred microliters of each bacterial host (10^5 CFU/ml) and their corresponding phage (10^5 PFU/ml) isolates were added to 10 ml. The tubes were incubated in a preset shaking incubator (80 rpm) at 37°C for 48 h. Samples were taken at 24 and 48 h of incubation, and the phage titer for each sample was determined using the standard plaque assay. Plaque assay was performed in triplicates for each sample, and the results were expressed as PFU per milliliter.

One-Step Growth Curve

A one-step growth curve experiment was performed to determine the latent period and burst size of the selected phages as previously described (21), with some modifications. Briefly, 5 ml of exponential-phase culture of each host was centrifuged at 8,000 × g for 5 min at 4°C. The pallet was resuspended in 10 ml of double-strength TSB supplemented with 2 mM of $CaCl_2$ to obtain an OD of 0.4–0.5 (600 nm). The bacterial concentration was adjusted using sterile double-strength TSB to obtain 1 × 10^8 CFU/ml. Each phage (10^8 PFU/ml) was added to its respective host bacterial suspension to achieve multiplicity of infection (MOI) 1.0. The mixture was left at room temperature for 10 min to allow phages to adsorb to the host bacteria. After 10 min, 1.5 μl of the mixture was transferred into 2-μl Eppendorf tubes and centrifuged at 11,000 × g for 10 min to remove unadsorbed phage particles. The pellet was resuspended in 100 μl of TSB supplemented with 10 mM of magnesium sulfate (mTSB) and transferred into 9.9 ml of prewarmed mTSB. The samples were incubated in a shaking incubator (160 rpm) at 37°C for 1 h.

Two hundred microliters was drawn from each sample at 5-min intervals for 60 min. Plaque assay was performed in triplicates for each samples to determine phage titer. The data generated were used to determine the latent period, burst time, and phage relative burst size per infected cell. The burst size was calculated as the ratio of the final count of released phage progeny to the initial count of infected bacterial host cell during the latent period using the following formula as previously described (28):

$$\text{Relative burst size} = \frac{\text{final titer (PFU)} - \text{initial titer (PFUs)}}{\text{initial titer (PFUs) (PFUs)}}$$

The relative burst size at different time points was plotted against time to determine the latent period and burst size of each phage isolate.

Statistical Analysis

The viability and stability of phages were tested at different temperatures and pH levels. The data were converted to $\log_{10}$ PFU per milliliter and analyzed using SAS (2010). The effect of temperature, time, and phage type on viability and stability of phages was analyzed using the general linear model (GLM) procedure of SAS (2010) for a 2 (temperature) × 3 (time) × 8 (phages) factorial treatment arrangement according to the following model:

$$Y_{ijkl} = \mu + T_i + S_j + V_k + (T \times S)_{ij} + (T \times V)_{ik} \\ + (S \times V)_{jk} + (T \times S \times V)_{ijk} + E_{ijkl}$$

where Y_{ijkl} is the observation of the dependent variable $ijkl$; μ is the fixed effect of population mean for the variable; T_i is the effect of temperature; S_j is the effect of time; V_k is the effect of phages; $(T \times S)_{ij}$ is the effect of interaction between temperature at level i and time at level j; $(T \times V)_{ik}$ is the effect of interaction between temperature at level i and phage at level k; $(S \times V)_{jk}$ is the effect of interaction between time at level j and phage at level k; $(T \times S \times V)_{ijk}$ is the effect of interaction between temperature at level i, time at level j, and phage at level k; and E_{ijkl} is the random error associated with observation $ijkl$.

Phage viability and stability data in response to incremental levels of pH were evaluated for linear and quadratic effects using polynomial contrasts. Response surface regression analysis (Proc RSREG; SAS 2010) was applied to describe the responses to pH according to the following quadratic model: $y = a + bx + cx^2$, where y is the response variables, b and c are the coefficients of the quadratic equation, a is the intercept, x is the pH level, and $-b/2c$ is the x value for maximum response. For all statistical tests, significance was declared at $p \leq 0.05$.

RESULTS

Isolation, Purification, and Propagation of Bacteriophages

Thirty-one lytic E. coli O177-specific bacteriophages were isolated from cattle feces. Phages were able to infect 15% of the E. coli O177 isolates used for isolation. Phage isolates were designated as ECPV, according to the genus of the host bacteria,

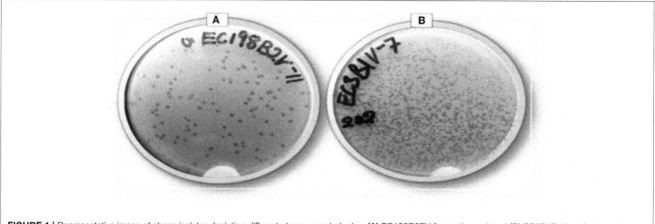

FIGURE 1 | Representative image of phage isolates depicting different plaque morphologies: **(A)** EC198B2PV (large plaques) and **(B)** EC3B1PV (small plaques).

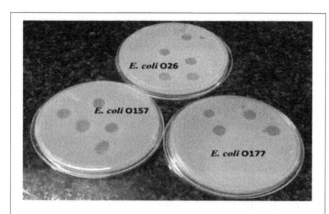

FIGURE 2 | Representative image depicting spot test results of phages on different *Escherichia coli* strains.

followed by the notation of phage virus and a numeric number as identity. Phage isolates revealed different plaque morphologies in terms of sizes, ranging from small to large (1–2 mm, respectively) plaques (**Figure 1**). A large proportion (71%) of the phage isolates revealed large plaques, while a small proportion (29%) showed small plaques on their preferred hosts. All the phages revealed clear (complete lysis) plaques, and no turbid plaques were observed. Phage titer after propagation ranged from 6.2×10^5 to 3.1×10^{13} PFU/ml. Phage EC3A2PV had the lowest titer, while phage EC198B1PV had the highest titer compared to other phage isolates.

Host Range of Phages and EOP Analysis Against Different *E. coli* Strains

A spot test was performed to determine the host range of eight selected lytic phage isolates against 50 bacterial hosts comprising different bacterial species. The results indicated that the phages were capable of infecting *E. coli* species (*E. coli* O177, *E. coli* 0157, and *E. coli* O26 environmental strains) tested (**Figure 2**). All phage isolates produced clear plaques against all *E. coli* O177 and 83–100% of *E. coli* O26 strains (**Table 1**). Three phages

(EC10C3PV, EC11B2PV, and EC12A1PV) were able to infect *E. coli* O157 (75–83%; **Table 2**). None of the phages could infect ATCC strains and environmental *Salmonella* species. The EOP analysis was performed on 15 (five *E. coli* O177, five *E. coli* O26, and five *E. coli* O157) isolates that were susceptible to phages on the spot test. Although spot test results revealed clear plaques on *E. coli* O177, EOP results exhibited various lytic patterns of the phages. Even though EOP analysis revealed high (EOP ≥ 0.5) productive infection on *E. coli* O177, moderate infections were observed (**Table 2**). Four phages revealed high EOP values (0.5–0.8) on *E. coli* O177 isolates. On the other hand, EOP analysis exhibited moderate and low productive infections on *E. coli* O26 and *E. coli* O157 isolates (EOP values range from 0.0 to 0.4 and 0.0 to 0.3, respectively).

Morphological Characterization of Phages Based on TEM

Eight selected phage isolates were subjected to TEM analysis to determine their morphotype. Transmission electron micrograph images of the phages and structural dimensions are shown in **Figure 3** and **Table 3**, respectively. Phage isolates were classified as per the International Committee on Taxonomy of Virus (ICTV) classification based on the three-dimensional structure observed. All phage isolates showed similar morphotype on TEM analysis. Structurally, the phages had an icosahedral head and a neck attached to a long contractile tail, with tail fibers, and they were classified under the order Caudovirales, *Myoviridae* family. The phage icosahedral heads ranged from 81.2 ± 6 to 95.6 ± 3 nm while the contractile tails ranged from 118.1 ± 0.3 to 135 ± 2 nm. Phage EC10C2PV had the longest icosahedral head with a diameter of 95.6 ± 3 nm and the longest contractile tail of 135 ± 2 nm with fibers. Phage EC10C3PV had the smallest icosahedral head with a diameter of 81.2 ± 6 nm and the shortest contractile tail of 118.1 ± 0.3 nm with fibers.

Phage Stability and Viability Against Different Temperatures

The results showed a significant ($p < 0.001$) time × temperature interaction effect on the stability and viability of the phages.

Characterization of Lytic Bacteriophages Infecting Multidrug-Resistant Shiga Toxigenic Atypical Escherichia coli...

209

TABLE 1 | Host range infection of the phages.

Host bacteria	No.	Phage host range (%)							
		EC366VPV	EC11B2PV	EC10C2PV	EC12A1PV	EC3A1PV	EC118BPV	EC366BPV	EC10C3PV
Pseudomonas aeruginosa[a]	1	1 (0%)	1 (0%)	1 (0%)	1 (0%)	1 (0%)	1 (0%)	1 (0%)	1 (0%)
Salmonella enterica[b]	1	1 (0%)	1 (0%)	1 (0%)	1 (0%)	1 (0%)	1 (0%)	1 (0%)	1 (0%)
Salmonella typhimurium[c]	1	1 (0%)	1 (0%)	1 (0%)	1 (0%)	1 (0%)	1 (0%)	1 (0%)	1 (0%)
Escherichia coli O177[d]	13	13 (100%)	13 (100%)	13 (100%)	13 (100%)	13 (100%)	13 (100%)	13 (100%)	13 (100%)
E. coli O26[d]	12	12 (100%)	10 (83%)	11 (92%)	11 (92%)	10 (83%)	11 (92%)	11 (92%)	11 (92%)
E. coli O157[d]	12	12 (0%)	9 (75%)	12 (0%)	10 (83%)	12 (0%)	12 (0%)	12 (0%)	10 (83%)
Salmonella species[d]	10	10 (0%)	10 (0%)	10 (0%)	10 (0%)	10 (0%)	10 (0%)	10 (0%)	10 (0%)

[a,b,c,d]ATCC 27853, ATCC 12325, ATCC 14028, and environmental strains, respectively.

TABLE 2 | Efficacy of plating of phages against different Escherichia coli serotypes.

Bacterial strain	Bacteria ID	EOP ratio of phage isolates							
		EC10C2PV	EC10C3PV	EC118BPV	EC11B2PV	EC12A1PV	EC366BPV	EC366VPV	EC3A1PV
E. coli O177	CF-D-D202	0.7	0.8	0.6	0.5	0.7	0.8	0.8	1.0[a]
	CF-A27	0.5	0.6	0.7	0.7	1.0[a]	0.8	0.7	0.6
	CF-H361	1.0[a]	1.0[a]	0.5	0.6	0.8	0.8	0.6	0.7
	CF-A28	0.4	0.7	0.5	1.0[a]	0.5	0.5	1.0[a]	0.8
	CF-D-D246	0.7	0.9	1.0[a]	0.8	0.8	1.0	0.8	0.7
E. coli O26	2A	0.3	0.2	0.4	0.1	0.0	0.4	0.2	0.0
	4C	0.3	0.2	0.2	0.1	0.1	0.1	0.3	0.1
	17E	0.2	0.2	0.1	0.1	0.3	0.3	0.2	0.3
	21F	0.1	0.1	0.3	0.3	0.2	0.2	0.1	0.1
	25H	0.3	0.3	0.1	0.3	0.1	0.3	0.2	0.1
E. coli O157	1A	0.1	0.1	0.2	0.1	0.0	0.1	0.3	0.3
	3B	0.2	0.2	0.1	0.1	0.0	0.1	0.1	0.1
	5D	0.3	0.1	0.1	0.2	0.1	0.1	0.1	0.2
	7F	0.1	0.1	0.1	0.1	0.1	0.2	0.1	0.1
	8G	0.1	0.3	0.1	0.3	0.1	0.2	0.1	0.1

ID, identity.
[a]Reference host.

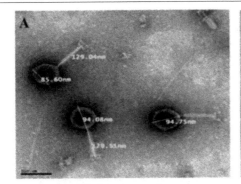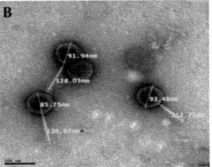

FIGURE 3 | Transmission electron micrograph images of representative phage isolates negatively stained with 1% ammonium molybdate. Both phages (**A**: EC11B2PV; **B**: EC118BPV) belong to the myoviridae family and are showing icosahedral capsid and long contractile tail with tail fibers. The bars indicate scale (100 nm).

Incubation of phages from 10 to 60 min resulted in significant phage growth at 37°C (**Figure 4**). The growth from 10 to 30 min ranged from 8.55 to 8.75 $\log_{10}$ PFU/ml (at 37°C).

Phage EC3A1PV revealed the lowest growth rate, while phage EC10C3PV exhibited the fastest growth rate from 10 to 60 min. Phage growth at 40°C when incubated for 10 to 60 min is

TABLE 3 | Phage dimensions based on transmission electron microscopy (TEM) analysis.

Phage ID	Phage morphotype				Order
	Head structure	Head dimensions (nm ± stdv)	Tail structure	Tail dimensions (nm ± stdv)	
EC366VPV	Icosahedral capsid	86.7 ± 2	Contractile sheath	120.3 ± 9	Caudovirales
EC11B2PV	Icosahedral capsid	91.5 ± 3	Contractile sheath	129.3 ± 0.2	
EC10C2PV	Icosahedral capsid	95.6 ± 3	Contractile sheath	135 ± 2	
EC366APV	Icosahedral capsid	88.5 ± 3	Contractile sheath	129.8 ± 3	
EC12APV	Icosahedral capsid	87.8 ± 2	Contractile sheath	121.9 ± 6	
EC118BPV	Icosahedral capsid	90.4 ± 3	Contractile sheath	123.9 ± 6	
EC3A1PV	Icosahedral capsid	85.6 ± 1	Contractile sheath	119.3 ± 1	
EC10C3PV	Icosahedral capsid	81.2 ± 6	Contractile sheath	118.1 ± 0.3	

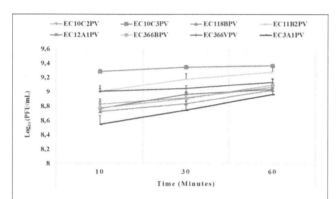

FIGURE 4 | Effect of time on persistence (stability/survivability) of individual phages at 37°C. The error bars represent the standard deviation. PFU, plaque-forming unit.

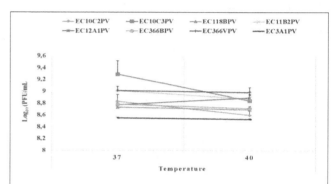

FIGURE 6 | Survival and stability of individual phages when exposed to different temperatures for 10 min. The error bars represent the standard deviation. PFU, plaque-forming unit.

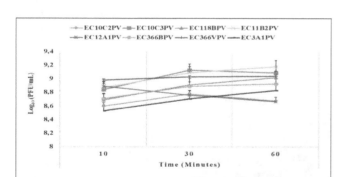

FIGURE 5 | Effect of time on persistence (stability/survivability) of individual phages at 40°C. The error bars represent the standard deviation. PFU, plaque-forming unit.

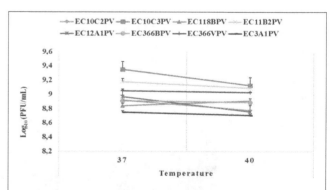

FIGURE 7 | Survival and stability of individual phages when exposed to different temperatures for 30 min. The error bars represent the standard deviation. PFU, plaque-forming unit.

depicted in **Figure 5**. From 10 to 30 min, seven phages revealed significant growth rates (ranging from 8.71 to 9.13 $\log_{10}$ PFU/ml). A decrease in phage EC12A1PV's growth rate was observed (from 10 to 60 min) while two phages (EC10C2PV and EC10C3PV) exhibited a decrease in growth rate from 30 to 60 min of incubation period.

An exposure of individual phages to 37°C for 10–30 min showed a significant increase in growth rate with time (0.4–2.3% growth rate at 37°C; **Figures 6, 7**). The average growth

rate of the phages increased from 0.2 to 0.17 $\log_{10}$ PFU/ml at 37°C (10–30 min of incubation period). Phages revealed various responses when incubated at 40°C. A decline in growth rate in other phages was observed. When incubated for 10 min at 40°C, EC10C3PV's growth rate declined the most by 4.8%, while phage EC3A1PV's growth rate was the least affected, showing only a 0.2% decline. After 30 min of incubation, a decline in growth rate was observed in phages EC366BPV (0.2%), EC366VPV (0.2%), and EC10C3PV (2.4%) (**Figure 7**). When incubated for 60 min at 40°C, phages EC10C2PV (0.28 $\log_{10}$ PFU/ml), EC10C3PV (0.39

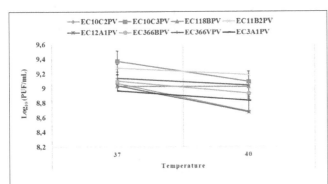

FIGURE 8 | Survival and stability of individual phages when exposed to different temperatures for 60 min. The error bars represent the standard deviation. PFU, plaque-forming unit.

$\log_{10}$ PFU/ml), and EC12A1PV (0.37 $\log_{10}$ PFU/ml) exhibited the greatest decline in growth rates when compared to their respective rates for 60 min at 37°C (**Figure 8**).

Phage Stability and Viability Against Different pH Levels

Response surface regression analysis revealed quadratic effects ($p < 0.0001$) of pH on phage stability when incubated for 24 and 48 h (**Figures 9A–H, 10A1–H1**, respectively). The pH optima for all the phages ranged from 7.6 to 8.0 with the R^2 values ranging from 0.90 to 1.0 when incubated for 24 h (**Figures 9A–H**). Three phages showed maximum stability at pH 8.0 determined from the following quadratic equations: $y = -13.9 (\pm 2.93) + 6.4 (\pm 0.98)x - 0.4 (\pm 0.07)x^2$ (EC10C2PV), $y = -13.9 (\pm 3.04) + 6.4 (\pm 1.01)x - 0.4 (\pm 0.08)x^2$ (EC366BPV), and $y = -13.9 (\pm 2.97) + 6.4 (\pm 0.99)x - 0.4 (\pm 0.08)x^2$ (EC366VPV). Phages EC10C3PV and EC11B2PV exhibited maximum stability at pH 7.6, which was determined from the following quadratic equations: $y = -13.4 (\pm 2.87) + 6.1 (\pm 0.95)x - 0.4 (\pm 0.07)x^2$ and $y = -13.5 (\pm 2.94) + 6.1 (\pm 0.98)x - 0.4 (\pm 0.07)x^2$, respectively. When incubated for 48 h, pH optima for phage stability ranged from 7.9 to 8.0 with R^2 values ranging from 0.90 to 1.0 (**Figures 10A1–H1**). Seven phages exhibited maximum stability at a higher (8.0) optimum pH while only one phage showed maximum stability at a lower (7.9) pH determined from the quadratic equation $y = -13.8 (\pm 3.10) + 6.3 (\pm 1.03)x - 0.4 (\pm 0.08)x^2$.

One-Step Growth Curve Bacteriophages

A one-step growth curve analysis for the eight phage isolates was performed to determine the latent period and relative burst size per infected bacterial cell. Data generated were analyzed and used to construct triphasic curves (**Figures 5–11A–H**). The latent period for all the phages ranged from 15 to 25 min (average = 20 ± 3.8 min). Phages EC11B2PV and EC3A1PV had the longest latent period (25 min), while phages EC118BPV and EC366VPV had the shortest (15 min) latent period. The latent period for the other four phages was 20 min. In terms of burst size, phages EC10C3PV and EC12A1PV had the largest burst size per infected cell (522 and 367 PFUs, respectively), while phage EC366VPV had the smallest burst size (91 PFUs) per infected cell.

DISCUSSION

The emergence of antibiotic resistance in foodborne pathogens has revitalized interest in the possible exploitation of lytic bacteriophages as an alternative biocontrol strategy. Because of their ability to lyse multidrug-resistant pathogens, lytic bacteriophages are considered as a natural and green technology for food preservation and safety (29). The isolation, identification, and full characterization of the bacterial host is a prerequisite for the successful isolation of suitable lytic bacteriophages intended for biocontrol of antimicrobial foodborne pathogens (30). Furthermore, reliable, reproducible, and efficient methods need to be employed for selection of suitable phage candidates for biocontrol application (31). In this study, 31 lytic E. coli O177-specific bacteriophage isolates were successfully isolated from cattle feces using multidrug-resistant atypical enteropathogenic E. coli O177 as a host. Since cattle are the main reservoirs of the atypical enteropathogenic E. coli O177 strain, this supports the idea that phages are present in every ecosystem where their hosts exist (4). The phages exhibited clear and discrete plaques with different sizes. The plaque size ranged between small and large (1–2 mm, respectively) sizes while phage titers ranged from 6.2×10^5 to 3.1×10^{13} PFU/ml. Interestingly, a large proportion (71%) of phage isolates produced large and clear plaques on their preferred hosts. These characteristics were similar to those reported for E. coli O157-, Listeria-, Pseudomonas-, Salmonella-, and Vibrio-specific phages (23, 32, 33). From a biocontrol point of view, strictly lytic phages with high titers are considered as ideal candidates for biocontrol application (4, 34).

Host range is one of the most important criteria when selecting phages intended for biocontrol of antimicrobial foodborne pathogens (35). Eight phages were selected to determine phage host range. The selection criteria were based on the lytic profiles, plaque clarity, and size of the phages. A spot test revealed that the phages were capable of infecting different E. coli strains from two different categories [environmental atypical enteropathogenic E. coli O177 and Shiga toxin-producing E. coli (E. coli O26 and E. coli O157)]. Clear plaques were predominantly observed on E. coli O177 and E. coli O26 serotypes. Interestingly, three phages exhibited clear plaques on E. coli O177, E. coli O26, and E. coli O157 strains, suggesting that these phages were polyvalent, infecting strains from two different categories. Despite this, no phage could infect all the ATCC strains and environmental Salmonella species tested in this study. This could be attributed to the fact that ATCC strains and Salmonella species lack specific receptors for phage attachment. Based on EOP analysis, phages revealed high efficiency (EOP ≥ 0.5) on the E. coli O177 strain. Despite the fact that all the phages revealed clear plaques on E. coli O26 and O157 strains on the spot test, only three phages exhibited medium to low EOP (<0.5) on E. coli O26 and O157 serotypes. This suggested that phages were highly specific to the E. coli O177 strain. Moreover, host specificity is regarded as a desirable characteristic for potent phage application, particularly in live animals to ensure that they have little or no impact on the beneficial gut microflora (2, 6). Furthermore, infectivity variation might be due to the

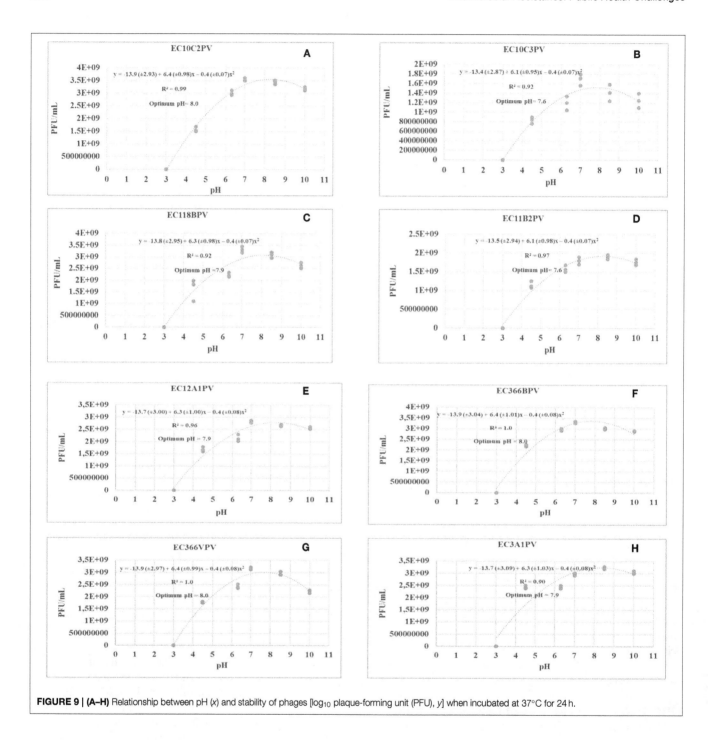

FIGURE 9 | (A–H) Relationship between pH (x) and stability of phages [$\log_{10}$ plaque-forming unit (PFU), y] when incubated at 37°C for 24 h.

non-specific binding receptors on the host cell wall or the presence of phage-resistant strains (6).

A negative staining procedure was used for TEM analysis. Based on TEM results, all eight phage isolates revealed a similar morphotype. Structurally, the phages had an icosahedral head and a neck attached to a long contractile tail with tail fibers connected to the baseplate. The icosahedral head of the phages ranged from 81.2 ± 6 to 95.6 ± 3 nm in size while the contractile tails ranged from 118.1 ± 0.3 to 135 ± 2 nm. Based on these characteristics, phage isolates were classified under the order Caudovirales and *Myoviridae* family (27). Moreover, these characteristics were similar to those of T1-7-like *E. coli* phages (4, 36). Given the fact that the *Myoviridae* family contains double-stranded DNA phages (4), all eight phages were presumptively classified under linear double-stranded DNA phages. The tail fibers contain proteins, which help the phage to recognize their specific receptors on the bacterial cell wall and thus restrict the phage from binding to non-specific bacterial cell (37). This explains the host specificity of the phages isolated in this study.

Characterization of Lytic Bacteriophages Infecting Multidrug-Resistant Shiga Toxigenic Atypical Escherichia coli...

213

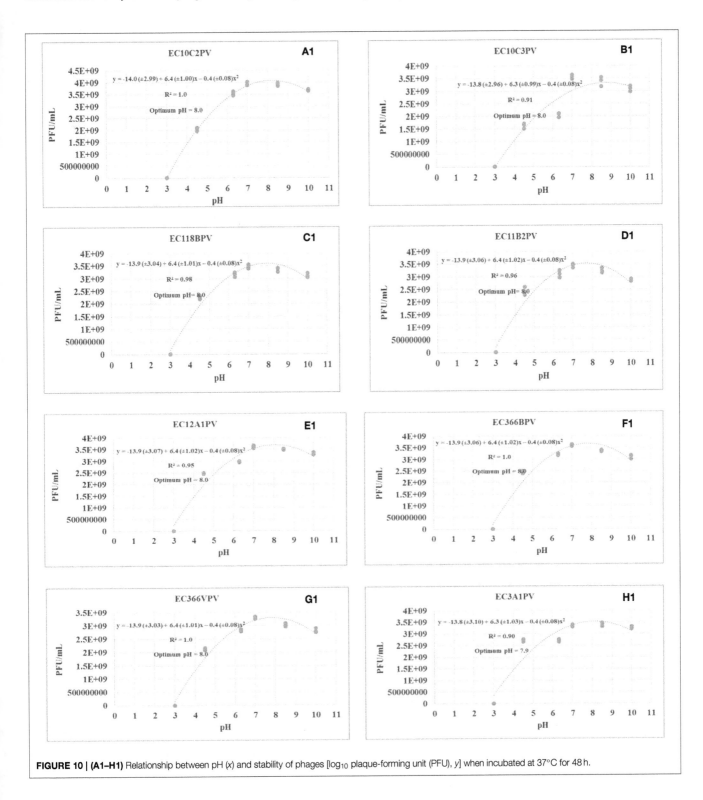

FIGURE 10 | (A1–H1) Relationship between pH (*x*) and stability of phages [log$_{10}$ plaque-forming unit (PFU), *y*] when incubated at 37°C for 48 h.

External factors such as pH and temperature may influence the stability and infectivity of the phages (7). These factors may fluctuate, particularly in live animals because of diet and/or ambient temperature. In view of this, phages intended for biocontrol application, particularly in live ruminants, must be tested against an appropriate range of pH and temperature. For this reason, the effect of exposure to different temperatures (37 and 40°C) for different times on infectivity and stability of eight phages was evaluated. Given that complete bacterial lysis by phage takes 20–40 min (33), phage growth at different temperatures was monitored after 10, 30, and 60 min. Furthermore, the incubation temperatures were selected because

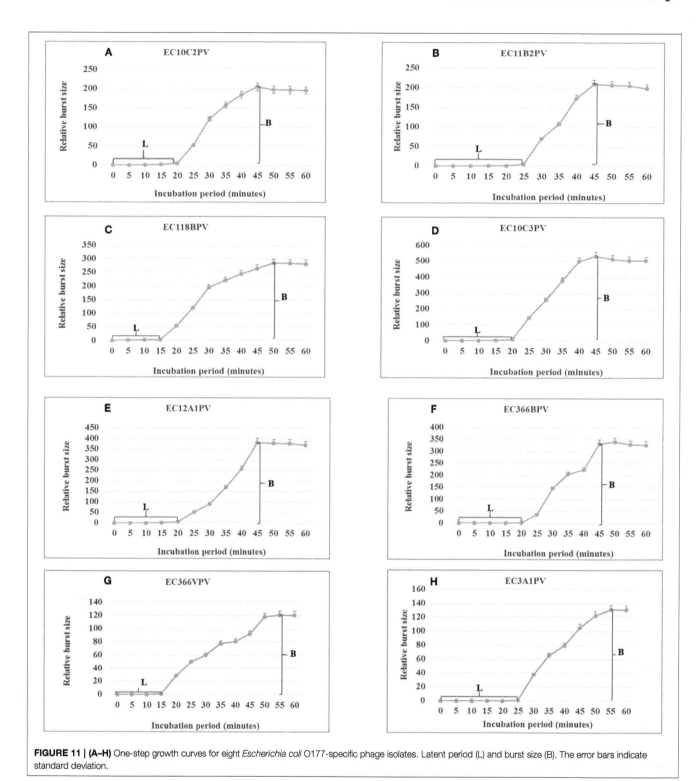

FIGURE 11 | (A–H) One-step growth curves for eight *Escherichia coli* O177-specific phage isolates. Latent period (L) and burst size (B). The error bars indicate standard deviation.

the temperature in the digestive system of the ruminant ranges from 37 to 40°C. The ability of phages to survive at these temperatures suggests that they can be applied in live animals as biocontrol agents. When incubated at 37°C, phages revealed a significant growth rate at each time point. Phages EC10C3PV, EC11B2PV, and EC366VPV revealed the fastest growth rates;

phage EC3A1PV showed the slowest growth rate from 10 to 60 min. These results are similar to those reported in previous studies (28).

Phages revealed variable growth patterns when exposed to 40°C. Generally, phages showed a decline in growth rate at 40°C when compared to their growth rate at 37°C. When exposed to 40°C for 10–30 min, seven phages exhibited a significant growth rate. However, one phage revealed a decline in growth rate after 30 min while two phages, EC10C2PV and EC10C3PV, only exhibited a decline in growth from 30 to 60 min at 40°C. This demonstrates that these three phages were less stable at high temperature and, therefore, their application in live animals is limited because the rumen temperature is 39°C. Despite this, the other five phages were fairly stable at 40°C, suggesting they may be suitable for biocontrol application in live animals.

The response surface regression analysis revealed a significant relationship between pH and phage stability. The optimal pH for phages at different incubation times ranged from pH 7.6 to 8.0 (24 h) and pH 7.9 to 8.0 (48 h). When incubated for 24 and 48 h, all phages exhibited similar growth trends and survival over a wide range of pH (4.5–10.0). Despite this, all the phages were sensitive to low pH (3.0) with no activity being observed after 24 and 48 h of incubation at this pH. This is consistent with previous studies, which reported that exposure of phages to pH 3.0 and below significantly reduced the viability and stability of phages (38, 39). Although the optimum pH for all the phages is 7.6–8.0, phages revealed good stability even at lower pHs of 6.3 and 7.0, which encompasses rumen pH values (6.5–6.9). And this indicates their potential suitability for use in preharvest intervention strategies that may be designed for application in ruminants.

Phage latent period and burst size are important parameters to consider when selecting phages for biocontrol purposes (5, 31). Phages with a short latent period and large burst size are more effective in inactivating bacteria and are thus considered to be suitable for biocontrol application (35). One-step growth curves revealed that the eight phages have different patterns of growth, suggesting that they have distinct genotypes. They displayed outstanding characteristics such as short latent periods and large bust sizes, which make them attractive for the control of the *E. coli* O177 strain. The latent period of phages ranged from 15 to 25 min, while the burst size ranged from 91 to 522 PFU per host cell. In addition, the average latent period for all the phages was 20 ± 3.8 min while the burst size was 260 ± 144 PFU per host cell. These results were consistent with those reported previously (35). Two phages, EC118BPV and EC366VPV, had the shortest latent period (15 min) while EC11B2PV and EC3A1PV had the longest latent period (25 min). Phages EC10C3PV, EC118BPV, and EC12A1PV had the largest burst size per infected cell (522 and 367 PFU per host cell, respectively). Interestingly, these three phages also showed broad host range in the spot test. This demonstrates that these phages are better suited for biocontrol application (40).

In conclusion, lytic bacteriophages infecting the *E. coli* O177 environmental strain were successfully isolated in this study. Furthermore, phages were capable of infecting three *E. coli* strains from two different categories, atypical enteropathogenic *E. coli* (*E. coli* O177) and Shiga toxin-producing *E. coli* (*E. coli* O26 and *E. coli* O157). Despite this, no phage could infect ATCC strains and environmental *Salmonella* species tested. Considering strong lytic activity, broad spectrum, and stability at different temperatures and pH levels, phages isolated in this study are considered as potential candidates for *in vivo* control of the *E. coli* O177 strain. However, further studies using appropriate *in vitro* and *in vivo* models are required to evaluate the efficacy of *E. coli* O177-specific phages in reducing *E. coli* O177 in live animals and meat products. Moreover, whole-genome sequence analysis is also required to determine the presence of undesirable genes in these phages.

ETHICS STATEMENT

The statement, Ethical clearance was obtained from the Faculty of Natural and Agricultural Sciences Ethics committee, North West University prior to the commencement of the study. An ethics number NWU-01223-19-S9 was assigned to the study.

AUTHOR CONTRIBUTIONS

VM and CA conceived and designed the experiments, contributed reagents, material, and analysis tools. PM performed the experiments. PM, VM, and CA wrote the paper and data analysis.

FUNDING

This research was supported financially by the National Research Foundation (Grant Number: 112543) and the North-West University Postgraduate Bursary.

ACKNOWLEDGMENTS

The authors wish to thank Dr. Anine Jordaan for her technical support during TEM analysis for bacteriophages and Mr. B. J. Morapedi for his assistance in sample collection.

REFERENCES

Akhtar M, Viazis S, Diez-Gonzalez F. Isolation, identification and characterization of lytic, wide host range bacteriophages from waste effluents against *Salmonella enterica* serovars. *Food Control*. (2014) 38:67–74. doi: 10.1016/j.foodcont.2013.09.064

Huang C, Shi J, Ma W, Li Z, Wang J, Li J, et al. Isolation, characterization, and application of a novel specific *Salmonella* bacteriophage in different food matrices. *Food Res Int*. (2018) 111:631–41. doi: 10.1016/j.foodres.2018.05.071

Sillankorva SM, Oliveira H, Azeredo, J. Bacteriophages and their role in food safety. *Int J Microbiol*. (2012) 2012:863945. doi: 10.1155/2012/863945

Harada LK, Silva EC, Campos WF, Del Fiol FS, Vila M, Dabrowska K, et al. Biotechnological applications of bacteriophages: state of the art. *Microbiol Res*. (2018) 212–3:38–58. doi: 10.1016/j.micres.2018.04.007

Niu Y, Johnson R, Xu Y, McAllister T, Sharma R, Louie M, et al. Host range and lytic capability of four bacteriophages against bovine and clinical human isolates of Shiga toxin producing *Escherichia coli* O157: H7. *J Appl Microbiol*. (2009) 107:646–56. doi: 10.1111/j.1365-2672.2009.04231.x

Akhtar M, Viazis S, Christensen K, Kraemer P, Diez-Gonzalez F. Isolation, characterization and evaluation of virulent bacteriophages against *Listeria monocytogenes. Food Control.* (2017) 75:108–15. doi: 10.1016/j. foodcont.2016.12.035

Yin Y, Liu D, Yang S, Almeida A, Guo Q, Zhang Z, et al. Bacteriophage potential against *Vibrio parahaemolyticus* biofilms. *Food Control.* (2019) 98:156–63. doi: 10.1016/j.foodcont.2018.11.034

Ateba CN, Bezuidenhout CC. Characterisation of *Escherichia coli* O157 strains from humans, cattle and pigs in the North-West Province, South Africa. *Int J Food Microbiol.* (2008) 128:181–8. doi: 10.1016/j.ijfoodmicro.2008.08.011

Akindolire M, Babalola O, Ateba C. Detection of antibiotic resistant *Staphylococcus aureus* from milk: a public health implication. *Int J Environ Res Public Health.* (2015) 12:10254–75. doi: 10.3390/ijerph120910254

Dlamini BS, Montso PK, Kumar A, Ateba CN. Distribution of virulence factors, determinants of antibiotic resistance and molecular fingerprinting of *Salmonella* species isolated from cattle and beef samples: suggestive evidence of animal-to-meat contamination. *Environ Sci Pollut Res.* (2018) 5:32694–708. doi: 10.1007/s11356-018-3231-4

WHO. *Listeriosis – South Africa.* (2018). Available online at: https://www.who. int/csr/don/28-march-2018-listeriosis-south-africa/en/ (accessed March 07, 2019).

Barilli E, Vismarra A, Villa Z, Bonilauri P, Bacci C. ESβL *E. coli* isolated in pig's chain: genetic analysis associated to the phenotype and biofilm synthesis evaluation. *Int J Food Microbiol.* (2019) 289:162–7. doi: 10.1016/j. ijfoodmicro.2018.09.012

WHO. *WHO's First Ever Global Estimates of Foodborne Diseases Find Children Under 5 Account for Almost One Third of Deaths.* (2015). Available online at: http://www.who.int/mediacentre/news/releases/2015/foodborne-disease-estimates/en/ (accessed February 25, 2019).

Farrokh C, Jordan K, Auvray F, Glass K, Oppegaard H, Raynaud S, et al. Review of Shiga-toxin-producing *Escherichia coli* (STEC) and their significance in dairy production. *Int J Food Microbiol.* (2013) 162:190–212. doi: 10.1016/j.ijfoodmicro.2012.08.008

Gould LH, Mody RK, Ong KL, Clogher P, Cronquist AB, Garman KN, et al. Increased recognition of non-O157 Shiga toxin–producing *Escherichia coli* infections in the United States during 2000–2010: epidemiologic features and comparison with *E. coli* O157 infections. *Foodborne Pathog. Dis.* (2013) 10:453–60. doi: 10.1089/fpd.2012.1401

Hungaro HM, Mendonça RCS, Gouvêa DM, Vanetti MCD, De Oliveira Pinto CL. Use of bacteriophages to reduce *Salmonella* in chicken skin in comparison with chemical agents. *Food Res Int.* (2013) 52:75–81. doi: 10.1016/j.foodres.2013.02.032

Chen J, Ren Y, Seow J, Liu T, Bang W, Yuk H. Intervention technologies for ensuring microbiological safety of meat: current and future trends. *Compr Rev Food Sci Food Safety.* (2012) 11:119–32. doi: 10.1111/j.1541-4337.2011.00177.x

Boatemaa S, Barney M, Drimie S, Harper J, Korsten L, Pereira L. Awakening from the listeriosis crisis: food safety challenges, practices and governance in the food retail sector in South Africa. *Food Control.* (2019) 104:333–42. doi: 10.1016/j.foodcont.2019.05.009

Sambrook J, Fritsch EF, Maniatis T. *Molecular Cloning: A Laboratory Manual.* 2nd Edn. Cold Spring Harbor, NY: Cold Spring Harbor Laboratory Press (1989).

Van Twest R, Kropinski AM. Bacteriophage enrichment from water and soil. In: *Bacteriophages. Methods in Molecular BiologyTM.* Humana Press (2009). p. 15–21. doi: 10.1007/978-1-60327-164-6_2

Adams MH, editor. Methods of study of bacterial viruses. *Bacteriophages.* New York, NY: Interscience Publishers (1959). p. 443–522.

Sambrook J, Russell DW. *Molecular Cloning: A Laboratory Manual.* 3rd Edn. Cold Spring Harbor, NY: Cold Spring Harbor Laboratory Press (2001).

Zhang H, Yang Z, Zhou Y, Bao H, Wang R, Li T, et al. Application of a phage in decontaminating *Vibrio parahaemolyticus* in oysters. *Int J Food Microbiol.* (2018) 275:24–31. doi: 10.1016/j.ijfoodmicro.2018.03.027

Kutter E. Phage host range and efficiency of plating. In: Clokie MRJ, Kropinski AME, editors. *Bacteriophages. Methods in Molecular BiologyTM.* New York, NY: Humana Press; Springer (2009). p. 501. doi: 10.1007/978-1-60327-164-6_14

Manohar P, Stalsby Lundborg C, Tamhankar AJ, Nachimuthu, R. Therapeutic characterization and efficacy of bacteriophage cocktails infecting *Escherichia coli, Klebsiella pneumoniae* and *Enterobacter* species. *Front Microbiol.* (2019) 10:574. doi: 10.3389/fmicb.2019.00574

Brenner S, Horne R. A negative staining method for high resolution electron microscopy of viruses. *Biochim Biophys Acta.* (1959) 34:103–10. doi: 10.1016/0006-3002(59)90237-9

Ackermann HW. Phage classification and characterization. In: Clokie MRJ, Kropinski AM, editors. *Bacteriophages: Methods and Protocols, Volume 1: Isolation, Characterization, and Interactions.* Totowa, NJ: Humana Press; Springer (2009). p. 127–40. doi: 10.1007/978-1-60327-164-6_13

El-Dougdoug NK, Cucic S, Abdelhamid AG, Brovko L, Kropinski AM, Griffiths MW, et al. Control of *Salmonella Newport* on cherry tomato using a cocktail of lytic bacteriophages. *Int J Food Microbiol.* (2019) 293:60–71. doi: 10.1016/j. ijfoodmicro.2019.01.003

Moye Z, Woolston J, Sulakvelidze A. Bacteriophage applications for food production and processing. *Viruses.* (2018) 10:205. doi: 10.3390/v10040205

Rao BM, Lalitha K. Bacteriophages for aquaculture: are they beneficial or inimical. *Aquaculture.* (2015) 437:146–54. doi: 10.1016/j.aquaculture.2014.11.039

Pereira C, Moreirinha C, Lewicka M, Almeida P, Clemente C, Cunha Â, et al. Bacteriophages with potential to inactivate *Salmonella Typhimurium*: use of single phage suspensions and phage cocktails. *Virus Res.* (2016) 220:179–92. doi: 10.1016/j.virusres.2016.04.020

Niu YD, McAllister TA, Nash JH, Kropinski AM, Stanford K. Four *Escherichia coli* O157: H7 phages: a new bacteriophage genus and taxonomic classification of T1-like phages. *PLoS ONE.* (2014) 9:e100426. doi: 10.1371/journal.pone.0100426

Perera MN, Abuladze T, Li M, Woolston J, Sulakvelidze A. Bacteriophage cocktail significantly reduces or eliminates *Listeria monocytogenes* contamination on lettuce, apples, cheese, smoked salmon and frozen foods. *Food Microbiol.* (2015) 52:42–8. doi: 10.1016/j.fm.2015.06.006

Snyder AB, Perry JJ, Yousef AE. Developing and optimizing bacteriophage treatment to control enterohemorrhagic *Escherichia coli* on fresh produce. *Int J Food Microbiol.* (2016) 36:90–7. doi: 10.1016/j.ijfoodmicro.2016.07.023

Duc HM, Son HM, Honjoh KI, Miyamoto T. Isolation and application of bacteriophages to reduce Salmonella contamination in raw chicken meat. *LWT.* (2018) 91:353–60. doi: 10.1016/j.lwt.2018.01.072

Truncaite L, Šimoliunas E, Zajancˇkauskaite A, Kaliniene L, Mankevicˇiute R, Staniulis J, et al. Bacteriophage vB_EcoM_FV3: a new member of "rV5-like viruses". *Arch Virol.* (2012) 157:2431–5. doi: 10.1007/s00705-012-1449-x

Singh A, Arya SK, Glass N, Hanifi-Moghaddam P, Naidoo R, Szymanski CM, et al. Bacteriophage tailspike proteins as molecular probes for sensitive and selective bacterial detection. *Biosens Bioelectron.* (2010) 26:131–8. doi: 10.1016/j.bios.2010.05.024

Hu Z, Meng XC, Liu F. Isolation and characterisation of lytic bacteriophages against *Pseudomonas* spp., a novel biological intervention for preventing spoilage of raw milk. *Int Dairy J.* (2016) 55:72–8. doi: 10.1016/j. idairyj.2015.11.011

Stalin N, Srinivasan P. Efficacy of potential phage cocktails against *Vibrio harveyi* and closely related *Vibrio* species isolated from shrimp aquaculture environment in the south east coast of India. *Vet Microbiol.* (2017) 207:83–96. doi: 10.1016/j.vetmic.2017.06.006

Kalatzis PG, Bastías R, Kokkari C, Katharios P. Isolation and characterization of two lytic bacteriophages, φSt2 and φGrn1; phage therapy application for biological control of vibrio alginolyticus in aquaculture live feeds. *PLoS ONE.* (2016) 11:e0151101. doi: 10.1371/journal.pone.01 51101

17

Prediction of Antimicrobial Resistance in Gram-Negative Bacteria from Whole-Genome Sequencing Data

Pieter-Jan Van Camp[1,2], David B. Haslam[3,4] and Aleksey Porollo[2,4,5]*

[1] Department of Biomedical Informatics, University of Cincinnati, Cincinnati, OH, United States, [2] Division of Biomedical Informatics, Cincinnati Children's Hospital Medical Center, Cincinnati, OH, United States, [3] Division of Infectious Diseases, Cincinnati Children's Hospital Medical Center, Cincinnati, OH, United States, [4] Department of Pediatrics, University of Cincinnati, Cincinnati, OH, United States, [5] Center for Autoimmune Genomics and Etiology, Cincinnati Children's Hospital Medical Center, Cincinnati, OH, United States

*Correspondence:
Aleksey Porollo
Alexey.Porollo@cchmc.org

Background: Early detection of antimicrobial resistance in pathogens and prescription of more effective antibiotics is a fast-emerging need in clinical practice. High-throughput sequencing technology, such as whole genome sequencing (WGS), may have the capacity to rapidly guide the clinical decision-making process. The prediction of antimicrobial resistance in Gram-negative bacteria, often the cause of serious systemic infections, is more challenging as genotype-to-phenotype (drug resistance) relationship is more complex than for most Gram-positive organisms.

Methods and Findings: We have used NCBI BioSample database to train and cross-validate eight XGBoost-based machine learning models to predict drug resistance to cefepime, cefotaxime, ceftriaxone, ciprofloxacin, gentamicin, levofloxacin, meropenem, and tobramycin tested in *Acinetobacter baumannii, Escherichia coli, Enterobacter cloacae, Klebsiella aerogenes,* and *Klebsiella pneumoniae.* The input is the WGS data in terms of the coverage of known antibiotic resistance genes by shotgun sequencing reads. Models demonstrate high performance and robustness to class imbalanced datasets.

Conclusion: Whole genome sequencing enables the prediction of antimicrobial resistance in Gram-negative bacteria. We present a tool that provides an *in silico* antibiogram for eight drugs. Predictions are accompanied with a reliability index that may further facilitate the decision making process. The demo version of the tool with pre-processed samples is available at https://vancampn.shinyapps.io/wgs2amr/. The stand-alone version of the predictor is available at https://github.com/pieterjanvc/wgs2amr/.

Keywords: antimicrobial resistance, antibiotic resistance, whole-genome sequencing, machine learning, prediction, genotype-phenotype relationship

---

Abbreviations: AB, antibiotic; ABR, antibiotic resistance; ARG, antibiotic resistance gene; ARGC, antibiotic resistance gene cluster; MCC, Matthew's correlation coefficient; MIC, minimum inhibitory concentration; WGS, whole genome sequencing.

INTRODUCTION

Since the discovery and widespread use of antibiotics (AB) in the early 20th century, resistance to those same AB has generally developed rapidly; often even within the first years of introduction (Marston et al., 2016). As a consequence, many bacteria have developed antibiotic resistance (ABR) to most of the major classes of AB, often seen in the Gram-negatives (Centers for Disease Control and Prevention, 2018). Effective treatment of these infections requires knowledge of the organism's susceptibility to the various AB, currently obtained by culturing bacteria in the clinical laboratory and subsequent testing for commonly used AB. Depending on the pathogen, this process may require 72 h or more. Drug susceptibility is usually reported to the clinician as either resistant or susceptible (sometimes intermediate is also used) with cut-offs based on the minimum inhibitory concentration (MIC) of an AB needed to halt growth or kill the pathogen in the lab. In serious systemic infections, early treatment with an effective antibiotic is paramount as unexpected resistance may lead to treatment failure, while fear of inadequate therapy may drive overly broad antibiotic use which contributes to extensively resistant and potentially untreatable bacteria (Marston et al., 2016).

With decreasing cost and increasing speed of high-throughput sequencing technology such as whole genome sequencing (WGS), in-depth analysis of pathogens is increasingly used in clinical decision-making. Studies already showed the potential of these techniques in ABR prediction in single, Gram-positive pathogens like *Staphylococcus aureus* and *Mycobacterium tuberculosis*. An example is the Mykrobe predictor that maps DNA sequencing data to a reference genome and a set of plasmid genes conferring ABR (Bradley et al., 2015). The model also accounts for polymorphism in select loci when predicting drug resistance. Data analysis and prediction is rapid, enabling it as a practical tool for clinical care during the decision-making process. PhyResSE is another tool that follows a similar strategy but may process data in minutes to a few days, attributing such time extension to more careful variant calling (Feuerriegel et al., 2015). Both tools report high accuracy of ABR prediction. However, their application to other pathogens like Gram-negative bacteria has not been described.

The prediction of ABR in Gram-negative bacteria, often the cause of serious systemic infections, is more challenging as the source of drug resistance is more complicated. For example, Gram-negative pathogens may possess one or more β-lactamases with similar amino acid sequences but various activity against β-lactam-based AB (Livermore, 1998). They are also more likely to develop mutations that result in lower membrane permeability, or increase the expression of a variety of genes for excreting xenobiotics (efflux pumps) and for inactivating β-lactam-targeting drugs (Marston et al., 2016). There have been a few clinical predictors reported for assessing the risk of infection with resistant Gram-negative bacteria but they solely rely on data from the electronic health record and just predict the likelihood of infection with a resistant strain rather than individual drug resistance (Martin et al., 2013; Vasudevan et al., 2014). Thus far, only a handful of studies were published

on the prediction of Gram-negative resistance using WGS data. These models were built for individual species, such as *Neisseria gonorrhoeae* or *Klebsiella pneumonia,* and were based on small sample sizes resulting in poor predictive accuracy (Eyre et al., 2017; Nguyen et al., 2018). A more extensive study recently published by Drouin et al. (2019) utilizes 107 machine-learning-based models, trained on WGS data, to predict ABR in 12 bacterial species, including six Gram-negatives, against a variety of AB with generally high accuracy. These models were trained without incorporating prior ABR knowledge as they were based on nucleotide k-mers from sequenced genomes of these pathogens, thus utilizing information from non-coding regions and polymorphism. Furthermore, their methodology produced small, human-interpretable decision trees, when the k-mers are mapped back to the respective genomes to make decisions interpretable (provided that k-mers belong to annotated genomic regions). However, the study was performed on heavily imbalanced datasets, while reporting only two-class accuracy, which could overestimate the real performance. Finally, isolates with intermediate resistance were excluded from the final predictors making the performance estimates on such samples uncertain. For more details on the bioinformatics approaches to the AMR analysis and prediction, the reader can refer to a recent review (Van Camp et al., 2020).

In this work, we present a machine learning-based method for the fast estimation of ABR in 5 Gram-negative species for 8 AB. The models were trained on WGS data and laboratory confirmed drug susceptibility. All isolates were assigned to either of two classes (susceptible or resistant) and subsequently used in the training and validation of binary predictors. Each model was evaluated using multiple performance measures. The presented workflow could inform early clinical decision-making on the choice of AB therapy (within a day) while waiting for the final antibiogram (typically 2–4 days) thereby decreasing the time to start effective therapy. A web-based demo application to show the potential clinical implementation is publicly available at https://vancampn.shinyapps.io/wgs2amr/. The stand-alone tool can be freely downloaded from https://github.com/pieterjanvc/wgs2amr/.

MATERIALS AND METHODS

Pathogens and Antibiotics of Interest

This study focused on five common nosocomial Gram-negative organisms that can cause sepsis (Vincent, 2003; Couto et al., 2007): *Acinetobacter baumannii, Escherichia coli, Enterobacter cloacae, Klebsiella aerogenes,* and *Klebsiella pneumoniae.* These specific Gram-negative pathogens were chosen because, in addition to clinical relevance, they are the most represented in terms of DNA-sequenced and AMR annotated samples available at NCBI. For machine learning, the larger the dataset to train on, the more accurate and generalized model can be achieved. *E. cloacae* is the major representative of *Enterobacter* species and therefore part of ESKAPE pathogens. Their antibiotic susceptibility was evaluated for cefepime, cefotaxime, ceftriaxone, ciprofloxacin, gentamicin, levofloxacin, meropenem, and tobramycin. This panel of AB covers those most commonly used to treat Gram-negative bacterial infections. Consequently, these AB are most frequently tested for susceptibility against bacterial isolates.

Public Data Collection

Meta-data for 6564 bacterial samples (isolates) were retrieved from the NCBI BioSample database using the "antibiogram" keyword filter. Of these, 4933 samples had the required information, such as bacterium name, antibiogram, and sequencing data accession number. For this work, all "intermediate" ABR levels were converted to "resistant" to project data to a binary classification problem (i.e., resistant versus susceptible). The list was subsequently refined to only include the bacteria and AB of interest (see section "Pathogens and antibiotics of interest") resulting in 2516 samples. Given the resistance to AB was highly imbalanced in the data (mostly skewed toward resistant phenotype), the samples were randomly chosen so that the number of susceptible, and resistant isolates for each antibiotic was as equal as possible in order to balance the input for machine learning models. This resulted in a final total of 946 samples (**Supplementary Table S1**). Of these, 3% of samples available for each species (total $n = 31$) were set aside to create a demo dataset to showcase the online application (see section "Preliminary pipeline implementation and evaluation" for details). The remaining 915 samples were used to build and evaluate eight XGBoost-based models, where available data for each antibiotic were randomly split in 70% training and 30% testing subsets. The overall flow of data collection is summarized in **Figure 1**. The counts of samples per species include: *A. baumannii* – 256; *E. cloacae* – 67; *E. coli* – 330; *K. aerogenes* – 51; and *K. pneumoniae* – 211. Of note, we did not stratify samples by different bacterial species during the model training as we intended our models to be species independent. **Table 1** shows the distribution of the 915 samples through the AB of interest.

Whole genome sequencing data for all samples were retrieved from the NCBI Sequence Read Archive (SRA) using the SRA toolkit (SRA Toolkit Development Team, 2019). In case multiple runs (SRR) of a sample (SRS) were available (e.g., sample was run through different sequencers or with different settings), the file

TABLE 1 | Summary of the 915 samples used to build and evaluate antimicrobial resistance prediction models.

Antibiotic	Resistant	Susceptible	Total
Cefepime	442	275	717
Cefotaxime	437	50	487
Ceftriaxone	671	133	804
Ciprofloxacin	577	335	912
Gentamicin	351	542	893
Levofloxacin	471	258	729
Meropenem	332	420	752
Tobramycin	354	320	674

Note that not all samples were tested for every antibiotic, thus the counts per AB do not add up to 915.

with the smallest size was selected. Smaller file size may frequently be attributed to lower sequencing depth and/or shorter shotgun reads. We reasoned that, if a model is able to make predictions on smaller sequence files, it will most likely be applicable to larger files with better gene coverage. List of all samples used can be found in **Supplementary Table S1**.

In-House Dataset of Samples

Gram-negative bacterial pathogens were collected from blood or urine of patients hospitalized at Cincinnati Children's Hospital Medical Center (CCHMC), 19 samples total. Organisms were identified to the species level and antimicrobial susceptibility testing was performed using the VITEK® 2 machine (Biomerieux) in the Diagnostic Infectious Diseases Testing Laboratory at CCHMC. Samples represent *A. baumannii* ($n = 1$), *E. coli* ($n = 11$), *K. aerogenes* ($n = 2$), and *K. pneumoniae* ($n = 3$). No in-house samples are available with *E. cloacae*. Two available samples of *Klebsiella oxytoca* are included. DNA was extracted from overnight liquid broth cultures using the QIAamp PowerFecal DNA Kit (Qiagen Inc, Germantown, MD, United States). Sequencing libraries were generated using the Nextera XT kit (Illumina Corporation, San Diego, CA, United States). Pooled libraries were sequenced on a NextSeq 500 (Illumina Corporation, San Diego, CA, United States) in the Microbial Genomics and Metagenomics Laboratory at

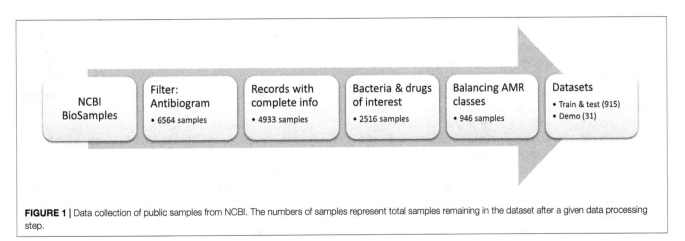

FIGURE 1 | Data collection of public samples from NCBI. The numbers of samples represent total samples remaining in the dataset after a given data processing step.

CCHMC using paired 150 bp reads to a depth of approximately 5 million reads per sample. Sample collection was approved by the Institutional Review Board (IRB) at CCHMC (IRB approval # 2016–9424: Molecular Epidemiology of Bacterial Infections). The in-house samples are available at the NCBI BioSample database (BioProject ID: PRJNA587095), where detailed metadata can be found (see **Supplementary Table S1** for sample IDs). Of note, the antimicrobial susceptibility testing with VITEK takes at least 72 h and generally requires a pure isolate, whereas sequencing preparation followed by the WGS data analysis can be completed under 48 h and does need to not rely on a pure colony (Scaggs Huang et al., 2019).

Analysis of WGS Data

The sequencing files in the FASTQ format were aligned to 4579 antibiotic resistance genes (ARG) found in the NCBI Bacterial Antimicrobial Resistance Reference Gene Database (NCBI Accession: PRJNA313047, version as of September 26, 2018) using DIAMOND (Buchfink et al., 2015), a greatly improved version of BLASTx (Altschul et al., 1990) with regards to speed, and on par sensitivity. Given the same ARG can be present in multiple species (e.g., plasmid DNA), no filtering was performed based on original bacterium in which the ARG was sequenced. The default settings of DIAMOND were used to map shotgun reads to ARGs.

Antibiotic resistance genes coverage (C) within a sample was quantified as follows. First, reads aligned by DIAMOND were discarded if the alignment to the gene covered <90% of the read's length or yielded <90% sequence identity. Second, a gene was discarded if all aligned reads covered <90% of its length (i.e., protein sequence). The cutoff was chosen as being suboptimal after probing 70, 80, 90, and 100% coverage (**Supplementary Table S2**). If a gene was retained in the hit list, the number of alignments (n) was adjusted for gene length (i.e., the number of amino acids, L), and sequencing depth (i.e., total number of reads in the file divided by 10^7, D). Such scaled data (Eq. 1) are better suitable for the machine learning.

$$C = \frac{n}{L \times D} \qquad (1)$$

Clustering Similar Antibiotic Resistance Genes

Many of the ARG in the NCBI database have a high sequence similarity (e.g., polymorphism in strains or sequences derived from closely related species) that cannot be discriminated by the alignment techniques used in this study. Therefore, antibiotic resistance gene clusters (ARGC) were created using the cluster_fast module of the USEARCH algorithm (Edgar, 2010) to group genes with ≥90% sequence identity together, naming them after the most representative gene as defined by USEARCH (i.e., cluster centroid). This threshold for grouping was chosen as a suboptimal compromise between balancing the number of genes per cluster, performance of the model, and the biological relevance of the genes grouped together (**Supplementary Table S3**). For cutoffs lower 85%, genes from different ABR classes started to group together, hence such cutoffs

were excluded from consideration. The clustering resulted in the reduction of the potential input space for the machine learning models from 4579 ARG to 1027 ARGC, with 410 clusters (40%) consisting of just a single gene. To represent the coverage of each ARGC, the average coverage (Eq. 1) of all ARG detected in this ARGC was taken. Finally, of the 1027 ARGC, only 152 were found in our data and thereby used for subsequent machine learning.

Building and Evaluating Machine Learning Models

Regression models are less stable on datasets where the input space is large, sparse, and the features are correlated (e.g., in the context of this work, drug resistance may be exerted by multiple ARGC; Farrar and Glauber, 1967; Devika et al., 2016). Using penalized regression (e.g., LASSO and Ridge regression) to reduce both the input space and select most important features can help increase performance of the model, but it still operates on the premise that input features are uncorrelated. In correlated datasets, feature selection will be distorted in this process resulting in less reliable model interpretation. Decision trees, on the other hand, inherently perform better in such cases as correlation does not influence the feature selection process (Piramuthu, 2008). In random forest models, hundreds to thousands of these trees are built, each with different subset of the input space, resulting in a more robust reporting of important features. Neural networks (NN), especially their currently popular application to deep learning, and require much larger training data-sets (tens of thousands to millions of input vectors/samples) than currently available for antimicrobial resistance (hundreds of samples) in order to demonstrate benefits of deep learning. Moreover, the resulting NN-based models represent a black box that would be difficult to dissect in order to see the decision making rules and factors influencing the decision (Van Camp et al., 2020).

XGBoost is an extreme gradient booster for decision trees that is capable of handling correlated inputs. It has innate support for sparse datasets (in our case, only a handful of ARGC are present in each sample) and can extract important features to provide additional insights in the decision-making process (Chen and Guestrin, 2016). Although XGBoost supports multi-class classification (i.e., model can choose between more than two classes), our samples can have resistance to multiple AB at the same time (i.e., multi-labeling classification), which is not supported and thus a separate, independent binomial model (resistance versus susceptible) was created for each antibiotic of interest (8 models total).

The input for each model was the list of ARGC and their presence ($C > 0$) or absence ($C = 0$) in each sample (Eq. 1). The output was binomial with label *resistant* (= 1) or *susceptible* (= 0) to the antibiotic of interest. The XGBoost models were trained with a learning rate of 0.1, maximum tree depth of 2, training subsampling of 0.8, and column subsampling of 0.8. All other parameters were kept default. The algorithm was run for a maximum of 300 iterations, but early stopping was done when no improvement was seen in 50 consecutive iterations using 10-fold cross-validation.

Despite the efforts to balance the number of samples with susceptible and resistant phenotypes per drug the final distributions on individual AB remained unbalanced (**Table 1**) because each sample was not tested for all drugs of interest. For two most imbalanced drugs, cefotaxime and ceftriaxone, an under-sampling was performed to reach 3:1 ratio and prevent the model overfitting toward the over-represented class. For heavily class-imbalanced data, standard performance measures like sensitivity or 2-class accuracy could overestimate the true performance. The Matthew's correlation coefficient (MCC) was therefore used as a more stringent performance statistic (Eq. 2). MCC measures binary classification in unbalanced datasets with range from -1 (inverse prediction) through 0 (random prediction) to 1 (perfect prediction).

$$MCC = \frac{TP^*TN - FP^*FN}{\sqrt{(TP + FP)(TP + FN)(TN + FP)(TN + FN)}} \quad (2)$$

where *TP*, *TN*, *FP*, and *FN* are true positive, true negative, false positive, and false negative instances, respectively.

For complete performance evaluation, two-class accuracy (Acc, Eq. 3), sensitivity (recall, R), precision (P), specificity (Sp), areas under ROC (AUC), and precision-recall (PR-AUC) curves are also provided.

$$Acc = \frac{TP + TN}{TP + FP + TN + FN} \quad (3)$$

where *Acc* is a two-class accuracy; *TP*, *TN*, *FP*, and *FN* are the same as in Eq. 2.

Reliability Index

To provide an additional assessment how certain the prediction is by a given model, we introduce a reliability index (RI). The RI is based on the observation that in classification models values closer to extremes (0 or 1) are more likely to yield a correct prediction compared to values hovering around 0.5. Using adjusted model output (AMO, Eq. 4), we computed a misclassification rate (MR, Eq. 5) for every AMO in the test subset of each model, defined as the percentage of incorrect predictions in test cases with AMO equal or higher than a given cutoff (Eq. 5). A regression model was fit to this MR distribution for each drug and then was used to calculate the MR for new model outputs (**Supplementary Figure S1**). The RI is the inverse of the MR and simply defined as 1 – MR.

$$AMO(x) = \begin{cases} x & ,x \geq 0.5 \\ 1-x & ,x < 0.5 \end{cases} \quad (4)$$

$$MR(c) = \frac{fp + fn}{tp + fp + tn + fn} \quad (5)$$

where tp, fp, tn, and fp are the number of true positive, false positive, true negative, and false negative instances, respectively, predicted with AMO $\geq c$.

Feature Importance

XGBoost, being a random forest-based algorithm, can provide important features from the model once it has been built in order to evaluate the individual feature impact in the decision-making process. In our case, XGBoost lists the most important ARGC for each model. By design, random-forest-based algorithms ignore strongly correlated features while using only one in the model, as adding redundant features will not provide extra discrimination capabilities (see section "Building and evaluating machine learning models"). From a biology standpoint, however, it is interesting to know all the ARGC that occur in high frequency. Thus, when the most important features are extracted from the models, we reviewed the correlated features ARGC as well.

In consideration that organism(s)/strain(s) composition in the sample should not be known *a priori*, whereas *de novo* genome assembly may be inefficient and inaccurate, no genome assembly from WGS data is conducted in this work. Therefore, the prediction model is agnostic to the source of the detected antimicrobial gene, as to whether it is inherent to an organism or acquired via mobile genetic element (plasmid). Hence, no weighting scheme for plasmid-derived genes was considered for the model.

Preliminary Pipeline Implementation and Evaluation

The long term goal of this project is to build a platform where prediction models like the ones presented here can be used in research or clinical practice to quickly estimate a bacterium's antibiogram from WGS data with sufficient accuracy, in order to inform early decisions about the correct AB use while awaiting the final antibiogram.

For illustration of developed models, an R-Shiny web-based application was developed where pre-processed samples from two datasets unseen in training (31 public, demo dataset, and 19 in-house samples, sections "Public data collection" and "In-house dataset of samples") can be individually submitted to the prediction models and subsequently compared to their actual ABR status. Furthermore, the application allows the user to explore the performance of the current ABR models in more detail, and review the important genes used in the decision-making process.

RESULTS

Data Collection and Pre-processing

After the processing and filtering (sections "Analysis of WGS data" and "Clustering similar antibiotic resistance genes"), of the 4579 ARG in the NCBI database 2605 (57%) were detected in at least one of the 946 samples. When clustered, only 152 ARGC (15%) were detected in the whole dataset. The median number of ARGC present in any sample is 10 resulting in a very sparse dataset. **Table 2** lists the most frequently found ARGC per species.

To review correlation between the 152 ARGC, a hierarchical clustering using Ward's algorithm (Ward, 1963) was performed (**Figure 2A**). An example of the strong correlation between several specific ARGC can be seen in **Figure 2B**. Even though some of the clusters have similar names, they represent different subtypes of the same gene (i.e., different enough in sequence to be placed in separate clusters, section "Clustering

TABLE 2 | Most common antibiotic resistance gene clusters per species detected from the WGS data.

Species (Total samples)	Most common gene (% occurrence)	Second most common gene (% occurrence)
A. baumannii (264)	Class C beta-lactamase ADC-98 (98.5)	OXA-51 family carbapenem-hydrolyzing class D beta-lactamase OXA-561 (98.5)
E. coli (341)	Class C extended-spectrum beta-lactamase EC-18 (99.4)	Aminoglycoside O-phosphotransferase APH(3″)-Ib (51.3)
E. cloacae (70)	Multidrug efflux RND transporter permease subunit OqxB21 (92.2)	Fosfomycin resistance glutathione transferase FosA2 (78.6)
K. aerogenes (53)	Multidrug efflux RND transporter permease subunit OqxB21 (100.0)	FosA family fosfomycin resistance glutathione transferase (100.0)
K. pneumoniae (218)	FosA family fosfomycin resistance glutathione transferase (100.0)	Class A beta-lactamase SHV-200 (96.3)

The occurrence refers to the percentage of samples, stratified by species, where a given ARGC is found in the WGS data.

TABLE 3 | Performance of final ABR prediction models.

Antibiotic	Acc	R	P	Sp	MCC	AUC	PR-AUC
Cefepime	0.82	0.86	0.86	0.77	0.62	0.89	0.92
Cefotaxime	0.83	0.93	0.86	0.53	0.52	0.80	0.92
Ceftriaxone	0.84	0.93	0.87	0.56	0.55	0.88	0.96
Ciprofloxacin	0.81	0.86	0.85	0.73	0.60	0.89	0.94
Gentamicin	0.91	0.90	0.89	0.93	0.82	0.96	0.95
Levofloxacin	0.81	0.87	0.84	0.70	0.58	0.89	0.94
Meropenem	0.89	0.82	0.92	0.94	0.78	0.94	0.94
Tobramycin	0.95	0.92	0.98	0.98	0.90	0.97	0.98

similar antibiotic resistance genes"). The full table with all ARGC pairwise correlation values can be found in supplements (**Supplementary Table S4**).

XGBoost Model Training and Testing

Since sparse input in machine learning models can bias performance (both under- or overestimating) depending on the split in training and testing data (Wu et al., 2013), we trained 51 independent models for each antibiotic (polling isolates of all species together). Each model was trained and validated with a different split in order to see the performance distribution (refer to **Supplementary Figure S2** for the overall flow of model training). **Figure 3** shows the distribution of AUC based on the testing subset for each individual split. The model with the median performance over all 51 splits for each antibiotic (represented by the thick line in the boxplots) is assumed to be the closest to real-life performance (i.e., the least biased) and was chosen as the final model. The performance of these final models are detailed in **Table 3** and **Figure 4** (see **Supplementary Table S5** for the performance of all other models).

Feature Importance

Regardless of fluctuations in model performance based on split in training and testing, the important features ARGC extracted from the models appeared to be largely the same per antibiotic prediction. **Table 4** shows the 5 most important ARGC (on average over the 51 models) for each ABR prediction model. The full table can be found in the supplements (**Supplementary Table S6**).

As mentioned in section "Feature importance", once a feature is chosen for the use in the decision-making, random forest-based methods often ignore other highly correlated features as they do not contribute to class discrimination. However, in the context of this study, when unused ARGC may provide additional biological

insights, we list all ARGC, chosen by the models and those correlated, in supplemental materials (**Supplementary Table S4**).

Comparison With Other Algorithms

XGBoost models were compared with those based on LASSO and Ridge regression, which also can deal with data sparsity and have built-in feature selection (**Supplementary Table S7**). In 6–7 (depending on the metric to compare) out of 8 AB, XGBoost models appear to be slightly better than linear regression models. The real advantage of XGBoost over the linear regression algorithms is the robustness in the important feature selection. **Table 5** in conjunction with **Supplementary Table S6** demonstrate that XGBoost yields the best consistency in selecting top informative features compared to LASSO and Ridge regression models.

Reliability Indexes

Figure 5 shows distributions of the RI for each final model based on the corresponding testing set. While there is no unified cut-off for RI across all models, there is a clear trend that correct predictions tend to have a higher RI.

Practical Implementation of Models

Demo dataset (section "Preliminary pipeline implementation and evaluation") is used to illustrate how new unseen samples could be run through the pipeline of preprocessing and subsequent prediction by the 8 models (**Figure 6**). For a given sample, each antibiotic is assigned a binary resistance prediction with a confidence (reliability index). For demonstration purposes, current implementation retrieves meta-data information for a given sample, such as species name (a header of the table), and known drug resistance status (last colored column).

Figure 6 shows how prediction results on novel samples could be presented to the clinician in the format of an antibiogram. The online application provides a more intuitive way to explore the results and use of this pipeline. The predicted antibiograms from all extra samples (the Demo set based on public samples and the In-house dataset) can be explored in detail, and an additional tab (not shown) provides more information about the models and the important features. The summary of all predictions for Demo and In-house datasets can be found in **Figure 7**. The web-based demonstration and stand-alone versions of the application can be found at https://vancampn.shinyapps.io/wgs2amr/ and https://github.com/pieterjanvc/wgs2amr/, respectively.

DISCUSSION

This work provides a framework wherein bacterial samples can be tested quickly to obtain a preliminary antibiogram to guide initial antibiotic selection for treatment. Culturing bacteria and getting a full antibiogram can take 2–4 days, whereas WGS and the computational pipeline presented here only takes around a day. At present, sequencing is taking up the majority of time but is likely to decrease significantly with the improvements in sequencing technologies.

Presenting the results as an early antibiogram estimate (**Figure 6**) instead of just individual predictions, provides clinicians with a clear and intuitive way to inform the choice of the otherwise empiric initial AB. The general resistance pattern of the whole antibiogram can be informative in itself, even if there may still be errors in individual predictions. The latter is further aided by the addition of the RI that indicates how certain the models are on individual predictions. While there is not a single clear cut for the RI, **Figures 5, 7** suggest that the majority of samples assessed with a high RI appear to have correct predictions. All of this helps early, informed AB choice that can decrease the time to start effective AB therapy while limiting the use of empiric broad-spectrum AB and slowing the development of new resistant strains. The predictions could become especially helpful in settings where resources do not permit the use of a full microbiology lab (e.g., in developing countries). Upcoming technologies, like the Nanopore MinION, (Z) (2019), will allow clinicians in the near future to sequence pathogens with smaller portable devices. This, coupled with analytical pipelines like the one presented here, could provide valuable information on pathogen resistance that would otherwise not be available. Regardless, the results will require clinical judgment.

All pathogens have several ARGC that are found in nearly every sample, regardless of its resistance status to the tested AB (e.g., *class C extended-spectrum beta-lactamase EC-18* cluster was detected in 99% of *E. coli* isolates, **Table 2**). This underlines that Gram-negatives have no easy one-to-one genotype-phenotype relationship for some ARG as their presence does not equal resistance *per se*. A well-studied example of this is the *AmpC* gene, which is expressed in many species or strains, even those fully susceptible to AB (Bajaj et al., 2016). The complex relationships between the ARG and phenotype dictated the application of more complex machine learning algorithms, such as random forest (the basis of XGBoost). An additional advantage of XGBoost is that it provides a glimpse into its decision-making process by reporting the list of features ARGC most often used when building the model as a proxy for key decisions. The downside of this simplification is that caution is warranted when interpreting these features. Finally, given that the datasets are sparse, models are prone to having to rely on different features depending on the split in training and testing. The higher the consistency in selecting important features across different independent models, the more robust the final model is anticipated to be (**Table 5**).

An intuitive example is the *class A extended-spectrum beta-lactamase* cluster as an important feature in the cephalosporin prediction models (**Table 4**). Other ARGCs seem less relevant

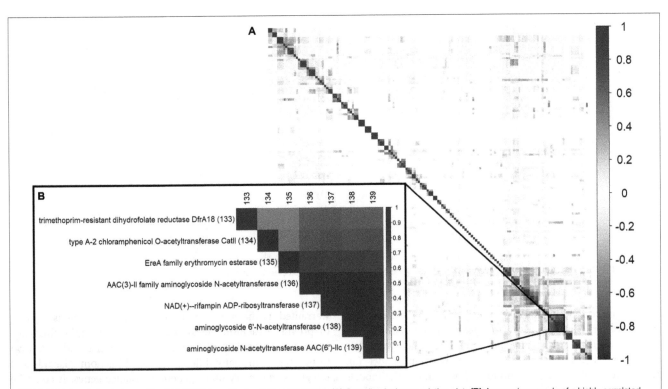

FIGURE 2 | Correlation between the 152 ARGC found in the analyzed samples. **(A)** Overall pairwise correlation plot. **(B)** A zoom-in example of a highly correlated group of ARGC. Numbers in parentheses are the same serial numbers as in columns provided for easy matching.

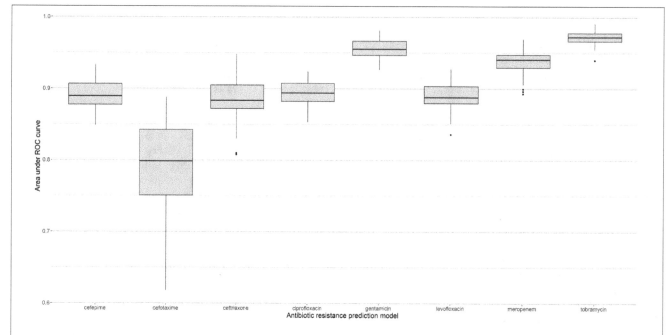

FIGURE 3 | Performance of XGBoost models based on 51 different splits of the data. Boxplots represent distribution of AUC for the corresponding testing subsets, with thick lines indicating the median performance.

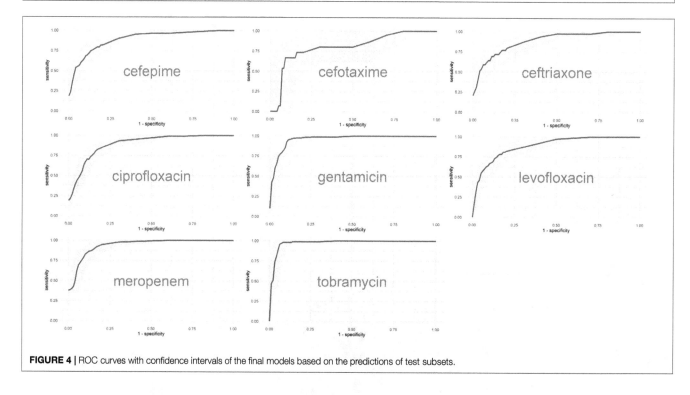

FIGURE 4 | ROC curves with confidence intervals of the final models based on the predictions of test subsets.

at first glance but might make more sense when interpreted in a broader context. *AAC(6′)-Ib family aminoglycoside 6′-N-acetyltransferase* is an aminoglycoside resistance gene, but apart from being important in the tobramycin model (an aminoglycoside), it is also found to be important in the models predicting cephalosporin and levofloxacin resistance. This is where a more careful interpretation of important features is

warranted as the non-linearity of XGBoost models is starting to provide less intuitive connections. For example, this gene is found in a variety of Gram-negative species and is known to be present in many different plasmids, genomic islands and integrons that carry other genetic resistance genes. It could be that this gene is a proxy for other, more relevant genes or even other genetic factors in the genome associated with resistance

TABLE 4 | Top 5 most important features for each antibiotic model.

ARGC	Gain
Cefepime	
AAC(6′)-Ib family aminoglycoside 6′-N-acetyltransferase	18.90 ± 3.27
Class A extended-spectrum beta-lactamase CTX-M-222	7.84 ± 1.07
Aminoglycoside O-phosphotransferase APH(3″)-Ib	6.44 ± 1.91
Class C extended-spectrum beta-lactamase EC-18	5.49 ± 1.30
Carbapenem-hydrolyzing class A beta-lactamase KPC-33	5.14 ± 1.32
Cefotaxime	
Aminoglycoside nucleotidyltransferase ANT(3″)-IIa	17.09 ± 7.27
AAC(6′)-Ib family aminoglycoside 6′-N-acetyltransferase	13.75 ± 7.65
Class C extended-spectrum beta-lactamase EC-18	13.16 ± 4.84
Multidrug efflux RND transporter permease subunit OqxB21	9.74 ± 4.27
OXA-51 family carbapenem-hydrolyzing class D beta-lactamase OXA-561	8.26 ± 3.86
Ceftriaxone	
AAC(6′)-Ib family aminoglycoside 6′-N-acetyltransferase	15.52 ± 4.35
Class C beta-lactamase CMY-163	8.76 ± 1.79
Class A extended-spectrum beta-lactamase CTX-M-222	8.37 ± 2.17
Class C extended-spectrum beta-lactamase EC-18	8.10 ± 1.99
Multidrug efflux RND transporter permease subunit OqxB21	7.00 ± 3.20
Ciprofloxacin	
AAC(6′)-Ib family aminoglycoside 6′-N-acetyltransferase	23.44 ± 4.94
Sulfonamide-resistant dihydropteroate synthase Sul1	10.29 ± 3.20
Tetracycline efflux MFS transporter Tet(B)	4.99 ± 1.71
Class A beta-lactamase TEM-219	4.93 ± 1.14
Aminoglycoside O-phosphotransferase APH(3″)-Ib	4.47 ± 1.63
Gentamicin	
Aminoglycoside N-acetyltransferase AAC(3)-IIc	28.79 ± 3.10
ANT(3″)-Ia family aminoglycoside nucleotidyltransferase AadA1	20.98 ± 2.52
Aminoglycoside nucleotidyltransferase ANT(2″)-Ia	17.79 ± 2.03
OXA-24 family carbapenem-hydrolyzing class D beta-lactamase OXA-25	4.15 ± 1.59
Mph(E) family macrolide 2′-phosphotransferase	2.07 ± 1.10
Levofloxacin	
AAC(6′)-Ib family aminoglycoside 6′-N-acetyltransferase	25.11 ± 6.17
Sulfonamide-resistant dihydropteroate synthase Sul1	7.72 ± 3.73
Tetracycline efflux MFS transporter Tet(B)	5.92 ± 1.67
Class A beta-lactamase TEM-219	5.89 ± 1.74
Class C extended-spectrum beta-lactamase EC-18	4.97 ± 1.73
Meropenem	
Carbapenem-hydrolyzing class A beta-lactamase KPC-33	30.09 ± 5.21
Bleomycin binding protein Ble-MBL	9.55 ± 2.02
OXA-23 family carbapenem-hydrolyzing class D beta-lactamase OXA-483	8.58 ± 3.25
Class C extended-spectrum beta-lactamase EC-18	5.79 ± 2.05
Class A beta-lactamase SHV-200	5.59 ± 2.74
Tobramycin	
AAC(6′)-Ib family aminoglycoside 6′-N-acetyltransferase	60.50 ± 5.02
Aminoglycoside nucleotidyltransferase ANT(2″)-Ia	17.91 ± 1.98
Aminoglycoside N-acetyltransferase AAC(3)-IIc	6.54 ± 1.24
Aminoglycoside 6′-N-acetyltransferase AAC(6′)-Iq	4.62 ± 1.51
ArmA family 16S rRNA [guanine(1405)-N(7)]-methyltransferase	1.89 ± 0.97

Gain is the relative importance of the ARGC in a prediction model, reported here as mean with standard deviation computed over 51 independent models for the same AB.

TABLE 5 | Counts of unique features found among top 5 across 51 independent models for each AB.

Antibiotic model	LASSO	Ridge	XGBoost
Cefepime	28	13	11
Cefotaxime	38	38	12
Ceftriaxone	25	29	12
Ciprofloxacin	30	16	13
Gentamicin	16	12	18
Levofloxacin	24	17	11
Meropenem	25	18	11
Tobramycin	14	16	14

The lower number signifies the more consistent feature selection across data resampling.

(Wilson et al., 2016; Lehtinen et al., 2017). Furthermore, this gene is prominent in *Klebsiella* species which could be used during decision-making to take advantage of innate differences in resistance between species. The fact that our prediction models are species independent could make them more powerful when focusing on resistance patterns in contaminated, mixed, and metagenomic samples. The latter is part of the future goals of this work. To show that the presence of ARG only could easily predict species, a model with the same input, but trained on predicting species instead of ABR, was built and had a near perfect accuracy (**Supplementary Table S8**).

The most striking discordance between an antibiotic and its model's important ARGC features was observed for levofloxacin. None of the most important ARGC picked up by the model are directly related to quinolone resistance. This is likely because levofloxacin resistance is largely based on mutations or small variations (e.g., gyrase gene; Chen and Lo, 2003). Given our models do not incorporate such information (section "Clustering similar antibiotic resistance genes"), all important ARGC in the levofloxacin resistance model appear to be proxies for these mutations. This illustrates both the strength and limitations of models like XGBoost. It can make accurate predictions (**Table 3**) on correlated and complex data by using non-linear logic, but the interpretation of such models can be obscure and could limit biological understanding of the underlying processes.

As any other previous work in this early-stage field of predicting ABR based on the WGS data, our study has several limitations. One of the main challenges was the sparsity of the model input, which may result in biased performance depending on the split in training and testing data. Even after clustering highly similar ARG in ARGC (hence no account for polymorphism), we still ended up with some ARGC only seen once in the whole dataset (median presence of 10 out of 152 clusters per sample). The sparsity is likely because some genes are rare, or the dataset is not fully representative of all evaluated resistances (limitation of using publicly available data). If we would only have used the genes originally sequenced in the bacteria of interest, we might have had less sparsity, but would likely be underestimating the presence of resistance as many species have developed similar resistance genes or exchanged them in processes like horizontal gene transfer. The

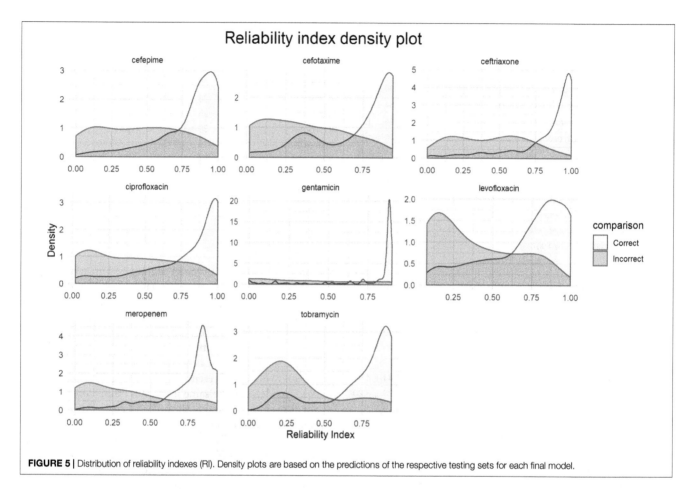

FIGURE 5 | Distribution of reliability indexes (RI). Density plots are based on the predictions of the respective testing sets for each final model.

Escherichia coli

antibiotic	prediction	reliability	reference
cefepime	Susceptible	0.24	Incorrect
cefotaxime	Resistant	0.86	Unknown
ceftriaxone	Resistant	0.86	Correct
ciprofloxacin	Resistant	0.96	Correct
gentamicin	Susceptible	0.88	Correct
levofloxacin	Resistant	1	Correct
meropenem	Susceptible	0.86	Correct
tobramycin	Resistant	0.66	Correct

FIGURE 6 | Example of the predicted antibiogram. An illustration of the output from the *R* shiny app using the sample SAMN07450853 from the Demo set. Other samples from the Demo and In-house datasets can be accessed through the app. The "reference" column compares the predicted resistance to the one confirmed in the clinical laboratory. This would normally not be present at the time the models do their prediction for *de novo* samples. Color coding used: green – correct, red – incorrect, and blue – unknown.

second reason performance suffered in some cases is the class imbalance between available susceptible and resistant samples, e.g., cefotaxime only has 50 susceptible samples (**Table 1**), and also the lowest performance (**Table 3**). By creating many independent models for each antibiotic and selecting the one with median performance, we ensured that the final model would be the closest estimate of the real-life performance (section "XGBoost model training and testing"). This technique is not to

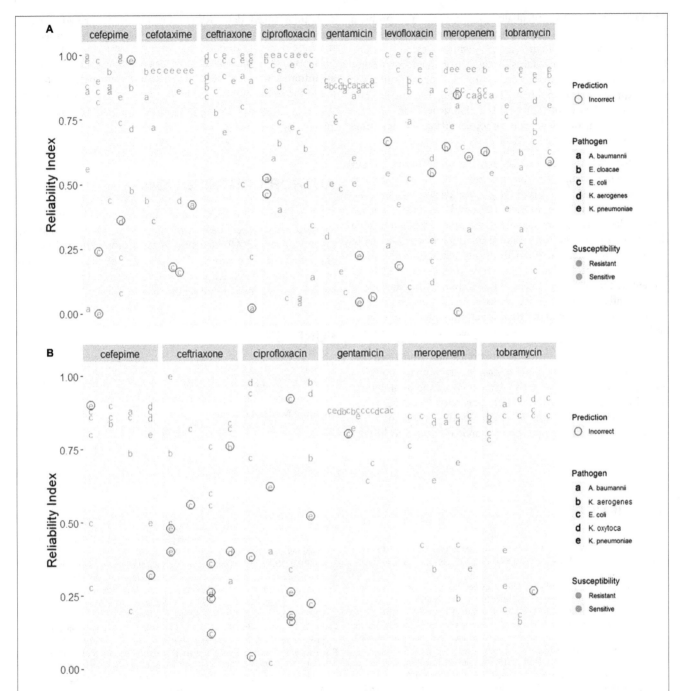

FIGURE 7 | Prediction of samples from the **(A)** Demo and **(B)** In-house datasets. Predictions are grouped by antibiotic and ordered by reliability index. Incorrect predictions encircled in red, predictions with no known resistance in the meta-data are not shown. In-house dataset was not tested for cefotaxime and levofloxacin, hence these two ABs are not shown.

be confused with model cross-validation, where different splits of data are used to enhance one final model, and additional validation data is needed to estimate the performance.

Other limitations are that the models cannot predict the level of resistance (i.e., as regression) as they were trained on a binary data (resistant versus susceptible). Using the MIC values as input could help in this case, but the data is not always available or may be inconsistent. Also, the

current predictor accounts for presence or absence of certain known drug resistance genes and hence cannot detect the presence of previously unseen genes conferring new drug resistance. In other words, the prediction of a sample being resistant has higher confidence than being susceptible. Furthermore, due to the nature of sequencing data (DNA-seq), the models cannot incorporate resistance originating from the over-expression of genes targeted by inhibitors. RNA-seq potentially could mitigate this problem but presents additional challenges. (Meta-)transcriptomics data, unfortunately, and remains mostly within research realm. Complexity of reference database, inference of organisms/strains, and their relative abundance data (Cox et al., 2017), dynamic gene expression profile upon different drug treatments, and overall complexity of data preparation/generation impede the application of meta-transcriptomics data for real-time predictions (Van Camp et al., 2020).

Finally, the models use sequencing data derived from isolates, but it remains to be seen how they would perform on contaminated or mixed (e.g., metagenomic) samples. All limitations will be further addressed in future studies. Nevertheless, this study has shown a great potential of sequencing data as a basis for the prediction of antimicrobial resistance in Gram-negative bacteria. We additionally focused on the more practical implementation of resistance prediction models by presenting the end-users (medical practitioners) with an easy to use and interpret interface where novel predictions on different AB are shown together as in a traditional antibiogram but with an additional RI to further assist during the decision making process.

To summarize, this work demonstrates that whole-genome sequencing coupled with modern machine-learning methods has great potential to deliver early estimations of the antibiogram for Gram-negative bacteria. The generated models, being trained solely on the presence-absence of the clusters of ARG, demonstrate promising performance and robustness to heavily class-imbalanced data. RI are introduced to provide further assessment of predictions and may be used in subsequent machine learning models to improve accuracy further. By presenting the results in the form of an antibiogram, we provide an intuitive way for the clinician to interpret predictions and guide the initial empiric antibiotic choice before the laboratory results are available. This may help in shortening the time to start effective AB treatment.

AUTHOR CONTRIBUTIONS

P-JV did the data collection and curation, model training and validation, developed the R shiny app, and stand-alone analytical pipeline. DH and AP conceived of the study, evaluated results, and supervised the project. DH provided clinical samples for the In-house dataset. AP provided computational resources. All authors participated in writing the manuscript.

FUNDING

This work was supported by the Centers for Disease Control (Contract Number OADS BAA 2016-N-17812) and funding from the Academic Research Committee at Cincinnati Children's Hospital Medical Center.

REFERENCES

Altschul, S. F., Gish, W., Miller, W., Myers, E. W., and Lipman, D. J. (1990). Basic local alignment search tool. *J. Mol. Biol.* 215, 403–410. doi: 10.1016/S0022-2836(05)80360-2

Bajaj, P., Singh, N. S., and Virdi, J. S. (2016). *Escherichia coli* β-Lactamases: what really matters. *Front. Microbiol.* 7:417. doi: 10.3389/fmicb.2016.00417

Bradley, P., Gordon, N. C., Walker, T. M., Dunn, L., Heys, S., Huang, B., et al. (2015). Rapid antibiotic-resistance predictions from genome sequence data for *Staphylococcus aureus* and *Mycobacterium tuberculosis. Nat. Commun.* 6:10063. doi: 10.1038/ncomms10063

Buchfink, B., Xie, C., and Huson, D. H. (2015). Fast and sensitive protein alignment using DIAMOND. *Nat. Methods* 12, 59–60. doi: 10.1038/nmeth.3176

Centers for Disease Control and Prevention (2018). *Antibiotic / Antimicrobial Resistance.* Available online at: https://www.cdc.gov/drugresistance/index.html (accessed March 20, 2019).

Chen, F.-J., and Lo, H.-J. (2003). Molecular mechanisms of fluoroquinolone resistance. *J. Microbiol. Immunol. Infect.* 36, 1–9.

Chen, T., and Guestrin, C. (2016). XGBoost: a scalable tree boosting system. *Proc. Int. Conf. Knowl. Discov. Data Min.* 16, 785–794. doi: 10.1145/2939672.2939785

Couto, R. C., Carvalho, E. A. A., Pedrosa, T. M. G., Pedroso, E. R., Neto, M. C., and Biscione, F. M. (2007). A 10-year prospective surveillance of nosocomial infections in neonatal intensive care units. *Am. J. Infect. Control* 35, 183–189. doi: 10.1016/j.ajic.2006.06.013

Cox, J. W., Ballweg, R. A., Taft, D. H., Velayutham, P., Haslam, D. B., and Porollo, A. (2017). A fast and robust protocol for metataxonomic analysis using RNAseq data. *Microbiome* 5:7. doi: 10.1186/s40168-016-0219-5

Devika, S., Jeyaseelan, L., and Sebastian, G. (2016). Analysis of sparse data in logistic regression in medical research: a newer approach. *J. Postgrad. Med.* 62, 26–31. doi: 10.4103/0022-3859.173193

Drouin, A., Letarte, G., Raymond, F., Marchand, M., Corbeil, J., and Laviolette, F. (2019). Interpretable genotype-to-phenotype classifiers with performance guarantees. *Sci. Rep.* 9:4071. doi: 10.1038/s41598-019-40561-2

Edgar, R. C. (2010). Search and clustering orders of magnitude faster than BLAST. *Bioinformatics* 26, 2460–2461. doi: 10.1093/bioinformatics/btq461

Eyre, D. W., De Silva, D., Cole, K., Peters, J., Cole, M. J., Grad, Y. H., et al. (2017). WGS to predict antibiotic MICs for *Neisseria gonorrhoeae. J. Antimicrob. Chemother.* 72, 1937–1947. doi: 10.1093/jac/dkx067

Farrar, D. E., and Glauber, R. R. (1967). Multicollinearity in regression analysis: the problem revisited. *Rev. Econ. Stat.* 49, 92–107. doi: 10.2307/1937887

Feuerriegel, S., Schleusener, V., Beckert, P., Kohl, T. A., Miotto, P., Cirillo, D. M., et al. (2015). PhyResSE: a web tool delineating *Mycobacterium tuberculosis* antibiotic resistance and lineage from whole-genome sequencing data. *J. Clin. Microbiol.* 53, 1908–1914. doi: 10.1128/JCM.00025-15

Lehtinen, S., Blanquart, F., Croucher, N. J., Turner, P., Lipsitch, M., and Fraser, C. (2017). Evolution of antibiotic resistance is linked to any genetic mechanism affecting bacterial duration of carriage. *Proc. Natl. Acad. Sci. U.S.A.* 114, 1075–1080. doi: 10.1073/pnas.1617849114

Livermore, D. M. (1998). Beta-lactamase-mediated resistance and opportunities for its control. *J. Antimicrob. Chemother.* 41(Suppl. D), 25–41. doi: 10.1093/jac/41.suppl_4.25

Marston, H. D., Dixon, D. M., Knisely, J. M., Palmore, T. N., and Fauci, A. S. (2016). Antimicrobial resistance. *JAMA* 316, 1193–1204. doi: 10.1001/jama.2016.11764

Martin, E. T., Tansek, R., Collins, V., Hayakawa, K., Abreu-Lanfranco, O., Chopra, T., et al. (2013). The carbapenem-resistant *Enterobacteriaceae* score: a bedside score to rule out infection with carbapenem-resistant *Enterobacteriaceae* among hospitalized patients. *Am. J. Infect. Control* 41, 180–182. doi: 10.1016/j.ajic.2012.02.036

MinION (2019). *Oxford Nanopore Technologies*. Available online at: http://nanoporetech.com/products/minion (accessed May 16, 2019).

Nguyen, M., Brettin, T., Long, S. W., Musser, J. M., Olsen, R. J., Olson, R., et al. (2018). Developing an in silico minimum inhibitory concentration panel test for *Klebsiella pneumoniae*. *Sci. Rep.* 8, 1–11. doi: 10.1038/s41598-017-18972-w

Piramuthu, S. (2008). Input data for decision trees. *Expert Syst. Appl.* 34, 1220–1226. doi: 10.1016/j.eswa.2006.12.030

Scaggs Huang, F. A., Mortensen, J., Skoch, J., Andersen, H., Staat, M. A., Schaffzin, J. K., et al. (2019). Successful whole genome sequencing-guided treatment of *Mycoplasma hominis Ventriculitis* in a preterm infant. *Pediatr. Infect. Dis. J.* 38, 749–751. doi: 10.1097/INF.0000000000002306

SRA Toolkit Development Team (2019). *SRA Toolkit NCBI - National Center for Biotechnology Information/NLM/NIH*. Available online at: https://github.com/ncbi/sra-tools (accessed March 15, 2019).

Van Camp, P.-J., Haslam, D. B., and Porollo, A. (2020). Bioinformatics approaches to the understanding of molecular mechanisms in antimicrobial resistance. *Int. J. Mol. Sci.* 21:1363. doi: 10.3390/ijms21041363

Vasudevan, A., Mukhopadhyay, A., Li, J., Yuen, E. G. Y., and Tambyah, P. A. (2014). A prediction tool for nosocomial multi-drug resistant gram-negative *Bacilli* infections in critically ill patients - prospective observational study. *BMC Infect. Dis.* 14:615. doi: 10.1186/s12879-014-0615-z

Vincent, J.-L. (2003). Nosocomial infections in adult intensive-care units. *Lancet* 361, 2068–2077. doi: 10.1016/S0140-6736(03)13644-6

Ward, J. H. (1963). Hierarchical grouping to optimize an objective function. *J. Am. Stat. Assoc.* 58, 236–244. doi: 10.2307/2282967

Wilson, B. A., Garud, N. R., Feder, A. F., Assaf, Z. J., and Pennings, P. S. (2016). The population genetics of drug resistance evolution in natural populations of viral, bacterial and eukaryotic pathogens. *Mol. Ecol.* 25, 42–66. doi: 10.1111/mec.13474

Wu, W., May, R. J., Maier, H. R., and Dandy, G. C. (2013). A benchmarking approach for comparing data splitting methods for modeling water resources parameters using artificial neural networks. *Water Resour. Res.* 49, 7598–7614. doi: 10.1002/2012WR012713

Permissions

All chapters in this book were first published by Frontiers; hereby published with permission under the Creative Commons Attribution License or equivalent. Every chapter published in this book has been scrutinized by our experts. Their significance has been extensively debated. The topics covered herein carry significant findings which will fuel the growth of the discipline. They may even be implemented as practical applications or may be referred to as a beginning point for another development.

The contributors of this book come from diverse backgrounds, making this book a truly international effort. This book will bring forth new frontiers with its revolutionizing research information and detailed analysis of the nascent developments around the world.

We would like to thank all the contributing authors for lending their expertise to make the book truly unique. They have played a crucial role in the development of this book. Without their invaluable contributions this book wouldn't have been possible. They have made vital efforts to compile up to date information on the varied aspects of this subject to make this book a valuable addition to the collection of many professionals and students.

This book was conceptualized with the vision of imparting up-to-date information and advanced data in this field. To ensure the same, a matchless editorial board was set up. Every individual on the board went through rigorous rounds of assessment to prove their worth. After which they invested a large part of their time researching and compiling the most relevant data for our readers.

The editorial board has been involved in producing this book since its inception. They have spent rigorous hours researching and exploring the diverse topics which have resulted in the successful publishing of this book. They have passed on their knowledge of decades through this book. To expedite this challenging task, the publisher supported the team at every step. A small team of assistant editors was also appointed to further simplify the editing procedure and attain best results for the readers.

Apart from the editorial board, the designing team has also invested a significant amount of their time in understanding the subject and creating the most relevant covers. They scrutinized every image to scout for the most suitable representation of the subject and create an appropriate cover for the book.

The publishing team has been an ardent support to the editorial, designing and production team. Their endless efforts to recruit the best for this project, has resulted in the accomplishment of this book. They are a veteran in the field of academics and their pool of knowledge is as vast as their experience in printing. Their expertise and guidance has proved useful at every step. Their uncompromising quality standards have made this book an exceptional effort. Their encouragement from time to time has been an inspiration for everyone.

The publisher and the editorial board hope that this book will prove to be a valuable piece of knowledge for researchers, students, practitioners and scholars across the globe.

List of Contributors

Ming-Hsien Chiang
Department and Graduate Institute of Biology and Anatomy, National Defense Medical Center, Taipei, Taiwan
Graduate Institute of Life Sciences, National Defense Medical Center, Taipei, Taiwan

Ya-Sung Yang and Yung-Chih Wang
Division of Infectious Diseases and Tropical Medicine, Department of Internal Medicine, Tri-Service General Hospital, National Defense Medical Center, Taipei, Taiwan

Jun-Ren Sun
Institute of Preventive Medicine, National Defense Medical Center, Taipei, Taiwan

Shu-Chen Kuo
National Institute of Infectious Diseases and Vaccinology, National Health Research Institutes, Zhunan, Taiwan

Yi-Tzu Lee
School of Medicine, National Yang-Ming University, Taipei, Taiwan
Department of Emergency Medicine, Taipei Veterans General Hospital, Taipei, Taiwan

Yi-Ping Chuang
Department and Graduate Institute of Microbiology and Immunology, National Defense Medical Center, Taipei, Taiwan

Te-Li Chen
Graduate Institute of Life Sciences, National Defense Medical Center, Taipei, Taiwan
Institute of Clinical Medicine, National Yang-Ming University, Taipei, Taiwan

Shifu Aggarwal, Smrutiti Jena and Sasmita Panda
Infectious Disease Biology, Institute of Life Sciences, Bhubaneswar, India

Savitri Sharma
Jhaveri Microbiology Centre, LV Prasad Eye Institute, Brien Holden Eye Research Centre, Kallam Anji Reddy Campus, Hyderabad, India

Benu Dhawan
Department of Microbiology, All India Institute of Medical Sciences, New Delhi, India

Kinshuk Chandra Nayak
Institute of Life Sciences, Bhubaneswar, India

Gopal Nath
Department of Microbiology, Institute of Medical Sciences, Banaras Hindu University, Varanasi, India

N. P. Singh
Department of Microbiology, Faculty of Medical Sciences, University of Delhi, New Delhi, India

Durg Vijai Singh
Infectious Disease Biology, Institute of Life Sciences, Bhubaneswar, India
Department of Biotechnology, Central University of South Bihar, Gaya, India

Roumayne L. Ferreira, Graziela S. Rezende, Marcelo Silva Folhas Damas, Eduardo Leonardecz, Emeline Boni Campanini, Iran Malavazi, Anderson F. da Cunha and Maria-Cristina da Silva Pranchevicius
Departamento de Genética e Evolução, Universidade Federal de São Carlos, São Carlos, Brazil

Mariana Oliveira-Silva and André Pitondo-Silva
Programas de Pós-graduação em Odontologia e Tecnologia Ambiental, Universidade de Ribeirão Preto, Ribeirão Preto, Brazil

Márcia C. A. Brito
Laboratório Central de Saúde Pública do Tocantins, Palmas, Brazil

Fabiana R. de Góes
Instituto de Ciências Matemáticas e de Computação, Universidade de São Paulo, São Carlos, Brazil

Elodie Olivares
University of Strasbourg, CHRU Strasbourg, Fédération de Médecine Translationnelle de Strasbourg, EA7290, Institut de Bactériologie, Strasbourg, France
BioFilm Pharma SAS, Saint-Beauzire, France

Stéphanie Badel-Berchoux
BioFilm Control SAS, Saint-Beauzire, France

Christian Provot and Thierry Bernardi
BioFilm Pharma SAS, Saint-Beauzire, France
BioFilm Control SAS, Saint-Beauzire, France

Gilles Prévost and François Jehl
University of Strasbourg, CHRU Strasbourg, Fédération de Médecine Translationnelle de Strasbourg, EA7290, Institut de Bactériologie, Strasbourg, France

Bing Bai, Zhiwei Lin, Guangjian Xu, Fan Zhang, Zhong Chen, Peiyu Li, Qiwen Deng and Zhijian Yu
Department of Infectious Diseases and Shenzhen Key Lab of Endogenous Infections, Shenzhen Nanshan People's Hospital and the 6th Affiliated Hospital of Shenzhen University Health Science Center, Shenzhen, China
Quality Control Center of Hospital Infection Management of Shenzhen, Shenzhen Nanshan People's Hospital, Guangdong Medical University Shenzhen, China

Zhangya Pu
Key Laboratory of Viral Hepatitis of Hunan Province, Department of Infectious Diseases, Xiangya Hospital, Central South University, Changsha, China

Xiang Sun and Jinxin Zheng
Department of Infectious Diseases and Shenzhen Key Lab of Endogenous Infections, Shenzhen Nanshan People's Hospital and the 6th Affiliated Hospital of Shenzhen University Health Science Center, Shenzhen, China

Paul Loubet and Albert Sotto
VBMI, INSERM U1047, Université de Montpellier, Service des Maladies Infectieuses et Tropicales, CHU Nîmes, Nîmes, France

Jérémy Ranfaing, Catherine Dunyach-Remy and Jean-Philippe Lavigne
VBMI, INSERM U1047, Université de Montpellier, Service de Microbiologie et Hygiène Hospitalière, CHU Nîmes, Nîmes, France

Aurélien Dinh
Service des Maladies Infectieuses, AP-HP Raymond-Poincaré, Garches, France

Louis Bernard
PRES Centre Val de Loire, Université François Rabelais de Tours, Tours, France
Service des Maladies Infectieuses, CHU Tours, Tours, France

Franck Bruyère
PRES Centre Val de Loire, Université François Rabelais de Tours, Tours, France Service d'Urologie, CHU Tours, Tours, France

Paulo J. M. Bispo, Lawson Ung and James Chodosh
Department of Ophthalmology, Massachusetts Eye and Ear, Harvard Medical School, Boston, MA, United States
Infectious Disease Institute, Harvard Medical School, Boston, MA, United States

Michael S. Gilmore
Department of Ophthalmology, Massachusetts Eye and Ear, Harvard Medical School, Boston, MA, United States
Infectious Disease Institute, Harvard Medical School, Boston, MA, United States
Department of Microbiology and Immunobiology, Harvard Medical School, Boston, MA, United States
Department of Ophthalmology and Department of Microbiology, Harvard Medical School, Boston, MA, United States

Shelley B. Gibson, Sabrina I. Green, Carmen Gu Liu, Keiko C. Salazar, Justin R. Clark, Austen L. Terwilliger, Anthony W. Maresso and Robert F. Ramig
Department of Molecular Virology and Microbiology, Baylor College of Medicine, Houston, TX, United States

Heidi B. Kaplan
Department of Microbiology and Molecular Genetics, McGovern Medical School, University of Texas Health Science Center at Houston, Houston, TX, United States

Barbara W. Trautner
Department of Molecular Virology and Microbiology, Baylor College of Medicine, Houston, TX, United States
Center for Innovations in Quality, Effectiveness and Safety, Michael E. DeBakey VA Medical Center, Houston, TX, United States
Department of Medicine, Baylor College of Medicine, Houston, TX, United States

Zahid Hayat Mahmud, Mir Himayet Kabir, Sobur Ali, M. Moniruzzaman, Khan Mohammad Imran, Tanvir Noor Nafiz, Md. Shafiqul Islam, Dilruba Ahmed, Arif Hussain and Niyaz Ahmed
International Centre for Diarrhoeal Disease Research, Dhaka, Bangladesh

Syed Adnan Ibna Hakim, Martin Worth and Dara Johnston
WASH Division, UNICEF Bangladesh, Dhaka, Bangladesh

Isidro García-Meniño, Dafne Díaz-Jiménez, Vanesa García, Saskia C. Flament-Simon, Jorge Blanco and Azucena Mora
Laboratorio de Referencia de Escherichia coli, Departamento de Microbiología y Parasitología, Facultad de Veterinaria, Universidad de Santiago de Compostela, Lugo, Spain

María de Toro
Plataforma de Genómica y Bioinformática, Centro de Investigación Biomédica de La Rioja, Logroño, Spain

Carolina Ferrari, Patrizia Cambieri, Piero Marone and Stefano Gaiarsa
Microbiology and Virology Unit, Fondazione IRCCS Policlinico San Matteo, Pavia, Italy

Marta Corbella
Microbiology and Virology Unit, Fondazione IRCCS Policlinico San Matteo, Pavia, Italy
Biometric and Medical Statistics Unit, Fondazione IRCCS Policlinico San Matteo, Pavia, Italy

Francesco Comandatore
Pediatric Research Center Romeo ed Enrica Invernizzi, University of Milan, Milan, Italy
Department of Biomedical and Clinical Sciences "L. Sacco", University of Milan, Milan, Italy

Erika Scaltriti
Risk Analysis and Genomic Epidemiology Unit, Istituto Zooprofilattico Sperimentale della Lombardia e dell'Emilia Romagna (IZSLER), Brescia, Italy

Claudio Bandi
Pediatric Research Center Romeo ed Enrica Invernizzi, University of Milan, Milan, Italy
Department of Biosciences, University of Milan, Milan, Italy

Davide Sassera
Department of Biology and Biotechnology "L. Spallanzani", University of Pavia, Pavia, Italy

Wenya Xu, Tao Chen, Huihui Wang, Qing Wu, Ye Xu, Xiucai Zhang and Tieli Zhou
Department of Clinical Laboratory, The First Affiliated Hospital of Wenzhou Medical University, Wenzhou, China

Weiliang Zeng and Kaihang Yu
School of Laboratory Medicine and Life Science, Wenzhou Medical University, Wenzhou, China

Marcus Ho-yin Wong, Bill Kwan-wai Chan and Edward Wai-chi Chan
State Key Laboratory of Chemical Biology and Drug Discovery, The Hong Kong Polytechnic University, Kowloon, Hong Kong

Sheng Chen
State Key Laboratory of Chemical Biology and Drug Discovery, The Hong Kong Polytechnic University, Kowloon, Hong Kong

Department of Infectious Diseases and Public Health, Jockey Club College of Veterinary Medicine and Life Sciences, City University of Hong Kong, Kowloon, Hong Kong

Lei Liu, Huai Lin, Ranjit Das, Siyi Wang, Hongmei Qi, Jing Yang and Yi Luo
College of Environmental Science and Engineering, Ministry of Education Key Laboratory of Pollution Processes and Environmental Criteria, Nankai University, Tianjin, China

Qing Wang
College of Environmental Science and Engineering, Ministry of Education Key Laboratory of Pollution Processes and Environmental Criteria, Nankai University, Tianjin, China
Hebei Key Laboratory of Air Pollution Cause and Impact (preparatory), College of Energy and Environmental Engineering, Hebei University of Engineering, Handan, China

Yingang Xue
Key Laboratory of Environmental Protection of Water Environment Biological Monitoring of Jiangsu Province, Changzhou Environmental Monitoring Center, Changzhou, China

Daqing Mao
School of Medicine, Nankai University, Tianjin, China

Mehdi Goudarzi, Mohammad Javad Nasiri and Hossein Goudarzi
Department of Microbiology, School of Medicine, Shahid Beheshti University of Medical Sciences, Tehran, Iran

Nobumichi Kobayashi
Department of Hygiene, School of Medicine, Sapporo Medical University, Sapporo, Japan

Masoud Dadashi
Department of Microbiology, School of Medicine, Alborz University of Medical Sciences, Karaj, Iran

Roman Pantůček
Department of Experimental Biology, Faculty of Science, Masaryk University, Brno, Czechia

Maryam Fazeli
Department of Virology, Pasteur Institute of Iran, Tehran, Iran

Ramin Pouriran
School of Medicine, Shahid Beheshti University of Medical Sciences, Tehran, Iran

Mirmohammad Miri
Department of Critical Care and Anesthesiology, Imam Hossein Hospital, Shahid Beheshti University of Medical Sciences, Tehran, Iran

Anahita Amirpour
Department of Internal Medicine, Shahid Beheshti University of Medical Sciences, Tehran, Iran

Sima Sadat Seyedjavadi
Department of Mycology, Pasteur Institute of Iran, Tehran, Iran

Peter Kotsoana Montso and Collins Njie Ateba
Bacteriophage Therapy and Phage Bio-Control Laboratory, Department of Microbiology, Faculty of Natural and Agricultural Sciences, North-West University, Mmabatho, South Africa
Food Security and Safety Niche Area, North-West University, Mmabatho, South Africa

Victor Mlambo
Faculty of Agriculture and Natural Sciences, School of Agricultural Sciences, University of Mpumalanga, Mbombela, South Africa

Pieter-Jan Van Camp
Department of Biomedical Informatics, University of Cincinnati, Cincinnati, OH, United States
Division of Biomedical Informatics, Cincinnati Children's Hospital Medical Center, Cincinnati, OH, United States

David B. Haslam
Division of Infectious Diseases, Cincinnati Children's Hospital Medical Center, Cincinnati, OH, United States
Department of Pediatrics, University of Cincinnati, Cincinnati, OH, United States

Aleksey Porollo
Division of Biomedical Informatics, Cincinnati Children's Hospital Medical Center, Cincinnati, OH, United States
Department of Pediatrics, University of Cincinnati, Cincinnati, OH, United States
Center for Autoimmune Genomics and Etiology, Cincinnati Children's Hospital Medical Center, Cincinnati, OH, United States

Index

Printed in the USA
CPSIA information can be obtained
at www.ICGtesting.com
JSHW051405091023
49903JS00006B/283